Rational-Emotive and Cognitive-Behavioral Approaches to Child and Adolescent Mental Health: Theory, Practice, Research, Applications

Michael Bernard • Mark D. Terjesen
Editors

Rational-Emotive and Cognitive-Behavioral Approaches to Child and Adolescent Mental Health: Theory, Practice, Research, Applications

Springer

Editors
Michael Bernard
Melbourne Graduate School of Education
University of Melbourne
Melbourne, VIC, Australia

Mark D. Terjesen
Department of Psychology
St. John's University
Jamaica, NY, USA

ISBN 978-3-030-53900-9 ISBN 978-3-030-53901-6 (eBook)
https://doi.org/10.1007/978-3-030-53901-6

This Springer imprint is published by the registered company Springer Nature Switzerland AG
The registered company address is: Gewerbestrasse 11, 6330 Cham, Switzerland

Preface

This book for professionals documents the evolution of Rational Emotive Behavior Therapy (REBT) practice with younger populations. It is the third in a series of books published by Springer commencing with the 1983 book I (Michael) edited with Albert Ellis and which we completely revised in 2006. Over 12 months ago, Mark put a call into me and said it was time for the next edition. Largely through his efforts, we assembled an amazing array of REBT-trained practitioners to write on their specialized applications of REBT in their field of endeavor. Only five of the 2006 group of contributors (Bernard, Doyle, Esposito, Terjesen, Vernon) have made contributions to this book with the remaining 36 authors/co-authors being new to the book. Many of our authors represent the current generation of young mental health practitioners all of whom share with us the passion for REBT. As REBT is an example of and is the earliest form of Cognitive Behavioral Therapy (CBT), this volume highlights the place of REBT within the broader clinical context of CBT, offering important discussions as to the overlap as well as unique applications of the practical and scholarly work of both REBT and CBT.

When I (Michael) began my professional career in 1979 employing REBT with children as young as five—with their families and teachers—there was a suspicion and distrust that REBT's verbal and cognitive form of therapy was not suitable for younger populations. Since then, REBT has become recognized as one of two (along with Beck's cognitive therapy) major schools of cognitive behavior therapy, and today, as illustrated throughout this book, cognitive restructuring using a variety of creative and experiential as well as traditional strategies can be readily employed with younger populations. Furthermore, the importance of strengthening children and adolescents' capacity for rational thought and teaching explicit rational beliefs (e.g., self-acceptance) is seen as more important to today's wholistic education of young people than it was in previous generations.

The type of social-emotional learning and psycho-education we employ with children and adolescents is partly based on a very intelligent and successful curriculum written by Bill Knaus, the psychologist of the Living School, that was situated at the Institute for Rational Living in NYC. Bill wrote *Rational Emotive Education: A Manual for Elementary School Teachers*. Additionally, in 1980, Ann Vernon wrote a beautiful little yellow-covered book, *Help Yourself to a Happier You*, that presented a wide variety of creative and experiential activities for teaching young people the ABCs of REBT. Ann's pioneering work is very well represented in Chap. 4 of this edition, "Teaching REBT to Children and Adolescents: Creative Techniques that Work." Another influential text that presented the strategies for using REBT with younger populations was the book I (Michael) wrote with Marie Joyce, *Rational Emotive Therapy with Children and Adolescents: Theory, Practice, Research* (John Wiley). I (Michael) was honored to have been asked by Janet Wolfe, who was at the time Executive Director of the Institute for Rational Emotive Therapy, to write *The REBT Therapist's Pocket Companion for Working with Children and Adolescents*. Over the years, the Institute's Director of Professional Training, Ray DiGiuseppe, added his creativity and ingenuity in demonstrating how to use REBT with younger populations.

We've organized this book into three parts. Part I, Foundations, covers the essentials of REBT and CBT theory and practice with younger populations. Part II, Childhood Disorders, Difficulties and Different Populations, contains chapters revealing the depth and breadth of REBT and the broader approach of CBT's uses to address mental health problems of childhood including integration with best-practices from allied fields. Part III, Applications, showcases how REBT and its educational derivative Rational Emotive Education has been used as preventative mental health education in coaching of children and adolescents, and how parents and teachers can use the ABCs and rational beliefs to manage stress and do their personal best. Finally, the last chapter addresses how latest advances in technology can help REBT and CBT ideas to be communicated to young people with challenges.

It is exciting to see how REBT practice and science with younger populations has evolved and flourished over the years from what it was in the late 1970s. The distinctiveness of REBT from allied CBT approaches still holds and it is a testimony to the brilliance of Al Ellis that it has stood the test of time and proven its clinical utility for helping young people and their significant others cope and live with mental health challenges.

Melbourne, VIC, Australia Michael Bernard
Jamaica, NY, USA Mark D. Terjesen

Contents

Contributors

Korrie Allen Department of Child, Family and School Psychology, University of Denver, Denver, CO, USA

Ennio Ammendola Fordham University, New York, NY, USA

Michael Bernard Melbourne Graduate School of Education, University of Melbourne, Parkville, VIC, Australia

Camille Bernstein Psychology Department, The Hagedorn Little Village School, New Rochelle, NY, USA

Caroline L. Boxmeyer Academic Affairs in the College of Community Health Sciences at The University of Alabama, Tuscaloosa, AL, USA

Department of Psychiatry and Behavioral Medicine, Tuscaloosa, AL, USA

Samantha Busa Department of Child and Adolescent Psychiatry, Hassenfeld Children's Hospital at NYU Langone, New York, NY, USA

Roxana A. I. Cardos Department of Clinical Psychology and Psychotherapy/The International Institute for the Advanced Studies of Psychotherapy and Applied Mental Health, Babeş-Bolyai University, Cluj-Napoca, Romania

Daniel O. David Department of Clinical Psychology and Psychotherapy/The International Institute for the Advanced Studies of Psychotherapy and Applied Mental Health, Babeş-Bolyai University, Cluj-Napoca, Romania

Department of Oncological Sciences, Icahn School of Medicine at Mount Sinai, New York, NY, USA

Oana Alexandra David Department of Clinical Psychology and Psychotherapy, Babes-Bolyai University, Cluj-Napoca, Romania

Tamara Del Vecchio Department of Psychology, St. John's University, Queens, NY, USA

Kristene A. Doyle Albert Ellis Institute, New York, NY, USA

Courtney Duhning St. John's University, Jamaica, NY, USA

Brooke Edelman St. John's University, Queens, NY, USA

Maria Esposito-Pickering Private Practice, Amityville, NY, USA

Olga Gulyayeva Fuller St. John's University, Queens, NY, USA

Nora Gerardi Psychologist at Cognitive & Behavioral Consultants, New York, NY, USA

Queens College, New York, NY, USA

Michael Hickey Center for Psychological Evaluation and the Center for Treatment and Research of Obsessive-Compulsive & Related Disorders, Albert Ellis Institute, New York, NY, USA

Oksana Huk Psychology Department, Iona College, New Rochelle, NY, USA

Shannon (Shane) Jones Center for Youth Development and Intervention, University of Alabama, Tuscaloosa, AL, USA

Jamie M. Joseph Cognitive Behavior Therapy & Evaluation, Coral Springs, FL, USA

Francesca Kassing Trauma and Grief Center at Baylor College of Medicine/Texas Children's Hospital, Houston, TX, USA

Demetris Katsikis Institute for Rational-Emotive and Cognitive Behavior Therapy, Athens, Greece

Chrysoula Kostogiannis Institute for Rational-Emotive and Cognitive Behavior Therapy, Athens, Greece

Robyn Kurasaki New Hyde Park School District, New Hyde Park, NY, USA

John E. Lochman Center for Prevention of Youth Behavior Problems at The University of Alabama, Tuscaloosa, AL, USA

Adrienne Matta School Psychologist, Wilton Public Schools, Wilton, CT, USA

Veronica Milito Department of School Psychology, St. Johns University, Queens, NY, USA

Alexa K. Pata St. John's University, Jamaica, New York, USA

Nicole P. Powell Center for Youth Development and Intervention at the University of Alabama, Tuscaloosa, AL, USA

Jessica K. Prizer School Psychology, St. John's University, Jamaica, NY, USA

Mayra Reyes-Ruiz St. John's University, Queens, NY, USA

Jaco Rossouw Centre for Cognitive-Behaviour Therapy, Cape Town, South Africa

Department of Psychiatry, Faculty of Medicine and Health Science, Stellenbosch University, Stellenbosch, South Africa

Robin J. Sakakini School and Clinical Psychologist, Oaks Christian School, West Lake Village, CA, USA

Stephanie Schwartz Anxiety Disorders Center, Child Mind Institute, New York, NY, USA

Silviu A. Matu Department of Clinical Psychology and Psychotherapy/The International Institute for the Advanced Studies of Psychotherapy and Applied Mental Health, Babeş-Bolyai University, Cluj-Napoca, Romania

Sara Stromeyer Department of Psychology, University of Alabama, Tuscaloosa, AL, USA

Breanne Taylor Nova Southeastern University, Fort Lauderdale, FL, USA

Angelica Terepka Columbia University Irving Medical Center, New York, NY, USA

Mark D. Terjesen Department of Psychology, St. John's University, Jamaica, NY, USA

Leonell Torres-Pagán New York Presbyterian Hospital, Columbia University Medical Center, Queens, NY, USA

Ann Vernon University of Northern Iowa, Tucson, AZ, USA

About the Editors

Michael Bernard, PhD, is an international consultant to universities, organizations, educational authorities, and governments. Since 2004, he has been a Professorial Fellow at the University of Melbourne, Melbourne Graduate School of Education, and an Emeritus Professor, California State University, Long Beach. He is the Founder of You Can Do It! Education (youcandoiteducation.com.au), a program for promoting student social-emotional well-being and achievement that is being used in over 6000 schools in Australia, New Zealand, Vietnam, Singapore, England, Romania, and North America. Michael was the first Sport Psychologist of the Collingwood Football Team. He is the author of over 50+ books, 30+ book chapters, and 30+ journal articles in areas associated with student well-being and achievement, peak performance, resilience, and positive parenting. With his business partner and wife, Patricia Bernard, he has created an online positive parenting program consisting of eLearning programs, articles, and audio-video motivational programs for young people (youcandoiteducation.com.au/parents). Michael has worked as a consultant school psychologist helping families and schools address the educational and mental health needs of school-age children. Over the past decade, he has focused on the design and conduct of high performance mindset and resilience professional development programs. Michael helped establish the Master of Educational Psychology program in the then Faculty of Education, University of Melbourne. A close colleague of Albert Ellis, Fellow of the Albert Ellis Institute, an approved supervisor, and Editor for 8 years of the *Journal of Rational-Emotive & Cognitive-Behavior Therapy*, Michael is Co-founder of the Australian Institute for Rational Emotive Behaviour Therapy and is the author of many books on REBT.

Mark D. Terjesen, PhD, is Professor of Psychology and Assistant Chairperson in the Department of Psychology at St. John's University in Queens, NY, USA. Dr. Terjesen has served as Program Director of the School Psychology (PsyD and MS) programs and has trained and supervised doctoral students throughout his tenure, having mentored over 100 doctoral dissertation research projects. Dr. Terjesen has studied, published, and presented at a number of national and international conferences on topics related to assessment and clinical work with children, adolescents, and families. He has trained many professionals internationally in the use of Rational Emotive Behavior Therapy (REBT) and cognitive-behavioral practices with children and families. Dr. Terjesen has served as President of the School Division of the New York State Psychological Association, President of the Trainers of School Psychologists, and is Past President of Division 52 (International Psychology) of the American Psychological Association of which he is also a fellow. Dr. Terjesen is a Fellow of the Albert Ellis Institute and an approved supervisor. He serves as the Clinical Director at North Coast Psychological Services in Syosset, NY. Dr. Terjesen and his wife, Dr. Carolyn Waldecker, are the proud parents of Amelia Grace who has taught them how to apply the principles of REBT in their role as parents.

Part I
Foundations

Chapter 1
Rational Emotive, Cognitive Behavioral Approaches to the Challenge of Child and Adolescent Mental Health

Michael Bernard and Mark D. Terjesen

The history of cognitive restructuring with children and youth doubtless goes back many centuries and may be traced to early philosophers and religious preachers (Robertson, 2010; Robertson & Codd, 2019). Socrates, let us remember, was persecuted by the Athenians for supposedly corrupting the youth of that ancient city. And the Greek-Roman Stoic Epictetus, who is often acknowledged as one of the main philosophical fathers of Rational Emotive Behavior Therapy (REBT) and Cognitive Behavioral Therapy (CBT), pioneered in conveying significant cognitive teachings to the young people as well as the adults of his time. Because of his influence, some 2000 years ago, the Roman Emperor Marcus Aurelius was raised from childhood in the Stoic tradition and consequently was later led to write his famous *Meditations*, one of the most influential books of all time, outlining the principles and practice of cognitive restructuring. One of the major proponents of Stoicism in the context of mental health was the Swiss psychiatrist Paul Dubois, who in his clinical work taught patients a Stoic philosophy of life (Robertson & Codd, 2019).

In modern times, methods of teaching children and adolescents to talk more sensibly to themselves, and thereby to make themselves individually and socially more effective, were pioneered by Alfred Adler. Not only was Adler (1927) probably one of the first cognitive therapists to specialize in direct psychological approaches to youngsters, but he and his associates, starting in the 1920s, saw the importance of using cognitive approaches in the school system and of teaching these skills to parents to employ in the rearing of children. Today, the field of psychotherapy has seen a decided shift to a more cognitive behavioral orientation

M. Bernard
Melbourne Graduate School of Education, University of Melbourne, Parkville, VIC, Australia
e-mail: m.bernard@unimelb.edu.au

M. D. Terjesen (✉)
Department of Psychology, St. John's University, Jamaica, NY, USA
e-mail: Terjesem@stjohns.edu

M. Bernard, M. D. Terjesen (eds.), *Rational-Emotive and Cognitive-Behavioral Approaches to Child and Adolescent Mental Health: Theory, Practice, Research, Applications*, https://doi.org/10.1007/978-3-030-53901-6_1

(Norcross & Karpiak, 2012; Norcross, Sayette, & Pomerantz, 2018) including child and adolescent therapy. This is further affirmed by the adoption of the definition of psychotherapy by the American Psychological Association (APA) (emphasis added):

> Psychotherapy is the informed and intentional application of clinical methods and interpersonal stances derived from established psychological principles for the purpose of assisting people to *modify their behaviors, cognitions, emotions*, and/or other personal characteristics in directions that the participants deem desirable. (Campbell, Norcross, Vasquez, & Kaslow, 2013)

History of Rational Emotive and Cognitive Behavioral Therapy with Children and Adolescents

Since the late 1950s there has been considerable conceptual and empirical theories as to the nature of emotional and behavioral disturbance from a cognitive/thinking perspective (Ellis, 1957, 1962). Among the original approaches is Rational Emotive Behavior Therapy (REBT) originally referred to as Rational Therapy and Rational Emotive Therapy (Ellis, 1995). Soon after he started to use REBT with adults, at the beginning of 1955, he saw that it could also be employed with children either directly by a therapist or indirectly by an REBT practitioner working with the children's parents. This was reflected in his first book on REBT, *How to Live with a "Neurotic"* (Ellis, 1957), where he offered some cognitive parenting techniques. When he began making tape recordings of REBT sessions, he recorded a series of sessions with an 8-year-old female bed-wetter (Ellis, 1959), which were widely circulated and encouraged many other therapists to use RET methods with children. In the 1960s, cognitive restructuring with youngsters was promoted by a number of REBT-oriented writers who showed how it could be effectively employed by therapists, parents, and school personnel (Doress, 1967; Ellis, 1967; Ellis, Wolfe, & Moseley, 1966; Glicken, 1967, 1968; Hauck, 1967; Lafferty, Dennell, & Rettich, 1964; McGory, 1967; Wagner, 1966).

By and large, the only cognitive restructuring approach being employed with school-age children through the late 1960s was REBT. A shift was seen in the late 1960s, where behavior therapists began to open their minds to cognition, and as a consequence, widely practiced and researched behavioral methods of helping youngsters overcome their emotional and behavioral problems began to be combined with REBT and other cognitive methods like Beck's cognitive therapy. During the 1970s, a large number of articles, chapters, and manuals appeared that explained the use of REBT with children and adolescents (e.g., Knaus, 1974). A review of these early pioneers of clinical models and outcome studies may be found in Bernard, Ellis, and Terjesen (2005). At the same time, cognitive behavioral therapy techniques were being implemented among youth; however, some early concerns were noted in the methodology of these studies (Hobbs, Moguin, Tyroler, & Lahey, 1980).

Indeed, because of the observed success of REBT that was found in early clinical and experimental investigations, the Institute for Rational-Emotive Therapy in New York started the Living School in 1970, a small private grade school where all the children were taught REBT along with the usual elementary-school curriculum. The school flourished for 5 years, in the course of which it was found that teachers (not therapists) could teach young children REBT in the regular classroom situation and thereby help them (and their parents) to improve their emotional health and to live more happily and efficiently. Publications on the use of REBT in this school setting were published by DiNubile and Wessler (1974), Ellis (1971a, 1971b, 1972, 1973, 1975), Gerald and Eyman (1981), Knaus (1974), Sachs (1971), and Wolfe and staff (1970). In order to have a greater impact in classrooms both in the community and across the country, the Living School was transformed in 1975 into the Rational-Emotive Education Consultation Service, which provided: (1) in-service workshops for teachers and counselors; (2) consultations to schools, classes, and teachers wishing to implement a program of RET; and (3) materials and techniques for use in classrooms and/or school counseling settings (Waters, 1981).

From the early 1980s with the publication of the first edition of this book, Rational Emotive Approaches to the Problems of Childhood (Ellis & Bernard, 1983) and Bernard and Joyce's (1984) "Rational Emotive Therapy with Children and Adolescents," through the 1990s and early part of the twenty-first century, clinical and educational applications of REBT have been written about extensively. A special issue of the School Psychology Review was devoted to the implications of REBT and REE for the role of school psychologists (Bernard & DiGiuseppe, 1990). Bernard and DiGiuseppe's book (1993) "Rational Emotive Consultation in Applied Settings" contained a variety of chapters detailing ways in which REBT could be used by practitioners to address the mental health needs of primary caregivers of young people (parents, teachers) with emotional and behavioral disorders as well as provided ways in which the ABCs and rational beliefs could be introduced by primary caregivers to young people. Similar to REBT, but perhaps somewhat later, the extension to the application of CBT in working with youth was seen both empirically as well as conceptually through the first major publications in the area (Craighead, Meyers, & Craighead, 1985; Meyers & Craighead, 1984). There were a number of early research reviews that supported the efficacy of REBT (Hajzler & Bernard, 1991) and CBT among youth (Weisz, Weiss, Alicke, & Klotz, 1987). A more current summary of the efficacy of the extant literature for REBT, CBT, and REE is offered in Chap. 2 of this edited volume.

Today, it is abundantly clear that within the fields of clinical psychology (child), school psychology, school counseling and guidance, REBT and CBT are preferred methodologies incorporated within the tool boxes of counselors and psychologists who work with children and adolescents. Further, in the field of school-wide prevention and promotion programming, REBT- and CBT-based applications are often seen in social-emotional learning curricula (Dayan, 2016). REBT-based programs such as the You Can Do It! Education (YCDI!) (e.g., Bernard, 2008, 2013, 2017, 2018a, 2018b; Bernard, Elias, Bell, Ferrito, & Langione, 2017; Bernard & Walton, 2011) (see Chap. 20 of this book). Over 100,000 3–6-year old children are learning rational, positive beliefs as a result of participating in the REBT-based YCDI early childhood program (Ashdown & Bernard, 2012; Bernard, 2018a). Over the past several decades, the Albert Ellis Institute in New York and affiliated training REBT centers throughout the world have offered the Child and Adolescent Certificate in Rational Emotive Behavior Therapy to large numbers of practitioners. Further, the Beck Institute offers a 3-day CBT with a Youth training program to teach clinicians developmentally appropriate and practical CBT skills in clinical work with caregivers, children, and adolescents.

Interestingly, despite REBT being considered to be the first formal system under the Cognitive Behavioral Therapy (CBT) spectrum (Hollon & DiGiuseppe, 2010; MacLaren, Doyle, & DiGiuseppe, 2015), in the field of cognitive behavioral child treatment, clinical psychologists have not embraced REBT as extensively as in other mental health professions. This may be due in part to a perception that REBT has no research base to speak of and, as a consequence, REBT has been ignored by CBTers (M. A. Reinecke, personal communication, 2005). Hopefully, the material presented in the subsequent chapters will dispel this notion.

Theoretical Considerations in Applications of RE-CBT to Childhood Disorders

In this section, we examine important theoretical foundations that underpin the practice of RE-CBT with younger populations.

REBT and CBT Developmental Model of Childhood Disorders

Grave and Blissett (2004) and Garber and colleagues (Garber, Frankel, & Herrington, 2016) offer some important developmental consideration in the application of RE-CBT among youth. The integration of the developmental level of the child with cognitive behavioral approaches is one that has been met with challenges (Ollendick, Grills, & King, 2001) that may preclude their participation in some of the more complex aspects of REBT and CBT (Grave & Blissett, 2004). In looking at both the theory and the science, there is little question that REBT and CBT are developmentally oriented and meets existing criteria for establishing a therapy's developmental credentials (e.g., Holmbeck, Greenley, & Franks, 2003; Shirk, 2001; Weisz & Hawley, 2002). It is important that REBT and CBT clinicians who work with children and adolescents take into account the critical developmental tasks and milestones relevant to a particular child's or adolescent's presenting problem (e.g., Bernard, 2004) and have the flexibility to be able to choose which presenting symptoms to prioritize, depending on the degree to which each of the symptoms is developmentally atypical. Further, being developmentally sensitive with assessment and treatment methods where clinicians to take into account the developmental levels of the child or adolescent has been a long-standing practice within REBT (e.g., Bernard & Joyce, 1984). Whereas most treatment models focus on the assessment of symptoms and diagnosis (Garber et al., 2016), we have found that REBT- and CBT-driven assessments have consideration of the strengths and weaknesses of the student and their developmental ability to benefit from specific cognitively oriented interventions. For example, REBT does little disputing of irrational beliefs in children younger than six and reserves more sophisticated disputing of general beliefs until after the age of 11 or 12. Table 1.1 developed by Ann Vernon, an innovator in the production of age-appropriate creative activities that teach children and adolescents the basics of REBT, has specified developmental issues to take into account when practicing REBT with younger populations.

As can be seen in the chapters of this book, REBT and CBT have always thought *multi-systemically* and always consider the need to involve peers, teachers, parents, and the whole family while treating the child. As reflected in this volume, REBT and CBT practitioners believe that emotional disorders and abnormal behavior in childhood can be best understood in terms of an interaction between "person" and environmental (e.g., parenting, peer) variables. Bernard and Joyce (1984) characterized this perspective as follows:

> Children demonstrate characteristic ways of thinking about and relating to their environment which exert an influence on their environment. Similarly, situations themselves modify the behavior and attitudes of people by providing (or not providing) appropriate learning experiences and enrichment opportunities as well as rewarding and punishing consequences for behavior within certain contexts. We believe that there is an almost inexorable reciprocal relationship between abnormal behavior and a deviant environment such that abnormalities in either the person or the environment of the person tend to bring out abnormalities in the other. It would seem, therefore, necessary to determine how persons and environments interact and covary together in analyzing childhood psychopathology.

This was further reflected in similar sentiments expressed by Bernard (2004):

> The extent to which children's thinking and associated beliefs are dominated by irrationality rather than rationality depends upon their age, their biological temperament (e.g., feisty, fearful, flexible), their home environment including their parent's style of parenting (e.g., firm/not firm, kind/unkind), the extent to which their parents model and communicate irrational or rational beliefs and whether there are negative events present in their lives (e.g., divorce, persecution). Children who manifest social-emotional- behavioral and achievement problems often present with developmental delays in their capacity to think rationally and logically concerning affective-interpersonal issues (e.g., have difficulty keeping things in perspective, personalize negative experiences) as well as in the development of other emotional self-management skills (e.g., relaxation, finding someone to talk with). They also are dominated by a range of irrational beliefs including self-downing, low frustration tolerance, and the lack of acceptance of others.

Child Factors

The ability to engage in the process of REBT and CBT is impacted by a number of factors, chief among them may be the child's cognitive developmental level (Garber et al., 2016; Shirk, 1999) engaging in cognitive therapy. According to REBT theory, children are born with an innate capacity to think irrationally and illogically. What moderates the influence of irrationality is the development of rationality and logical

Table 1.1 Developmental milestones (Vernon, 2004)

Early childhood (4–5 years) (pre-concrete operational thinking; the world of pre-school, play/fantasy)	
Difficult in distinguishing real from make believe Egocentric Perspective-taking impossible Self-esteem quite high Overestimate ability to do things Beginning to develop impulse control High self-efficacy Pre-concrete operational thinking Through play, children learn how to be cooperative and take turns Solve problems using information from what they see or hear rather than using logical reasoning Difficulty with abstract concepts like death and divorce	Aspect of their cognitive style is centration – inability to view a situation/person from multiple perspectives Because of difficulty in understanding intentionality, they are likely to misinterpret other's behavior and respond inappropriately Cannot understand it is possible to experience multiple emotions at the same time Toward the end of the stage, children begin to develop a sense of empathy acquiring a better understanding of other people's feelings
Typical problems: difficulties in cooperative play and fears due to tendency to take things literally and failure to distinguish reality from fantasy. Situational problems.	
Middle childhood (6–10 years) (developing a sense of belongingness with friends – socialization – and teachers)	
Prone to misinterpretations of reality. Prone to make faulty inferences concerning the motives of others (if their best friend does not sit next to them, likely to assume friend is angry with them rather than consider other alternative explanations) Lack of ability to generate problem-solving alternatives (alternative solution generation, consequential thinking, cause-effect) when faced with adversity Development of impulse control necessary to cope with the structure of schooling Adult and peer approval important At age 8, children enter the concrete operational stage that aids problem-solving; they are able to think more logically but cannot reason abstractly (use concrete logical disputes) Problem-solving is limited by the inability to consider alternative courses of action before approaching a situation Self-understanding improves Developmental trend toward internal locus of control	Become more self-critical comparing self with others and may tend to experience low self-esteem in comparison to children in early childhood period Children evaluate their degree of success in making friends and or at risk for rejection, peer pressure, and conformity as socialization becomes central developmental task Children begin to develop perspective-taking skills and, as a consequence, are better able to resolve interpersonal conflict Cannot understand possible to experience multiple emotions at the same time Adept at hiding emotions More able to recognize and communicate feelings to others than before Aware that they are not the sole cause of another's feelings They are also better able to recognize feelings more effectively that contributes to improved problem-solving skills
Typical problems: anxiety associated with issues surrounding peer approval (being chosen for a team, anxiety about not being liked or ridiculed by classmates); anxiety associated with school performance (grades, being liked by teacher; being disciplined by teacher). Situational problems.	

(continued)

Table 1.1 (continued)

Early adolescence (11–14 years) (middle school, grades 6–8) (emotional roller coaster)	
Heightened anxiety due to a variety of factors (self-consciousness of differences with others brought about by puberty/physical development, shift focus to peer group and adolescents want to be like everyone else, accepted); imaginary audience (increase in anxiety) Mood fluctuations Overly sensitive to performance and appearance (increase in low self-esteem) Push for independence leads to changes in parent-child relationship (increase in home problems including anger and rebelliousness) Formal operational thinking Imaginary audience – assume everyone is looking at them – on display Personal fable – mistaken beliefs that because they are unique and invulnerable, bad things happen to others but not to them (unprotected sex) – leads to high incidence of risk-taking behavior (increase in risk-taking behaviors)	Peers play a more important role (increase in peer conforming behavior; increase in down feelings due to peer rejection) Young people feel increasingly vulnerable due to push for independence but lack of experiences and reliance on parents (tension) Rapid physical changes; physical/hormonal changes lead to discomfort, confusion as sexual thoughts arouse accompanied by guilt and embarrassment Shift from concrete to formal operational thinking begins at 12, complete by 15 Think more abstractly, can hypothesize, predict consequences (not in emotional domain); difficulty making logical cause-effect connection when applied to self (failing a test results from not having studied) Do not assume these children are capable of mature cognition Unable to generate alternatives for dealing with emotions
Typical problems: easily overwhelmed by feelings, problems arise when feeling overwhelmed; anger, depression, and mood swings are common. Oversensitivity in relationships with friends/family. Excessive worry about how they look, act, and belong. And their sexuality. Anger with family due to striving for independence. Emotional reactions to adults' over-reactions; anger may cover up feelings of inadequacy, depression; increased intensity of emotions.	
Mid-adolescence (high school, 15–18 years.) (independence/emotional maturity-stepping stone to world of young adult) (Vernon, 1993)	
Formal operational thinking continues to evolve – new cognitive abilities Lack of experience to make appropriate choices Interests are in exploring different roles and achieving independence Friendships continue to be important but change; may not be as dependent on friends as more emotionally mature; intimate relationships bring with them challenges of dating/sexual experimentation	Experimentation increases More able to deal with emotional issues although wide individual differences Self-confidence increases
Typical problems: problems arise (anxiety) due to issues inherent in more intimate relationships and uncertainties about the future including transition to post-secondary education and work. Push for more independence from parents (anger) and anxiety about being too independent. Experience more loneliness than before as their needs/interests and friends change. Self-doubt concerning themselves grows if they perceive shortcoming in skills/knowledge to get into university or job of their choice.	

reasoning abilities which emerge around the age of six (Piaget's concrete operational stage of development) with abstract reasoning abilities developing more fully around the age of 11 or 12 (Piaget's formal operational stage of development). Clinical approaches seek to consider a child's level of cognitive development as defined by Piaget's stages and therapeutic methods offered by REBT and CBT. The prerequisite skill of connecting thoughts and emotions requires both meta-cognition and causal reasoning (Garber et al., 2016) and clinicians would be wise to consider the developmental stage of the child before engaging in RE-CBT. As an example, whereas we employ rational self-statements with children of all ages, we generally do not dispute irrational beliefs with children who are less than 7 years old, and we do not often logically dispute irrational beliefs in the abstract with children much below the age of 11 or 12.

There are a number of interesting overlaps between the theories of Ellis and those of Piaget. Both share the assumption of constructivism. They also place great "faith" in the scientific reasoning method of investigation and the power of formal logical reasoning.

Sandberg and McCullough (2010) describe the systematic approach toward gathering evidence against a testable hypothesis during scientific reasoning. This is quite analogous to REBT and CBT clinicians working with students to "test" their irrational beliefs or automatic thoughts that are impacting their affective and behavioral states. Both appear to be in agreement concerning the importance of cognition in the experience and expression of emotions. Piaget (1952) wrote that "it is, in fact, only a romantic prejudice that makes us suppose that affective phenomena constitute immediate givens or innate and ready-made feelings similar to Rousseau's 'conscience'" (p. 12).

In his writings, Ellis (e.g., 1994) discusses the idea that the strength of one's propensity for irrational thought and the strength of conviction one has in one's irrational beliefs is heavily influenced by genetics (MacLaren et al., 2015). Podina and colleagues (Podina, Popp, Pop, & David, 2015) offer some preliminary evidence as to a genetic marker for predicting irrationality when stressed. Ellis recognized that while parenting practices, peers, and one's culture may condition the beliefs of young people through modeling and direct communication, the tendency for beliefs to be fully integrated within a young person's view of the world and the extent to which a young person's cognitive processing is characterized by absolutism is not learned but is biologically determined (Bernard et al., 2005). The evidence provided by Ellis to substantiate nature over nurture when it comes to the origins of an individual's irrational thinking is partly found in the many instances of families seen by Ellis where only one child presented with an internalizing or externalizing problem but their sibling did not, despite the parenting styles having remained constant. Some children who experience distress and demonstrate maladaptive behaviors have parents who appear to be reasonably well adjusted, who have positive attitudes toward their child, and whose child-rearing practices appear to be sound.

As already indicated, REBT and CBT have historically recognized the importance of the young person's cognitive developmental level of maturity in treatment. On the assessment side, a recognition of child development enables the practitioner to judge whether a presenting problem is a transient and/or a normal developmental phenomenon (i.e., fear of the dark) or whether it represents something more serious. The level at which the cognitively-based intervention is used (rational self-statements, disputing of inferences, or abstract disputing of irrational beliefs) depends on the linguistic and cognitive maturity of the young client.

REBT and CBT recognize, as do the proponents of many different approaches to childhood psychopathology, that there is a reciprocal relationship between mental and emotional development. When children are very young, the quality of their subjective emotional experience is very much limited by their capacity to think about and understand the meaning of their experience. The cognitive limitations of the early childhood period can often result in children's acquiring beliefs about themselves and their surrounding world that are untrue and irrational and that if not corrected can have an extremely deleterious effect on their future wellbeing. That is, children construct their own theories and arrive at their own conclusions based on inferences from what they have observed. The child's conception of the world is idiosyncratically organized and derives from the child's limited capacity to make observations and draw logical conclusions.

In working with children, we are struck by the pervasive influence that their ideas and beliefs have on their emotions and behavior. These beliefs are often implicit and frequently result from the child's having formed a conclusion based on limited evidence and having used the conclusion as an "unquestioned" rule for guiding subsequent behavior. The beliefs, be they rational, or irrational, that are formed early in life may become firmly fixed, and they represent part of the phenomenological framework of children that provides the basis for self-evaluation, for the demands they place on others, and for the interpretation they make of the behavior of others. Young children's incapacity for rational and logical thought limits the types of ideas that they acquire and frequently reinforces a variety of irrational beliefs which take many years to overcome.

A cognitive analysis of maladjustment in children and adolescents frequently reveals beliefs about themselves, others, and the world, as well as logical reasoning processes that appear to be either a holdover from or a regression to pre-concrete operational levels of thinking and primitive belief systems. Characteristics of pre-concrete operational thought include:

1. Drawing arbitrary inferences – conclusions not based on evidence or when evidence contradicts conclusion
2. Selective abstraction – focusing on a detail taken out of context, ignoring salient features of the situation
3. Magnification/minimization – errors in evaluating the significance of an event
4. Personalization – tendency to relate external events to themselves when no basis for making connection

5. Overgeneralization – drawing a conclusion based on limited and isolated events
6. Dichotomous thinking – tendency to place events into opposite categories (e.g., good-bad)

The advent of formal operational thought capacities in adolescents also brings with it its own problems. Adolescents in their early teens begin to experience a form of egocentrism (Remmel & Flavell, 2004), a "naive, idealism" (not dissimilar in effect from the egocentrism of the early childhood period), that frequently leads to a variety of emotional and behavioral problems. The struggle for a personal identity and for new definitions of social relationships that accompanies the increased capacity for reflective and abstract thought often results in adolescents' acquiring sets of beliefs concerning themselves (self-rating) and others (demandingness) that accompany some people throughout life.

Parental Factors Parents may serve as role models and reinforcing-punishing agents and can play a major part in preventing, minimizing, or exacerbating emotional and behavioral problems in their children. The role of parenting cognitions, affect, and behavior as they relate to child adjustment are elaborated on in Chaps. 6 and 22 of this volume. In considering the role of parenting in adjustment, we agree with Bard's (1980) comments:

> Some children seem especially prone to make themselves miserable about their parent's relatively minor imperfections. I emphasize this point at the onset to attack the myth that parents are always to blame and to alert practitioners to the fact that parent-child problems may be extremely complex. (p. 93)

Ellis (1973) posited that the worst thing that parents can do to their children is to blame them for their mistake making and wrongdoing. Such blaming encourages children to continue to blame themselves and inevitably leads to chronic feelings of anxiety, guilt, and low self-esteem for some children and hostility and bigotry in others.

Irrational beliefs of parents can influence their parenting behavior in two basic ways. One is through their emotions.

> Parents frequently get very upset when their child breaks a rule because they believe that: (a) "My child must be good all the time"; (b) "I find it awful or horrible when my child is not-I can't stand it," and (c) "My child deserves punishment because he has made me so angry and for being such a bad child." The belief that children must never break a rule leads to extreme anger which produces intense and non-constructive disciplinary action. (Bernard & Joyce, 1984)

Alternatively, parents may employ inappropriate and counterproductive methods of child management because of ignorance. That is, they believe that what they are doing is the correct thing to do, and often, it is the only way that they can conceptualize relating to their children. Their maladaptive behavior is not associated with extreme emotional arousal but motivated directly by their "unjustified" and "outdated" assumptions.

Conceptualization of an Emotional Episode

Incidents of emotional upset are complicated psychological phenomena. The theoretical approaches of REBT, CT, and CBT are grounded in the role of cognitions, beliefs, evaluations, and perceptions in contributing to unhealthy negative affective states and behaviors (Beck & Dozois, 2011; DiGiuseppe, Doyle, Dryden, & Backx, 2014). The CBT umbrella attempts to group a number of therapies together that share common elements and clinical applications. While approaches such as Cognitive Therapy, Dialectical Behavior Therapy, and Problem-Solving Therapy share similarities, there are some unique aspects to each of them. As an example, the Beck Cognitive Therapy model proposes that faulty information processing and biased perceptions lead to the development of ineffective cognitive schemas (Beck & Haigh, 2014; Buschmann, Horn, Blankenship, Garcia, & Bohan, 2018). Similarly, REBT has very unique distinctive features. In this section, we will discuss the theory of REBT in explaining an emotional episode among youth and where appropriate highlight the distinctive components of other models. For a thorough review of the distinctiveness of these models, refer to Dryden (2015).

Ellis (1994) has provided his now famous ABC model (outlined below) to help clients grasp the role of their thoughts in causing emotional disturbance. Wessler and Wessler (1980) expanded the ABC model to help therapists to a fuller understanding of these complex psychological events. At the start of every emotional event, a stimulus is presented to the child:

Step 1: Stimuli are then sensed by the person's eyes, ears, sense of smell, touch, etc.

Step 2: Sensory neurons process the stimuli and transmit them to the CNS.

Step 3: Not all sensations enter consciousness. Some are filtered out and others are perceived. Perception is Step 3. Perception, however, is not an exact replication of reality. Perceptions consist of equal parts of information provided by the senses and information provided by the brain. At this point, all information is organized, categorized, and defined. Perception is as much a peripheral as a CNS function.

Step 4: People usually do not stop thinking after they have perceived information. In most cases, they attempt to extract more information than is present in the perception, so some interpretations or inferences are likely to follow perceptions.

Step 5: Humans are not just passive processors of information. Inferences and conclusions usually have some further meaning associated with them. Conclusions and inferences may vary in their importance to an individual. Almost all inferences are appraised by the person either positively or negatively in relation to the person's life. Irrational appraisals consist of *absolutes* (shoulds, oughts, musts, needs) and *evaluations* (awfulizing, I can't standit-it-is, global rating of self, others, the world).

Step 6: According to rational emotive behavior therapy, affect or emotion accompanies appraisal. We feel happy or sad or mad at Step 6, after we have appraised something as being beneficial, threatening, etc.

Step 7: Emotional states are not separate psychological phenomena. Emotions have evolved as part of the flight-fight mechanism and exist primarily to motivate adaptive behavior. Therefore, emotions usually include not only the reactions of the autonomic nervous system and the phenomenological sensations, but action tendencies or behavioral response sets that are learned.

Step 8: Responses, once they are made, usually have some impact on the external world. This effect can be desirable or undesirable, and feedback of our action tendencies serves as a reward to strengthen or extinguish a response set.

Given this model, emotional disturbance develops because of one or two types of cognitive errors: empirical distortions of reality that occur at Step 4 (inferences) and irrational, exaggerated, and distorted appraisals of inferences at Step 5. According to REBT, it is primarily the appraisal that is necessary for emotional disturbance. This is the B in Ellis's ABC. Ellis has noted, however, that, many times, the appraisals are about distortions of reality. Faulty inferences usually do accompany exaggerated appraisal, but the appraisal alone is sufficient to arouse disturbed affect.

We have found that visuals can assist in clinical work in communicating the relationship among beliefs/thoughts and emotions and behaviors. The iceberg metaphor (see Fig. 1.1), so often used in explaining the psychoanalytic model of psychotherapy, can really be quite helpful in understanding the role of cognitions and how while they may not be observable are very powerful in terms of behavioral and affective expression. Much like the vast majority of an iceberg's volume is underwater (not seen) and guides an iceberg's movement, one's emotions and behaviors

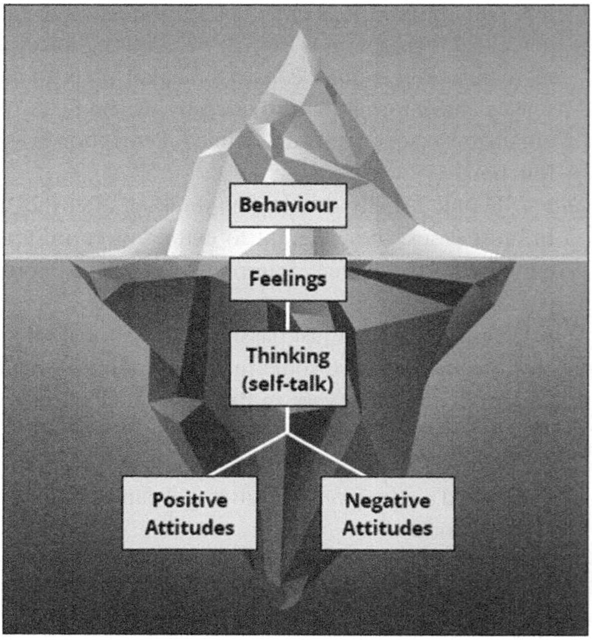

Fig. 1.1 The iceberg model in explaining the RE-CBT model. (Bernard, 2018a, 2018b)

are strongly influenced by their self-talk (beliefs). Clinical work that focuses on understanding how that which is observable (emotions and behaviors) are influenced by these unseen elements, whether they are under the influence of positive of negative ones is important. We also think this visual may be helpful in distinguishing between more just below the surface level beliefs often seen in Cognitive Therapy ("I am going to fail") and the deeper beliefs ("If I fail, that means I am a failure.") that may contribute to more profound negative affect. These distinctions will be elaborated on in the below.

Let's take a hypothetical clinical example to explain how these two cognitions operate. George, a 14-year-old, has moved to a new neighborhood and has not met new friends. He is sitting quietly in the neighborhood playground while the other teenagers are talking among themselves or playing basketball. He feels very anxious and his associated action potential is withdrawal. He sits alone leaning up against a wall, reading a book. As he sees others gather nearby, George thinks, "They'll never like me, they'll think I'm weird, and they won't want to speak with me no matter what I do." George has drawn these inferences from his peer's behavior. In fact, they are predictions about what might happen but never actually has happened. Inferences alone are not sufficient to arouse high levels of anxiety. Some adolescents, although not George, might be perfectly happy to sit by themselves and read books, but George appraises this situation quite negatively and irrationally. His implicit absolute "I need people to like and approve of me" leads him to catastrophize "It's awful that I don't have anyone to play with" and, then, to put himself down "I must be a jerk if they won't play with me."

Hot and Cold Cognitions

Prior to discussing specific automatic thoughts and irrational beliefs that are consistent with the RE-CBT model, it may be important to highlight the differences between cold and hot cognitions to guide clinical work. Although the concept of hot and cold cognitions is often used in RE-CBT, its history can be traced back to the work of Abelson and Rosenberg (1958) who used the concepts of hot and cold cognitions to make the distinction between facts/knowledge (cold) and appraisals (hot). Cold cognitions may be considered to be the first level of cognition and reflects how one may process information independent of emotion. Hot cognitions are the more emotional of the two, where the manner in which we think about an event is influenced by our emotions (David & Szentagotai, 2006; Gavita & Joyce, 2008).

While cold cognitions (e.g., no one in my class likes me) may be incorrect and we would look at challenging those inferences, they may not lead to an emotional response unless they are negatively appraised (e.g., "They SHOULD like me! It's TERRIBLE that they don't. I am a loser"). Gavita and Joyce posit that when classifying cognitions clinicians may want to distinguish between the knowing (cold) and appraising (hot) thoughts. They also suggest clinicians be mindful of the surface cognitions (inferences) which are easier for clients to be aware of and the more deep cognitions (beliefs or schemas) which can be a challenge to access without support.

Defining Thoughts, Schemas, and Beliefs

While the different CBT approaches all highlight the importance of thinking, the terminology used and specific types of beliefs vary somewhat dependent on the model. The Beckian model of cognitive therapy focuses on automatic thoughts (ATs) that relate to a specific situation and may take the form of inferences or evaluations (Soflau & David, 2017). These beliefs are generally considered to focus on three types or levels of cognitions: automatic thoughts (ATs), intermediate beliefs, and core beliefs (Leder, 2017). These ATs are considered to be surface level and are fairly accessible specific beliefs about a past, present, or future stimuli (e.g., "He hated my presentation"; "I am being boring"; "I will fail") and have been linked to emotions among children (Beck, 2005; Hogendoorn et al., 2010; Schniering & Rapee, 2002). The intermediate beliefs are often considered to be conditional statements that are distorted and overly rigid in nature (Leder, 2017). An example would be when students think: "If I don't make the big shot in the game, people will be mad at me." Finally, the core beliefs/schemas are proposed to be more challenging to access and are highly generalized beliefs about oneself and the world and form the basis for all other cognitions (Leder, 2017). An example would be: "I am a loser" or "Things will never go my way".

In REBT, the terms *belief* and *belief system* refer to that aspect of human cognition that is responsible for the mental health and the psychological well-being of the individual. Beliefs are a central explanatory construct of REBT, and it is important that the meaning of the term be as clear as possible.

Ellis (e.g., 1977) developed an ABC (DE) theory of emotional disturbance that describes how a person becomes upset. REBT starts with an emotional and behavioral consequence (C) and seeks to identify the activating event (A) that appears to have precipitated (C). While the commonly accepted viewpoint is that, (A) caused (C), REBT steadfastly maintains that it is the individual's beliefs (B) about what happened at (A) that more directly "create" (C). Disputation (D), one of the cornerstones of the REBT practice of therapeutic change, involves employing the scientific method of challenging and questioning anti-empirical and untenable hypotheses that are illogical and dysfunctional, as well as imperative and absolutistic assumptions (irrational beliefs) that individuals may hold about themselves, about others, and about the world, which lead to the particular interpretations and appraisals that the individual forms about the activating event. When individuals who hold irrational beliefs begin to change their unsound assumptions, to reformulate them into more empirically valid statements, and to believe strongly in the validity of the new ideas, they now have developed new cognitive (philosophical), emotive, and behavioral effects (E's).

Belief may be viewed as a very broad hypothetical construct that embraces at least three distinct subclasses of cognitive phenomena: (1) thoughts that an individual is thinking and is aware of at a given time about A; (2) thoughts about A that the individual is not immediately aware of; and (3) more abstract beliefs that the individual may hold in general (Bernard, 1981; David, Freeman, & DiGiuseppe, 2010). Eschenroeder (1982) was in essential agreement with this analysis when he wrote that the ABC scheme is a simplification of the complex processes of the perception, interpretation, and evaluation of events and the activation of emotional reactions and behavioral responses:

> The B-element of the ABC refers to rather different phenomena: (1) *thoughts and images*, which can be observed through introspection by the individual; (2) *unconscious processes*, which can be inferred post hoc from the individual's. feelings and behavior ("unconscious verbalizations"); (3) the *belief system* underlying the person's thoughts, emotions, and behaviors. (p. 275)

The more abstract beliefs that people hold are unspoken and constitute the assumptive framework by which they evaluate, appraise, and form conclusions about what they observe to be happening to themselves, to others, and in the world around them. These abstract beliefs are not expressed in the self-talk of people but can be considered relatively enduring personality traits that affect people's interpretations of reality and often, in so doing, guide subsequent behavior. They are inferred from the types of thought statements that clients are able to articulate to themselves and to the practitioner as well as from their pattern of behavior. For example, students who strongly hold the belief that they desperately need others to depend and rely on, tend to interpret situations in terms of whether they offer that level of personal security and also may seek out environments and relationships that satisfy this self-perceived need.

Abstract beliefs can be differentiated on the basis of whether they reflect absolutistic and imperative qualities (irrational) or relativistic and conditional qualities (rational). Those beliefs that lead to self-defeating emotional and behavioral consequences are almost always expressed as unqualified shoulds, oughts, musts, commands, and demands and are deemed "irrational." Ellis has indicated that if people hold rigid views and beliefs about how they, others, and the world *should* or *must* be under all circumstances, then they are likely to experience some form of disturbance. Beliefs that are expressed not as commands but as more healthier preferences and that are viewed as conditional on and relative to a set of circumstances are defined as rational and lead to more adaptive levels of emotionality and appropriate behavior.

In terms of the ABC model, rational beliefs generally lead to moderate emotions that enable clients to achieve their future goals by facilitating constructive behavior, although rational beliefs may result in extreme levels of some emotions that are contextually appropriate, such as extreme sadness and regret. Irrational beliefs lead to extreme emotional consequences (intense anxiety, anger, or depression) and behavioral reactions (aggression or withdrawal) that are not consistent with the context and interfere with the ability of the individual to improve the situation (Fig. 1.2).

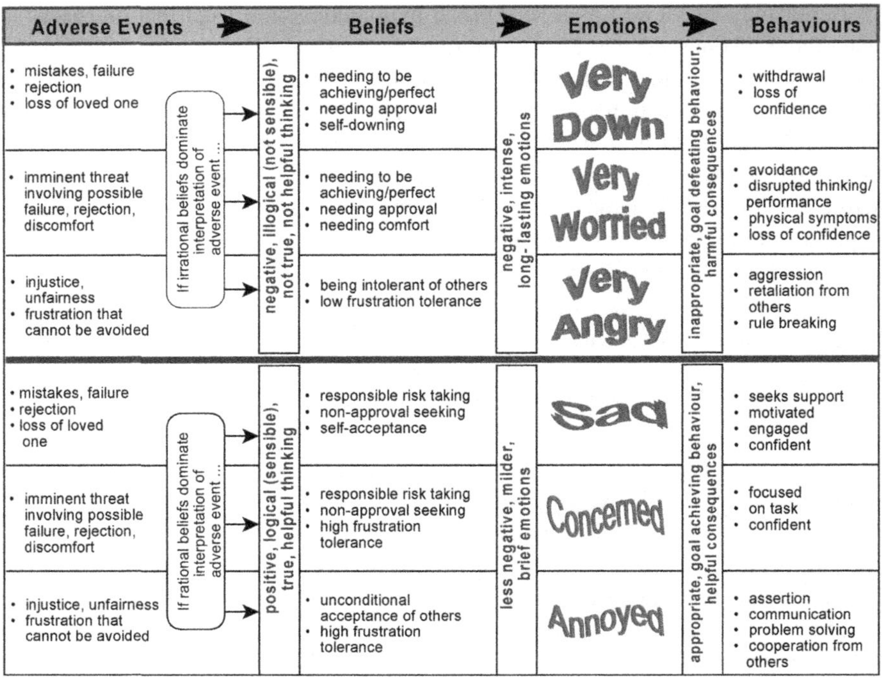

Fig. 1.2 The relationship of children's irrational beliefs to their emotions and behaviors. (Bernard, 2004)

Rational emotive behavior theory states that irrational beliefs in the form of *absolutes* (shoulds, oughts, musts, needs) are the psychological core of children and adolescent emotional and behavioral problems (see Bernard, 2004). For example,

- I must be successful.
- I need love and approval.
- The world should give me what I want comfortably, quickly, and easily.
- People must treat me fairly and considerately.

Ellis indicates that there are a number of derivatives of absolutes that also contribute to the intensity of emotional problems including *awfulizing*, *I can't-stand-it-it is* and *global rating* (self, others, world). For example,

- It's awful to make mistakes.
- I can't stand to be criticized.
- I can't stand having to do boring homework.
- People who treat me badly are bad people and deserve severe punishment.
- School is stupid.
- I'm stupid.

As a result of their rigidly held irrational beliefs, young people are prone to misrepresent reality (errors of inference including faulty conclusions, predictions).

Sometimes, these inferences are referred to as *automatic thoughts* and are consistent with the Beck model of CT. For example,

- I will always make mistakes.
- My teacher doesn't like me.
- All homework is boring.
- People always act unfairly to me.
- I'm a hopeless student.

The tendency for young people to selectively attend to and remain over-focused on the negative aspects of their environment is strongly influenced by their core irrational beliefs and feelings. That is, they may look to "gather data" that is consistent with their faulty belief system.

For example, they pay attention to:

- Children who are not wanting to play with them.
- Mistakes and other negative comments offered by their teacher concerning school work.
- The boring aspects of homework.
- Classmates who are mean to them.
- Negative aspects of the way they look.

Common Irrational Beliefs of Children include (Waters, 1982):

1. It's awful if others don't like me.
2. I'm bad if I make a mistake.
3. Everything should always do my way: I should always get what I want.
4. Things should come easy to me.
5. The world should be fair and bad people should be punished.
6. I shouldn't show my feelings.
7. Adults should be perfect.
8. There's only one right answer.
9. I must win.
10. I shouldn't have to wait for anything.

Common irrational beliefs of adolescents include (Waters, 1982):

1. It would be awful if my peers didn't like me. It would be awful to be a social loser.
2. I shouldn't make mistakes, especially social mistakes.
3. It's my parents' fault I'm so miserable.
4. I can't help it. That's just the way I am, and I guess I'll always be this way.
5. The world should be fair and just.
6. It's awful when things don't go my way.
7. It's better to avoid challenges rather than risk failure.
8. I must conform to my peers.
9. I can't stand to be criticized.
10. Others should always be responsible.

While Ellis proposed that demandingness was the core belief that all other derived from, Bernard and Joyce (1984) have offered the view that the irrational tendency of self-downing/self-depreciation rather than being derivative of core absolutes is primary. They argued that children and adolescents who have this trait put themselves down when they are faced with a variety of negative events be they mistakes, rejection, and unfairness of "bad hair" days. A factor analysis of the Child and Adolescent Scale of Irrationality (Bernard & Cronan, 1999) yielded "Self-Downing" as one of a number of distinct factors representing different patterns of irrational thinking. Chapter 2 in this edited volume summaries the research on measures of irrationality and automatic thinking among youth.

Distinctiveness of REBT and CBT in Clinical Work with Youth

While this edited volume aims to present the theory, science, and applications of REBT and CBT, the use of REBT is not synonymous with the use of CBT (Bernard et al., 2005). Ellis (1980) argued that although general or non-preferential REBT is virtually synonymous with CBT, specific or preferential REBT is not. Preferential REBT includes a deep philosophical emphasis, a humanistic outlook, the seeking of a profound and maintained personality change, the use of active disputing techniques, the teaching of clients how to give up any kind of rating of their egos or their selves (and, instead, only how to rate their acts and performances), and the getting at and eliminating of secondary as well as primary sources of unhealthy negative affect (e.g., anxiety, anger, and depression).

Although preferential REBT is highly suitable for many bright adolescents, it may require too much philosophical analysis. and more of an application of rigorous scientific method than many average youngsters, not to mention most young children, are capable of fulfilling. In the case of younger children, non-preferential REBT, or general cognitive behavioral therapy, is usually employed. This is also consistent with the developmental considerations addressed earlier. These students are shown how they upset themselves with irrational and unrealistic beliefs; how to identify or catch these thoughts and ideally they are taught how to actively discuss, debate, and dispute beliefs and to develop more rational and helpful philosophies by which to run their lives. Students often resist this kind of teaching, and especially the internalization of a scientific way of thinking, and as such, they are frequently provided with rational or coping statements (as is explained in several of the succeeding chapters of this book) and are encouraged and reinforced for believing these more sensible beliefs.

CBT subsumes a variety of methods that attempt to modify cognitive content and processes that support problem behavior. The main difference between CBT and REBT is that CBT does not attempt to modify the overall philosophy and assumptive world of clients through the use of disputational methods and other more didactic forms of direct discussion and psychoeducation. It appears that CBT is more problem-focused (or behavior-focused) and defines goals of treatment in terms of specifiable behavior change. REBT views problem behavior (and emotions) as symptomatic of an underlying belief system that constitutes the core of maladjustment. An effective REBT solution is conceived of as having been achieved when the client has adopted a more flexible, relativistic, and conditional outlook on life, which manifests itself in a more objective and empirically based reality-testing approach, in emotional reactions that are consistent with reality, and in self-enhancing, goal-directed behavior.

A CBT solution involves the client's acquiring cognitive and metacognitive strategies not only for dealing with a presenting problem, but also for dealing with a range of stressful situations that may confront the client in the future. These general and conceptually based strategies may involve the client's learning to think (and act) more reflectively and to adopt a more systematic problem-solving approach to life's difficulties.

Given the intersection of beliefs, affect, and behavior in the development of client difficulties, REBT interventions are also cognitive, emotive, and behavioral (and not *strictly* cognitive) in its treatment methods. That is, as their beliefs influence their feelings and behaviors, their emotions influence their thoughts and behaviors, and their behaviors influence their thoughts and feelings, REBT encourages the use of a wide variety of intellectual, affective, and activity-oriented techniques that will be demonstrated throughout this edited volume. Figures 1.3 and 1.4 represent all elements of the REBT model in a more pictorial, metaphorical format. These may be useful visuals to share with clients with the key takeaway from the house is that Attitudes are the foundations that determine the extent to which students experience positive wellbeing and flourishing or social-emotional and mental health problems (or blockers).

When a house (or student's life) is built on a rocky, unstable, weak foundation of negative attitudes (or ways that they view themselves and life), the house (the student) will have more chance of experiencing the 5 blockers, plus have weaker character, leading to non-achievement and unhappiness (Fig. 1.3). Alternatively, when a house (or student's life) is built on a firm, stable, strong foundation of positives attitudes (or ways of viewing themselves and life), the house (student) will have more chance of possessing the 5 SELs, plus have a stronger character, leading to achievement and happiness (see Fig. 1.4).

RE-CBT Model of Assessment and Treatment of Children and Adolescents

Chapter 3 in this volume provides extensive details of RE-CBT work with young people summarized in four stages (RATE): Relationship Building, Assessment, Treatment, and Evaluation. The following figure encapsulates and summarizes systematic steps to take when working with a young person. As you will see in the other problem-specific chapters in this edited volume, many integrate multiple components of these steps with appropriate modification as it relates to the areas of concern (Fig. 1.5).

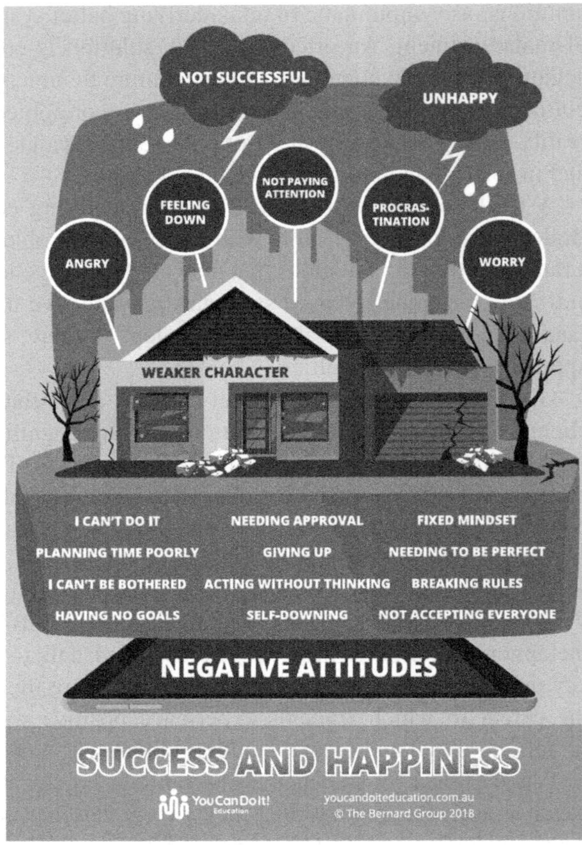

Fig. 1.3 Negative attitudes lead to poor social-emotional difficulties and mental health issues. (Bernard, unpublished)

Allied Cognitive Behavioral Theories

While REBT is generally considered to be the initially developed theory and clinical approach under the CBT tent, there are other complimentary cognitive behavioral theories and techniques that help define additional aspects of cognitive processing and functioning of young people that influence their mental health. Some of these are discussed more in-depth in subsequent chapters, and we will highlight some of these here.

The Interpersonal Cognitive Problem-Solving View of Maladjustment While REBT views irrational beliefs and cognitive processing errors as the source of childhood disorders, other cognitive behavioral theorists have taken a different perspective and see emotional disturbance as resulting from a deficit in the cognitions that are usually present in well-functioning children. Spivack, Platt, and Shure (1976) and Shure (1996) have identified several interpersonal cognitive problem-solving skills. Their research identified several skills in solving social problems that consistently

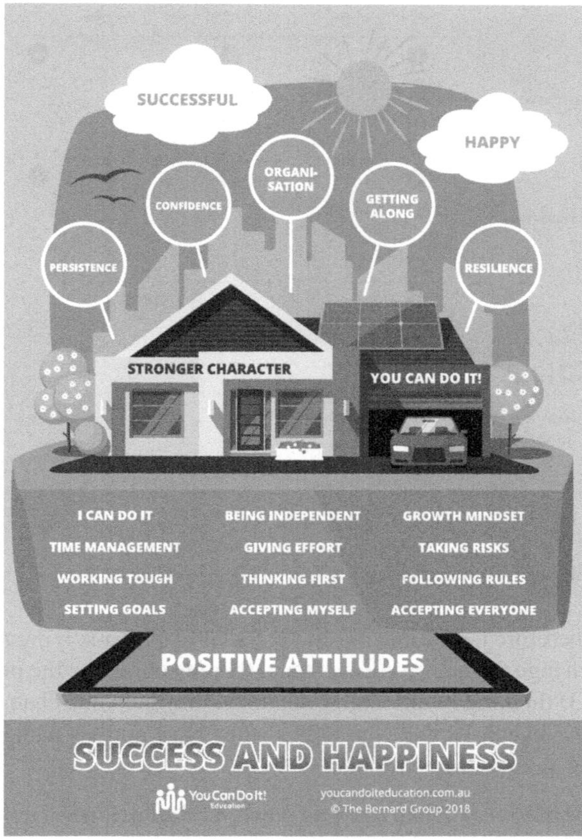

Fig. 1.4 Positive attitudes lead to success and happiness. (Bernard, unpublished)

distinguish psychopathological from normal populations. The most important skill they have uncovered is alternative-solution thinking (i.e., the number of different solutions that a child can generate to solve a specific practical problem). The second most important skill, consequential thinking, measures children's ability to predict the social consequences or results of their actions. Once children can generate alternatives and predict sequences, the next skills that seem to be important are the ability to anticipate problems and the implementation of a solution to plan around them. Spivak and his colleagues have termed these "means-end thinking."

Research suggests that attempts to teach children interpersonal, cognitive problem-solving skills can lead to reduced emotional upset and more adaptive behavior (e.g., Hess, 2014; Urbain & Kendall, 1980). Interpersonal, cognitive problem-solving skills can be effective for several reasons within the context of Wessler and Wessler's emotional episode model. Problem-solving could occur after the inferences, the appraisals, or the affect. Effective problem-solvers may experience disturbed affect less often because (1) they distract themselves from the appraisal and thereby lift affect—as long as one is thinking about how to go about solving a problem, one is less likely to be entertaining catastrophizing ideas and

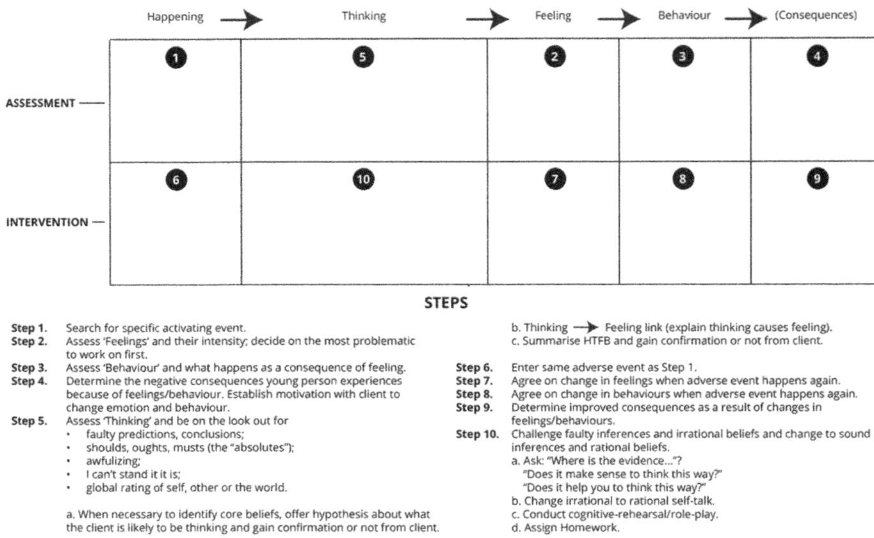

Fig. 1.5 10 steps for RE-CBT assessment and intervention

therefore to become upset; (2) social-problem-solving may bring about solutions to change the activating event and thereby eliminate the problem in the first place; and (3) thinking of alternative solutions may help one change one's appraisal of a negative event. People who believe they have options may be less likely to view events as awful or catastrophic.

Behavioral Disorders as Verbal Mediational Deficits Meichenbaum (1977, 2017) characterized the thinking styles of children with affective and behavioral difficulties in terms of three mediational deficiencies: (1) they may not comprehend the nature of the problem or the task and thus cannot discover what mediators to produce—a "comprehension" deficiency; (2) they may have the correct mediators within their repertoire but may fail to produce them spontaneously and appropriately—a "production" deficiency; and (3) the mediators that children produce may not guide their ongoing behavior—what a "mediational" deficiency.

Cognitive self-verbalization treatment programs are designed to foster the acquisition both of specific skills and of more general reflective thinking strategies including those processes involved in the treatment of a variety of behavior disorders such as attention-deficit/hyperactivity disorder (e.g., Hinshaw, 2000) and aggression (e.g., Lochman, Whidby, & FitzGerald, 2000). By providing the child with skills that can be employed in problem situations, these programs appear to influence the inferences made (Step 4) by the child when initially faced with a difficult impersonal or interpersonal task. Equipped with a task-specific skill, the child may no longer underestimate his or her coping resources; a result would be a reduction in the affective stress that presumably would previously have been experienced (Step 6). Alternatively, adaptive task performance brings about self-perceived "need satisfaction," thereby reducing the frequency with which the child's demands are not fulfilled. It can be seen that both the interpersonal cognitive problem-solving and the verbal mediational perspectives tend to emphasize direct cognitive behavioral solutions to childhood problems, whereas REBT and CBT are very much oriented toward emotional problem-solving.

The Future

While RE-CBT has demonstrated support in the prevention and treatment of the emotional and behavioral problems of children and youth, there are a number of trends from a scientific as well as applied perspective that we can anticipate in this area. As indicated earlier, there is little question that the understanding of how the cognitive developmental status of children relates to maladjustment will serve as a background to determining the type of cognitive intervention that is best suited to children who manifest different levels of mental and emotional maturity. More than 5 decades ago, Gordon Paul (1967) prompted researchers to transition away from asking "What treatments work?" to asking "*What* treatment, by *whom*, is most effective for *this* individual, with *that* specific problem, and under *which* set of circumstances?" (p. 111). Understanding what RE-CBT techniques work for which students, with what diagnoses/problems, and under which school, family, and peer conditions will lead to greater refinement of the science and practice of RE-CBT.

The use of cognitively oriented preventive mental health programs such as REE and You Can Do It! Education will proliferate as the research presented in this chapter and others in this edited volume supports their use as an evidence-based intervention.

The extent to which faulty thinking processes and the irrational beliefs of parents and teachers influence childhood maladjustment will be more fully analyzed. There are chapters in this volume that discuss the role of irrationality among both of these important groups. The role that significant others can play in correcting the maladaptive thinking patterns and beliefs of younger populations will be of increasing interest. The popularity of cognitively oriented parent and teacher education programs will grow.

The behaviorally oriented cognitive practitioners will begin to recognize (assess and treat) more fully that children and their significant others have emotions that influence both behavioral dysfunctions and the potential effects of treatment. Cognitively oriented practitioners working with children in families and in classroom settings will conduct more systematic assessments of behavioral problems so that the benefits of treatment can be more fully and objectively verified.

There will be an increasing cross-fertilization of cognitive approaches to the problems of childhood. As the contributors to this volume attest, there is a greater acceptance within the cognitive behavioral school of the utility of cognitive practices that have originated in different psychological theories and traditions. It is hoped that this trend will continue.

Test Yourself Questions

1. Discuss some of the philosophical underpinnings to RE-CBT and how this may be integrated into clinical work?
2. How would you describe the primary differences in the application of REBT and CBT?
3. Developmentally, what are important factors to consider before engaging in RE-CBT in clinical work with youth?

References

Abelson, R. P., & Rosenberg, M. J. (1958). Symbolic psychologic: A model of attitudinal cognition. *Behavioral Science, 3*(1), 1–13.
Adler, A. (1927). *Understanding human nature*. New York: Garden City Publishing.
Ashdown, D. M., & Bernard, M. E. (2012). Can explicit instruction in social and emotional learning skills benefit the social-emotional development, well-being, and academic achievement of young children? *Early Childhood Education Journal, 39*, 397–405.
Bard, J. A. (1980). *Rational-emotive therapy in practice*. Champaign, IL: Research Press.
Beck, A. T. (2005). The current state of cognitive therapy: A 40-year retrospective. *Archives of General Psychiatry, 62*(9), 953–959. https://doi.org/10.1001/archpsyc.62.9.953
Beck, A. T., & Dozois, D. J. A. (2011). Cognitive therapy: Current status and future directions. *Annual Review of Medicine, 62*(1), 397–409. https://doi.org/10.1146/annurev-med-052209-100032
Beck, A. T., & Haigh, E. A. P. (2014). Advances in cognitive theory and therapy: The generic cognitive model. *Annual Review Clinical Psychology, 10*(1), 1–24.
Bernard, M. E. (1981). Private thought in rational-emotive psychotherapy. *Cognitive Therapy and Research, 5*, 125–142.
Bernard, M. E. (2004). *The REBT therapist's pocket companion for working with children and adolescents*. New York: Albert Ellis Institute.
Bernard, M. E. (2008). The effect of You Can Do It! Education on the emotional resilience of primary school students with social, emotional, behavioral and achievement challenges. *Proceedings of the Australian Psychological Society Annual Conference, 43*, 36–40.
Bernard, M. E. (2013). You Can Do It! Education: A social-emotional learning program for increasing the achievement and well-being of children and adolescents. In K. Yamasaki (Ed.), *School-based prevention education for health and adjustment problems in the world*. Tokyo: Kaneko Shobo.
Bernard, M. E. (2017). Impact of teaching attitudes and behaviors for learning on the reading achievement of students falling behind. *International Journal of Learning, Teaching and Educational Research, 16*, 51–64.
Bernard, M. E. (2018a). *You Can Do It! Early childhood program achieve* (3rd ed.). East Melbourne, Australia: The Bernard Group. https://youcandoiteducation.com.au/
Bernard, M. E. (2018b). *NEW Program Achieve (years 1–6; years 7–12). A social-emotional learning curriculum*. East Melbourne, Australia: The Bernard Group. https://youcandoiteducation.com.au/
Bernard, M. E., & Cronan, F. (1999). The child and adolescent scale of irrationality. *Journal of Cognitive Psychotherapy, 13*, 121–132.
Bernard, M. E., & DiGiuseppe, R. (1990). Rational-emotive therapy and school psychology. *School Psychology Review (Mini-Series), 19*, 267–321.

Bernard, M. E., & DiGiuseppe, R. (Eds.). (1993). *Rational-emotive consultation in applied settings* (p. 210). Hillsdale, NJ: Erlbaum.

Bernard, M. E., Elias, M. J., Bell, P. J., Ferrito, J. J., & Langione, K. (2017). Social and emotional learning: Role of school psychologists in Australia. In M. Thielking & M. Terjesen (Eds.), *Handbook of Australian school psychology international research, practice and policy* (pp. 503–519). Cham, Switzerland: Springer.

Bernard, M. E., Ellis, A., & Terjesen, M. D. (2005). Rational emotive behavior approaches to childhood disorders: History, theory, practice and research. In A. Ellis & M. E. Bernard (Eds.), *Rational emotive behavior approaches to childhood disorders*. New York: Springer.

Bernard, M. E., & Joyce, M. R. (1984). *Rational emotive therapy with children and adolescents: Theory, treatment strategies, preventative methods*. New York: Wiley.

Bernard, M. E., & Walton, K. E. (2011). The effect of You Can Do It! Education in six schools on student perceptions of wellbeing, teaching-learning and relationships. *Journal of Student Well-Being, 5*, 22–37.

Buschmann, T., Horn, R. A., Blankenship, V. R., Garcia, Y. E., & Bohan, K. B. (2018). The relationship between automatic thoughts and irrational beliefs predicting anxiety and depression. *Journal of Rational – Emotive & Cognitive – Behavior Therapy, 36*(2), 137–162.

Campbell, L. F., Norcross, J. C., Vasquez, M. J., & Kaslow, N. J. (2013). Recognition of psychotherapy effectiveness: The APA resolution. *Psychotherapy, 50*(1), 98–101. https://doi.org/10.1037/a0031817

Craighead, W. E., Meyers, A. W., & Craighead, L. W. (1985). A conceptual model for cognitive-behavior therapy with children. *Journal of Abnormal Child Psychology, 13*(3), 331. Retrieved from https://jerome.stjohns.edu/login?url=https://search-proquest-com.jerome.stjohns.edu/docview/1300107511?accountid=14068

David, D., Freeman, A., & DiGiuseppe, R. (2010). Rational and irrational beliefs: Implications for mechanisms of change and practice in psychotherapy. In D. David, J. Lynn, & A. Ellis (Eds.), *Rational and irrational beliefs. Research, theory, and clinical practice* (pp. 195–217). New York: Oxford University Press.

David, D., & Szentagotai, A. (2006). Cognition in cognitive-behavioral psychotherapies; toward an integrative model. *Clinical Psychology Review, 26*(3), 284–298.

Dayan, T. (2016). Cognitive strategies in social emotional learning programs and review of. In *You can do it! education (Doctoral Dissertation)*. New York: St. John's University.

DiGiuseppe, R. A., Doyle, K. A., Dryden, W., & Backx, W. (2014). *A practitioner's guide to rational emotive behavior therapy* (3rd ed.). Oxford: Oxford University Press.

DiNubile, L., & Wessler, R. (1974). Lessons from the living school. *Rational Living, 9*, 29–32.

Doress, I. (1967). The teacher as therapist. *Rational Living, 2*, 27.

Dryden, W. (2015). *Rational emotive behaviour therapy*. London: Routledge. https://doi.org/10.4324/9781315749433

Ellis, A. (1957). *How to live with a "neurotic."* New York: Crown, 1957. Rev. ed., New York: Crown, 1975 and North Hollywood: Wilshire.

Ellis, A. (1959). *Psychotherapy session with an eight-year-old female bed wetter.* Cassette recording. New York: Institute for Rational-Emotive Therapy.

Ellis, A. (1962). *Reason and emotion in psychotherapy*. Secaucus, NJ: Citadel.

Ellis, A. (1967). Talking to adolescents about sex. *Rational Living, 2*, 7–12.

Ellis, A. (1971a). An experiment in emotional education. *Educational Technology, 11*, 61–64.

Ellis, A. (1971b). *Rational-emotive therapy and its application to emotional education*. New York: Institute for Rational-Emotive Therapy.

Ellis, A. (1972). Emotional education in the classroom: The living school. *Journal of Child Psychology, 1*, 19–22.

Ellis, A. (1973). Emotional education at the living school. In M. M. Ohlsen (Ed.), *Counseling children in groups*. New York: Holt, Rinehart and Winston.

Ellis, A. (1975). Rational-emotive therapy and the school counselor. *School Counselor, 22*, 236–242.

Ellis, A. (1977). The basic clinical theory of rational-emotive therapy. In A. Ellis & R. Grieger (Eds.), *Handbook of rational-emotive therapy* (p. 1977). New York: Springer.
Ellis, A. (1980). Rational-emotive therapy and cognitive behavior therapy: Similarities and differences. *Cognitive Therapy and Research, 4*, 325–340.
Ellis, A. (1994). *Reason and emotion in psychotherapy* (Rev. ed.). Secaucus, NJ: Lyle Stuart and Citadel Press.
Ellis, A. (1995). Changing rational-emotive therapy (RET) to rational emotive behavior therapy (REBT). *Journal of Rational-Emotive & Cognitive-Behavior Therapy, 13*(2), 85–89. https://doi.org/10.1007/BF02354453. ISSN 0894-9085.
Ellis, A., & Bernard, M. E. (1983). An overview of rational-emotive approaches to the problems of childhood. In A. Ellis & M. E. Bernard (Eds.), *Rational-emotive approaches to the problems of childhood*. New York: Plenum Press.
Ellis, A., Wolfe, J. H., & Moseley, S. (1966). *How to raise an emotionally healthy, happy child*. New York/Hollywood, CA: Crown/Wilshire.
Eschenroeder, C. (1982). How rational is rational-emotive therapy? A critical appraisal of its theoretical foundations and therapeutic methods. *Cognitive Therapy and Research, 6*, 274–282.
Garber, J., Frankel, S. A., & Herrington, C. G. (2016). Developmental demands of cognitive behavioral therapy for depression in children and adolescents: Cognitive, social, and emotional processes. *Annual Review of Clinical Psychology, 12*, 181–216. https://doi.org/10.1146/annurev-clinpsy-032814-112836
Gavita, O. A., & Joyce, M. R. (2008). A review of the effectiveness of group cognitively enhanced behavioral based parent programs designed for reducing disruptive behavior in children. *Journal of Cognitive and Behavioral Psychotherapies, 8*(2), 185–199.
Gerald, M., & Eyman, W. (1981). *Thinking straight and talking sense*. New York: Institute for Rational-Emotive Therapy.
Glicken, M. (1967). Counseling children: Two methods. *Rational Living, 1*, 27–30.
Glicken, M. D. (1968). Rational counseling: A dynamic approach to children. *Elementary School Guidance and Counseling, 2*, 261–267.
Grave, J., & Blissett, J. (2004). Is cognitive behavior therapy developmentally appropriate for young children? A critical review of the evidence. *Clinical Psychology Review, 24*(4), 399–420.
Hajzler, D. J., & Bernard, M. E. (1991). A review of rational emotive outcome studies. *School Psychology Quarterly, 6*, 27–49.
Hauck, P. A. (1967). *The rational management of children*. New York: Libra Publishers.
Hess, R. E. (2014). Interpersonal Cognitive Problem Solving (ICPS): Competence-building primary prevention program. In *The National Mental Health Association* (pp. 163–236). London: Routledge.
Hinshaw, S. P. (2000). Attention deficit/hyperactivity disorder: The search for viable treatments. In P. C. Kendall (Ed.), *Child & adolescent therapy* (2nd ed.). New York: Guilford Press.
Hobbs, S. A., Moguin, L. E., Tyroler, M., & Lahey, B. B. (1980). Cognitive behavior therapy with children: Has clinical utility been demonstrated? *Psychological Bulletin, 87*, 147–165.
Hogendoorn, S. M., Wolters, L. H., Vervoort, L., Prins, P. J. M., Boer, F., et al. (2010). Measuring negative and positive thoughts in children: An adaptation of the children's automatic thoughts scale (CATS). *Cognitive Therapy and Research, 34*(5), 467–478.
Hollon, S. D., & DiGiuseppe, R. (2010). Cognitive psychotherapies. In J. C. Norcross & G. VandenBos (Eds.), *History of psychotherapy: Continuity and change* (2nd ed.). Washington, DC: American Psychological Association.
Holmbeck, G. R., Greenley, R. N., & Franks, E. A. (2003). Developmental issues and considerations in research and practice. In A. E. Kazdin & J. R. Weisz (Eds.), *Evidence-based psychotherapies for children and adolescents*. New York: Plenum Press.
Knaus, W. J. (1974). *Rational-emotive education: A manual for elementary school teachers*. New York: Institute for Rational-Emotive Therapy.
Lafferty, G., Dennell, A., & Rettich, G. (1964). A creative school mental health program. *National Elementary Principal, 43*, 28–35.

Leder, G. (2017). Know thyself? Questioning the theoretical foundations of cognitive behavioral therapy. *Review of Philosophy and Psychology, 8*(2), 391–410. http://dx.doi.org.jerome.stjohns.edu:81/10.1007

Lochman, J. E., Whidby, J. M., & FitzGerald, D. P. (2000). Cognitive-behavioral assessment and treatment with aggressive children. In P. C. Kendall (Ed.), *Child & adolescent therapy* (2nd ed.). New York: Guilford Press.

MacLaren, C., Doyle, K. A., & DiGiuseppe, R. (2015). Rational emotive behavior therapy: Theory and practice. In H. Tinsley, S. H. Lease, & N. S. Giffin-Wiersma (Eds.), *Contemporary theory and practice in counseling and psychotherapy* (pp. 233–263).

McGory, J. E. (1967). Teaching introspection in the classroom. *Rational Living, 2*, 23–24.

Meichenbaum, D. (1977). *Cognitive-behavior modification: An integrative approach*. New York: Plenum Press.

Meichenbaum, D. (2017). Teaching thinking: A cognitive behavioral perspective. In *The evolution of cognitive behavior therapy* (pp. 85–104). New York: Routledge.

Meyers, A. W., & Craighead, W. E. (1984). *Cognitive behavior therapy with children*. New York: Plenum Press.

Norcross, J. C., & Karpiak, C. P. (2012). Clinical psychologists in the 2010s: 50 years of the APA Division of Clinical Psychology. *Clinical Psychology: Science and Practice, 19*(1), 1–12.

Norcross, J. C., Sayette, M. A., & Pomerantz, A. M. (2018). Doctoral training in clinical psychology across 23 years: Continuity and change. *Journal of Clinical Psychology, 74*(3), 385–397. https://doi-org.jerome.stjohns.edu/10.1002/jclp.22517

Ollendick, T. H., Grills, A. E., & King, N. J. (2001). Applying developmental theory to the assessment and treatment of childhood disorders: Does it make a difference? *Clinical Psychology and Psychotherapy, 8*, 304–314.

Paul, G. L. (1967). Strategy of outcome research in psychotherapy. *Journal of Consulting Psychology, 31*(2), 109–118. https://doi.org/10.1037/h0024436

Piaget, J. (1952). *The origins of intelligence*. New York: Norton.

Podina, I., Popp, R., Pop, I., & David, D. (2015). Genetic correlates of maladaptive beliefs: COMT VAL158MET and irrational cognitions linked depending on distress. *Behavior Therapy, 46*(6), 797–808. https://doi.org/10.1016/j.beth.2015.06.004

Remmel, E., & Flavell, J. H. (2004). Recent progress in cognitive developmental research: Implications for clinical practice. In H. Steiner (Ed.), *Handbook of mental health interventions in children and adolescents: An integrated developmental approach* (pp. 73–97). San Francisco: Jossey-Bass.

Robertson, D. J. (2010). *The philosophy of Cognitive-Behavioural Therapy (CBT): Stoic philosophy as rational & cognitive psychotherapy*. London: Karnac.

Robertson, D., & Codd, R. T. (2019). Stoic philosophy as a cognitive-behavioral therapy. *The Behavior Therapist, 42*(2), 42–50.

Sachs, N. J. (1971). Planned emotional education: The living school. *Art in Daily Living, 1*, 8–13.

Sandberg, E. H., & McCullough, M. B. (2010). The development of reasoning skills. In E. H. Sandberg & B. L. Spritz (Eds.), *A clinician's guide to normal cognitive development in childhood* (pp. 179–198). New York: Routledge/Taylor & Francis Group.

Schniering, C. A., & Rapee, R. M. (2002). Development and validation of a measure of children's automatic thoughts: The children's automatic thoughts scale. *Behaviour Research and Therapy, 40*(9), 1091–1109.

Shirk, S. (1999). Developmental therapy. In W. K. Silverman & T. H. Ollendick (Eds.), *Developmental issues in the clinical treatment of children* (pp. 60–73). Needham Heights, MA: Allyn & Bacon.

Shirk, S. R. (2001). Development and cognitive therapy. *Journal of Cognitive Psychotherapy, 15*, 155–163.

Shure, M. (1996). *I can problem solve: An interpersonal cognitive problem-solving program*. Champaign, IL: Research Press.

Soflau, R., & David, D. O. (2017). A meta-analytical approach of the relationships between the irrationality of beliefs and the functionality of automatic thoughts. *Cognitive Therapy and Research, 41*(2), 178–192.

Spivack, G., Platt, J., & Shure, M. (1976). *The problem-solving approach to adjustment*. San Francisco: Jossey-Bass.

Urbain, E. S., & Kendall, P. C. (1980). Review of social-cognitive problem-solving interactions with children. *Psychological Bulletin, 88*, 109–143.

Vernon, A. (1993). *Developmental assessment with children and adolescents*. Alexandria, VA: American Counseling Association.

Vernon, A. (2004). Counseling children and adolescents: Developmental considerations. In A. Vernon (Ed.), *Counseling children and adolescents* (3rd ed., pp. 1–31). Denver, CO: Love Publishing.

Wagner, E. E. (1966). Counseling children. *Rational Living, 1*(26), 28.

Waters, V. (1981). The living school. *RETwork, 1*, 1.

Waters, V. (1982). Therapies for children: Rational-emotive therapy. In C. R. Reynolds & T. B. Gutkin (Eds.), *Handbook of school psychology*. New York: Wiley.

Weisz, J. R., Weiss, B., Alicke, M. D., & Klotz, M. L. (1987). Effectiveness of psychotherapy with children and adolescents: A meta-analysis for clinicians. *Journal of Consulting and Clinical Psychology, 55*(4), 542–549. http://dx.doi.org.jerome.stjohns.edu:81/10.1037/0022-006X.55.4.542

Weisz, J. R., & Hawley, K. M. (2002). Developmental factors in the treatment of adolescents. *Journal of Consulting and Clinical Psychology, 70*, 21–43.

Wessler, R. A., & Wessler, R. L. (1980). *The principles and practices of rational-emotive therapy*. San Francisco: Jossey-Bass.

Wolfe, J., & Staff. (1970). Emotional education in the classroom: The living school. *Rational Living, 4*, 23–25.

Chapter 2
The Current Status of Rational Emotive and Cognitive Behavioral Therapy (RE-CBT) Research with Children and Adolescents

Mark D. Terjesen, Courtney Duhning, Alexa K. Pata, and Jessica K. Prizer

The Current Status of Rational Emotive and Cognitive Behavioral Therapy (RE-CBT) with Children and Adolescents

Measurement of Beliefs and Thoughts

Referrals for clinical services among youth often focus on behavioral or affective areas of concern. This is also true for both diagnostic and progress-monitoring assessment measures as well. Although cognitions have been recognized as a central factor in the development and maintenance of emotional and behavioral problems in children (Bernard, Ellis, & Terjesen, 2005), and alterations in cognitions have been shown to be vital for treatment, few self-report measures have been designed to specifically assess irrational beliefs, self-statements, or automatic thoughts in children and adolescents (Schniering & Rapee, 2002; Terjesen, Kassay, & Anderson, 2017).

Several questionnaires have been developed to assess maladaptive beliefs in adults, such as the Cognitions Checklist (CCL; Beck, Brown, Steer, Eidelson, & Riskind, 1987), the Automatic Thoughts Questionnaire (ATQ; Hollon & Kendall, 2007, as cited in Schniering & Rapee, 2002), the Anxious Self-Statements Questionnaire (ASSQ; Kendall & Hollon, 1989, as cited in Schniering & Rapee, 2002), and the Rational and Irrational Beliefs Scale (RAIBS; Mogoașe, Ștefan, & David, 2013). In addition, while some irrational belief measures such as the Rational Behavior Inventory (RBI; Shorkey & Whiteman, 1977) and Irrational Beliefs Test (IBT; Jones, 1968) have been written to include indicators of emotional distress, other measures such as the General Attitude and Belief Scale II (GABS; DiGiuseppe

M. D. Terjesen (✉) · C. Duhning · A. K. Pata · J. K. Prizer
St. John's University, Jamaica, NY, USA
e-mail: Terjesem@stjohns.edu

M. Bernard, M. D. Terjesen (eds.), *Rational-Emotive and Cognitive-Behavioral Approaches to Child and Adolescent Mental Health: Theory, Practice, Research, Applications*, https://doi.org/10.1007/978-3-030-53901-6_2

et al. 1989, as cited in Terjesen, Salhany, & Scuitto, 2009), Survey of Personal Beliefs (SPB), Attitude and Belief Scale (ABS), and Irrational Belief Scale (IBS) contain exclusively cognitive items (Terjesen et al., 2009; Vîslă, Flückiger, & grosse Holtforth, M.,, & David, D., 2016). Building off of this research, a large proportion of questionnaire measures for youth that target beliefs and cognitions have been created as downward extensions of instruments originally developed for adults (e.g., ATQ-C, CTI-C, CCL-C; Hogendoorn et al., 2010; Schniering & Rapee, 2002). However, items originally designed for adults may not necessarily be appropriate for measuring similar beliefs in youth (Schniering & Rapee, 2002). This is because the language and concepts used within adult measures may not be directly applicable to youth and may be interpreted differently due to their different levels of understanding (Hogendoorn et al., 2010; Schniering & Lyneham, 2007). The reason that this is potentially limiting is because downward extensions may not accurately measure the specific beliefs or maladaptive thoughts that children or adolescents engage in and may not adequately assess their internal experience (Hogendoorn et al., 2010; Schniering & Rapee, 2002). Because of these concerns, it is important for researchers to design, and clinicians to choose, measures specifically designed for children and adolescents with consideration for developmental level and items that reflect youth-friendly language and appropriate reading levels.

Similar to selecting behavioral and affective rating scales, it is important to consider whether a broad-band measure that evaluates a range of unhealthy cognitions or a more narrow-band approach that targets specific thoughts related to a specific affective or behavioral state would be most appropriate. There are a number of self-report measures developed to assess thoughts associated with different disorders in youth. In the area of depression, measures of thinking among youth include the Automatic Thoughts Questionnaire for Children (ATQ-C; Stark et al., 1990, as cited in Schniering & Rapee, 2002), the Cognitive Triad Inventory for Children (CTI-C; Kaslow, Stark, Printz, Livingston, & Tsai, 1992), and the Hopelessness Scale for Children (HPLS; Kazdin, Rodgers, & Colbus, 1986). In the area of anxiety disorders, measures include The Children's Cognitive Assessment Questionnaire (CCAQ; Zatz & Chassin, 1983) which measures automatic thoughts on test anxiety, and the Social Anxiety Scale for Children (SASC; Dandes et al., 1986, as cited in Schniering & Rapee, 2002). One of the few measures designed to assess cognitions related to both anxiety and depression in youth is the Negative Affect Self-Statement Questionnaire (NASSQ; Ronan, Kendall, & Rowe, 1994) which was developed to measure the self-statements that are associated with negative affect common to both anxiety and depression (Schniering & Rapee, 2002).

Although there has been some research surrounding cognitions and self-statements related to assessing automatic thoughts for specific affective states (e.g., anxiety or depression), the research surrounding more general measures of irrationality and automatic thoughts among children and adolescents, and more specifically their psychometric properties, is lacking (Terjesen et al., 2017). We agree with the assertion of Terjesen and colleagues over a decade ago (Terjesen et al., 2009), that within existing measures of beliefs, there is considerable variation among the psychometric properties, utility for assessment, and quality of standardization samples for each measure which influences the ability to draw normative conclusions. This is concerning because measures of irrational beliefs are central to assessing presenting problems in psychotherapy as well as for guiding clinical decision making (Terjesen et al., 2009). Additionally, these measures can be helpful for identifying changes in irrational beliefs and measuring the effectiveness of specific interventions over time (Terjesen et al., 2009).

Research has also suggested that the content of cognitions and their themes can be related to the expression of psychopathology, for example, while beliefs of personal failure, loss, and hopelessness are typically associated with depression, thoughts of physical or psychological threat are typically associated with anxiety, and thoughts of being wronged or transgressed are typically associated with anger (Schniering & Rapee, 2002). Additionally, children with anxiety disorders tend to report self-talk that is future-oriented, unstable, and focused on threat while children demonstrating depressive symptoms tend to report self-talk that is past-oriented, stable, and focused on loss or failure (Hogendoorn et al., 2010). The difference in cognitions reported can be utilized to not only differentiate typically developing children and adolescents from those with clinically significant difficulties but can also be utilized to differentiate between different childhood disorders by analyzing the *number* of negative or irrational cognitions as well as the *type* of cognitions.

In looking at measures developed based on the model of REBT, Terjesen and colleagues (Terjesen et al., 2017) expressed some concerns about early measures of irrational beliefs in youth that included the Children's Survey of Irrational Beliefs (Knaus & Eyman, 1974), the Idea Inventory (Kassinove et al., 1977; Wasserman & Vogrin, 1979), the Rational Behavior Inventory (Shorkey & Saski 1983; Shorkey & Whiteman, 1977), and a modified version of Ellis's Irrational Belief Scale (Haase et al., 1979; Lee et al., 1979). Shortcomings of these measures included that they were not appropriate for a wide age range, did not achieve adequate reliability or validity, and many were not developed past their initial conceptions (Terjesen et al., 2017). Existing scales of irrational beliefs also contain some conceptual flaws (Terjesen et al., 2009). For example, many purported measures of irrational beliefs assess beliefs embedded with emotional distress (e.g., "I often get excited or upset when things go wrong"; Shorkey & Whiteman, 1977) or behavioral consequences (e.g., "I avoid facing my problems"; Jones, 1968) rather than exclusively assessing the irrational beliefs independently. When this occurs, it may obscure the meanings of the results by artificially inflating the reported correlations between cognition, emotion, and behavior and make it more difficult to evaluate change when items labeled as beliefs are not actually measuring beliefs (Hogendoorn et al., 2010; Terjesen et al., 2009). Another major weakness of these measures of childhood irrationality included that they did not fully reflect updated developments in REBT's conceptualization of irrationality (Bernard & Cronan, 1999; Terjesen et al., 2017).

One measure of irrational beliefs among youth that has been revised and efforts made to continue to improve it psychometrically is the Child and Adolescent Scale of Irrationality (CASI) which was developed by Bernard and Laws (1988) to measure the irrational beliefs of children and adolescents between the ages of 10 and

18 years old. In the development of the CASI, Bernard and Laws (1988) aimed to overcome the flaws associated with existing measures of childhood irrationality by removing the emotional or behavioral components within the existing items in order to create exclusively cognitively worded items and prevent confounding the correlations with other measures of emotional or behavioral functioning (Terjesen et al., 2017). Bernard and Cronan (1999) later revised the measure again to make its items more reflective of Ellis's newer conception of irrationality and more consistent with REBT theory (Terjesen et al., 2017). The CASI assesses five irrational processes: (1) demandingness, such as "must," "need," or "should" statements, (2) awfulizing, such as "It's awful," or "it is the end of the world" types of statements, (3) low frustration tolerance, such as "I can't stand it" or "It's intolerable" statements, (4) global rating of others or the world, such as "The world is horrible," or "Others are worthless" types of statements, and (5) self-global rating such as "I'm worthless" or "I'm no good" types of statements (Bernard & Cronan, 1999). In a validation study conducted by Bernard and Cronan (1999), researchers found significant correlations between scales of irrationality and behavior and emotional problems in a large sample of Australian youth, reporting that total irrationality scores were associated with scores of anxiety, anger, and teacher ratings of emotional problems (Terjesen et al., 2017).

Through a series of studies consisting of over 1000 participants, Terjesen and colleagues (Terjesen et al., 2017) sought to evaluate the factor structure, reliability, construct validity, and discriminative validity for the 49-item revised CASI (Bernard & Cronan, 1999). Their results showed strong correlations among measures of affective and behavioral functioning with the CASI and differences were demonstrated between clinical and school-based samples providing evidence of validity for the CASI (Terjesen et al., 2017). Regarding reliability of the measure, while the CASI was considered reliable as a whole, there was some variability in the internal consistency of the irrational belief subscales which ranged from 0.62 (Awfulizing) to 0.86 (Self Ratings of Worth; Terjesen et al., 2017). Additionally, although expert validation for a revised factor structure was provided, identifying an underlying factor structure for the CASI in this research was not successful (Terjesen et al., 2017). That is, in these studies, the statistically clustered factors did not appear to lend to any particular pattern of responding based on beliefs, content, or theory. One interpretation of these results is that children's thought patterns may not differentiate into clear domains as predicted and that children may be more likely to generalize their irrationality rather than adhere to consistent, categorized irrationality (Terjesen et al., 2017). In addition, it is possible that subtle differences in the language used or content areas of items may have reflected how youth previously thought but may not reflect how youth currently think (Terjesen et al., 2017). This would in turn result in children not understanding the meaning of the items as intended as well as lower reliability and consistency (Terjesen et al., 2017). Terjesen and colleagues (Terjesen, Kassay, Anderson, & O'Brien, 2020) have since revised the CASI and have conducted focus groups of students as well as obtained expert feedback as to the items and language. Efforts to create a more balanced approach toward types of beliefs as well as content areas (e.g., peers, parents, school) are reflected and some international data have been published (Bernardelli & Terjesen, 2018). Sample items are seen in Table 2.1.

Another measure available for evaluating negative self-statements and automatic thoughts in children includes the Children's Automatic Thoughts Scale (CATS; Schniering & Rapee, 2002). One of the unique features of the CATS is that it was designed to assess negative beliefs across both internalizing and externalizing difficulties in children and adolescents using developmentally sensitive items (Schniering & Rapee, 2002). Items focused exclusively on cognitions rather than emotional or behavioral indicators of distress and were developed by interviewing clinically depressed, anxious, or behavior disorder children and adolescents aged 6–16 years about the self-statements that they experience across various situations (Schniering & Rapee, 2002).

Confirmatory factor analyses with the resulting items showed that negative automatic thoughts in youth load on four distinct factors including physical threat, social threat, personal failure, and hostility, which then load onto a single higher order factor (Schniering & Rapee, 2002). This factor structure was later replicated with new samples of clinical and non-clinical children and adolescents (Schniering & Rapee, 2002). Regarding psychometrics, internal consistency for the total scale and subscales was high and test–retest reliability for a subsample of children and adolescents demonstrated good retest reliability in children's total scores at 1 and 3 months after the initial testing (Schniering & Rapee, 2002). The questionnaire is considered a stable measure of automatic thoughts in children and adolescents, and discriminant validity for the CATS was obtained by comparing subscale and total score differences between non-clinical youth and clinically depressed, anxious, and behavior disorder youth (Schniering & Rapee, 2002). In 2010, a further adaptation of the CATS was developed, the Children's

Table 2.1 Directions and sample items from the child and adolescent scale of irrationality

	Strongly disagree				Strongly agree
1. Parents who are too strict are total idiots.	1	2	3	4	5
2. I think others are better than me.	1	2	3	4	5
3. The worst thing is to have your friends mistreat you.	1	2	3	4	5
4. I must get good grades.	1	2	3	4	5
5. I think I'm pathetic when people don't like me.	1	2	3	4	5

When you are ready to begin, please reach each sentence below and pick your answer by ***circling a number from "1" to "5."*** The five possible answers for each sentence are:

1 = Strongly Disagree

2 = Disagree

3 = Not Sure

4 = Agree

5 = Strongly Agree

For example, if you were given the sentence "*I like to read comic books*," you would circle a "**1**" if you ***Strongly Disagree***. If you were given the sentence "*I like to keep my room neat and tidy*," you would circle a "**5**" if you ***Strongly Agree***. Please be sure to answer all of the questions.

Automatic Thoughts Scale-Negative/Positive (CATS-N/P), to incorporate both positive and negative self-statements (Hogendoorn et al., 2010).

While both the CASI and the CATS are promising measures in evaluating unhealthy thoughts among youth, measures that tap into additional domains of responding or measures that provide greater context for items may be beneficial. Other measures assessing cognitive, emotional, behavioral, and physiological responses in different ways could also inform therapeutic approaches. One example is through the use of situational vignettes that create the context for the irrational belief items. Vignettes help young people to feel more engaged, especially when discussions surround sensitive topics, while allowing them to retain a high level of control over the process of responding (Barter & Renold, 2000). In contrast to measures such as the CASI which use individual, isolated items that ask for the level of agreement, measures which use vignettes may provide more of an opportunity to evaluate multiple domains of responses (i.e., choices of cognitive, emotional, behavioral, and physiological responses) and may appear more relatable or realistic to children and adolescents. However, from a review of the literature, no questionnaires to date have been designed to assess thoughts along with emotions, behaviors, and physiological responses together, using situational written vignettes. This approach would be an important next step to allow for assessment of the broad range of responses (i.e., cognitive, emotive, behavioral, and physiological) that young people may experience in different situations which parallel potential real-life scenarios. One assessment tool that is currently in the preliminary stages of being developed for this purpose is the Children's Irrational Response Checklist (CIRCL) which utilizes written vignettes to aid in the acceptability and comprehension of the measure items for children and offers youth the ability to provide responses in multiple domains (Pata, O'Brien, & Terjesen, 2018). By linking reported thoughts to emotional, behavioral, and physiological responses, this would likely assist practitioners in assessing patterns of beliefs and responses among youth for use with case conceptualizations and treatment planning. Preliminary analyses of the factors for this measure and results of an initial expert review indicated that 90.4% of the total cognitive and behavioral response options achieved expert consensus regarding the type of belief or response that it was meant to represent which suggests that the measure aligns closely with REBT theory and its core concepts (Pata et al., 2018).

Clinical Effectiveness of RE-CBT

A complete review and modular approach that examines the research on the clinical applications of Rational Emotive Behavior Therapy and Cognitive Behavioral Therapy among youth is beyond the scope of this chapter. To guide the reader in understanding the science as it relates to the practice and effectiveness of these clinical approaches, we have broken down the research on application into three sections: REBT, CBT, and School-Based Curricula Interventions that integrate the RE-CBT model.

REBT in the Treatment of Clinical Problems

Rational Emotive Behavior Therapy (REBT), introduced by Albert Ellis in the late 1950s, is one of the main pillars of Cognitive Behavioral Therapy. It has been successfully applied to a wide array of psychological disturbances and has been used within various domains including clinical psychology, education, and organizational settings (David, Cotet, Matu, Mogoase, & Stefan, 2017). Since its creation, several hundred papers have been published focusing on the theory and practice of REBT (David, Szentagotai, Eva, & Macavei, 2005). However, there are a handful of inconsistencies as well as gaps found in the REBT literature with regard to its effectiveness with children and adolescents (Bernard et al., 2005). These problems stem from a failure to report the specific characteristics of studies, the therapeutic settings, and the specific treatments utilized (Bernard et al., 2005). Traditionally, because the details of the research are often poorly reported, it has been difficult to determine the effectiveness of the therapy and what factors are influencing therapeutic change (Bernard et al., 2005). Therefore, due to the inconsistent reporting of research study characteristics, it is difficult to determine whether the research is poorly conducted or poorly reported (Bernard et al., 2005). However, there have been a number of recent reviews of the science of REBT among youth that we will briefly highlight below.

In their meta-analysis of the use of REBT with children and adolescents, Gonzalez et al. (2004) looked at 19 studies and made several interesting conclusions. The authors' analyses revealed that, overall, REBT was more effective than an alternative treatment (Weighted Effect Size [WES] of 0.57) and more effective than a no-treatment control (WES of 0.49). Specifically, REBT was most effective in its reduction of disruptive behaviors (WES of 1.15) followed by irrationality (WES of 0.51). This is interesting in the fact that REBT interventions target the irrational beliefs which may influence the presentation of unhealthy negative emotions or behaviors. As such, one would assume beliefs would change at a much higher rate than disruptive behaviors. This may also reflect, as discussed earlier, the importance of developing psychometrically sound measures of irrationality among youth. Two important points to consider: a) this was based on a total of 7 effect sizes and b) there were no significant differences between studies that were identified as well-designed compared to those that were not. This both provides a rationale for a needed increase in the number of treatment outcome studies, as well as an examination of what components of treatment lead to clinical change. Gonzalez et al. (2004) identified a number of limitations which may impact the social validity of their findings including a smaller number of studies analyzed, the exclusion of all dissertations, and the fact that the vast majority of studies were conducted in the same setting (e.g., school).

Subsequent to the work of Gonzalez et al. (2004), Esposito (2009) reviewed 72 studies, more than twice the number of studies identified by previous quantitative meta-analyses of REBT with youth populations (Gonzalez et al., 2004, $n = 19$; Trip, Vernon, & McMahon, 2007, $n = 26$). This is largely due to differences in inclusion criteria across reviews as Esposito (2009) included dissertations and did not require studies to include a control or comparison group as previous reviews did. Results of the studies indicate that REBT is an effective form of psychotherapy for use with children and adolescents as there was a large positive overall within-group effect size (M = 0.85) and a moderate positive effect size between REBT and control groups (M = 0.63). This indicates that children and adolescents who received REBT demonstrated greater positive changes than those in the control groups. Additionally, a small positive effect size (M = 0.32) was found for the comparison of REBT to alternative conditions, indicating that REBT is as effective, if not slightly more effective than other forms of treatment (e.g., psychoanalytic treatment, other forms of CBT, relaxation, Gestalt therapy, behavior therapy, self-instructional therapy, social problem solving, and psychoeducation) for children and adolescents with various presenting problems. However, it should be noted that in most of the research, samples consisted of generally non-clinical students and most research was conducted in schools.

In comparison to the work of Gonzalez et al. (2004), when examined by construct, the largest effect sizes for REBT treatment groups were found for changes in automatic thoughts followed by irrational beliefs as opposed to disruptive behavior (Esposito, 2009). Further, REBT was found to be moderately effective in targeting anxiety whereas small to moderate effect sizes were found for the reduction of depressive symptoms. Interestingly, REBT was found to be more effective for adolescents than for children. This finding supports the need for a possible change in the clinical approach of REBT as a function of age such that strategies are employed to better target younger age groups. Esposito (2009) noted a handful of limitations which were similar to those reported by Gonzalez et al. (2004) with most reflecting the outcome studies failure to report specific important variables. For example, only six out of the 72 usable studies reported a mean age of participants.

In their recent meta-analysis of 82 articles on the use of REBT across all ages, David et al. (2017) aimed to provide a more comprehensive and up-to-date quantitative review of REBT expanding on the extant literature. The authors aimed to both examine the empirical evidence supporting the efficacy and effectiveness of REBT interventions for children, adolescents, and adults as well as REBT's effect on mechanisms of change (i.e., rational and irrational beliefs) and the relation between alleged mechanisms of change and intervention outcomes.

Overall, results showed, in most cases, REBT had medium and significant effect sizes in both between- and within-groups for outcome measures at post-intervention (within-groups d = 0.56; between-groups d = 0.58) and follow-up (within-groups d = 0.46; between-groups d = 0.66). Similar effect sizes were found for between- and within-groups for REBT interventions on both rational and irrational beliefs at post-intervention (within-groups d = 0.61; between-groups d = 0.70) and follow-up (within-groups d = 0.33; between-groups d = 0.57). Exceptions to this were the within-groups outcome and mechanism analyses at follow-up which were still significant but small in magnitude. Analyses suggest that, overall, REBT is an effective treatment across various conditions. However, it is important to note that participants' age category moderated post-intervention effect sizes for within-groups. For example, studies conducted on adults yielded a medium effect size (d = 0.59) as well as those conducted on adolescents (d = 0.46) while those conducted on children yielded a small effect size (d = 0.20). This is related to findings reported in Esposito (2009) and similarly suggest the need for a possible reevaluation in the clinical approach of REBT for younger ages.

When comparing REBT interventions to a control group, David et al. (2017) found that REBT generated high effect sizes for distress (d = 0.94) and school performance (d = 0.86) at post-test and high effect sizes for behavioral outcomes, health outcomes, and school performance at follow-up indicating that REBT is greatly effective in targeting these variables for change. Further, REBT generated medium effect sizes for anger, behavioral outcomes, depression, emotional outcomes, health outcomes, and quality of life at post-test, and for distress, depression, and overall emotional outcomes at follow-up. REBT generated small but significant effect sizes for anxiety, cognitive outcomes, and other types at post-test and quality of life at follow-up. When comparing pre- to post-test REBT intervention measures, within-groups, authors reported an overall medium effect size in symptoms measured at post-intervention. Specifically, a high effect size for REBT was found for anger (d = 0.88) at post-test and psychophysical symptoms at follow-up. These results suggest that that REBT is highly effective in treating these outcome variables. Authors acknowledge that some outcome categories (e.g., anger) included a limited number of studies which does not allow for resulting strong conclusions. Taken together, based on the analyses included in the review, REBT interventions are efficacious and effective for various conditions regardless of clinical status, age of sample, and delivery format. Additionally, REBT interventions are effective when analyzing their effect on proposed mechanisms of change including irrational and rational beliefs.

Of note, among the studies included in the David et al. (2017) review, randomized trails obtained higher effect sizes when compared to nonrandomized studies. Furthermore, the quality of the studies negatively predicted effect sizes at post-intervention and at follow-up. This somewhat makes sense as studies with more scientific and clinical rigor have often been linked to smaller effect sizes. Interestingly, the year of publication was a positive predictor at both post-intervention and follow-up. It is possible that more current studies yielded higher effect sizes because they focus on more clinical populations or use more effective procedures as research in this area has recently expanded. However, it is important to note the effect size of REBT in the studies reviewed was moderated by the type of comparison condition.

We support the recommendations of David et al. (2005, 2017) in the need for developing new methods for evaluating rational and irrational beliefs to better understand their role in clinical targets of emotion and behavior. At this point in time, most measures of irrational beliefs are based on self-report scales which are sensitive to coping and prove difficult to measure the true nature and extent of irrational beliefs. Having more psychometrically sound instruments to uniformly measure REBT mechanisms of change (e.g., irrational and rational beliefs) will serve to employ mechanisms of change analyses to further test the REBT change theory. Furthermore, while the David et al. (2017) review may be the most current and extensive as it includes different settings, treatment modalities, and clinical presentations, unlike previous meta-analyses, their review did not conduct analyses solely pertaining to children and adolescents. Future research should continue to examine the extant literature pertaining to the effectiveness of REBT on exclusively children and adolescents.

Cognitive Behavioral Therapy in the Treatment of Clinical Problems The broader term of Cognitive Behavioral Therapy (CBT) encompasses many different clinical approaches that are often integrated together (Higa-McMillan, Francis, Rith-Najarian, & Chorpita, 2016). These may include more traditional Beck-ian Cognitive Therapy (CT; DeRubeis, Keefe, & Beck, 2019), Behavioral Therapy (BT; Weisz et al., 2017), and even some of the "third wave" interventions (Hetrick, Cox, Witt, Bir, & Merry, 2016) as well as more integrated approaches that target specific clinical problems (e.g., trauma-focuses CBT; Cohen & Mannarino, 2019) or work with parents (Perihan et al., 2019). This often seems to be the case in CBT treatment outcome studies where clinicians may either not specify what clinical interventions are used or provide descriptions that reflect an integration of a number of different approaches. While the prior section made efforts to focus on studies that specifically identified REBT as the intervention approach, here we attempt to provide an overall summary of the effectiveness of CBT in the treatment of clinical problems among youth.

In a meta-analysis consisting of 447 studies summarizing 50 years of research, Weisz and colleagues (Weisz et al., 2017) reported that youth-focused CBT produced the strongest treatment effects across youth, parent, and teacher informants for a wide array of psychological disorders and target behaviors. It is important to look more closely at the differential effects for specific types of presenting problems as Hofmann and colleagues (Hofmann, Asnaani, Vonk, Sawyer, & Fang, 2012) found significant support for treating internalizing disorders with CBT and mixed support for externalizing disorders.

The efficacy of CBT for depression varies with some studies reporting strong evidence and others suggesting little improvement (Hofmann et al., 2012; Kazantzis, 2018). In a meta-analysis with 106 studies on youth CBT in the treatment of depression, 77.11% of youths improved at post-treatment and 81.92% of youth had improved outcomes at follow-up in comparison to a random youth sample (Sun, Rith-Najarian, Williamson, & Chorpita, 2019). In more significant cases of depression, CBT has been effective in reducing suicidal ideation and self-harm (Labelle, Pouliot, & Janelle, 2015). Building coping skills and improving emotion regulation skills in adolescents is a promising form of treatment; not only does it help decrease suicidal and self-harm behavior, but it provides constructive feedback for ways to cope in the future (Labelle et al., 2015). Overall, CBT is considered to be an effective treatment for depression (Weersing, Jeffreys, Do, Schwartz, & Bolano, 2017) with a greater understanding as to what specific CBT factors best lead to clinical change for depression among youth is warranted.

Research also suggests strong efficacy of CBT for anxiety disorders (Comer, Hong, Poznanski, Silva, & Wilson, 2019) with medium to large effect sizes reported for social anxiety disorder, panic disorder, and post-traumatic stress disorder among youth (Hofmann et al., 2012). Evidence consistently supports the effectiveness of CBT and SSRIs for decreasing anxious symptomology individually (Wang et al., 2017); however, the combination of CBT and SSRIs not only reduces symptoms quickly, but also improves response to treatment (Wang et al., 2017).

Due to the high level of comorbidity among childhood anxiety disorders (Leyfer, Gallo, Cooper-Vince, & Pincus, 2013), a transdiagnostic approach is often applied by therapists to address common concerns as it is more practical (Ewing, Monsen, Thompson, Cartwright-Hatton, & Field, 2015). A transdiagnostic approach assumes that similar psychological processes maintain symptoms across conditions; therefore, emotional and behavioral change occurs through a common approach (Chalder et al., 2019). CBT effects show generality as anxiety also decreased after a series of CBT sessions targeting depression (Weisz, McCarty, & Valeri, 2006). Simultaneously, CBT effects also show specificity as externalizing problems did not decrease when targeting an internalizing disorder like depression (Weisz et al., 2006). Treatment of multiple problems concurrently also appears to produce significantly smaller mean effect sizes than treatment of a single target problem (Weisz et al., 2017). Providing children and adolescents with transdiagnostic CBT is very efficacious and can be utilized when resources (i.e., manualized treatment programs, resources in different languages) are unavailable to tailor interventions to the child (Ewing et al., 2015). Further, Ewing et al. (2015) found that children in the transdiagnostic CBT group were 3.99 times more likely to remit from their anxiety disorder in comparison to the control group suggesting generalized CBT treatment is better than no treatment at all. This is particularly helpful for school professionals to know as manualized treatment programs can sometimes be more feasibly implemented, yet still effective (Schwartz, Chambless, McCarthy, Milrod, & Barber, 2019). Manualized CBT treatment programs have reduced anxiety symptomology in children from early preschool through late adolescence. Programs of note include *Cool Kids, Cool Little Kids Plus Social Skills, Coping-Cat, Coping Koala, One-Session Treatment, Strongest Families, and Timid to Tiger* (Schwartz et al., 2019).

There has been a recent expansion in the application of CBT for anxiety in clinical work in children with autism spectrum disorder (ASD; McConachie et al., 2014; Perihan et al., 2019). This approach is discussed in the chapter on working with students with ASD in this edited volume. While it is clear that CBT may be beneficial in helping children with ASD manage their thoughts and emotions, Perihan et al. (2019) argue that children need time to learn and implement these novel cognitive skills for coping with their anxiety.

Clinical interventions for the treatment of anger and aggression often are integrated with systemic approaches (McCart & Sheidow, 2016) and have shown medium to large effects after CBT treatment (Hofmann et al., 2012). In studies with treatments identified as behavioral therapy in combination with CBT or solely CBT, the decrease in conduct problems and aggression was significantly large in comparison to other therapeutic models (Fossum, Handegård, Adolfsen, Vis, & Wynn, 2016; Smeets et al., 2015).

The front-line treatment for child and adolescent OCD is CBT (Smeets et al., 2015) and large effect sizes have been reported for treatment outcomes (Freeman et al., 2018; Hofmann et al., 2012). CBT is so effective for OCD that researchers have suggested comparable outcomes to SSRIs when examining symptom severity (Smeets et al., 2015). In a meta-analysis including eight randomized controlled trials for obsessive–compulsive disorder, exposure–response prevention (ERP) was also effective (Ale, McCarthy, Rothschild, & Whiteside, 2015). This finding is interesting as ERP does not include relaxation and implements exposure earlier in treatment indicating that there is no evidence that introducing anxiety management strategies like relaxation or cognitive strategies before beginning exposure improves outcomes (Ale et al., 2015). Therefore, introducing exposure earlier in CBT treatment can likely be tolerated and effective with anxious individuals (Ale et al., 2015; Gryczkowski et al., 2013; Voort, Svecova, Jacobson, & Whiteside, 2010).

Regardless of psychological disorder or target behavior, larger outcome effects have been indicated for interventions with parental involvement compared to child-only treatments. This supports the idea that family participation plays a significant role in the efficacy of CBT (Perihan et al., 2019). Parental involvement was also significantly related to larger effect sizes post-treatment as well as at follow-up suggesting that parental involvement is not only associated with better outcomes, but also with sustainably better outcomes (Manassis et al., 2014; Sun et al., 2019). Although there may be some barriers to parental involvement or obstacles preventing a child's access to treatment, in a world filled with technological growth, CBT is now also being delivered through online means in order to enhance the accessibility of treatment (Rooksby, Elouafkaoui, Humphris, Clarkson, & Freeman, 2015). Studies have shown that computer-delivered CBT is similarly effective in reducing symptomology compared to in-person CBT (Rooksby et al., 2015; Vigerland et al., 2016). Internet-delivered CBT is effective for psychiatric and somatic conditions in children and adolescents (Vigerland et al., 2016). Of the three studies that directly compared in-person CBT with internet-based CBT, results did not significantly differ and the effectiveness of the intervention was comparable. Internet-based CBT may be a more feasible way of delivering treatment across a wide range of disorders.

Overall, CBT has been shown to be effective in the treatment of clinical problems among youth. CBT treatments have successfully targeted anxiety, depression, OCD, ASD, and other disorders often seen in children and adolescents. While tailored and individualized interventions are beneficial, research also shows that transdiagnostic approaches are also efficacious (Chalder et al., 2019). CBT is continuously expanding and being delivered through means such as treatment manuals and the internet to further disseminate evidence-based practices.

Social-Emotional Learning and RE-CBT

Social and emotional learning (SEL) programs are regularly implemented within schools and have been linked to positive academic, affective, and behavioral outcomes (Zins & Elias, 2007). As clinical work that utilizes RE-CBT promotes the development of effective problem-solving skills through cognitive strategies, it makes sense that these CBT strategies are built into some of the SEL curricula (Dayan, 2016).

Rational Emotive Education (REE), also referred to as Rational Emotive Behavioral Education (REBE), aims to help children understand how their behaviors are the consequences of their beliefs (Trip, McMahon, Bora, & Chipea, 2010). We will use the term REE based on the initial model of the program (Knaus, 1974) but where specific researchers report using REBE we will use their terminology. As there is another chapter in this edited volume that discusses REE as a social-emotional curriculum, we aim to highlight the research efficacy behind it.

REBE works to promote an understanding among children of how they are both responsible for and can change their dysfunctional behavior (Trip et al., 2010). REBE uses games and plays to approach aspects of irrational beliefs (e.g., awfulizing, absolutistic demands, low frustration tolerance, inferential behaviors, etc.) and to illustrate their negative effect on emotions and behaviors (Trip et al., 2010). REBE activities demonstrate the relationship between cognitions and emotional/behavioral consequences and aim to differentiate between dysfunctional and functional positive/negative emotions (Trip et al., 2010). The use of REBE as an educational off-shoot of REBT has a lengthy history and has been shown to improve children's self-concept, levels of aspiration, leadership skills, and development of an internal locus of control (Knaus & Bokor, 1975; Omizio, Cubberly, & Omizio, 1985; Rosenbaum et al., 1991, as cited in Trip et al., 2010). Other positive areas of clinical change have been seen in both affective states like anxiety and neuroticism (DiGiuseppe & Kassinove, 1976) as well as in irrational beliefs and failure attribution (Popa, 2004).

REE is promoted as an efficient prophylactic against emotional and behavioral difficulties among non-clinical populations of children and adolescents (DiGiuseppe et al., 1977, as cited in Trip et al., 2007). Other studies have argued that by participating in REE programs, children are able to learn the REBT assumptions, modify their irrational beliefs, and have more functional emotions/behavior than before (Trip et al., 2007). In an earlier review of REE studies, DiGiuseppe and Bernard (1990) found that more than 90% of the studies supported REE efficiency in diminishing irrational beliefs and 50% of studies supported a decrease in anxiety levels and an increase in self-esteem. This information was further corroborated by Hajzler and Bernard (1991) who asserted that irrational beliefs and anxiety decreased in 88% of studies surveyed and self-esteem improved in 50% of studies.

In their quantitative meta-analytical review, Trip et al. (2007) aimed to further investigate the effectiveness of REE and results generally supported its efficacy and effectiveness. Specifically, REE had a powerful effect on lessening irrational beliefs and dysfunctional behaviors along with a moderate effect regarding changing inferences and decreasing negative emotions (Trip et al., 2007). These results are consistent with conclusions drawn by DiGiuseppe and Bernard (1990) who argued that REE was more efficient than other interventions concerning irrational belief modifications (Trip et al., 2007). Taken together, Trip et al. (2007) concluded that REE is a viable approach that can lessen irrational beliefs and dysfunctional behaviors as well as affect negative emotions and behaviors. This is contradictory to other researchers who argued that REE did not offer enough data to support the possible efficiency with school populations (Gossette & O'Brien, 1993). However, many of the aforementioned methodological challenges noted in reviews of REBT as a clinical intervention also were areas of concern in the REE/REBE literature. That is, not all studies employed a control/comparison group, specificity as to curricula and interventions used was lacking, and choice of measures of clinical impact were flawed.

Some of the prior limitations were addressed in a study conducted by Trip et al. (2010). The researchers aimed to assess the efficiency of an REBE program for children (ages 10–11 years old) in the reduction of irrational beliefs, dysfunctional inferential beliefs, maladaptive emotions, and behaviors. The results of the study suggest that REBE is an efficient way to decrease irrational beliefs in children (Trip et al., 2010). Specifically, unconditional self-acceptance appeared as a singular benefit that was maintained during the follow-up phase (Trip et al., 2010). Low frustration showed a moderate decline as a result of REBE but slightly increased again in the follow-up phase (Trip et al., 2010). Additionally, REBE training had little to moderate influence on absolutistic demands for fairness (Trip et al., 2010). Overall, irrationality significantly decreased following the intervention but moderately increased in the follow-up phase (Trip et al., 2010). These findings corroborate those confirmed by Trip et al. (2007) in their meta-analysis which indicated the main effect of REBE in modifying irrational beliefs.

Conclusion

Based on the summary of the current measurement tools in practice and empirical studies conducted so far, RE-CBT may be considered to be an efficacious form of psychotherapy for a wide range of presenting problems and clinical disorders among youth. The overall quantity of the CBT outcome studies is considerably noteworthy in comparison to those studies that specifically utilize REBT as an intervention. However, some of the meta-analytic reviews indicate that REBT is as effective as the CBT interventions in clinical work with youth. Further, there is considerable variability in terms of quality of measurement development and intervention methodologies reported. As noted earlier, there exist a number of methodological concerns that may warrant attention in order to accurately determine which specific components of interventions are effective under what conditions, and with what populations. When scholarly work is used to guide clinical practice and the authors indicate that the intervention was REBT or CBT, without a sufficient description of the exact treatment strategies utilized, it leads to a further dilution of the ability to draw conclusions. We believe that as the science and practice of RE-CBT continues to develop, that future research may wish to develop measures that are more psychometrically sound to target the mechanism of change (i.e., irrational beliefs or automatic thoughts) and integrate the relationships among cognitive, affective, and behavioral constructs. Further, a sufficient description of specific clinical interventions that are consistent with the theoretical approach under examination as well as an assessment of clinician competency is warranted. Finally, additional research that examines variables that may predict which students are not responsive to RE-CBT as a clinical intervention may help clinicians consider alternative treatment approaches.

Test Yourself Questions

1. What measures may be helpful to consider in the evaluation of the mechanism of change (e.g., irrational and rational beliefs) among children and adolescents?
2. What are some of the challenges in linking the science of RE-CBT to clinical practice?
3. How might REBE be used to promote social-emotional learning among youth in schools?

References

Ale, C. M., McCarthy, D. M., Rothschild, L. M., & Whiteside, S. P. (2015). Components of cognitive behavioral therapy related to outcome in childhood anxiety disorders. *Clinical Child and Family Psychology Review, 18*(3), 240–251.

Barter, C., & Renold, E. (2000). "I wanna tell you a story": Exploring the application of vignettes in qualitative research with children and young people. *International Journal of Social Research Methodology, 3*(4), 307–323. https://doi-org.jerome.stjohns.edu/10.1080/13645570050178594

Beck, A. T., Brown, G., Steer, R. A., Eidelson, J. I., & Riskind, J. H. (1987). Differentiating anxiety and depression: A test of the cognitive content-specificity hypothesis. *Journal of Abnormal Psychology, 96*(3), 179–183. https://doi-org.jerome.stjohns.edu/10.1037/0021-843X.96.3.179

Bernard, M. E., & Cronan, F. (1999). The child and adolescent scale of irrationality: Validation data and mental health correlates. *Journal of Cognitive Psychotherapy, 13*(2), 121–132.

Bernard, M. E., Ellis, A., & Terjesen, M. D. (2005). Rational emotive behavior approaches to childhood disorders: History, theory, practice and research. In A. Ellis & M. E. Bernard (Eds.), *Rational emotive behavior approaches to childhood disorders*. New York: Springer.

Bernard, M. E., & Laws, W. (1988). Childhood irrationality and mental health. In *Paper presented at the 24th International Congress of Psychology*. Sydney, Australia.

Bernardelli, S., & Terjesen, M. (2018). The child and adolescent scale of irrationality: Preliminary validation for an Italian population. *International Psychology Bulletin (IPB), 22*(4), 28–39.

Chalder, T., Patel, M., James, K., Hotopf, M., Frank, P., Watts, K., et al. (2019). Persistent physical symptoms reduction intervention: A system change and evaluation in secondary care (PRINCE secondary)–a CBT-based transdiagnostic approach: Study protocol for a randomised controlled trial. *BMC Psychiatry, 19*(1), 307.

Cohen, J. A., & Mannarino, A. P. (2019). Trauma-focused cognitive behavioral therapy for childhood traumatic separation. *Child Abuse & Neglect, 92*, 179–195.

Comer, J. S., Hong, N., Poznanski, B., Silva, K., & Wilson, M. (2019). Evidence base update on the treatment of early childhood anxiety and related problems. *Journal of Clinical Child and Adolescent Psychology, 48*(1), 1–15. https://doi.org/10.1080/15374416.2018.1534208

David, D., Szentagotai, A., Eva, K., & Macavei, B. (2005). A synopsis of rational-emotive behavior therapy (REBT); Fundamental and applied research, Journal of Rational-Emotive & Cognitive-Behavior Therapy., *23*(3), 175–221. https://doi.org/10.1007/s10942-005-0011-0

David, D., Cotet, C., Matu, S., Mogoase, C., & Stefan, S. (2017). 50 years of rational-emotive and cognitive-behavioral therapy: A systematic review and meta-analysis. *Journal of Clinical Psychology, 74*(3), 304–318. https://doi.org/10.1002/jclp.22514

Dayan, T. (2016). *Cognitive strategies in social emotional learning programs and review of "You Can Do It! Education" (Doctoral Dissertation).* New York: St. John's University.

DeRubeis, R. J., Keefe, J. R., & Beck, A. T. (2019). Cognitive therapy. In K. S. Dobson & D. J. A. Dozois (Eds.), *Handbook of cognitive-behavioral therapies* (pp. 218–248). The Guilford Press.

DiGiuseppe, R., & Bernard, M. (1990). The application of rational-emotive theory and therapy to school-aged children. *School Psychology Review, 19*, 268–286.

DiGiuseppe, R., & Kassinove, H. (1976). Effects of rational-emotive school mental health program on children's emotional adjustment. *Journal of Community Psychology, 4*, 382–387.

Esposito, M. A. (2009). *REBT with children and adolescents: A meta-analytic review of efficacy* (Publication No. 3361233*)* [Doctoral Dissertation, St. John's University]. ProQuest Dissertations Publishing.

Ewing, D. L., Monsen, J. J., Thompson, E. J., Cartwright-Hatton, S., & Field, A. (2015). A meta-analysis of transdiagnostic cognitive behavioural therapy in the treatment of child and young person anxiety disorders. *Behavioural and Cognitive Psychotherapy, 43*(5), 562–577.

Fossum, S., Handegård, B. H., Adolfsen, F., Vis, S. A., & Wynn, R. (2016). A meta-analysis of long-term outpatient treatment effects for children and adolescents with conduct problems. *Journal of Child and Family Studies, 25*(1), 15–29.

Freeman, J., Benito, K., Herren, J., Kemp, J., Sung, J., Georgiadis, C., et al. (2018). Evidence base update of psychosocial treatments for pediatric obsessive-compulsive disorder: Evaluating, improving, and transporting what works. *Journal of Clinical Child and Adolescent Psychology, 47*(5), 669–698. https://doi.org/10.1080/15374416.2018.1496443

Gonzalez, J. E., Nelson, J. R., Gutkin, T. B., Saunders, A., Galloway, A., & Shwery, C. S. (2004). Rational emotive therapy with children and adolescents: A meta-analysis. *Journal of Emotional and Behavioral Disorders, 12*(4), 222–235. https://doi.org/10.1177/10634266040120040301

Gossette, L. R., & O'Brien, M. R. (1993). Efficacy of rational emotive therapy with children: A critical reappraisal. *Journal of Behavior Therapy and Experimental Psychiatry, 24*, 15–25.

Gryczkowski, M. R., Tiede, M. S., Dammann, J. E., Brown Jacobsen, A., Hale, L. R., & Whiteside, S. P. (2013). The timing of exposure in clinic-based treatment for childhood anxiety disorders. *Behavior Modification, 37*(1), 113–127.

Hajzler, J. D., & Bernard, E. M. (1991). A review of rational-emotive education outcome studies. *School Psychology Quarterly, 6*, 27–49.

Hetrick, S. E., Cox, G. R., Witt, K. G., Bir, J. J., & Merry, S. N. (2016). Cognitive behavioural therapy (CBT), third-wave CBT and interpersonal therapy (IPT) based interventions for preventing depression in children and adolescents. *Cochrane Database of Systematic Reviews, 8*, CD003380. https://doi.org/10.1002/14651858.CD003380.pub4

Higa-McMillan, C. K., Francis, S. E., Rith-Najarian, L., & Chorpita, B. F. (2016). Evidence base update: 50 years of research on treatment for child and adolescent anxiety. *Journal of Clinical Child & Adolescent Psychology, 45*(2), 91–113. https://doi.org/10.1080/15374416.2015.1046177

Hofmann, S. G., Asnaani, A., Vonk, I. J., Sawyer, A. T., & Fang, A. (2012). The efficacy of cognitive behavioral therapy: A review of meta-analyses. *Cognitive Therapy and Research, 36*(5), 427–440.

Hogendoorn, S. M., Wolters, L. H., Vervoort, L., Prins, P. J. M., Boer, F., Kooij, E., et al. (2010). Measuring negative and positive thoughts in children: An adaptation of the children's automatic thoughts scale (CATS). *Cognitive Therapy & Research, 34*(5), 467–478. https://doi-org.jerome.stjohns.edu/10.1007/s10608-010-9306-2

Jones, R. G. (1968). *A factored measure of Ellis' irrational belief system with personality, maladjustment correlates* (Doctoral Dissertation, Texas Tech University, 1969). Dissertations Abstracts International B, 29, 4379.

Kaslow, N. J., Stark, K. D., Printz, B., Livingston, R., & Tsai, S. L. (1992). Cognitive triad inventory for children: Development and relation to depression and anxiety. *Journal of Clinical Child Psychology, 21*, 339–347.

Kazantzis, N. (2018). Introduction to the special issue on processes of cognitive behavioral therapy: Does "necessary, but not sufficient" still capture it? *Cognitive Therapy and Research, 42*, 115–120. https://doi.org/10.1007/s10608-018-9891-z

Kazdin, A. E., Rodgers, A., & Colbus, D. (1986). The hopelessness scale for children: Psychometric characteristics and concurrent validity. *Journal of Consulting and Clinical Psychology, 54*, 241–245.

Knaus, W. J. (1974). *Rational emotive education: A manual for elementary school teachers*. Institute for Rational-Emotive Therapy.

Knaus, W. J., & Bokor, S. (1975). The effects of rational-emotive education lessons on anxiety and self-concept in sixth grade students. *Rational Living, 11*, 25–28.

Labelle, R., Pouliot, L., & Janelle, A. (2015). A systematic review and meta-analysis of cognitive behavioural treatments for suicidal and self-harm behaviours in adolescents. *Canadian Psychology/Psychologie Canadienne, 56*(4), 368.

Leyfer, O., Gallo, K. P., Cooper-Vince, C., & Pincus, D. B. (2013). Patterns and predictors of comorbidity of DSM-IV anxiety disorders in a clinical sample of children and adolescents. *Journal of Anxiety Disorders, 27*(3), 306–311.

Manassis, K., Lee, T. C., Bennett, K., Zhao, X. Y., Mendlowitz, S., Duda, S., et al. (2014). Types of parental involvement in CBT with anxious youth: A preliminary meta-analysis. *Journal of Consulting and Clinical Psychology, 82*(6), 1163.

McCart, M. R., & Sheidow, A. J. (2016). Evidence-based psychosocial treatments for adolescents with disruptive behavior. *Journal of Clinical Child and Adolescent Psychology, 45*(5), 529–563. https://doi.org/10.1080/15374416.2016.1146990

McConachie, H., McLaughlin, E., Grahame, V., Taylor, H., Honey, E., Tavernor, L., et al. (2014). Group therapy for anxiety in children with autism spectrum disorder. *Autism, 18*(6), 723–732.

Mogoaşe, C., Ştefan, S., & David, D. (2013). How do we measure rational and irrational beliefs? The development of rational and irrational beliefs scale (RAIBS) – a new theory-driven measure. *Journal of Cognitive & Behavioral Psychotherapies, 13*(2a), 529–546.

Omizio, M. M., Cubberly, W. E., & Omizio, S. A. (1985). The effects of Rational-Emotive Education groups on self-concept and locus of control among learning disabled children. *Exceptional Child, 32*, 13–19.

Pata, A. K., O'Brien, C., & Terjesen, M. (2018, November 16). *The development of the children's irrational response checklist.* [Poster session]. ABCT 52nd Annual Convention, Washington, DC.

Perihan, C., Burke, M., Bowman-Perrott, L., Bicer, A., Gallup, J., Thompson, J., et al. (2019). Effects of cognitive behavioral therapy for reducing anxiety in children with high functioning ASD: A systematic review and meta-analysis. *Journal of Autism and Developmental Disorders*, 1–15.

Popa, S. (2004). Rational emotive education efficacy in children irrational and inferential beliefs modification. *Romanian Journal of Cognitive and Behavioral Psychotherapies, 4*, 53–67.

Ronan, K. R., Kendall, P. C., & Rowe, M. (1994). Negative affectivity in children: Development and validation of a self-statement questionnaire. *Cognitive Therapy and Research, 18*, 509–528.

Rooksby, M., Elouafkaoui, P., Humphris, G., Clarkson, J., & Freeman, R. (2015). Internet-assisted delivery of cognitive behavioural therapy (CBT) for childhood anxiety: Systematic review and meta-analysis. *Journal of Anxiety Disorders, 29*, 83–92.

Schniering, C. A., & Lyneham, H. J. (2007). The Children's Automatic Thoughts Scale in a clinical sample: Psychometric properties and clinical utility. *Behaviour Research and Therapy, 45*(8), 1931–1940. https://doi-org.jerome.stjohns.edu/10.1016/j.brat.2006.09.009

Schniering, C. A., & Rapee, R. M. (2002). Development and validation of a measure of children's automatic thoughts: The children's automatic thoughts scale. *Behaviour Research and Therapy, 40*(9), 1091. https://doi-org.jerome.stjohns.edu/10.1016/S0005-7967(02)00022-0

Schwartz, R. A., Chambless, D. L., McCarthy, K. S., Milrod, B., & Barber, J. P. (2019). Client resistance predicts outcomes in cognitive–behavioral therapy for panic disorder. *Psychotherapy Research, 29*(8), 1020–1032.

Shorkey, C. T., & Whiteman, V. L. (1977). Development of the Rational Behavior Inventory: Initial validity and reliability. *Educational and Psychological Measurement, 37*(2), 527–534.

Smeets, K. C., Leeijen, A. A., van der Molen, M. J., Scheepers, F. E., Buitelaar, J. K., & Rommelse, N. N. (2015). Treatment moderators of cognitive behavior therapy to reduce aggressive behavior: A meta-analysis. *European Child & Adolescent Psychiatry, 24*(3), 255–264.

Sun, M., Rith-Najarian, L. R., Williamson, T. J., & Chorpita, B. F. (2019). Treatment features associated with youth cognitive behavioral therapy follow-up effects for internalizing disorders: A meta-analysis. *Journal of Clinical Child & Adolescent Psychology, 48*(sup1), S269–S283.

Terjesen, M. D., Kassay, K. S., & Anderson, D. L. (2017). Evaluation of the psychometric properties of a measure of child irrationality. *Journal of Rational-Emotive & Cognitive-Behavior Therapy, 35*(4), 413–431. https://doi-org.jerome.stjohns.edu/10.1007/s10942-017-0269-z

Terjesen, M. D., Kassay, K. S., Anderson, D. L., & O'Brien, C. (2020). *A revised measure of irrational thinking among youth.* [Unpublished manuscript]. Department of Psychology, St. John's University, New York, USA.

Terjesen, M. D., Salhany, J., & Scuitto, M. J. (2009). A psychometric review of measures of irrational beliefs: Implications for psychotherapy. *Journal of Rational-Emotive & Cognitive Behavior Therapy, 27*(2), 83–92.

Trip, S., Vernon, A., & McMahon, J. (2007). Effectiveness of rational-emotive education: A quantitative meta-analytical study. *Journal of Cognitive and Behavioral Psychotherapies, 7*(1), 81–93.

Trip, S., McMahon, J., Bora, C., & Chipea, F. (2010). The efficiency of a Rational Emotive and Behavioral Education program in diminishing dysfunctional thinking, behaviors and emotions in children. *Journal of Cognitive and Behavioral Psychotherapies, 10*(2), 173–186.

Vigerland, S., Lenhard, F., Bonnert, M., Lalouni, M., Hedman, E., Ahlen, J., et al. (2016). Internet-delivered cognitive behavior therapy for children and adolescents: A systematic review and meta-analysis. *Clinical Psychology Review, 50*, 1–10.

Vîslă, A., Flückiger, C., & grosse Holtforth, M., & David, D. (2016). Irrational beliefs and psychological distress: A meta-analysis. *Psychotherapy and Psychosomatics, 85*(1), 8–15. https://doi-org.jerome.stjohns.edu/10.1159/000441231

Voort, J. L. V., Svecova, J., Jacobson, A. B., & Whiteside, S. P. (2010). A retrospective examination of the similarity between clinical practice and manualized treatment for childhood anxiety disorders. *Cognitive and Behavioral Practice, 17*(3), 322–328.

Wang, Z., Whiteside, S. P., Sim, L., Farah, W., Morrow, A. S., Alsawas, M., et al. (2017). Comparative effectiveness and safety of cognitive behavioral therapy and pharmacotherapy for childhood anxiety disorders: A systematic review and meta-analysis. *JAMA Pediatrics, 171*(11), 1049–1056.

Weersing, R. V., Jeffreys, M., Do, M. T., Schwartz, K. T. G., & Bolano, C. (2017). Evidence base update of psychosocial treatments for child and adolescent depression. *Journal of Clinical Child and Adolescent Psychology, 46*(1), 11–43. https://doi.org/10.1080/15374416.2016.1220310

Weisz, J. R., Kuppens, S., Ng, M. Y., Eckshtain, D., Ugueto, A. M., Vaughn-Coaxum, R., et al. (2017). What five decades of research tells us about the effects of youth psychological therapy: A multilevel meta-analysis and implications for science and practice. *American Psychologist, 72*(2), 79.

Weisz, J. R., McCarty, C. A., & Valeri, S. M. (2006). Effects of psychotherapy for depression in children and adolescents: A meta-analysis. *Psychological Bulletin, 132*(1), 132.

Zatz, S., & Chassin, L. (1983). Cognitions of test-anxious children. *Journal of Consulting and Clinical Psychology, 51*, 526–534.

Zins, J. E., & Elias, M. J. (2007). Social and emotional learning: Promoting the development of all students. *Journal of Educational & Psychological Consultation, 17*, 233–255. https://doi.org/10.1080/10474410701413152

Chapter 3
A Compendium of REBT Principles and Best Practices for Working with Children and Adolescents

Michael Bernard

As a lot of REBT practice is theory, hypothesis-driven. To be effective, you need to know the REBT theory of childhood emotional and behavioral problems. And without a doubt, effective REBT assessment requires practitioners to know what the theory of REBT offers as the likely irrational beliefs contributing to anxiety (e.g., performance, social), depression (including depression about depression), anger, procrastination, and the like. And to be effective in modifying irrationality, practitioners need to be conversant with different styles of disputing (Socratic, didactic) and disputing techniques (e.g., logical, empirical semantic, rational emotive imagery) as well as how to design in collaboration with younger clients meaningful between-session, homework activities.

Know Your Theory

- The extent to which children's thinking and associated beliefs are dominated by irrationality rather than rationality depends upon their cognitive-developmental status, their biological temperament (e.g., feisty, fearful, flexible), their home environment including their parent's style of parenting (e.g., firm/not firm, kind/unkind), the extent to which their parents model and communicate irrational or rational beliefs and whether there are negative events present in their lives (e.g., divorce, persecution).
- Children who manifest social-emotional-behavioral and achievement problems often present with developmental delays in their capacity to think rationally and logically concerning affective-interpersonal issues (e.g., have difficulty keeping

M. Bernard (✉)
Melbourne Graduate School of Education, University of Melbourne, Parkville, VIC, Australia
e-mail: m.bernard@unimelb.edu.au

M. Bernard, M. D. Terjesen (eds.), *Rational-Emotive and Cognitive-Behavioral Approaches to Child and Adolescent Mental Health: Theory, Practice, Research, Applications*, https://doi.org/10.1007/978-3-030-53901-6_3

things in perspective, personalize negative experiences) as well as in the development of other emotional self-management skills (e.g., relaxation, finding someone to talk with). They also are dominated by a range of irrational beliefs including self-downing, low frustration tolerance, and the lack of acceptance of others.

- Older children and adolescents in the face of adverse events have a tendency to revert to cognitive functioning that is characteristic of the pre-concrete operational stage of development. Characteristics of pre-concrete operational thought include:

  1. Drawing arbitrary inferences – conclusions not based on evidence or when evidence contradicts conclusion
  2. Selective abstraction – focusing on a detail taken out of context, ignoring salient features of the situation
  3. Magnification/minimization – errors in evaluating the significance of the event
  4. Personalization – tendency to relate external events to themselves when no basis for making connection
  5. Overgeneralization – drawing a conclusion based on limited and isolated events
  6. Dichotomous thinking – tendency to place events into opposite categories (e.g., good-bad)

- Rational emotive behavior theory states that irrational beliefs in the form of *absolutes* (shoulds, oughts, musts, needs) are the psychological core of children and adolescent emotional and behavioral problems.
  For example,
  I must be successful.
  I need love and approval.
  The world should give me what I want comfortably, quickly, and easily.
  People must treat me fairly and considerately.

- Ellis indicated that there are a number of derivatives of absolutes that also contribute to the type and intensity of emotional problems including *awfulizing*, *I can't-stand-it-it is* and *global rating* (self, others, world).
  For example,
  It's awful to make mistakes.
  I can't stand to be criticized.
  I can't stand having to do boring homework.
  People who treat me badly are bad people and deserve severe punishment.
  School is stupid.
  I'm stupid.

- As a result of their irrational beliefs, young people are prone to misrepresent reality (errors of inference including faulty conclusions, predictions). Sometimes, inferences are referred to as *automatic thoughts*.

For example,
I will always make mistakes.
My teacher doesn't like me.
All homework is boring.
People always act unfairly to me.
I'm a hopeless student.

- The tendency for young people to selectively attend to and remain over-focused on the negative aspects of their environment is also strongly influenced by their core irrational beliefs.
  For example, they pay attention to:
  Children who are not wanting to play with them.
  Mistakes and other negative comments offered by their teacher concerning schoolwork.
  The boring aspects of homework.
  Classmates who are mean to them.
  Negative aspects of the way they look.

- Common Irrational Beliefs of Children (Virginia Waters)

  1. It's awful if others don't like me.
  2. I'm bad if I make a mistake.
  3. Everything should always do my way: I should always get what I want.
  4. Things should come easy to me.
  5. The world should be fair and bad people should be punished.
  6. I shouldn't show my feelings.
  7. Adults should be perfect.
  8. There's only one right answer.
  9. I must win.
  10. I shouldn't have to wait for anything.

- Common Irrational Beliefs of Adolescents (Virginia Waters)

  1. It would be awful if my peers didn't like me. It would be awful to be a social loser.
  2. I shouldn't make mistakes, especially social mistakes.
  3. It's my parents' fault I'm so miserable.
  4. I can't help it. That's just the way I am, and I guess I'll always be this way.
  5. The world should be fair and just.
  6. It's awful when things don't go my way.
  7. It's better to avoid challenges rather than risk failure.
  8. I must conform to my peers.
  9. I can't stand to be criticized.
  10. Others should always be responsible.

- While other forms of child- and adolescent-oriented cognitive behavioral therapy focus on changing automatic thoughts including misrepresentations of reality and developing positive self-talk (as does REBT), distinctive to REBT assessment and treatment is the focus on assessing, disputing, and restructuring of children's and adolescent's irrational beliefs (absolutes and derivatives) into rational beliefs.

- REBT encourages parents and teachers as well as practitioners to promote the development in young people of an explicit set of rational beliefs considered as central to young people's positive social-emotional well-being: self-acceptance, high frustration tolerance, acceptance of others (Table 3.1).

Relationship Building

- Don't preach or give young clients a sermon on the need for them to change.
- Do not act like a teacher or parent. For example, do not communicate a negative tone about their behavior. Do not try to coerce change.
- Be empathic no matter how trivial your young client's concerns/problems appear to be ("That must be hard."). Do not be too quick to move into problem analysis/solving.
- Be non-judgmental (unconditionally accepting) of young clients when you hear about problems even when you disapprove of their behavior (if client broke law, engaged in sexual behavior). Do not let them feel you are judging them.
- Respect resistance and move forward to build trust. When you experience resistance, move slower and back off from interpretation. Use more indirect methods (e.g., puppets; reference to problems of a friend).
- Be patient as trust can be a slow process.
- With younger clients, sit alongside them rather than across the desk from them.
- Show genuine interest in young clients. Have them share personal stories. Invite them to bring in work and other valued possessions to show you (e.g., CDs, books, yearbooks, artwork).
- Build trust through mutual self-disclosure.
- In early sessions, listen, and reflect back feelings and information.
- Do not become over-involved emotionally; maintain objectivity. However, it is good to emotionally desire to help children.
- Especially with adolescents, work on winning their respect rather than their approval. You may have to ask them to do things they do not want to do.
- Use language appropriate to the age and cultural background of the young client.
- Deal directly with young clients' anxieties about why they are in therapy or receiving counseling ("Am I crazy?").
- Don't be afraid to communicate with humor (e.g., exaggeration). It is okay to laugh about a young client's or your own behavior, but never at the client.
- Help young clients develop the sense that you are on their side (not the side of parents or teachers).

Table 3.1 Typical ABC's of common childhood mental health problems

Typical ABC's of Anger in Children and Adolescents
*A*ctivating events: unfairness, inconsideration, disrespect, being picked on, not listened to, not getting one's way
*B*eliefs: Inferences (predictions, conclusions): This is unfair. I am never able to do what I want. Everyone else gets what he or she wants. Absolutes (shoulds, oughts, musts, needs): People should treat me fairly, considerately and with respect. I must have what I want. Evaluations (derivatives of the absolutes): This is awful, terrible...the worst thing in the world. I can't stand it...I shouldn't have to obey rules all the time. This person is totally bad and deserves to be punished.
*C*onsequences (emotions, behaviors): anger, aggressive behavior (physical, verbal), rule breaking, power struggles, defiance, and procrastination
Typical ABC's of Bullying in Children and Adolescents
Type 1: Children Who Bully Because They Feel Inferior
*A*ctivating events: peers who cannot defend themselves
*B*eliefs: Inferences (conclusions, predictions): I will be perceived by my peers as strong and "cool" if I can bully and intimidate others. Absolutes (shoulds, oughts, musts, needs): To be approved of and to feel worthwhile, I must be the strongest. I need my peers to think highly of me. Evaluations (derivatives of the absolutes): It is awful to be seen as weak. I can't stand it if my peers think they are stronger than me.
*C*onsequences (emotions, behaviors): underlying inferiority, anger, verbal/physical abuse
Type 2: Children Who Bully Because They Need to Be Seen as the Best in Everything including having to Control Others
*A*ctivating events: peers who cannot defend themselves Inferences (conclusions, predictions): Muscle power rather than brain power is the key to my success in school. The way to show others I am a man/woman is by showing my classmates through my fists and harsh words that I can control others and make the world run my way. Absolutes (shoulds, oughts, musts, needs): I must be successful and all-powerful in all areas of my life. I must be the best in all my academic and social activities and be seen by others as the strongest too. People should do my bidding. Evaluations (derivatives of the absolute): It is awful to be beaten by anyone. I can't stand losing. Coming in second means you are a loser.
*C*onsequences (emotions, behaviors): overconfidence, controlling behavior, victimization, and anger
Typical ABC's of Cheating in Children and Adolescents
*A*ctivating events: upcoming test, papers, assignments
*B*eliefs: Inferences (conclusions, predictions): Because I have always cheated on tests and have somehow managed to pass and not get caught, I will never be able to pass unless I continue to cheat. Absolutes (shoulds, oughts, musts, needs): I need to achieve well and be seen to be among the best in my schoolwork. Evaluations (derivatives of the absolute): It is terrible and awful for me to fail on an exam. I would be a total idiot if I did fail.
*C*onsequences (emotions, behaviors): anxiety, guilt, cheating, pressurizing friends to copy

(continued)

Table 3.1 (continued)

Typical ABC's of Feeling Down in Children and Adolescents
*A*ctivating Events: loss of parental love through desertion/abandonment/ neglect or death
*B*eliefs Inferences (conclusions, predictions): My parent doesn't love me. It's my fault my parent never wants to see me. I cannot do anything to get his/her to love me. I cannot be happy without his/her love. Life is not worth living if I cannot have his/her love. Absolutes (shoulds, oughts, musts, needs): I need my parent's love. Evaluations: I cannot bear to live without her love. This proves how unlovable and hopeless I am. This is terrible.
*C*onsequence (emotional, behavioral): down, crying, periods of inactivity, avoidance of people and tasks, tiredness, irritability
*A*ctivating Events: poor school performance
*B*eliefs Inferences (conclusions, predictions): I'm not good at any of my schoolwork and never will be. I am hopeless in everything I do. Absolutes (shoulds, oughts, musts, needs): I should/must achieve in my schoolwork. Evaluations: It is awful to make mistakes and do so poorly, I really can't stand it. This proves I am really a total failure.
*C*onsequence (emotional, behavioral): down, crying, periods of inactivity, avoidance of people and tasks, tiredness, irritability
*A*ctivating events: social rejection, teasing, no one to play with, not being invited, loss of boyfriend/girlfriend
*B*eliefs Inferences (conclusions, predictions): Everyone is against me. Everyone is teasing me. No one likes me. I'll never have any friends. I can't be happy without his/her love or attention. Absolutes (shoulds, oughts, musts, needs): I need people to like and approve of me. Evaluations: It is awful to be criticized, laughed at and alone. I can't stand it. This proves that I really am a hopeless person.
*C*onsequence (emotional, behavioral): down, crying, periods of inactivity, avoidance of people and tasks, tiredness, irritability
Typical ABC's of Procrastination/Under-Achievement in Children and Adolescents
*A*ctivating events: chores, homework
*B*eliefs: Inferences (conclusions, predictions): Difficult tasks are impossible. Everything will turn out okay whether I work or not. To do this work would be a violation of my personal integrity. Nothing I do at school will benefit me. Absolutes (shoulds, oughts, musts, needs): I shouldn't have to do things I do not feel like doing. Life should be comfortable and fun and never boring. Evaluations: This work I have to do is the worst thing in the world. I can't stand having to do it. The world is crap in forcing me to do this work.
*C*onsequences (emotions, behaviors): forgetfulness, daydreaming, delays in getting started and finishing schoolwork and chores, anger when forced to do things s/he doesn't feel like doing, impatience, impulsiveness, avoidance tactics, laziness, diffuse anxiety
Typical ABC's of Perfectionism in Children and Adolescents
Type 1: Compulsive Effort
*A*ctivating events: any work/activity/task deemed important to do and difficult to accomplish

(continued)

Table 3.1 (continued)

*B*eliefs: Inferences (conclusions, predictions): I will not be able to do this successfully. By putting in maximum effort, I can be perfect. Mistakes show that I cannot do things perfectly. Absolutes (shoulds, oughts, musts, needs): I really should do things perfectly. Evaluations: It would be a catastrophe to not to be able to do this perfectly…too unbearable to tolerate. It is awful to make mistakes. To be imperfect would prove I am a failure.
*C*onsequences (emotions, behaviors): generalized anxiety, excessive effort, depression when one fails
Type 2: Lack of Effort
*A*ctivating events: any work/activity/task deemed important to do and difficult to accomplish
*B*eliefs: Inferences (conclusions, predictions): I will not be able to do this perfectly. By putting in minimum effort, I have a ready-made excuse for not doing things perfectly (I didn't try). Why bother doing things if I cannot do them perfectly? Absolutes (shoulds, oughts, musts, needs): I really should do things perfectly. Evaluations: It would be a catastrophe not to be able to do this perfectly…too unbearable to tolerate. It is awful to make mistakes. To be imperfect would prove I am a failure.
*C*onsequences (emotions, behaviors): underlying anxiety, lack of effort, choosing not to participate in new activities where success is not guaranteed, choosing not to compete
Typical ABCs of Social Anxiety in Children and Adolescents
*A*ctivating events: being in social situations, meeting new people, having to give a speech
*B*eliefs: Inferences (conclusions, predictions): I'll say something stupid or not know what to say. People will think I'm stupid. No one will want to speak with me. I'll be too uncomfortable. Absolutes (shoulds, oughts, musts, needs): I need people to like and approve of me. I need to be comfortable. Evaluations: It is awful to be laughed at or criticized by others.
*C*onsequences (emotions, behaviors): social anxiety, discomfort anxiety, avoidance, blushing, physical signs of nervousness, stammering, mumbling
Typical ABCs of Performance Anxiety in Children and Adolescents
*A*ctivating events: having to take a test, give a speech
*B*eliefs: Inferences (conclusions, predictions): I'll make mistakes. I have no talent in doing this and never will have. Absolutes (shoulds, oughts, musts, needs): I must perform well at all times. Evaluations (derivatives of the absolutes): It would be a catastrophe and intolerable to not perform well.
*C*onsequences (emotions, behaviors): tenseness, high anxiety/panic attack, forgetfulness, procrastination in preparation, shaky performance, careless mistakes, physical symptoms of nervousness (e.g., sweaty palms, muscle tenseness)
Typical ABC's of School Phobia in Children and Adolescents
*A*ctivating events: having to go to or stay at school
*B*eliefs: Inferences (conclusions, predictions): Something bad will happen to me at school. I might even be killed. I will go to school and everyone will laugh at me. The teacher will think there is something wrong with me. I will not know what to do. I am too far behind to catch up. I will not understand what to do. It will be totally uncomfortable and unpleasant to be in class and with my classmates. They'll tease me and think I'm a total loser.

(continued)

Table 3.1 (continued)

Absolutes (shoulds, oughts, musts, needs): I should/must achieve in my schoolwork. I need be to be liked and approved of. I need to be comfortable.
Evaluations: To be laughed at by my classmates and thought badly of by my teacher is awful and terrible. I cannot stand feeling so uncomfortable. Showing people how weak I am will prove that I am hopeless.
*C*onsequences (emotions, behaviors): discomfort anxiety, social/performance anxiety, refusal to attend school or go to class, clinginess to mother, avoidance of children who attend school.
Typical ABC's of Secondary Emotional Distress in Children and Adolescents
*A*ctivating events: procrastination, depression, angry, anxiety
Inferences (conclusions, predictions): I am the only person with this problem. There must be something wrong with me. I'll always have this problem.
Absolutes (shoulds, oughts, musts, needs): I shouldn't have this problem. I need people to think highly of me.
Evaluations: It's awful to have this problem. I can't stand it if people see I have a problem. I cannot stand myself for having this problem. I must be a real loser.
*C*onsequences (emotions, behaviors): guilt, down, denial of primary problem

- For young clients referred for educational under-achievement, explain to young clients that the reason they have been referred to you by their teacher(s) or parent(s) is that they have a lot more potential that they have been showing and that with a little coaching from you, they can learn skills to help them develop their potential and to be successful.
- In working with clients who have anger problems, be tactful in indicating that the cause of their problems are their attitudes/beliefs and if they would only change their attitudes, they would not have current problems. Such a tactic may lead to young clients feeling blamed, a lack of bonding and to them choosing not to return for further sessions.

Suggestions for Your First Session

- Define the role of therapist/counselor (problem solver: "I am good at helping you if you have hassles with others, worries about the future, hurt feelings.") Reassure young clients that they are not crazy and that having a problem is not "bad" everyone has problems – especially when growing up. Explain that just as they go to a medical doctor when they have a cold, break a leg, etc., they go to someone when they have a social, behavioral or emotional problem. Explain that counseling is a safe place to explore feelings and thoughts.
- Establish confidentiality limits with parents, teachers, and young client. Ask whether there is anything they have shared with you that they do not want someone else to know.
- Share reason for referral.
- If you sense a young client's reluctance/resistance to being referred, normalize feelings ("It seems that you don't want to be here and that's all right. However,

someone who cares about you thinks there is something wrong, maybe I can help."). Share information about the counseling/therapy process you are using.

- Explain that the two of you will be working together helping the young person deal with particular problems. Indicate that for most sessions, you will be asking them to talk about their thoughts, feelings, behaviors and you will be showing them different ways to manage their feelings so that when something bad happens, they do not feel so upset and how to feel better. Indicate you will be asking them to perform various "experiments" during the week that can provide them with additional ways to solve problems. Stress that it is very important that the young client carry through with the practice involved in conducting the experiments. Indicate the number of sessions.
- Normalize problem and communicate hope ("Lots of kids lose their temper a lot, have big worries, get very down." And lots of kids learn how to feel better and not be so upset. We can come up with some ideas to deal with this.") (With adolescents, share information about typical adolescent development).
- Start off by finding out about interests/hobbies/skills/talents of young client including pets/family members ("teach me about you"). Ways to do this: write a story; draw a picture of family, an acrostic poem. Consider using a "get acquainted" structured activity (share something personal).
- Ask one question about the presenting problem ("I heard you are being treated badly by a classmate?") and then paraphrase/summarize the answer. Gain agreement. Do not minimize the problem nor dramatize.
- Indicate that you would like to be able to talk with the young client about ways to make things better.
- Review what young clients can to say to their classmates in response to the question: "Where were you?" during time client was with you (possible answer: "I was getting extra help with my homework"). Have clients select what they feel comfortable saying.
- Inform the child how you will be communicating with parents.
- Young clients present with different degrees of willingness to change. Some may be so caught up in their personal issues (e.g., abuse) they may be unaware of the need for therapy and the need for them to work on changing themselves. Said another way, you may be ready to do REBT, but they might not. In these cases, be patient. Work on developing their self-awareness and readiness to change as a prerequisite to REBT.

Assessment

- Remind yourself to differentiate in your assessment the young clients' *emotional problems* (e.g., problems on the inside) such as anger, anxiety, feeling down and their *practical problems* (e.g., problems on the outside) such as making friends, how to get someone to stop teasing, organizational skills deficits, lack of assertion skills.

- When a young client describes a negative activating event, ask: "How did that feel?" Then, help them to clarify whether they were angry, anxious and/or down.
- To elicit problems, say: "Some kids in your situation might feel ___________." Then check with client.
- Let young clients know that having strong negative feelings is normal and OK. Say: "You know, lots of kids from time-to-time have strong feelings about things. Some can get really furious about what other people do, some worry a great deal, sometimes, kids get very down about things."
- Teach young clients two pre-requisites skills.

  1. An *emotional schema* for conceptualizing their feelings. Many young people have an "all or none" view of their emotions. For example, they believe they can either be angry or happy. You can use a 10-point scale from "Feeling nothing at all" to "Could not be any more upset" to illustrate to young people they have options in terms of how upset they become when faced with negative events. Help them see that moderate levels of anger, anxiety and feeling down are not only normal but also helpful in solving problems but extreme levels are harmful and can lead to self-defeating behavior on their part. An Emotional Thermometer can be used for this purpose.
  2. Help develop in young clients an *emotional vocabulary* for describing and differentiating their feelings. Many young people are aware that they are upset but may lack the linguistic tools for analyzing their different emotional states.

- Assess the following emotions and behaviors:

  – Feeling down (including feeling angry with self)
  – Feeling anxious (worried): social anxiety, performance anxiety (including perfectionism, test anxiety), discomfort anxiety (anxious about being anxious)
  – Feeling angry with another
  – Low frustration tolerance/procrastination (work avoidance, angry about having to do something that is boring)
  – Relationship problems
  – Secondary emotional problems: feeling down about primary emotional/behavioral problem (e.g., being down, procrastination)

- Sometimes, when you ask young clients about the degree of emotional upset they experienced when they were confronted with a negative event in the recent past, they might say: "Medium upset. Maybe a 5 out of 10 on the Emotional Thermometer." Unless you can identify a time when your client was extremely upset (e.g., 8–10 on the Emotional Thermometer) it is unwise to conclude that the client has an emotional problem or harbors irrational beliefs. To "get at" a more extreme emotional reaction of young clients, ask: "When was the last time you got extremely upset (really angry, anxious or down) – a time when you were getting close to the top of the Emotional Thermometer?"

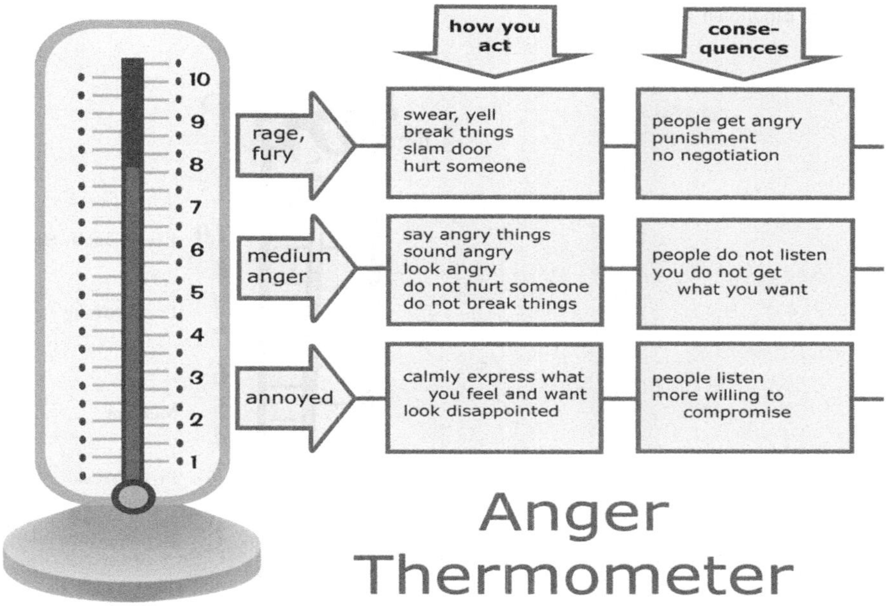

Fig. 3.1 Anger thermometer

- In assessing anger, identify the negative consequences for young clients in terms of the environmental response to your client (what people say or do) when your client behaves in a very aggressive fashion. Negative consequences are the prime factors for angry young clients to be motivated to change their emotions, behaviors and anger-creating beliefs. You can use the Anger Thermometer to represent these relationships to your client (Fig. 3.1).
- Once you have identified different emotional-behavioral problems of a young client, determine which shall be the first problem to work on. Indicate that problems will be worked on one at a time.
- Help client to set a goal for emotional-behavioral change. Ask: "The next time ________________ occurs, rather than feeling extremely (down/anxious/angry) how would you rather feel and behave?" Seek agreement from client that rather than feeling extremely down/anxious/angry (8–10 on the Emotional Thermometer), it would be better to feel only moderately down/anxious/angry and for his/her behavior to change from negative to positive (Fig. 3.2).

Fig. 3.2 Emotional Thermometer

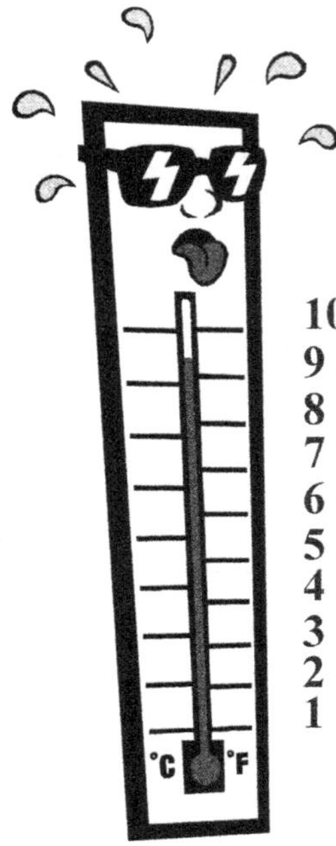

Methods and Techniques for Assessing Thinking

- Standardized self-report surveys: CASI-3 (Terjesen, M.D., Kassay, K., & Anderson, D. (2017). Evaluation of the psychometric properties of a measure of child irrationality. *Journal of Rational-Emotive & Cognitive-Behavior Therapy*. https://doi.org/10.1007/s10942-017-0269-z)
- Thought clouds (e.g., cartoon characters in various problematic situations with empty thought clouds above their head for young clients to write in their thinking).
- Incomplete sentences (e.g., "When your father swore at you, you thought to yourself, ______________________").
- Instant Reply (e.g., "Can you replay in your mind what happened last Saturday when your father swore at you? What time of day was it, who was around, what exactly did he say and do, and what did you think?").
- When ____________ happened, you felt ____________, because______________ (what were you thinking?)?
- With younger clients, instead of using the traditional ABC framework to represent and explain important relationships, the HTFB framework is frequently employed to make more concrete these same relationships.

Happening → Thinking → Feeling → Behaving

- It is often a good idea to write down for young clients a summary of the assessment data you are gathering. The following headings that can be written on the board or a piece of paper:

Happening →	Thinking →	Feeling →	Behaving
John teases me	Everyone teases me. I have no friends. I'll never have friends. This is terrible. I'm a loser	Down (9/10)	Withdraw
John teases me	This is unfair. He shouldn't do this. I can't stand this. He's a real ___.	Anger (10/10)	Fight

- The order of assessment questions is as follows:

  1. Identify a specific Happening (day, place, person, task).
  2. Assess different feelings the client had about the Happening and assess using the Emotional Thermometer, the intensity of each.
  3. Assess behavioral reactions that accompany feelings.
  4. Select one feeling at a time to work on. Then, assess what client was thinking looking for errors of inference (faulty conclusions, predictions), absolutes (shoulds, oughts, musts, needs) and derivative evaluations (awfulizing, I-can't-stand-it-it is, global rating). Be thorough in eliciting absolutes and derivative evaluations using *inference chaining* and *deductive interpretation* questioning.

- *Inference chaining* is a common strategy for assessing irrational beliefs. Assume the young client's inferences (e.g., predictions, conclusions) are true and ask young client what would it mean to him/her if his/her inference were true.
- An example of inference chaining used with a boy with learning disabilities who was depressed (Ray DiGiuseppe):

  Client: "I know I'll fail today's test."
  Therapist: "And what do you think would happen if you did fail it?"
  Client: "Well, I might fail all the tests."
  Therapist: "Well, let's suppose that would happen. What might you think? then?"
  Client: "I guess I would think that I'd be stupid or dumb."
  Therapist: "Well, what would it mean to you if you were not as smart as you would like to be?"
  Client: "I'd be no good."

- Remember that irrational beliefs – especially the absolutes – are frequently out of conscious awareness of young clients as well as other irrational evaluations. For young clients who have difficulty reporting on their thinking, you will need to use directive questioning and probing to get at these core irrationalities. Do not expect your clients to always provide them for you when you ask: "What else were you thinking."

- When children are unaware of their irrational beliefs, you can use a hypothesis-testing form of questioning sometimes called *deductive interpretation* as can be seen in the following. "When people get angry, they often think to themselves that people really *should* act respectfully and fairly. Did you have this idea when your father refused to listen to your point of view?" If the client agrees, use client's verbal and non-verbal language to validate whether client is merely agreeing to agree and please you or whether client really had the irrational thought during the time he/she was upset. If the young client gives you negative feedback, start over again to formulate a new hypothesis.
- Once you have identified a specific Activating event and Consequence (emotional) to work on, assess client's thinking. You will want to "gather" as many examples of client's inferences (conclusions, predictions), absolutes (shoulds, oughts, musts, needs) and evaluations (e.g., awfulizing, I-can't-stand-it-itis, global rating of self, another, world).
- To assess thinking, ask: "When ____________ happened, you felt ____________ because…?" When client provides answer (e.g., "I was angry because he acted so unfairly") elicit additional cognitions by asking "and" and "because" questions.
- Once you have assessed the full range of inferences, absolutes and evaluations, summarize and validate the information you have gathered. Say: "So let me get this straight, you have said that when ____________ happens and you think ____________, ________________, ______________, and ____________________, you get very ______________ (feeling) and you behave ____________________." Is that right?
- If young client does not agree with your summary, return to conduct further assessment.

Treatment

- For children the goals of REBT can be expressed as follows (Virginia Waters):

  1. Correctly identify emotions.
  2. Develop an emotional vocabulary.
  3. Distinguish between helpful and hurtful feelings.
  4. Differentiate between feelings and thoughts.
  5. Tune into self-talk.
  6. Make the connection between self-talk and feelings.
  7. Learn rational self-talk.

- For older children and adolescents, a more complex set of goals may be pursued in addition to the ones already listed (Howard Young):

  1. Teach the ABCs (Happening → Thinking → Feeling → Behaving)

2. Dispute shoulds, oughts, musts and needs.
3. Dispute awfulizing.
4. Dispute I-can't-stand-it-it is.
5. Dispute self- and other-downing.

- Teach self-acceptance, high frustration tolerance and acceptance of others.
- Collaborate with your client on goals for emotional and behavioral change. Ask: "The next time _______________ happens, rather than getting extremely angry/anxious/down, what would be a better emotional reaction from you? How would you like to feel and behave the next time ___________ happens?
- You can sometimes use the HTFB model to help young clients to select goals and to focus on how their thinking can help them accomplish their goals.
For example,

Now

Happening	→	Thinking	→	Feeling	→	Behaving
John teases me		Everyone teases me. I have no friends. I'll never have friends. This is terrible. I'm a loser.		Down (9/10		Withdraw

---

In Future

Happening	→	Thinking	→	Feeling	→	Behaving
John teases me		?????		Down (3/10) Confident		Ignore Assertive

Do not forget to ask about what changes they would like to see in any practical problems (e.g., getting better grades, stopping someone from bullying).

Explain to young clients that they can change how they feel when something bad happens.

- Before disputing, make sure you repeatedly teach the B-C link.
- One of the important ideas that you want to explicitly teach young clients is that it is not what happens to you that causes your feelings, it is your thinking that causes you to feel the way you do. In REBT, we sometimes call this insight "Emotional Responsibility." Emotional responsibility is at the core of gaining emotional self-control and the development of an internal locus of control.
- You can teach the B-C link in a number of ways. You can ask your young client: "If 100 young people were called a bad name by their brother, would they all be as angry as you? I think you'll agree that some would be even angrier and some less angry? Why do you think people feel differently about the same event? Can you see that the reason people feel differently is because they are thinking different thoughts about the event?"

- Using a Happening → Thinking → Feeling → Behaving diagram elicited from your client concerning an event in his/her life, point out that between what happens and his/her feelings is thinking.
- The B-C link can be taught explicitly. Summarize as follows: "When __________ happened, you were thinking __________________, and as a result, you felt __________________." Can you see how your thinking rather than what happened determines how upset you get?"
- Before you begin disputing your young client's irrational thinking, explain to your client the difference between facts (supported by factual evidence) and guesses or assumptions (something we guess or believe to be true but may or may not be supported by evidence).
- For example, you can say "Years ago, people had the assumption that the world was flat and as a result, they did not sail very far from home fearing they would fall off the edge of the world. Years later, as a result of early explorers taking foolish chances and sailing all around the world without falling off, people changed their assumption about the shape of earth."
- "When we have a look at what you are thinking, we shall be on the lookout for thoughts you have that are true, "I made a mistake" and those thoughts, "I am no good for making a mistake" and assumptions that are false. This is because false assumptions can cause all sorts of problems."
- In order to help your young clients understand the process of disputing (sometimes called "challenging") and to soften the impact of your disputes so that your clients do not feel you are attacking/criticizing them—you can explain that sometimes you play the role of a "thought detective." In this role, you are on the lookout for any thoughts that your client may have that are not true, not sensible and not helpful. Depending on the age of your clients, you can define this type of thinking as "irrational."
- The five main REBT intervention strategies used with young clients to restructure faulty inferences (predictions, conclusions), absolutes (shoulds, oughts, needs, musts) and evaluations (awfulizing, I can't stand it, global rating of self, other, world) are:

  1. Empirical disputation
  2. Logical disputation
  3. Semantic disputation
  4. Rational self-statements (with/without disputing)
  5. Rational emotive imagery

- There are two main disputational styles you can use to help young clients change their irrational beliefs into more rational ones (Ray DiGiuseppe).

  Didactic Style. This method involves you directly explaining to young clients where their emotions come from and the differences between rational and irrational beliefs. This will include a mini-lecture as to why a belief is irrational. An example of a didactic dispute is as follows:

  "You are saying that you can't stand it when your brother chooses not to play with you. Now, you have survived up into today even after being excluded by your brother. I think you can see there is no evidence to support your idea."

- *Socratic Style.* This method involves you drawing information from young clients using a series of leading questions rather than by direct lecturing. This method helps young clients think through things themselves rather than just accept the therapist's viewpoint. Examples of such questions are:
  "In looking over your 12 years of life, is there any evidence you can think of that shows that you cannot stand it when your brother chooses not to play with you? If there is no evidence, what can you conclude?
- *Empirical disputation* involves an examination of evidence to determine whether the client's inferences and evaluation are reality based "Where is the evidence to support your idea that no one likes you?" "Where is the evidence that you are an idiot because you received a poor grade?" "Where is it written that you must do everything perfectly?" "Is it true that you must?"
- *Empirical analysis* is a common form of empirical disputation and involves you and the young client designing a simple experiment to gather data to test the client's interpretation of reality (conclusions, predictions). For example, in the case of George, a 10 year old, who is quite down about being teased by a few of his classmates, one of his faulty inferences contributing to him feeling so down is: "No one likes me."

  – To use empirical disputation, you can provide George with a class list and have him go down the list noting those classmates whom he thinks like him or could be friends with him. If the list contains a few check marks, such data provides the evidence to George that his assumption of "No one likes me" is false. He can then be helped to generate a new rational self-statement such as: "Even though people are teasing me, I still have friends."
  – Another example of *empirical analysis and disputation* that you could utilize to help George cope with teasing and his belief "No one likes me" is as follows. You could have George conduct the following experiment. You could generate a list of common peer behaviors that are indicative that someone is liked (e.g., people say hello, invited to play at recess, someone helps you with your work, someone sits by you at lunch). You could then assign George the task of recording each instance during the ensuing week when he notices one of his classmates engaging in behaviors on the list. If over a week's time, George has recorded instances of positive peer behavior directed towards him, he would, once again, have evidence to dispute his thinking that "No one likes me."
  – You would then go on to dispute his deeper irrational evaluations: "I need to be liked by everyone. It is awful to be teased. I can't stand it. I'm a nobody."

- *Logical disputation* involves an examination of whether the conclusions the client is drawing and the expectations clients formulate are sensible and logically follow from the facts ("Does it make sense to conclude you are never going to be able to pass a math exam?" "Does it follow that because someone acts badly towards you from time to time that he is a totally bad person in every respect?" "Just because to want to succeed in your schoolwork, does it follow logically that it must happen?").

- *Semantic disputation* involves you providing young clients with an objective definition of the words and phrases they employ in thinking about and evaluating their world.
  For example, if you have determined through your assessment that your client believes that "It is awful to be thought badly of by my peers," you can semantically dispute this using a Socratic style as follows: "Well, 'awful' really means the very worst things that could happen to you. Is being thought badly of by one or more of your classmates really the worst thing that could happen to you?"
  Another example of *semantic disputation* is seen in the following exchange between a therapist and young client.

  T: So, let me get this straight. When, you were not invited to the party at Mary's house and your friend was, you thought of yourself as a 'loser.' Is that what you thought?
  C: Yeah, I mean like Dina and Stephanie were invited.
  T: Well, I would upset myself about what happened, too. But, if you don't want to get so down, let's examine what you were telling yourself and see if it is rational.
  C: OK.
  T: When you think of yourself as a loser, the word 'loser' means more than "I am not popular enough with Mary to get invited to her party."
  The word 'loser' means loser in everything you have done, are doing and will be doing. It means your total essence is one of being a loser. Now, is your use of the word "loser" really true to this meaning?

- Empirical, logical, and semantic disputing can be used to dispute both inferences and evaluations.
- In teaching your young clients about the process of disputing, you can explain that disputing involves asking three questions about one's thinking:

  1. Is what I am thinking true? Is there evidence to support what I am thinking?
  2. Is my thinking logical? Does it make sense to think this way?
  3. Does it help me to think this way? Does my thought help me to achieve my goals and manage my emotions?

- You can explain that when a client answers "No" to any one of these questions, s/he should with your help, try to change the thought to one that is true, sensible, and helpful.
- As clients become familiar with disputing, move from a Didactic style of disputing where you explain to the client why his/her thinking is irrational, to a more Socratic style of disputing where you ask the client questions about a specific thought they have:

  1. Is there evidence to support this idea?
  2. Is it logical to think this way?
  3. Does it help you to think this way?

- Be clear that the irrational beliefs (inferences, absolutes, evaluations) that you dispute are only those that you have initially identified and validated when you assessed your young client's thinking. Make sure your young client accepts that s/he possesses the specific irrational belief you are disputing.
- In disputing young clients' "shoulds", validate their "preferences." Say, for example, "While I quite agree with you that it is preferable that your brother treats you nicely, I'm not sure that it makes sense to believe he should and must always be that way and that you can't stand it when he is unfair."
- Avoid the mistake of providing clients with new rational self-statements and beliefs without first showing them how their original irrational thoughts and beliefs were not true, sensible, and helpful.
- *Disputing "Needs"*
  - Young clients prone to anxiety oftentimes mistakenly believe that they *need* to be successful and/or *need* the approval of others. As success and acceptance ebbs and flows, such clients will experience frequent periods of uncertainty and anxiety in growing up. And if they have a tendency to put themselves down, they will also experience episodic periods of feeling down and depressed.
  - A standard REBT didactic dispute used with these clients involves you explaining the difference between "wants" and "needs." You can ask your client to identify real human needs (e.g., food, water, clothing, shelter). You can ask young clients whether achievement and approval are things people need for survival or are merely desirable.
  - Once your client can differentiate true needs from wants, you can help them re-structure their beliefs to:
  - While I would prefer to be successful, I don't need to be successful.
  - While I prefer to be liked and approved of, I don't need to be liked and approved of.
- *Disputing "Self-Downing"*
  - To dispute self-downing, you will want to show young clients how their thinking "I'm hopeless, a loser" does not make sense and is not true. You can begin by having your young client come up with a range of positive and negative traits using a self-concept circle divided into segments with pluses and minuses in each segment. Once completed, ask young client "Does it make sense to think because something bad happened (e.g., poor grade, teased, rejection) that you are totally bad?" "Do you lose all your positive qualities when you make something bad happen?"
  - Discuss the concept of *human fallibility*. Indicate that everyone is born as a mistake maker and, as such, it never makes sense to think "I must not make mistakes" as mistakes are inevitable.
  - Teach the following ideas to help engender both *self-acceptance* and *other-acceptance*: (1) Every person is complex, not simple, (2) I am complex, not simple, (3) Every person is made up of many positive and negative qualities, (4) I am made up of many positive and negative qualities, (5) A person is not

all good or all bad because of some of his or her characteristics, (6) I am not all good or all bad, (7) When I only focus on the negative characteristics of a person, I feel worse about the person, (8) When I only focus on my negative qualities, I feel worse about myself, (9) Focusing only on the negative qualities of someone else and thinking he is totally bad is irrational. People who do the wrong thing also have other positive qualities. (10) Only focusing on my negative qualities and concluding "I am hopeless" is irrational. Even when I do the wrong thing, I still retain my positive qualities."

- Ask a young client: "Would you put a friend of yours down because she didn't do well in a subject or wasn't invited to a party? Would it make sense to think that she was a total loser?" Once young client agrees ask: "Well then, why are you putting yourself down because of what happened. If you would not put your friend down, does it make sense to put yourself down?"
- Explain that a person's worth cannot be calculated from a person's performance.
- Use an analogy. Ask: "Would you junk a car if it had a flat tire?" When the young client can see that it would not make sense to do so, you can help him begin to see that junking himself when something bad happens does not make sense.
- For children who are depressed due to perceived loss of love from a parent through divorce, abuse or abandonment, gather evidence (instances of loving behavior) to prove or disprove the automatic thoughts "My parent doesn't love me." If it appears that there is no evidence of loving behavior on the part of the child's parent, be prepared to dispute the child's irrational belief that he needs his parents love, that he will not be able to be happy without it and that he is unlovable.

• *Disputing Low Frustration Tolerance/I Can't Stand-it-It is*

  - If you discover in your assessment that your client believes she/cannot stand an event occurring (e.g., specific homework to be done, being criticized by a teacher, staying in on a Saturday night), combine semantic with empirical disputing.
  - Semantic disputing: Explain to your client that "I can't stand it" literally means – dictionary definition – that s/he cannot exist, live in the presence of the negative activating event.
  - Combine with Empirical Disputing: "Now, do you have any evidence that you cannot survive in the presence of ___________? Will it kill you? Will you have a heart attack? Will your eyeballs fall out? Will you faint? Have you survived so far?"
  - Discuss with your young client that thinking "I can't stand it" often enough creates a situation where s/he starts believing it without question. You can say: "Sometimes, you react physically as though you will actually die. Now, where is the evidence you cannot stand it? How often have you said, 'I can't stand it' – and yet you're still alive?"

- Explain to your young client that if the statement "I can't stand it" is repeated often enough, s/he may feel something awful is going to happen. Indicate that s/he cannot trust this feeling or feeling you cannot stand it.
- Help your young clients come up with rational self-statements to replace their "I can't-stand-it-it is": "Even though I do not like this, I can put up with the situation and feeling this way."
- Use the phrase, "end of the world" to show the client s/he is awfulizing. Ask: "Would it be the end of the world?" results in young clients seeing that while the event might be bad and a disadvantage, it is not the worst thing that could happen. And "It's awful" means that it is *so* bad that it absolutely must not happen. But it *must* happen if it actually does happen, no matter how bad it is.

• *Disputing "Awfulizing"*

- The tendency to blow things out of proportion, to make mountains out of molehills, is characteristic of people of all ages. Make young clients aware that they are "awfulizing".
- Use the "catastrophe scale" exercise (see next page). On a blackboard or large sheet of paper, have the young client list all the catastrophes s/he can think of (given the current state of catastrophic events in the world, this should be easy). After listing, 9/11, other terrorist attacks, war, natural disasters, you can bring up one more event; the young client's complaint (e.g., Horace called my mother a bad name). It may not be necessary to point out that the event while bad, does not belong on the same list.

• *Disputing Global Rating of Another*

- There are a number of irrational beliefs of young clients that contain the component of "mistake-making" ("I'm a failure if I make a mistake." "Adults should be perfect." "I shouldn't make mistakes, especially social mistakes."). It is often the case that young clients referred for anger management and behavioral problems believe that people who are in positions of authority (parents, teachers) *should* never make mistakes (act unfairly). Any child referred for perfectionism and low self-esteem mistakenly equate mistakes with self-worth.
- You will want to explain what Ellis calls "human fallibility" by making the following points: (a) All human being including adults and young people make mistakes, (b) No one is perfect, (c) Mistakes do not take away from a person's good qualities, (d) A person is not the same as his/her performance, (e) People are not totally bad because they make mistakes, (f) People who make mistakes do not deserve to be blamed and punished as people, and (g) The reasons why people make mistakes are: lack of skill, carelessness or poor judgment, not having enough information, unsound assumptions, feeling tired or ill, different opinion, and their own irrational thinking.

- Draw a circle and divide it into eight pie-shaped wedges. Label every other pie wedge with a (+) or a minus (−). Have your young client complete this circle with regards to someone who they believe is a total no-good-nik for acting so badly.
- Once completed, discuss whether having one or more (-)s indicates that the person is *totally* bad. Explain that it does not make sense to think that because a person acts badly, s/he is without any positive qualities. Encourage the young client to separate judgments of another person's behavior from judgments of their overall worth and value as a human being.

- *Tips for Disputing*
  - Be animated when disputing.
  - For children aged 8–12 years old, make sure your disputes are concrete and tied to specific events. Rather than asking: "Where is the evidence you cannot stand people's disapproval?', it is more developmentally appropriate to ask: "Where is the evidence that you cannot stand being teased by Warren at 8.30 am on Thursday morning?".
  - You will need to go over the same disputes over successive sessions.
  - Be patient. Sometimes, it takes a client three sessions before he can employ a dispute and new rational effect to modify his feelings in a problematic situation.
  - Check to make sure that your young client is not just agreeing with you for the sake of agreeing.
  - Ask young clients to put in their own words their understanding of one of your didactic disputes.

- *Rational Self-Statements*
  - Rational self-statements are provided to young clients for rehearsal and for use in subsequent situations that tend to occasion in the young client high levels of emotionality. The use of rational self-statements is the preferred cognitive intervention for use with clients younger than the age of 8. For young clients, you can use "green light" and "red light" or "positive thinking" and "negative thinking" rather than "rational thinking" and "irrational thinking."
  - For clients older than 8, rational self-statements also are generated collaboratively between you and your client *after* disputing has occurred and are the main techniques for developing in clients new rational Effects (beliefs).
  - Examples of rational self-statements a young client can use to modify anger include: "People make mistakes. I can stand it when people call me names. It's not the end of the world. I don't have to get angry even though someone is angry with me or is acting badly. Nobody makes me angry. I make myself angry—when I could only make myself sorry with people's behavior. Anger is not cool."
  - Examples of rational self-statements a young client can use to modify feeling down include: "I have talent and am capable. I have friends. I am still me even

Table 3.2 The catastrophe scale

Directions: Think back to the last time you were *extremely* angry, worried, and/or down about something that had happened or was about to happen. Using your Emotional Thermometer, think of a time when you were 8, 9, or 10. Write the event in the space below:

____

At the time you were extremely upset, how bad was it for you that the event or situation had happened or was about to happen? Place a mark to show how you were thinking *at the time* you were very upset. On a scale of 1 to 100, how bad was it for you at the time the bad event was happening or was about to happen?

0	10	20	30	40	50	60	70	80	90	100
	not bad		bit bad		bad		very bad		awful, terrible	

Now, come up with a list of things that could happen to you or in the world that you would consider to be: catastrophic (awful terrible), very bad, bad, and a bit bad. Write them in the spaces below.

"Catastrophic" Events	**"Very Bad" Events**	**"Bad" Events**	**"A Bit Bad" Events**

Think again about the bad event that you listed in the first part of this activity. Which category would you now place it in? – catastrophic, very bad, bad, a bit bad

Important Point: We all sometimes make things worse than they are in our own thinking. Learning to keep things in perspective by not thinking that something is worse than it is helps you cope with bad events that can happen to you.

when bad stuff happens. I don't need to be successful in everything I do. I'll just do the best I can. I don't need everyone to like me all the time. I can survive and still be happy."

- Examples of rational self-statements a young client can use to modify anxiety include: "It's OK to mistakes. It does not have to be perfect. It's not the end of the world if someone does not want to play with me. I can handle getting nervous."
- Examples of rational self-statements a young client can use to modify fear include: "I can be brave. I can take care of myself in the dark. The dark is a fun place to be. There are many good things in the dark (Table 3.2)."

- *Rational Emotive Imagery (REI)*
  - REI involves asking the young client to recreate as vividly as possible in his/her mind a mental picture of a situation in which s/he experiences a very strong emotional response. When the feeling is as strong as possible, the young client is asked to change the feeling from being extreme (8, 9, or 10 on

the Emotional Thermometer) to a more moderate level (3, 4, or 5); for example, from extreme worry to moderate worry and concern.
  - When the young client indicates he was able to reduce the intensity of his emotional response, you can ask: "How were you able to do so?" (For example): "What did you do to change your anger to feeling sorry or disappointed about the bad things that people did?" Emphasize how changing thinking helped the young client reduce the level of upset.

- *Use Cognitive Behavior Rehearsal and Role Play*
  - No matter how effective you have been in disputing, many clients of any age when they return to their real world tend to fall back into using their old habitual irrational beliefs and self-talk when confronted with difficulty. To assist clients to be successful in applying new rational beliefs and self-talk in their problematic environment between sessions, it is good for you to give them practice in role-playing their use within the therapy session.
  - If you are working on helping a young client manage his anger when being teased by a classmate, you could have the young client pretend to verbally harass you and you, playing the role of your client, would think out loud rational self-statements (e.g., "I prefer him not to act this way. I don't like this but I can stand it. This isn't the worst thing that could happen. I can tolerate this. He's not a totally no good kid.") while at the same time ignoring him. You can then reverse roles with you playing the role of the "teaser" and your client thinking out loud the rational self-statements while ignoring you. This can be repeated with the client progressively internalizing the rational self-statements into his/her thinking.

- *Practical Problem Solving*
  - Many young clients are in trouble or are less than happy because they do not have the skills to handle a situation. If someone teases them, they may not know of any way to handle the situation than to fight. Many young clients would like to make more friends but do not know how to get them. Clients who would like to achieve better results in school may be lacking in academic confidence, persistence and organizational skills. In your REBT assessment, you will want to assess deficits in their practical skills and spend time during your sessions developing them.
  - *Helping Young Clients Solve Interpersonal Problems*
    Instruct young clients in the following steps:

    1. Define the problem in concrete, behavioral terms.
    2. Generate as many alternative solutions as you can without evaluating them. Remember, quantity is more important than quality; the more solutions the better.
    3. Go back and evaluate each alternative solution, giving both positive and negative consequences and eliminating absurd solutions.
    4. Choose one or two of the best solutions and plan your procedures step by step.

5. Put your plan into action and evaluate the results.

- *Homework*
  - You will want to explain to all your young clients that as a part of your work with them in helping them solve problems and to overcome difficulties as well as to feel better, it is vital that they put into practice the ideas you will be discussing with them during your sessions. These "homework activities" are crucial in helping them move from cognitive insight to active practice and application of new ways of thinking, feeling and behaving.
  - Be prepared for your young clients to "forget" or otherwise fail to perform weekly homework assignments. This is especially likely for young clients with low frustration tolerance who routinely procrastinate doing chores and/or homework.
  - Assign homework that you are reasonably sure your young client can perform. Do not assign too many tasks and activities for your client to accomplish. If your client fails to perform homework, identify the excuse(s) and help eliminate the reasons your client offers for not doing homework before assigning new homework.
  - *Examples of cognitive homework assignments*

    Each day rehearse rational self-statements (write rational statements on card for young client to remember and practice).

    For young clients who get angry, have them rehearse rational self-talk when they do not get their way (e.g., "Nobody can do everything they want whenever they want." "It is disappointing when I can't do what I want, but it isn't terrible and awful." "Talking back only makes things worse." "I still love them anyway even though I do not like the way they are acting.").

    Have clients bring in songs that illustrate irrational thinking.

    For clients subjected to peer group pressure, provide them with a list of phrases dealing with how to say "No" and have the client practice their use during the week (e.g., "No thanks, I don't want to, if you want to, go ahead. I don't." ""I don't think we should be doing this." "Please don't touch me like that!").

    Record sessions and have young client listen to the tape during the week to reinforce rational thinking.

    Assign stories to read that illustrate rational thinking of the protagonist.

    Present clients with thought clouds above illustrations of characters that are experiencing problems similar to theirs. Have them write in examples of irrational and rational self-talk that will help the character deal with a difficult situation.

    Present young clients with a blank Happening → Thinking → Feeling → Behaving chart and have them complete one that illustrates how they dealt with a problematic situation during the week.

    Invite young clients to teach their parents what they have been learning about rational thinking.
  - *Examples of Emotive Homework Assignments*

Suggest that the client gather data about his anger by keeping track of its frequency, location, outcome, as well as who else was involved (self-monitoring).
Have clients practice rational emotive imagery during the week.
Have clients practice rational self-statements using evocative and forceful language ("I *can* stand it when my brother teases me!!").
Have young clients agree to working on getting only moderately upset (angry, anxious, worried) during the forthcoming week.

– *Examples of Behavioral Homework Assignments*
Design an experiment where young clients agree to do something during the week they do not believe they can stand doing (e.g., working 10 minutes on their math homework).
For perfectionists, gain agreement on something they will do during the week where they have a high likelihood of failing (risk taking exercise).
For approval seekers, design a shame attacking exercise where they agree to engage in a behavior that will with high likelihood invite negative comments and laughs from peers/family members. The fact that they survive the episode will provide evidence to dispute their belief that they need people's approval and it would be awful to be criticized or thought badly of.
Design an experiment where the client agrees to gather evidence to support or contradict a belief they have that is more than likely irrational. For example, if a child believes as a result of repeated criticism from his mother "My mother doesn't love me," help the child agree upon a list of maternal loving behaviors (e.g., cooks for me, picks me up from school, asks me about my date, gives me a hug/kiss, buys me something I need). Then, provide the child with a chart that lists these behaviors and have the child record the number of times each day he observes his mother engaging in the behavior. Once the child can see that despite his mother's criticism, she still engages in different loving behaviors, the child will have concrete evidence to dispute his belief about his mother not loving him (not to be used in cases where you believe that the child will not observe any loving behaviors).

Evaluation

- From time to time during the course of therapy, contact your young client's teacher(s) and parents to ask about any positive changes that they are observing and determine whether their reports confirm what your client has been saying.
- You can ask about any problems they have observed during the week with particular reference to instances when your client appeared very angry, down or worried.
- On a regular basis, does your young client report to you at the beginning of a new session that s/he is better able to manage his/her emotions when s/he confronted difficulty during the previous week?
- Does your young client appear to successfully complete therapeutic homework assignments on a regular basis?

- Does your young client have more self-acceptance, frustration tolerance and acceptance of others than when s/he began therapy?
- As you are deciding about when to terminate therapy, ask yourself the following questions:
- Is your young client able to manage his/her emotional upsets?
- Is your young client able to solve his/her practical problems?
- Are your young client and his/her parents satisfied with progress?

Conclusion

My view is that REBT is significantly different from other forms of CBT including Beck's especially when practiced with younger populations. I think a primary reason is that it is very psycho-educational having its' origins in a curriculum (Rational Emotive Education) developed by Bill Knaus, *Rational-Emotive Education: A Manual for Elementary School Teachers* (1974), consultant psychologist at the Living School located at the time at the Institute for Rational Emotive Therapy, in New York City.

Test Yourself

1. In thinking about a youngster that you have recently worked with, identify specific inferences and evaluations that they may have had and what strategies you would use to change them?
2. How would you work to differentiate a practical problem from an emotional problem? What questions might you ask during the assessment phase to help establish the A-B-C model?
3. Complete the HTFB sheet for one of the youngsters you work with and consider what disputations you think would be helpful to change their belief system that contributes to their negative affect and behavior.

Recommended REBT Readings for Mental Health Practitioners

Cristea, I. A., Stefan, S., David, O., Mogoase, C., & Dobrean, A. (2015). *REBT in the treatment of anxiety disorders in children and adults*. New York: Springer.

Ellis, A., & Bernard, M. E. (Eds.). (2006). *Rational emotive behavioral approaches to childhood disorders*. New York: Springer.

Knaus, W. J. (1974). *Rational-emotive education: A manual for elementary school teachers*. New York: Albert Ellis Institute.

Vernon, A. (2009). *More what works when with children and adolescents: A handbook of individual counseling techniques*. Champaign, IL: Research Press.

Waters, V. (1980). *Rational stories for children*. New York: Albert Ellis Institute.

Chapter 4
Teaching REBT to Children and Adolescents: Creative Techniques that Work

Ann Vernon

Although REBT began as a form of therapy intended for use with adults, early in the practice of REBT, Ellis and his colleagues began applying the theory to children and adolescents, finding it to be highly effective with this population (Vernon, 2019). In particular, Ellis stressed the importance of teaching young clients positive mental health concepts that are the foundation of rational emotive behavior therapy to promote their social, emotional, behavioral, and cognitive development. Although REBT has been practiced very successfully with young clients, one of the misconceptions is that it is simply a "downward extension of REBT adult methods" (Ellis & Bernard, 2006, p. xi). In fact, there are numerous specific techniques that have been adapted to complement the developmental levels of children and adolescents, helping them learn REBT concepts in their "own language" (Vernon, 2019). These adaptations are crucial, because until around age 11 or 12 when the gradual shift from concrete to formal operational thinking begins, school-age children have difficulty thinking logically, hypothesizing, seeing things from multiple perspectives, and testing inferences (Arnett, 2014). Because most adolescents do not reach formal operational thinking until mid to late adolescence, it is important to take these developmental limitations into consideration (Berk, 2017).

In the foreward to my book, *What Works When with Children and Adolescents: A Handbook of Individual Counseling Techniques* (Vernon, 2002), Albert Ellis stated that the techniques in this book confirmed his original hypothesis that "REBT can be used effectively, in relatively few sessions, with moderately and more seriously disturbed children and adolescents" (p. x). His prediction was that techniques such as those described in that book will contribute to the popularity of this approach with young clients.

That has been my hope as I have worked over many years to develop age-appropriate techniques to explain the principles of REBT to children and adolescents,

---

A. Vernon (✉)
University of Northern Iowa, Tucson, AZ, USA

M. Bernard, M. D. Terjesen (eds.), *Rational-Emotive and Cognitive-Behavioral Approaches to Child and Adolescent Mental Health: Theory, Practice, Research, Applications*, https://doi.org/10.1007/978-3-030-53901-6_4

in individual counseling settings, as well as in prevention programs that are typically implemented in school classrooms or small groups. Because REBT has always had a psychoeducational emphasis which involves active teaching of the principles of the theory, it is especially appropriate for use with school-age children. In fact, an integral part of this theory is the emphasis on teaching and prevention (Vernon & Bernard, 2017). In 1971, The Living School was established at the Albert Ellis Institute to help young people learn rational principles. Although the Living School no longer exists, the concepts introduced in that setting have been promoted worldwide through programs such as *Thinking, Feeling, Behaving: Emotional Educational Curriculums for Children and Adolescents* (Vernon, 2006a, 2006b) and *You Can Do It! Education* (Bernard, 2013, 2018). These programs teach young people the skills necessary for dealing with current problems, as well as giving them attitudes and skills they can use to prevent or minimize problems that arise in the future. This self-help/preventive focus is extremely important given that children and adolescents face numerous challenges as they struggle to grow up in an increasingly complex society.

As you will read throughout the chapter, the REBT concepts as adapted for children and adolescents are presented with a strong emphasis on the creative arts because based on my clinical experience, it is essential to "think outside the box" when working with young clients. Following are several compelling reasons for considering this approach (Vernon, 2019):

1. The wide variety of techniques that you can draw from address different learning styles. Counseling has typically been characterized as an auditory/verbal approach, but that can be very limiting for young children in particular who developmentally may not be capable of verbally expressing themselves. It is also more appropriate for those who are more visual or kinesthetic.
2. These techniques are more impactful because they involve movement, music, games, drama, art, literature, and the use of concrete objects as metaphors. They facilitate expression of thoughts and feelings, and because children are actively involved in the intervention, their retention is far better. In fact, children will remember 5–15% of what they hear, 10–20% of what they see, and 40–50% if they hear it and see it. If they have some personal involvement, the retention rate climbs to 90% (Vernon & Barry, 2013). Certainly these statistics speak for themselves.
3. Because their thinking progresses from concrete to abstract, interventions with young clients need to be creative so that they can understand and apply the concepts. For example, I was working with a 16-year-old who was angry because his girlfriend hadn't called him the night before as promised. He was thinking the worst, convinced that she didn't want to go out with him anymore because he was such a loser, that this was the worst thing he could imagine happening to him, and that he would never be happy again. Since he was looking out the window as he fumed about his situation, I called his attention to the bug zapper hanging from a tree and asked him what the zapper did. "It kills the bugs," he said. I said, "So maybe it would help if you pretended that your head is a giant

bug zapper and every time you assume the worst or overgeneralize about things related to your girlfriend or other issues you could just 'zap' those thoughts, check out the facts before upsetting yourself further, and think more rationally." This concrete technique really resonated with him and he used it for many different problems.
4. Explaining REBT concepts through various creative arts approaches not only helps children be more attentive in the session, but it also helps them remember concepts between sessions. Because they are engaging and non-threatening, children are less resistant about being in counseling, which strengthens the therapeutic relationship.
5. Creative arts techniques are culturally responsive, which is imperative in today's multicultural world.

Self-Acceptance

From a developmental standpoint, one of the major tasks for children and adolescents is to develop a sense of self: identifying strengths and weaknesses, understanding how they are unique, expanding their self-understanding, seeing themselves as more complex personalities, and developing a personal/sexual/moral/social/ethnic identity (Vernon & Chen, 2019). From an REBT perspective, self-acceptance is based on the notion that people are worthwhile just because they exist and that there is no such thing as a perfect person because everyone is fallible and will make mistakes. For children and adolescents who are actively engaged in mastery and performance throughout their school-age years and beyond, this notion of self-acceptance is especially important because the concept implies that self-worth is not based on performance or others' opinions, and that global rating of self as good or bad is counterproductive (Vernon, 2009).

Techniques to Develop Self-Acceptance in Young Children

Can Do, Can't Do, Sort of Can Do

This is a simple intervention that helps young clients learn to accept themselves with strengths as well as weaknesses. It can be used with children who expect to do everything well and don't understand the idea of personal strengths *and* weaknesses. This intervention can readily be adapted for more than one child by having multiple copies of the paper strips and multiple sets of cans. It can also be used in a classroom by selecting 5 or 6 students to participate in the activity and then the entire class discusses what they learned and how it applies to them.

Materials needed include 3 empty soup or vegetable cans with the labels off and re-labeled as "Can Do," another as "Can't Do," and another as "Sort of Can Do."

In addition, you will need 10–12 strips of paper with different challenges written on each strip. These should include things that you think the children you are working with could do, things you think they can't do, and some things that might be do-able to an extent. Examples include: jumping up and down on one foot for 20 seconds, singing a simple song, writing their name with their less dominant hand, counting backward from 20-1, crawling under a tight space, putting something high up on a shelf, and so forth. Put these strips of paper in a small paper bag. Invite the client to draw one of the strips from the paper bag, read it, and perform the task. If it is something the child could do quite well, he or she puts it in the *can do* can; if he or she could not do it, the strip goes into the *can't do* can, and if it was something the child could sort of do, the child places the strip into the appropriate can and draws another strip.

Once the activity has been completed, it is important to debrief with the client, asking questions such as the following: what were things you could do? Couldn't do? Sort of could do? Do you think you should have been able to do everything? What does it say about you if there were some things you couldn't do or couldn't do very well? Is it really possible to do everything well? Suppose you couldn't do any of these things? What does that say about you and your value or worth as a person? The point to emphasize is that everyone has things they can do, can't so, or can do to some extent, but regardless, it has no bearing on their worth as a person. Using a concrete visual technique such as this is good because the next time the child engages in self-downing, you can refer to the three cans and remind him or her that it is natural to not be able to do all things well (Vernon, 2002, p. 71).

Perfectly, Perfectly

This intervention was developed for a perfectionistic 9-year-old who threw temper tantrums whenever he didn't perform perfectly on school work or in sports. The day before one of his scheduled therapy appointments, his teacher contacted me and told me that Phillip's behavior in the classroom was getting out of hand because if he got a less-than-perfect score, not only did he throw a tantrum, but lately he had been running out of the room in tears. His classmate was beginning to make fun of him and didn't want to work with him on classroom projects or play with him during recess.

When Philip came for his appointment, we first talked about how things were going and he was very open about how upset he got when he got a paper back with a less-than-perfect score. He said his brothers were really smart and got all A's and he thought he needed to be just like them. Rather than challenge his assumption that his brothers were perfect, I invited him to participate in a short experiment. I handed him a tennis ball and asked him to juggle it. Of course he could do this. I then gave him another ball and he tossed both balls back and forth. Then I introduced a third ball and asked him to juggle it, but he couldn't do it. I told him that I would try it next, and my results were the same as his. I asked him to go to the waiting room and ask the receptionists if they could do juggle all 3 balls, which of course they couldn't. We talked about this experience and the fact that it is difficult to do everything perfectly and what it means if someone can't. I followed this up with a reverse role play, a highly effective strategy with young clients. I played the role of Philip and asked him to pretend to be me, the therapist. I pretended that the teacher had handed a paper back to me and I missed several, so I threw a fit like Philip did, tearing up my paper and throwing it on the floor and crying. Philip, in his role as a therapist, asked me why I was so upset and I said it was because I didn't get a perfect score. He said, "You don't always have to get things perfect." I replied that I did because it meant that I was really stupid if I missed any questions. He said that it was ok to miss a few and that I wasn't stupid if I did. He said that I didn't need to be perfect. This was the point I was trying to make with him, so the combination of the tennis ball activity and the reverse role play was effective (Adapted from Vernon, 2006a, p. 107).

Techniques to Develop Self-Acceptance in Adolescents

Don't Soak It Up

This is a simple intervention that helps adolescents who are prone to self-downing learn that they don't have to be like sponges and soak up criticism and put-downs. A large sponge and a small bucket of water are needed.

When adolescents describe how upset they get when others criticize their looks, their actions, or other aspects about them, hand them a sponge. Ask them to hold the sponge so they can see how light it is, then ask them to dip the sponge in the water and note how heavy it is when it is water soaked. Explain that when others say negative things about them and they get upset, it is like they are a sponge, soaking up all the negative. Encourage them to look for evidence and ask themselves if they are what others say they are. If the negative label doesn't really apply to them, they need to "wring out the sponge" and not soak it up. If some of what is said about them is true, they can wring out some of the water. If they think that what others have said does apply to them, they don't wring out the sponge, but you help them see that just because this may be true about them, does this make them a bad, worthless person? Invite the client to share things others have said that are so upsetting and to practice "wringing out" the sponge by thinking about the evidence (is what they are saying true?), how it helps them to think that they are worthless just because someone else says bad things about them, what it says about them as a person if someone else criticizes them, and so forth. Help them understand that while they can't control what others say about them, they can control how they respond by changing the way they think, which in turn helps them change the way they feel.

Based on experience, this is a very good concrete technique to help clients remember not to let negative things others say or do get them down. It has also proven to be very effective with adults (Vernon, 2002, p. 77).

USA

This technique teaches adolescents about the concept of unconditional self-acceptance—accepting themselves as they are and avoiding global self-rating of self. You will need a paper bag labeled *USA* that contains 8 strips of paper, each with one of the following terms written on it: *peer relationships; relationships with parents; school performance; performance in music, sports, or drama; performance in a job or with chores; being responsible; being caring and kind; being respectful.*

When adolescents engage in self-downing, complaining about what a failure they are in school, sports, or relationships, ask them to draw a slip of paper out of the bag. Using a 1–5 scale (1 = low, 5 = high), invite them to rate themselves with respect to the term they drew, thinking about their performance in general as opposed to one or two isolated incidents. After they have done this for each term, discuss their ratings—were there some that were higher than others? Lower than others? Is it accurate to say that they are a complete failure in everything when they do better in some contexts than in others? Help them learn to accept themselves unconditionally as people with strengths as well as weaknesses, emphasizing that they are not "all good" or "all bad" (Vernon, 2002, p. 78).

Emotions

Emotional development is a gradual process that begins with developing a feeling vocabulary and understanding what emotions are appropriate in specific situations. Young children have a limited vocabulary for expressing how they feel, so they often express their feelings behaviorally (Vernon & Chen, 2019). As they mature, they are better able to recognize emotions in themselves and others and are better able to control their own emotions and communicate about them verbally and expressively (Glowiak & Mayfield, 2016). During middle childhood (ages 6–11), children understand that they can have more than one emotion at a time and their emotional expression becomes more complex. During early adolescence (ages 11–14), there is a great deal of emotional volatility and moodiness, and troublesome emotions such as anxiety, shame, depression, guilt, and anger occur more frequently than at any other age (Avenevoli, Swendsen, He, Burstein, & Merikangas, 2015; Broderick & Blewitt, 2014). These negative feelings can be overwhelming and often mask vulnerability and anger. This emotional roller coaster gradually subsides during mid-adolescence (ages 15–18) and adolescents are more capable of expressing their feelings effectively, being empathic, and dealing with emotionally charged issues.

Understanding how emotional development progresses is important to consider in introducing children and adolescents to the REBT conceptualization of emotions. The psychoeducational aspect of this theory readily lends itself teaching young clients what feelings are, how to identify and express them, how feelings can change, and the connection between feelings, thoughts, and behaviors. According to REBT theory, there is a distinction between healthy and unhealthy negative emotions, with the goal being to help children and adolescents change their thinking so that they experience healthy negative emotions (DiGiuseppe, Doyle, Dryden, & Backx, 2014). Especially during adolescence, it is important to help clients deal with the troublesome negative emotions that often result in self-defeating behaviors, including self-harm, suicide ideation or attempts, substance abuse, and other ineffective ways of coping.

Techniques to Promote Emotional Development in Children

Feel Wheel

The purpose of this intervention is to help young children develop a feeling vocabulary and understand how feelings are expressed. Make a feel wheel by taking a paper plate and dividing it into 10–12 pie shapes. Label each shape with feeling words such as happy, sad, mad, scared, excited, worried, grouchy, disappointed, angry, and frustrated. (These words can be adapted depending on the age of the client.) Make a paper arrow and attach it to a brass fastener which is attached to the middle of the wheel so that it can spin.

When working with clients who may express feelings behaviorally instead of emotionally, as younger children tend to do, it is important to teach them about different feelings they may experience and how they can express them with words as well as appropriate actions. Invite them to spin the spinner and when the spinner stops, read the feeling word and ask them to share an example of a time they felt this way. If they are unable to do this, you can model it, sharing an example of the feeling as you experienced it at their age. After the examples have been shared, ask them how they expressed that feeling…if they were happy, did they smile, laugh, or tell someone they were happy? If they were mad, did they yell, scream, or throw a tantrum? Continue spinning for feeling words, asking for examples of when they experienced this feeling and how they expressed it (Vernon, 2006a, pp. 25–26).

Adios, Anxiety

Anxiety is caused by our perception of events, but for children, this idea can be complicated by their limited cognitive skills which may interfere with their ability to perceive events correctly, making it difficult for them to distinguish between the possibility and probability of something happening (Vernon & Chen, 2019). When children are anxious, they assume something bad might happen and if it did, it would be so terrible that they wouldn't be able to stand it. They not only minimize their ability to cope, but they catastrophize and overgeneralize, which only increases their anxiety.

For this intervention you will need to take a large plain plastic tablecloth or a bedsheet and draw a hopscotch board on it. The squares should be large enough for the child to jump on. When your client describes what she is anxious about, discuss the A (what she perceives will happen), how she feels about this (C), and what thoughts are going on inside her head. Write these thoughts on paper. Then invite her to stand on the hopscotch board and read the first thought. For example, suppose she is anxious about playing in a piano recital because she is sure she will make lots of mistakes, which proves that she can't play the piano; that others will laugh at her and that would be awful; that she will start to cry and others would point fingers at her, which would be so embarrassing she couldn't stand it, and so forth. Challenge each irrational belief, one at a time, using logical, empirical, functional disputes. Then ask her if she can think of another way to think that wouldn't make her so anxious. When she is able to do this, she can hop to the next set of squares. Continue in this manner with all of her thoughts. When she reaches the end of the hopscotch board she can shout "Adios (goodbye) anxiety!" (Vernon, 2002, pp. 25–26).

Techniques to Promote Emotional Development in Adolescents

As previously noted, early adolescence in particular can be a difficult time for young teens whose emotions tend to be confusing, intense, volatile, and overwhelming (Vernon & Chen, 2019). Helping them learn effective ways of managing their unhealthy negative emotions is extremely important because they are also impulsive at this age, and if they are overwhelmed by intense negative emotions that they don't know how to handle, they may engage in self-defeating behaviors that have long-term negative consequences. The following interventions address two predominant emotions during adolescence: anxiety and depression.

Let It Go

For this intervention, you will need several balloons, pieces of string to tie on each balloon, very narrow strips of paper, several sheets of blank paper, and a pen. When clients present with anxiety, have them write what they are anxious about on separate strips of paper and place them in rank order from most to least anxiety-provoking. Next, help them identify the specific beliefs related to each of these anxiety-provoking situations and write them on separate sheets of paper. Then ask them to pick one of the identified situations (typically the least anxiety-provoking since it will be easier to work on) and teach them how to dispute the thoughts they had about that particular situation: is there evidence to support your prediction? How does it help you to think this way? Is it logical to think that what you are assuming will happen and if it does, it will be horrible? Once they have successfully disputed their irrational beliefs and identified a more rational way of thinking, invite them to fold that strip of paper and slip it into a balloon, blow up the balloon and tie it with a string, and if they feel like they are able to "let go" of that anxiety, they can let the balloon go. Continue in the same manner with the other anxiety-provoking thoughts. This is a very concrete way of reminding clients how they can "let go" of their anxiety by learning to think more rationally (Vernon, 2002, p. 93).

Depression Can Weigh You Down

Depression is a serious problem that impacts adolescents in multiple ways and is compounded by irrational thinking—believing that they will never feel better, that it's too difficult to fight it, and that there's no point in going on. Self-downing is also associated with depression (Vernon, 2019). This concrete intervention is designed to help teens identify and dispute irrational beliefs associated with depression. You will need a paper bag and 8–12 potatoes, as well as 16–24 strips of paper, a marker, and 8–12 straight pins.

When an adolescent client presents with depression and you and the client have identified irrational beliefs associated with feeling depressed in general, feeling depressed about being depressed, or beliefs about specific events that they attribute to depression, ask them to write each of these beliefs on individual strips of paper and pin them on the potatoes (one belief per potato). Put the potatoes in a bag and ask them to walk around the room with the bag, explaining the metaphor of depression as "weighing you down." Invite them to take out one potato at a time and work with them to dispute the irrational beliefs. After successfully disputing the belief, help them identify a more rational thought or a rational coping self-statement, write that on a strip of paper and put it in the bag and throw the potato with the irrational belief away. Continue with the other irrational beliefs. When the bag is empty except for the strips of paper with new rational beliefs and coping statements, ask them how they feel now that they aren't being weighed down by irrational beliefs that contribute to their depression (Vernon, original, unpublished).

Beliefs and Behaviors

From a developmental standpoint, younger children may lack the capacity for expressing their feelings verbally and instead, act out behaviorally (Vernon & Chen, 2019). In fact, it is often easier to ask children what they *did* relative to an activating event and then deduce the feeling. Furthermore, it can also be challenging to help them identify their beliefs that, from an REBT perspective, play such a pivotal role relative to their emotional and behavioral reactions. For example, simply asking "What did you *think* when you felt angry" will most likely be ineffective, so it is imperative to employ specific techniques to help them identify troublesome (irrational) beliefs, inappropriate or unhelpful behaviors, and understand the connection between what they think, feel, and behave.

Techniques to Promote Awareness of Beliefs and Behaviors in Children

Choosing to Behave

How many times have you heard children say that somebody else made them do something or that they can't help the way they behaved? This simple intervention can help them learn that others cannot control their behavior; they can choose how to behave.

I used this technique with 7-year-old Amelia who had a tendency to act out, both at home and at school. I asked her if she knew what a robot was and discussed the fact that robots really don't think for themselves—we wind them up and program them to do what we tell them to do. I invited her to do an experiment, which she was eager to do. First, I asked Amelia to stand up. Then I waved a "magic wand" and told her that she was now a robot who had to do everything I told her to do. I gave her some simple instructions, such as walking backward across the room, counting to 10, jumping up and down 5 times, etc. Then I pointed out that she did everything I asked her to do. I explained that in real life, there are definitely times when someone asks you to do something and you choose not to do it. I invited her to share other examples of when this has happened to her, such as a parent asking her to stop yelling at her brother, stop kicking the table, study her spelling words, and so forth. We discussed whether or not she had a choice about whether or not to yell at her brother, kick the table, or study her spelling words. She seemed to understand that she did have a choice about studying or kicking the table, but she said she didn't have a choice about yelling at her brother because he made her mad. To help her see that she did have a choice, I used puppets—the brother puppet who teased her, and the sister puppet who turned away and ignored the brother. We discussed the fact that even though she might feel like yelling, did it really do any good? Didn't it just get her in further trouble? Does she actually have a choice about how she behaves even when someone "starts it" like she said her brother did? I also reinforced the idea that even though others might *tell* us to do something, it is still our choice to do it or not, even though there may very well be consequences. I asked her for examples of this in the classroom and she readily agreed that sometimes even when the teacher told her to do something she chose not to. This concrete analogy served as a good reminder for Amelia that how she behaves is her choice (Adapted from Vernon, 2006a, p. 43).

Fact Fling

One of the important aspects related to helping children and adolescents understand how beliefs impact their feelings and behaviors is helping them distinguish between facts and assumptions. With younger children especially, cognitive limitations may make it more difficult to identify facts, which in turn can exacerbate problems (Vernon, 2009). For this intervention you will need several bean bags and 2 small buckets, one labeled *Facts* and one labeled *Assumptions/Beliefs*. You will also need a set of index cards with one statement (such as the following) per card and a basket to put the cards in.

Everyone likes science.
Kids who go to this school are awesome.
Girls are smarter than boys.
Most balls are round.
There are 365 days in a year.
If you don't get invited to a party it's because the kid having the party doesn't like you.
If your sister leaves her bike in the yard instead of putting it away, you think it's because she is lazy.
Dogs have 4 legs.
Candy can be bad for your teeth.
Drinking milk helps build strong bones.

After explaining the difference between a fact and a belief or an assumption, invite the client to draw one of the cards, read it, and then fling a bean bag into either the *Facts* bucket or the *Assumptions/Beliefs* bucket. After each fling, discuss why he or she chose that bucket and whether or not it was a correct choice. Discuss the importance of checking out facts and not acting on assumptions and what happens if they do act on an assumption, thinking it is a fact, but it isn't. Reinforce this idea by telling a short story:

Two kids were sitting in the cafeteria and one of their best friends walked into the room. Instead of coming to sit with them, which she usually did, she went to another table. What do you think these two kids were thinking? Maybe that she was mad at them, that she liked the others better, or that she was tired of being friends with them? What if these two kids got mad and stopped speaking to the girl who didn't sit with them because they thought she liked the others better? What might happen then? Discuss how this could start a whole chain of negative events just because they acted on an assumption that may or may not be true (Vernon, original, unpublished).

Techniques to Promote Awareness of Beliefs and Behaviors in Adolescents

Chain Reaction

I developed this intervention for a 16-year-old who was failing most of his school subjects because he thought the subjects were boring, he didn't like the teachers, and he didn't feel like studying because he had better things to do. What prompted me to use this intervention with him was when he complained about having a major exam to study for but he didn't feel like studying for it. Given that he had a bad grade in this class, failing the exam would probably mean that he would fail the course, but I was quite sure that he had not thought about consequences. This intervention helps clients identify behavioral consequences and how to change them by changing the way they think. For this intervention you will need a stapler, a pen, and 24 strips of paper.

After Ian told me that he didn't feel like studying for the exam, I told him that I understood that studying isn't what most teenagers necessarily like to do and that it was totally up to him whether he studied or not. "However," I said, "Let's take a look at the consequences of not studying versus what might happen if you did study." I took a strip of paper, numbered it #1, and wrote: having to study for a major exam. Then I asked him to identify how he feels when he thinks about having to study for the exam. He said he was a little angry about having to do something that he didn't want to do. I then asked him to identify the beliefs that come into his head when he thinks about having to study for the exam. As he verbalized these, I wrote them down on numbered strips of paper: It's too boring, I can't stand studying, I shouldn't have to do things I don't want to do, it's no big deal if I don't study, etc. After he had identified his beliefs, I looped the feeling strip (anger) and stapled it to the first strip, having to study for an exam. Then I took each of the beliefs he identified and looped these and stapled them, forming a chain. Then I asked him what he would probably do based on his thinking, and he said he probably wouldn't study. So then I asked him to identify consequences of not studying: probably failing the exam, having to retake it, his parents would be mad and ground him, he would miss out on things with his friends, and he might fail the course.

I then suggested that we do another chain with the same activating event, having to study for an exam. "But this time," I said, "Instead of feeling angry, maybe you are just a little irritated. If you were just a little irritated, would your thinking change?" He said that even though he didn't want to study, it would be an inconvenience, but he supposed he could tolerate it. I asked if he would make a different choice about studying if he had these thoughts instead of his thoughts on the first chain. He agreed that even though he didn't want to study, he probably would. I asked what the consequences would be if he chose to study, and he said he would probably pass the exam, pass the course, and not be grounded. I stapled all of these into a much shorter chain and then held the two of them up, asking which chain he wanted. The visual aspect of this intervention helped him see that by changing his thoughts he could change his behavior and prevent negative consequences from affecting his future (Adapted from Vernon, 2006b, p. 35).

I'm a Believer

A major focus in REBT is understanding the distinction between rational and irrational beliefs. When attempting to teach this concept to adolescents, it is first important to explain that rational beliefs are reasonable, logical, and can be empirically verified. They are consistent with reality and help people achieve their goals. They also result in healthy negative emotions. Irrational beliefs are illogical, unrealistic, and inflexible. They consist of demanding, catastrophizing, frustration intolerance, global rating of self and others, and result in unhealthy negative emotions (DiGiuseppe et al., 2014). Share an example with the client, using the same activating event so he or she can readily see the difference between the two sets of beliefs: You applied for a job but did not get it. If you are thinking rationally, you feel disappointed, but you don't put yourself down; you realize that there must have been other well-qualified applicants and that it isn't possible to get everything you want. If you are thinking irrationally, you are angry, thinking that it wasn't fair that you didn't get this job, that things should always be fair, that you won't be able to get a job as good as this one, and that it's not worth applying for other jobs because you probably won't get them anyway. Then give the client a list of his or her irrational beliefs, as well as other examples of both rational and irrational beliefs. These should be written on individual strips of paper. In addition, give him or her a sorting board, which is a sheet of paper divided down the middle with one side labeled *Rational Beliefs* and the other side *Irrational Beliefs*. Invite the client to sort the strips on the sorting board and then discuss how he or she decided where to place the strips and if they were correct, using a psychoeducational approach to help the client learn to distinguish between these two types of beliefs and the emotional and behavioral consequences of rational versus irrational thinking (Vernon, 2006b, pp. 151–153).

Techniques to Help Children Challenge Irrational Beliefs and Develop Problem-Solving Skills

Race to Be Rational

The purpose of this intervention is to help children identify how to think rationally instead of irrationally. For this activity you need two long strips of masking tape placed on opposite sides of a room and a paper bag containing strips of irrational beliefs such as the following (adapt to match your client's irrational beliefs): if everything I do isn't perfect, I'm a not a good kid; it's the end of the world if my parents don't let me do something I really want to do because I should be able to do whatever I want; I shouldn't ever make mistakes and if I do, it proves I'm stupid; I shouldn't have to work too hard at anything; everything should always be fair; it's awful if everyone doesn't like me; I'll never have any friends; it's terrible if others call me names; I should always get my way.

After first discussing the fact that there are two kinds of beliefs: rational (sensible) and irrational (insensible) and the difference between the two, I share an example: "Suppose someone calls me a name and I think that's terrible because kids shouldn't call others names, what would you say to me to help me think more sensibly?" After the client has come up with several questions to help me think more sensibly and when I am sure the client understands the distinction, I invite him or her to play a game. I explain that I will read an irrational (insensible) statement. The client stands on a masking tape line on one end of the room, thinks about how to respond to the irrational belief, and then races to the other end of the room and stands on the tape and challenges (out loud) the irrational belief. Although they may have some difficulty with this, you can give prompts, such as "Is it really possible to be able to do whatever you want to do? What if no one wanted to take a bath and they would stink up the world? Or what if everyone in the world thought they didn't need to work too hard at anything…would we have any inventions? Would men and women go to space? Is it realistic to think that you don't have to work hard on some things?" These types of prompts help the client learn more about challenging beliefs and think more rationally (Vernon, original, unpublished).

Search for Solutions

Given that children between the ages of 6 and 11 are still, for the most part, concrete operational thinkers, it is often difficult for them to identify multiple solutions to a problem and how to identify and assess consequences (Vernon & Chen, 2019). This is a simple strategy that promotes the development of problem-solving skills. You will need a sheet of paper and a pencil.

When young clients present with a problem, such as a friend starting a fight or calling them names, draw a circle on a sheet of paper and write this activating event in the center. Then like spokes on a wheel, draw several small circles around the larger circle. After discussing how they felt about the activating event, ask for the behavioral C—how did they react? Write this in one of the circles on the outside of the larger circle. Then ask if there was a positive (labeled +) consequence that resulted from this behavior and write it on a line drawn under the smaller circle. Then ask if there was a negative consequence (labeled −) and write that on a second line.

Ask if there were other things they could have done: what other options did they have? This may be more of a brainstorming as you guide them into identifying other alternatives, positive and negative consequences (there may not be positive or negative consequences for each solution/it may be one or the other) (Vernon, original, unpublished).

Techniques to Help Adolescents Challenge Irrational Beliefs and Develop Problem-Solving Skills

Up for the Challenge

This intervention is a visual way of helping adolescents learn to challenge irrational beliefs. You will need several balloons, a marker, and a straight pin. I used this intervention with a 15-year-old who was having difficulty challenging her irrational beliefs about a relationship break up initiated by her former boyfriend. Maria was very upset that Marcos had broken off the relationship and said she had actually been depressed all week, especially after she heard a rumor that he was interested in one of her best friends. After talking more about how she felt and how this related to how she was behaving, I asked her to identify what she had been thinking that contributed to her depressed mood. She identified several irrational beliefs: I'm nobody because he broke up with me; I'll never have another boyfriend and that will be awful; there must be something wrong with me or he wouldn't have broken up with me; he shouldn't have broken up with me to date one of my best friends, etc. As she stated them, I wrote them (one per balloon) on the balloons and blew them up and tied them. We then talked about how these beliefs were only making her more depressed. I modeled the process of disputing one of these beliefs using several different types of disputes: how is this type of thinking helping you? Where is the evidence that just because your boyfriend broke up with you that you are nobody? If your best friend came to you and said she is nobody because her boyfriend broke up with her, would you agree with her? Why or why not?

Once she had an idea of how to challenge her beliefs, we addressed each of them. When she was able to do this and identify a new, more rational way of thinking, she was invited to toss the balloon in the air and pop it (Vernon, original, unpublished).

Picture This

It is not uncommon during adolescence for clients to ignore consequences of their behavior and continue to behave in self-defeating ways. This intervention is good for clients who are "immune" to traditional forms of disputing because while they can admit that it isn't helping them to think that they shouldn't have to work hard to get good grades or that it isn't logical to think that they can graduate without passing all their subjects, they still cling to the belief that they shouldn't have to work hard and that there shouldn't be negative consequences. I developed this intervention for one such adolescent who up until this year had been doing very well in school and had already been accepted into college. However, recently her grades had dropped dramatically because she was skipping school, refusing to study, associating with a bad crowd, and drinking and partying most nights. Her parents sent her to therapy and she was not happy about that. My efforts to help her evaluate consequences of her behavior and dispute her irrational beliefs got me nowhere. Her parents were pressuring me to "make her change," so I told my client that I really couldn't do that…that she alone was in charge of what she chose to do. I told her that if she didn't want to change, she didn't have to, but that I would like her to take some pictures of what her life might be like 3 months from now (graduation) if she continued to make the choices she was now making. The next week she came with pictures of a torn up high school diploma, a pyramid of beer cans and a wrecked car, a picture of a low-income housing development, etc. When asked how she felt about this "picture" of her future, she said she thought it was ok. Then I said that it might be helpful to pretend that she didn't like that picture…that she did in fact decide to change, emphasizing that of course that was up to her. I invited her to take pictures of what this might look like, and when she came back the following week she had taken pictures of a high school diploma, a college campus, a dormitory, and a new car that her parents had promised her if she graduated. When asked which "picture" she wanted for her future, she said that she wanted to graduate, and it was at this point that I was able to do some effective disputing. Together we worked on establishing realistic goals that would help her get back on track (Vernon, original, unpublished).

Techniques for Teaching the A-B-C Model to Children

The A, B, C's

After verbally explaining the ABC model to young clients, one of the best ways to teach it is through games because by participating in something they like, they are more likely to retain the concepts. This is a game like musical chairs. You will need 5 chairs, each one labeled with either A (something that happened or might happen or you think happened), B (what you think about A), C (how you feel about A and how you behave when you feel that way), D (asking yourself questions to make sure your beliefs make sense), and E (finding a new way to think so you will feel better and act differently). You will need a basket containing examples of different activating events, feelings, behaviors, irrational beliefs, and disputes. These should be based on the client's ABC's. For example, the A might be missing problems on a math assignment, the B's would relate to how awful it is or how it proves he or she is stupid, and the C would be feeling angry and tearing up the paper. The D's would be asking for evidence that he or she is stupid just because some problems were missed, whether it makes sense to put yourself down for missing some problems, and so forth. The E cards can be examples of healthy negative emotions and more effective ways to think. Explain to the client that you will play some music and he or she should walk around the circle of chairs. When the music stops, the client will draw a card from the basket and read it. Then he or she needs to decide if it describes and activating event, a feeling or behavior, beliefs, asking questions to make sure the beliefs make sense, or feeling and thinking differently.

After playing several rounds of the game with different activating events (they could even be fictitious), you can teach the client the following song as a way of reinforcing the ABC model.

A-B-C Song (Tune: Now I Know My ABC's)

A is for something that is happening to me
C is how I feel and how I act about A

B is for thoughts that rumble in my head
D is for changing the thoughts that make me feel bad
E is for new ways to think, feel, and behave so now I am happier in so many ways (Vernon, original, unpublished).

Think, Feel, Behave

Helping children understand the connection between thinking, feeling, and behaving is a critical aspect of the ABC model. It can be introduced to young clients by telling them a story such as the following and then engaging them in a short experiment.

"Just imagine that you have a twin. You and your twin spend a lot of time together and like to do a lot of the same things. But just pretend that tomorrow your parents tell you that they are taking you to an amusement park and they show you a picture of a brand new roller coaster that you can ride on. Although you and your twin have ridden on a small roller coaster, you didn't like it very much and you are really scared to ride on this new one because it is so huge. But as soon as your twin sees the picture she is super excited, jumping up and down and saying that she can't wait. The next day comes and your twin lines up to get on the ride and you tell your parents you don't want to do it." Discuss with your client: If it is the very same event, riding on the roller coaster, why is your twin feeling excited and can't wait to get on the roller coaster and you are feeling scared and tell your parents you don't want to go?

Elicit the notion that it is what each one thinks that accounts for the differences in the way they feel and behave. After discussing this concept so that they understand that their feelings and behaviors are a direct result of how they think, invite the client to play a game that is like Concentration. First, develop some situation cards on red tag board that represents actual client situations or typical developmental situations. For example, a situation card might be: did not get invited to a friend's birthday party. Next, develop some thought cards on green tag board. Thought cards could be that this is awful, this friend must not like me, or she should have invited me. Then develop feeling cards on blue tag board. Examples might include sad, disappointed, or angry. Finally, develop some behaving cards on yellow tag board. Behaving cards could be cried, yelled, or said mean things. It is important that there are feeling, behaving, and thought cards to represent each situation card. Lay the cards face down on a flat surface in random order. Ask the client to first draw a red situation card and read it out loud. Then ask him or her to draw a green thought card. If it corresponds to the situation card, leave both cards face up. If not, leave the situation card up and draw another thought card until there is a match. Then leave both cards up and draw a blue feeling card, continuing in the same manner until there is a match, and do the same for the yellow behaving card. As the client plays the game, discuss how the emotional and behavioral reactions are based on beliefs, not the situation itself (Vernon, original, unpublished).

Techniques for Teaching the A-B-C Model to Adolescents

Learning the A, B, C's

It is much easier to teach the ABC model to adolescents who are in the process of developing more formal operational thinking abilities and are therefore better able to understand the theory behind REBT. At the same time, psychoeducation is important because many adolescents still believe that they aren't in control of how they think, feel, and behave. To introduce them to the model, use the following example: "You and your friend are at the mall just hanging out. Suddenly your friend pushes you back into a corner. You are angry and yell at her to stop pushing you. She puts her finger to her lips and whispers that she just saw a man with a gun coming close to where they were hiding." Ask your client if her feelings changed once her friend shared this information. Discuss the fact that when she thought that the friend was pushing her to be mean, she was angry, but when she thought it was because they could be in danger she felt differently. Next, explain the concept of rational and irrational beliefs by using the following example: "You and your friend have both had a steady boyfriend for about 6 months. In the last two weeks, your boyfriend broke up with you and her boyfriend broke up with her. You are devastated because you really liked this guy and you don't think you will ever be able to find someone like him. You put yourself down, thinking there must be something wrong with you—and that without him, you are nothing. Your friend is disappointed that her boyfriend broke up with her, but she tells you that there is nothing wrong with her; she's not a loser just because he broke up with her. She says she will eventually find someone else to date and doesn't think it is the end of the world." Discuss these different ways of thinking, introducing the terms rational and irrational and explaining the characteristics of each. Then introduce the concept of disputing by explaining that it is a bit like arguing with yourself, asking yourself whether it is logical to think this way, is there evidence to prove that what they are thinking is correct, and it is helping them to think irrationally? Give several examples and explain that the goal of disputing is to be able to think, feel, and behave differently as a result of disputing irrational beliefs. This information can be reinforced by selecting irrational songs and having them rewrite more rational lyrics, discussing how their feelings and behaviors would be impacted by thinking more rationally.

Change the Lens

This visual technique is an effective way to teach the A-B-C model to adolescents. Begin by handing the client a pair of dark glasses and asking him or her to put them on and imagine that there is a party this weekend and he/she is invited. Ask the client to "look" at this party through the dark/gloomy lens; in other words, everything about the event will be negative. Ask the client to verbalize how terrible this party will probably be. Then ask the client to take off the dark glasses and exchange them for a pair of glasses with a clear lens. Ask the client to "look" at the party from a clearer, more realistic perspective and verbalize what the party might be like. Explain that changing the lens from dark and gloomy, which resulted in negative, pessimistic thinking, to clearer thinking that is more rational and optimistic is like changing the way they think about an event. In other words, if he or she thinks the party will be fun, that there will be lots of friends to talk to, and that the music will be great, he or she probably feels excited. But if the event being mediated by the beliefs (explain the terms rational and irrational) which in turn affect feelings and behaviors, you can introduce the idea of "changing the lens" through disputing: asking questions to challenge the beliefs that result in the negative emotions.

Homework

Most children and adolescents don't like doing homework, so it is better to avoid using that term if you want them to do something in between sessions to reinforce concepts introduced during the sessions. I often invite them to participate in an "experiment" or a short project. A few homework suggestions are subsequently described.

1. When trying to help younger children differentiate between facts and assumptions, you can invite them to pretend to be fact "detectives," looking for facts when they are watching a television show, listening for assumptions when they are in a conversation, or pointing out facts about something when they are playing or going to a movie.
2. Invite children and adolescents to make rational posters or banners to hang in their rooms or in their school lockers.
3. Encourage them to make up rational songs, which young children enjoy doing. Suggest that they take a familiar tune and make up words that convey a rational or irrational point. Here is an example related to frustration tolerance (tune: "Where is Thumpkin?"):

   I can't stand it, I can't stand it, no I can't, no I can't
   This is just too boring, I just feel like snoring, I can't stand it, I can't stand it.

   The rational counterpart is:

   I can stand it, I can stand it, yes I can, yes I can,
   I don't have to like it, I just have to do it, I can stand it, I can stand it (Vernon, 2009, p. 177).

   Adolescents can rewrite lyrics to popular songs to make them more rational.
4. Suggest that they read rational stories and then write their own.
5. Invite them to interview others about how they tolerate frustration, what they tell themselves when they make mistakes, or how to set realistic goals and develop the persistence to achieve them.

6. Suggest that they do surveys to help them gain perspective. For example, one of my adolescent clients thought her parents were the worst in the world, so I invited her to make up a survey about what parents did or didn't allow their teenager to do and survey her friends. She quickly learned that her parents were no different than most others! Another client thought that adults never had to do anything they didn't want to do, so I had him do a survey to find out if this was true. After learning that his thinking was incorrect, we were able to work on his demand that he shouldn't have to do anything he didn't like to do.
7. Encourage younger children to pretend they are teachers who are teaching their parents or siblings about aspects of the A-B-C model, such as examples of sensible versus insensible behavior, what "makes" kids feel the way they do, or why different people feel differently about the same situation.
8. Invite adolescents to write their own problem with their irrational beliefs and then pretend to be an "expert" who writes some advice about how to deal with the problem by thinking more rationally.
9. With adolescents, use the AEI self-help form for those who are motivated to do so.

Test Yourself

1. In consideration of the developmental age of the child, what factor(s) would you want to consider as you design a creative intervention?
2. As identifying and changing beliefs are among the KEY approaches in work with youth, how would you modify your techniques/approaches as a function of presenting problem?
3. Why is it important to work on helping students manage their emotions *before* you teach them practical problem-solving?

References

Arnett, J. J. (2014). *Adolescence and emerging adulthood*. Boston: Pearson.

Avenevoli, S., Swendsen, J., He, J. P., Burstein, M., & Merikangas, K. R. (2015). Major depression in the National Comorbidity Survey–Adolescent Supplement: Prevalence, correlates, and treatment. *Journal of the American Academy of Child & Adolescent Psychiatry, 54*(1), 37–44. https://doi.org/10.1016/j.jaac.2014.10.010

Berk, L. (2017). *Development through the lifespan* (7th ed.). Upper Saddle River, NJ: Pearson.

Bernard, M. E. (2013). You Can Do It! Education: A social-emotional learning program for increasing the achievement and well-being of children and adolescents. In K. Yamasaki (Ed.), *School-based prevention education for health and adjustment problems in the world*. Tokyo: Kaneko Shobo.

Bernard, M. E. (2018). *NEW program achieve (years 1–6; years 7–12). A social-emotional learning curriculum*. East Melbourne: The Bernard Group. https://youcandoiteducation.com.au/

Broderick, P. C., & Blewitt, P. (2014). *The life span: Human development for helping professionals* (4th ed.). Upper Saddle River, NJ: Pearson.

DiGiuseppe, R., Doyle, K. A., Dryden, W., & Backx, W. (2014). *A practitioner's guide to rational emotive behavior therapy* (3rd ed.). New York: Oxford University Press.

Ellis, A., & Bernard, M. E. (Eds.). (2006). *Rational emotive behavioral approaches to childhood problems: Theory, practice, and research*. New York: Springer.

Glowiak, M., & Mayfield, M. A. (2016). Middle childhood: Physical and cognitive development. In D. Capuzzi & M. D. Stauffer (Eds.), *Human growth and development across the lifespan: Applications for counselors* (pp. 251–275). Hoboken, NJ: Wiley.

Vernon, A. (2002). *What works when with children and adolescents: A handbook of individual counseling techniques*. Champaign, IL: Research Press.

Vernon, A. (2006a). *Thinking, feeling, behaving: An emotional education curriculum for children* (2nd ed.). Champaign, IL: Research Press.

Vernon, A. (2006b). *Thinking, feeling, behaving: An emotional education curriculum for adolescents* (2nd ed.). Champaign, IL: Research Press.

Vernon, A. (2009). *More what works when with children and adolescents: A handbook of individual counseling techniques*. Champaign, IL: Research Press.

Vernon, A. (2019). Rational emotive behavior therapy. In A. Vernon & C. L. Schimmel (Eds.), *Counseling children and adolescents* (5th ed., pp. 222–257). San Diego, CA: Cognella.

Vernon, A., & Barry, K. D. (2013). *Counseling outside the lines: Creative arts interventions for children and adolescents. Individual, small group, and classroom applications*. Champaign, IL: Research Press.

Vernon, A., & Bernard, M. E. (2017). Rational emotive behavior in schools. In M. E. Bernard & W. Dryden (Eds.), *Rational emotive behavior education in schools*. New York: Springer.

Vernon, A., & Chen, P. C. (2019). Working with children, adolescents, and their parents: Practical applications of developmental theory. In A. Vernon & C. L. Schimmel (Eds.), *Counseling children and adolescents* (5th ed., pp. 1–36). San Diego, CA: Cognella.

Chapter 5
Rational Emotive and Cognitive Behavioral Group Therapy with Children and Adolescents

Mark D. Terjesen, Maria Esposito-Pickering, and Adrienne Matta

Childhood consists of a number of official (academic, club membership, sports team) and unofficial groups (peer play-groups) and we begin functioning as members of groups the moment we are born. The natural experience of existing in groups has logically led to group therapy being a popular treatment for over half a century. There are a number of notable considerations and challenges that warrant attention in setting up and running group therapy when providing clinical work with children and adolescents. This chapter will focus on the application of Rational Emotive and Cognitive Behavioral change methods in a group setting.

Approximately one in every five children will exhibit a mental, emotional, or behavioral health problem that will have a functional impact on them socially, academically, and in the home (Merikangas et al., 2010; National Council for Community Behavioral Healthcare, 2009; National Federation of Families for Children's Mental Health, 2008). Addressing these needs can occur through a number of different clinical approaches (Esposito, 2009). Group therapy with children and adolescents is a frequently utilized approach in both clinical and school-based settings (Terjesen & Esposito, 2006). Conducting therapy in groups allows for the direct impact of group members on one another and as Yalom and Leszcz (2005) posited "it is the group that is the agent of change" (p. 120). Groups may provide a meaningful way to address some of these clinical concerns, and schools may be a key setting in which to address these mental health problems

M. D. Terjesen (✉)
Department of Psychology, St. John's University, Jamaica, NY, USA
e-mail: Terjesem@stjohns.edu

M. Esposito-Pickering
Private Practice, Amityville, NY, USA

A. Matta
School Psychologist, Wilton Public Schools, Wilton, CT, USA

M. Bernard, M. D. Terjesen (eds.), *Rational-Emotive and Cognitive-Behavioral Approaches to Child and Adolescent Mental Health: Theory, Practice, Research, Applications*, https://doi.org/10.1007/978-3-030-53901-6_5

given that most children and adolescents spend a significant portion of their day in this setting (Matta, 2014; The President's New Freedom Commission on Mental Health, 2003). Economical factors combined with the current health care system have placed a greater emphasis on both clinical efficiency and cost-effectiveness (Matta, 2014). Group therapy is considered to be a viable and cost-effective intervention (Burlingame, Strauss, & Joyce, 2013). As such, implementing interventions in a group format seems to be a desirable alternative to individual treatment approaches (Hales, 2008).

Rational Emotive and Cognitive Behavioral Therapy

Rational Emotive Behavior Therapy (REBT) is considered to be the original form of cognitive behavioral therapy and was developed by Albert Ellis in the 1950s (David, Cotet, Matu, Mogoase, & Stefan, 2018). The theory and practice of REBT is based on the premise that when people engage in faulty, illogical, irrational, and unhealthy ways of thinking, they may experience unhealthy negative affective states and as such engage in unhealthy behaviors. The clinical approach entails having clients become aware of these unhealthy thoughts and then challenge them behaviorally, cognitively, and affectively to develop newer ways of thinking and experience healthier emotions and behaviors (DiGiuseppe, Doyle, Dryden, & Backx, 2013).

Ellis (1997, 2002) argued that REBT and Cognitive Behavior Therapy (CBT) lend themselves particularly well to use in group settings. Ellis (2002) stated that:

> Rational-Emotive Behavior Therapy (REBT) and Cognitive-Behavior Therapy (CBT) are efficient kinds of group therapy, because they involve people who regularly meet together with a leader in order to work on their psychological problems, they focus on the members' thoughts, feelings and behaviors, and they encourage all the participants to help each other change their cognitions, emotions and actions. (p. 51)

Ellis reported that he had been successfully using REBT in groups since 1959 (Ellis, 2002), sometimes with more effectiveness than individual REBT, yet the use of REBT in groups with youth has not often been systematically evaluated. Description of REBT in child and adolescent groups is found in the literature (e.g., Elkin, 1983). Esposito (2009), in her meta-analytic review of REBT, found that group treatment is just as effective as individual treatment.

Building off of an earlier version of this chapter (Terjesen & Esposito, 2006) we will present an overview of group therapy development and application among youth, discuss the integration of RE-CBT in group work with children and adolescents, summarize the research regarding the effectiveness of group therapy, and offer future considerations in RE-CBT group therapy.

General Considerations in Group Therapy with Children and Adolescents

The advantages of and disadvantages of group therapy with children and adolescents will now be briefly reviewed.

Advantages

Group therapy is a common method used with children and adolescents due to its numerous advantages over individual therapy. Corey and Corey (2013) outline a number of distinct advantages seen during group therapy that may be considered to be advantages in group work with youth: increase in self-awareness, provide an awareness of and changes in beliefs about themselves and others, examine how they relate to others, and offer a structured, guided context to learn new skills.

In their earlier work, Corey and Corey (1997) refer to these factors as "the special forces within groups that produce constructive changes" (p. 239). The concept of "Universality" is a powerful factor that cannot occur during individual therapy. Here, students relate to and recognize that other members of the group share in some of the same challenges that they are experiencing and as a result it may lead them to feel less isolated in their struggle. The support that they may receive can be both direct and indirect in this regard. That is, students in group therapy may receive verbal support but also may perceive support by the Universality of what others in the group are experiencing. Further, when other group members have demonstrated progress toward overcoming challenges (e.g., divorce of parents or death of a loved one) this may also provide hope and inspiration for those who are still struggling.

Students participating in a group receive direct feedback from both the group leader and the other group members, which may be an additional advantage of group therapy for children and adolescents. First, they may get multiple perspectives and solutions to a particular challenge. Second, if the problem they are experiencing relates to dealing with peers, feedback from fellow group members may be more valued. Group members may be direct and also may be more adept at "calling out their friends" when they believe that they are not being forthright, a skill that group leaders may not always have. In addition, offering and receiving feedback may assist group members to understand "the impact they have on others and decide what, if anything, they want to change about their interpersonal style" (Corey & Corey, 1997, p. 243).

This type of feedback may be seen in an RE-CBT based group, where in-between group meetings "homework" is assigned. Group leaders will check in as to completion of homework as well as any beliefs (e.g., "It was TOO difficult to do!") that may have interfered with completion. Feedback from other members of the group as to their homework completion as well as having group members actively participate in reviewing the work of others, can facilitate increased awareness and improved critical thinking. Further, in group treatment there is the possibility of a "mild competition" developing among group members which may be beneficial, especially in its ability to motivate members to work harder toward their goals.

Therapy skill acquisition may also be enhanced in a group setting as some group members may tend to learn therapeutic techniques better than those in individual therapy. We believe that this may be particularly true for children and adolescents especially as it relates to problem-solving techniques and treatment components of RE-CBT. To begin, students may learn some of these techniques vicariously through group work with a peer. As an example, in discussing specific beliefs that a student may hold and how these beliefs are linked to unhealthy affective states and behaviors, a student during individual therapy may experience discomfort as they are in "the hot seat" and not wish to discuss this issue. Further, they may worry about being wrong in answering the clinicians' questions. Alternatively, in group therapy, they may learn the RE-CBT model better by watching the group leader and other group members help tease out the beliefs, emotions, and behaviors of another group member. In addition, RE-CBT techniques are modeled by the therapist as well as by other group members. Modeling provided by other members of the group can be particularly advantageous as children and adolescents may be more likely to identify with their peers than with the group leader. Modeling of other group members may also promote overcoming any discomfort in sharing and disclosure. Oftentimes, when one group member opens up to the group, other members open up as well. Modeling within RE-CBT groups may be an effective approach to teaching group members how to challenge unhealthy thinking and develop logical, rational thoughts.

Members of a group may also benefit in a manner that is beyond the structured intent of the group. For example, in a task-oriented group (i.e., RE-CBT group for overcoming test anxiety) having a mixed-gender group may allow students an opportunity to interact with members of the opposite gender, and develop more effective social skills. In addition, groups may also be a source of school environmental knowledge, where group members learn about various aspects of the school (classroom, teachers, etc.) that other group members have experienced. While not the intention of the group, group members may benefit from this social component of the group.

Perhaps most importantly, groups provide a safe environment for members to share and grow. The group context offers an opportunity for group members to practice and receive constructive feedback from the group leader and their peers as they try to alter some aspects of their behavior or way of thinking. For the group leader, it also provides an opportunity to observe the group members in action interacting with one another and perhaps examine if the presenting issue is a skill deficit or a performance deficit. That is, do they lack the skills to demonstrate a behavior (e.g., social skills) or do they have the skills but something (e.g., anxiety) interferes with the skill performance. The group context provides the group leader with important information on members' interpersonal skills and styles, which may be more accurate and helpful than self-reports of behavior offered during in individual therapy.

Disadvantages

While there are a number of benefits for group therapy and it may be considered to be a time and cost-effective approach, group therapy is not for everyone, and it certainly has its limitations in clinical work with youth. Given that treatment is occurring through a group modality, logically it reduces the amount of time spent addressing the needs of each group member, as compared to individual work. As such, some may consider group therapy to be an inefficient method for the individual. As will be addressed later on in the chapter, it is important for the group leader to consider whether the degree of impairment that the client is experiencing would warrant more intensive, individual work. In some cases, this may be true. However, it is important to recognize that many, if not most, groups are comprised of clients with similar needs or complaints. As a result, while only one group member's specific needs are addressed at a time, other group members may benefit from the general information offered.

A valid concern about group therapy is that just the idea of therapy in a group format may intimidate a student who could benefit from the approach. This may be true for students who are socially anxious but also concerned about airing personal issues to their peers. The challenges of confidentiality cannot be guaranteed, and as such some children may be wary of the group setting for therapy. During individual therapy, students are reassured that for the most part everything they reveal (excepting child abuse and the intention to harm oneself or others) will remain confidential by the fact that the therapist is bound to legal and ethical codes and could face severe consequences for breaking confidentiality. These assurances become more complicated when therapy is conducted in a group with children and adolescents. One way to address the issue of confidentiality in groups is to create written contracts that all members must sign at the start of the group (see Appendix A). While these contracts are not legally or ethically binding, their existence may help ease the minds of those who may be hesitant to enter the group due to fears about confidentiality.

The structure of the group is important and providing the opportunity for all group members to be heard and valued is essential to group engagement and participation. This can be challenged by compulsive talkers or interrupters as group members. Group leaders can reduce the risk of constant interruption by certain group members by setting up specific "ground rules" for the group during the initial session. We encourage the group leader to facilitate the development of group rules. Rules that stress the importance of being respectful when each member is speaking and recognition of specific times when it is appropriate and inappropriate for members to make comments should be offered. In our experience, group members may police one another and offer feedback when they think that other members may be monopolizing the group. This may be particularly true for adolescents and this feedback may be used as part of the therapy process ("Robyn, how did you feel when Sean told you he thought you cut him off and would not let him finish his story?"). We also suggest that to avoid embarrassment, group leaders may wish to pull a student aside at a later time and offer feedback that they may be monopolizing the group process and encourage them to self-monitor their behavior.

Another important factor for group leaders to consider is that there may be a high level of suggestibility of some members in that they readily agree to the suggestions of other group members even if it is not in their best interest. It is important for group leaders to recognize the specific needs and persona of individual group members and consider how they may be affected by group participation. For example, some students may only do their group assignment because they think "It would be AWFUL to disappoint the group leader and/or group members." While this does lead to the group assignment being completed, it would be important to address the motive, or potential irrationality, behind their behavior. In addition, group leaders would benefit from considering and correcting members when they give bad advice or provide the wrong solution. This can be detrimental to highly suggestible members.

Overall, we have found that groups can be an important resource in working with children and adolescents and that the advantages outweigh the disadvantages. We believe that the structure of the REBT and CBT lends itself nicely to the format of group therapy for working with youth. We will briefly discuss the theory of REBT and its core assumptions as they relate to groups and then present some general guidelines for running groups with children and adolescents.

RE and Cognitive Behavioral Approaches Applied to Child and Adolescent Groups

At this point in the book, readers will be fairly familiar with the RE-CBT model and how it is applied when working with children, adolescents, and parents. However, we would like to provide a brief review of the model as it pertains to group therapy when working with these populations.

REBT in Child and Adolescent Groups

The broad umbrella of Cognitive Behavioral Therapy includes a number of clinical approaches among which is REBT. REBT operates under the premise that individuals possess disruptive, dysfunctional/irrational cognitions about events, which negatively impact their behavior and affect (DiGiuseppe et al., 2013). The cognitive *dysfunction* model differs from a cognitive *defici*t model, which implies that normal development involves the acquisition of certain cognitive processes. Some students may have failed to develop these skills or experience difficulty in applying them proficiently. This distinction between dysfunction and deficit is important to consider in determining what type of group to assign a student. To clarify the distinction, we will consider the case of a child who is socially anxious from that of a child who has social deficits as a function of their being diagnosed with autism spectrum disorder (ASD).

In order to meet the diagnostic criteria for autism spectrum disorder (ASD), a child must have "persistent deficits in social communication and social interaction" (American Psychiatric Association, 2013, p. 50). The difficulty in engaging in appropriate social interaction with others is a skill that failed to develop in the student with autism spectrum disorder. Alternatively, students who are socially anxious may in fact have acquired the appropriate social behaviors and know what the correct behavior to engage in is, but fail to do so. This may be due to any number of dysfunctional cognitions that the student may endorse: "If I say something and mess up and others think poorly of me …it would be terrible" or "I have to/must have approval of others, because not to would be intolerable." These dysfunctional cognitions are irrational in nature and would interfere with the students' ability to execute a socially appropriate behavior. That is, their performance of the behavior is impeded by these not-helpful styles of thinking.

This distinction is important to consider in that the type of therapy group a student may be assigned to may vary depending upon whether they (a) never acquired/learned the appropriate cognitive, social, and behavioral processes (deficit) or (b) they engage in distorted interpretations and perceptions of reality (dysfunction). If the presenting difficulties are a function of cognitive deficits, the best type of therapy group may be one that is more skills focused; that is, teaching students what they failed to develop. These groups may be staggered in terms of skill acquisition level, to allow other students who have demonstrated some level of competency in skill acquisition to provide a model for their peers. In our experience, these deficit-driven groups appear to be more often focused on behaviors that are externalizing in nature as here students can receive direct feedback from others about the performance of their behavior. The dysfunction-driven groups may focus more on internal cognitions/beliefs that may interfere with the performance of adaptive behaviors. Here the groups may take more of an RE-CBT approach and teach strategies to challenge unhealthy cognitions and develop and apply healthier alternatives. During these groups, the group leaders are able to see the interaction of the students' cognitions, their behaviors, and the environment (their peers) in which these behaviors occur. This allows for a greater understanding for the group leader and group members of the dynamic interaction of these variables and for an opportunity to practice/rehearse effective cognitions and behaviors in more natural contexts than may be present during individualized therapy.

Some Distinctive Features of RE-CBT Groups

RE-CBT group therapy with children and adolescents, much like individual therapy, is more psycho-educational than motivational. That is, the group leader's role is not to just inspire the group members but rather to provide them with knowledge and information within the Re-CBT framework to help them in achieving goals. Group leaders inform and educate members of the group on the dysfunctionality of their present cognitive schemas, teach them strategies to actively challenge these beliefs, and work with them on developing healthier and more realistic ways of thinking which will lead to more appropriate affective and behavioral responses.

RE-CBT proposes that the clinical approach of the group begins with a focus on the irrational beliefs and cognitive processing underlying emotions. Through a group format, peers may help group members readily identify the cognitive schemas/irrational beliefs that may be maintaining their affective and behavioral disturbance. This is a unique benefit of the group format, as compared to the group leader, peers may be better able to relate to understanding some of the underlying cognitions that lead to the unhealthy emotions experienced. In RE-CBT groups, there typically are a number of exercises, which will be detailed later, that assist to directly challenge unhealthy cognitions that will help facilitate emotional and behavioral change.

Early on in groups with children we focus on the RE-CBT theory of emotions, and assist students in understanding the differences between functional (healthy) and dysfunctional (unhealthy) emotions. Here it is important that clinicians consider the developmental level of functioning of the group members and cater their language in therapy to a level that the student will understand. While the more traditional RE-CBT language consisting of words like "functional", "dispute", "automatic thoughts", and "irrational" may be appropriate for older students, their use may serve to hinder the understanding of some of the core principals of RE-CBT with younger children. We suggest more "user-friendly" terms that share the same content/message. As such, we use "helpful", "challenge", and "healthy thinking" in place of the terms above. For a greater review of developmental consideration in the application of RE-CBT among youth the reader is referred to Grave and Blissett (2004) and Garber, Frankel, and Herrington (2016).

Developing an emotional vocabulary is an important aspect of RE-CBT psychoeducation in both individual and group treatment. The group leader may wish to determine members' emotional vocabulary, especially with younger children. We have found many students, when asked what they feel, will offer "bad" as a response or may in fact offer what they are thinking (i.e., "I feel like she doesn't like me"). The group leader, through didactic instruction as well as experiential exercises, will help students see a range of feelings (anger, sadness, frustration, anxiety) across an emotional continuum. At the same time, the group leader and group members may assist students in understanding the four aspects of every emotion:

Phenomenological—how the emotion feels.

1. Social Expression—how we communicate our goals and upset others.
2. Physiological Arousal—biological response.
3. Behavioral Predisposition—emotions are often important cues that we must act on problems. They may lead to behavior coping strategies that may be adaptive or dysfunctional in nature.

Consistent with the models of RE-CBT, group leaders work on teaching students that irrational beliefs/automatic thoughts are what lead to these dysfunctional, disturbed emotions. Using the Happening-Thinking-Feeling-Reaction/Behavior framework, students are taught the connection between thoughts and responses (i.e., behaviors and emotions) and learn the differences between irrational beliefs and the more rational, healthy cognitions that can lead to healthier, more functional negative emotions. However, before one begins an RE-CBT group, or any group for that matter, there are a few things that we believe warrant consideration.

General Guidelines for Forming RE-CBT Groups

The screening and selection of individuals to participate in the group is a very important aspect of group therapy, especially in RE-CBT, which follows a specific model with very specific goals. We have found that one of the earlier guidelines for group formation offered by Elkin (1983) still warrant consideration today. We discuss and expand on these guidelines in consideration of the development of RE-CBT groups.

To begin, we suggest that group leaders conduct a preliminary session with potential members either prior to the start of the group (in the case of a closed group) or before a new person joins the group (in the case of an open group). This preliminary session is basically a "goodness of therapeutic fit" to determine whether the goals of the potential member are consistent with the goals of the group. It also provides an opportunity for the potential group member to learn more about the group and interview the group leader, which may assist them in deciding whether or not to join the group. Group screenings of youth may also wish to involve the parents/caregivers in the initial meeting. During this meeting group goals are discussed, as well as group expectations and confidentiality. Group leaders may also wish to consider a screening instrument like the Group Selection Questionnaire (GSQ; Burlingame, Cox, Davies, Layne, & Gleave, 2011).

In consideration of admitting a student to a counseling group, group leaders may want to develop inclusionary and exclusionary criteria of the group. The exclusionary criteria of any group are entirely dependent upon the group, its leaders, and its goals. RE-CBT groups often have exclusionary criteria that may be more stringent than other groups. This may include ruling out potential members with severe pathology (i.e., psychotic, suicidal, brain damaged, or sociopathic) as well as those who may be uncommunicative or silent, as neither they nor other students will benefit from their participation (or the lack thereof). At the same time, leaders may wish to exclude students with some of the more extreme external disorders (conduct disorder, oppositional defiant disorder). Given the importance of in-between session work in RE-CBT groups, group leaders may exclude members who appear unwilling to do group assignments or therapy homework.

Inclusionary criteria, much like the exclusionary criteria, are dependent on the specific goals of the group. In order to be included in an RE-CBT group, potential members are provided information about the general structure and model of RE-CBT to ensure that this is something in which they wish to participate. As group activities are focused around this model, potential members agree to work on assignments and actively participate in all aspects of the group, especially disputing their own and other members' irrational beliefs. Given the goal-directed nature of RE-CBT, potential group members are to have very specific goals they want to work on during the group. We find that the ability to set therapy goals is more likely to be better developed in adolescents than in younger children. Younger children are often told by their parents or teachers what their goals are to be and leaders may expect that to continue to be the case for some in group therapy.

During the initial meeting of an RE-CBT group, group leaders may wish to provide a brief history of RE-CBT and review a number of the different techniques that will be used in the group. This helps prepare students for what is to be expected and may make them informed and ready to work. As discussed earlier, setting ground rules is quite important in group therapy. Group leaders may have specific rules about attendance, socializing outside the group, etc., and it is expected that all potential members agree to abide by these rules prior to joining the group. Providing students with a written list of the rules, or even having them sign a contract in which they agree to abide by the rules may also be helpful.

Finally, the preliminary meeting also provides the group leader with the opportunity to discuss and reinforce the important issue of confidentiality. Group members are informed of both their rights and limitations regarding confidentiality, including the circumstances in which group leaders are mandated to break confidentiality. Emphasizing the responsibility of all group members for assuring that all information revealed by fellow group members remains confidential is also promoted and reinforced. Group leaders would benefit from recognizing that given the social nature of a school, unfortunately confidential issues are not always kept secure. When this occurs, we recommend that the group leader addresses this individually with the student and in the group as well to review the rules of confidentiality. It is also at this time that the decision to allow a student to remain in the group following this breach of confidentiality is discussed.

Additional practical issues that must be decided before beginning a group include the time, dates, and location of group meetings as well as the group size. While these decisions will vary dependent upon setting, typically we have found that groups of younger students (up to age 7) should have no more than 4–5 members, while groups of older students (ages 8+) should have a 7–8 member maximum. Further, groups held in school should not be during major academic areas nor should they compete with other school-related activities that students find desirable (i.e., gym class). Marketing a group may also be an important variable to consider. As an example, Flanagan, Povall, Dellino, and Byrne (1998) held their group during a lunch period, provided popcorn, and called it a "popcorn club". If the group is going to set and evaluate specific goals, group leaders will want to determine in advance what methods/measures will be used for data collection to evaluate change and what the process will be for measure administration.

Another practical and clinical decision the group leader has to make is to determine the group type: open or closed. In an open group, students can join the group at any point provided that there is space in the group. As a result, there will be students in the group with different levels of skills. An advantage of this type of group is that it allows students to remain in the group until they have attained their goals. A potential disadvantage of this method is what Corey and Corey, Corey, Callanan, and Russell (1992) refer to as the "cozy-nest syndrome," in which group members are, "always 'working' and perhaps never changing" (p. 35). Alternatively, closed groups have a pre-determined number of sessions and all members begin and finish the group together. The disadvantage of a closed group format is that the group may conclude whether or not the student has reached his or her goals. However, having an end date can also act as an advantage and serve as a source of motivation to begin actively making changes (Corey et al., 1992). Another advantage of closed groups is that they are more cost-effective than groups lasting for over a year.

Types of RE-CBT Groups for Children and Adolescents

While RE-CBT groups are based on an evidence-based approach to psychotherapy, considering the content and factors that best lend themselves to a group format to lead to positive clinical outcomes is important. Yalom (1995) had originally proposed 11 therapeutic factors that were considered to be essential for treatment outcome via a group therapy approach. From these 11 factors, Fuhriman, Burlingame, Seaman, and Barlow (1999) reported that group cohesiveness, catharsis, and interpersonal learning were considered to be the most helpful by clients. While these factors have been debated (see Shechtman & Gluk, 2005), we think the proposed cluster by Lieberman and Golant (2002): affective insight, affective supportive, cognitive supportive, and cognitive insight (Shechtman & Gluk, 2005) may be among the most helpful in consideration of an RE-CBT group with youth.

Where RE-CBT groups with children and adolescents may differ from RE-CBT groups with adults is the fact that with adult RE-CBT groups, the goal may be to provide individual therapy within a group setting. While this can and does occur in child and adolescent therapy groups, in our experience these groups appear to involve more group tasks with less boundaries/structure than those that exist in the adult groups. That is, RE-CBT groups with youth may involve more group experiential exercises focusing on interaction and development of healthy thinking and appropriate behaviors as compared to adult groups.

RE-CBT groups for children and adolescents involve both content and process focus. That is, teaching RE-CBT content is important to facilitate change but RE-CBT groups are also process-oriented in that many of the in-group exercises will ask students to address how they are feeling and thinking at that moment. By identifying in session thoughts this may also assist in generating alternative healthy ways of thinking and the accompanying adaptive emotions and behaviors.

Smead (1995) discussed three different types of groups for children and adolescents that we believe are applicable to RE-CBT. We briefly discuss these types of groups and the role that RE-CBT can potentially play in facilitating emotional and behavioral change.

Counseling/Therapy Groups

In these groups, the focus is on behavioral and emotional change and they may be groups that are more general with a wide range of problems or they may be geared toward specific issues, such as dealing with a divorce, relationship issues, or grief. These groups are most closely aligned with the RE-CBT model and may assist students in developing better coping strategies. Groups that are more general may be for the students who regularly experience difficulty, while in the issue-driven groups, students are aware of the content focus of the groups (e.g., stress management). Vicarious learning may have a delayed effect in general groups as students get to hear peers work through an area of difficulty (e.g., college selection) that may not be an issue for them at present, but may become one in the future. Hopefully, at that point they will be able to recall the effective solutions of their peers. With content-specific groups, students listen and learn to help others who are at varying stages of distress when they are exposed to similar environmental stressors. As mentioned earlier, the universality aspect of these groups is at play here as students see that they are not alone and they are not the only ones experiencing difficulty. Participation may help normalize their affective experiences and may provide a resource for support outside the structure of the group.

Task-Oriented Groups

Task work group members strive toward a specific goal that is not necessarily emotional in nature, but may be more of the academic/achievement sort. These may be specific group tasks (e.g., create a school-wide bullying program), or one task that all members of the group may be working toward (e.g., SAT preparation). While this type of group is seen to be more practical in nature, we also focus on the emotional components that may interfere with students' ability to work toward the task. RE-CBT may assist in helping clarify which goal(s) to work on (e.g., college applications) and identifying potential practical and cognitive/emotive blocks ("it's too difficult") to goal attainment. Establishing a clear objective and a limited time frame in which to achieve that objective is helpful. Group leaders may help facilitate goal identification, explore the irrational beliefs that may impede goal achievement through extreme negative emotions and behaviors, restructure irrational to rational beliefs, and brainstorm effective strategies to meet this goal. When students may wish to select strategies that are impractical in nature, the RE-CBT group leader may engage in brainstorming and help them examine all potential solutions and evaluate which ones have the highest degree of success, are practical, and are acceptable. Additionally, the RE-CBT group leader will work to make sure the tasks chosen have a high degree of acceptability on the part of the group members, as low acceptability will lead to poorer effort toward goal attainment.

In task-oriented groups, group leaders may encourage students to go "out of their comfort zone." Students are encouraged to select a task they are not necessarily comfortable with, which helps promote risk-taking. At the same time, we want group members' efforts to be reinforced so we do not have group members select tasks that have a low probability for success.

If groups, either as a whole or individually, fail to achieve the selected goal(s), the RE-CBT group leader will use this as an opportunity to discuss feelings and cognitions related to the lack of task achievement, differentiating between healthy and unhealthy responses. That is, working toward more self-acceptance and avoiding self-defeating beliefs.

Psycho-Education/Guidance Groups

These groups generally constitute clinical work with "at-risk" populations. This may involve students who are at risk for a number of potential problems/disorders and may take on less of an academic focus than the task groups. Group members could be students who are at risk for eating disorders or drug and alcohol abuse. These may be students who are sub-clinical and have shown some of the early warning signs of developing a disorder but may not be eligible for formal services at this point. Here, RE-CBT group leaders assist students in overcoming faulty thinking that may put these students at risk. Promoting frustration tolerance and increasing their ability to engage in consequential thinking can be quite helpful in these groups. Education is a major part of these groups and the group leader can better serve these groups if they have a good balance of knowledge of the theory of RE-CBT along with knowledge about the specific area that students are determined to be at-risk for. Additional work with family members may be beneficial and help reduce the exposure to factors that may elicit risk-taking behavior. As an example, RE-CBT groups for students who are at risk for drug and alcohol abuse may focus on helping students express their feelings, develop effective coping skills to resist peer pressure and learn strategies on how to interact more effectively with others. At the same time, children and families will also receive comprehensive information on drugs and alcohol and learn about the dangers associated with them. In family-based sessions, these programs may involve parent training, family skills training, and family self-help groups to learn how to reinforce the lessons at home.

Engaging Children and Adolescents in Groups

Among the larger challenges facing group leaders working with children and adolescents in groups is to establish a therapeutic alliance. Despite the importance paid to the topic of the therapeutic alliance (also referred to as the working relationship) with children, very few empirical studies on the topic exist as it relates to group work. DiGiuseppe, Linscott, and Jilton (1996) proposed two main barriers to forming the therapeutic alliance with children and adolescents: (1) most children and adolescents are mandated to therapy; and (2) children and adolescents usually enter therapy in a pre-contemplative stage. That is, they are not even thinking about changing their behavior.

The level of motivation for change of children and adolescent in RE-CBT group therapy may be an important moderator of treatment effectiveness. With most children and adolescents entering therapy against their will, they generally do not believe they have a problem, do not wish to change, and may be completely unmotivated for treatment. This presents a major obstacle to the process of establishing therapeutic goals with children and adolescents, which is the first aspect of developing the therapeutic alliance (DiGiuseppe et al., 1996).

DiGiuseppe et al. (1996) have developed a cognitive behavioral approach toward motivating children/adolescents to change based on Prochaska and DiClemente's Stages of Change Model (1988; as cited in DiGiuseppe et al., 1996). We believe that this approach has important implications when working with children and adolescents in group therapy as well. The Stages of Change Model lists the five stages of change a person goes through as (1) pre-contemplative; (2) contemplative; (3) preparation; (4) action; and (5) maintenance. Students in the pre-contemplative stage have no intention of changing and usually do not recognize the issue at hand as problematic. This may be an accurate stage to consider most group members to be at. Once the student reaches the contemplative stage, he or she is beginning to perceive a problem and may be seeking help.

Entering a group at the pre-contemplative stage, when they do not perceive any problems, may be especially problematic in a group setting, as groups rely on the active participation of members. While we recognize the importance of the development of the relationship bond between the group leader and client, we think that in RE-CBT we can motivate students to change and build an alliance discussing goals with group members in a direct and open manner. Examining how the group members feel about these goals and target behaviors is a crucial step, especially considering that these goals are almost always set by others and are likely to be different from, or even completely contradictory to, the child or adolescent's own internal goals.

By having students explore the consequences of their behavior, this can be an important step toward bringing children and adolescents from the pre-contemplative stage into the contemplative stage. In a group setting, this provides a unique interactive opportunity for other group members, as they may be able to point out consequences that the child or the therapist may not have been able to identify.

Assessment in RE-CBT Child and Adolescent Groups

We propose that assessment should be an on-going part of the group therapy experience for youth both from a diagnostic as well as a progress-monitoring perspective. Involvement of data collection at multiple data points increases the responsiveness of the intervention to meet the needs of the students, assesses the effectiveness of intervention, and examines the stability over time and situations. We will briefly discuss some recommendations for standardized mental health batteries that we have found useful in working with children and adolescents, followed by more specific recommendations for RE-CBT groups.

Standardized Batteries for Assessment

A review of all evaluation measures that may be beneficial for children and adolescents in group therapy is beyond the scope of this chapter. However, we would suggest that for general problem groups, the group leader considers a broad-based measure, like the Behavioral and Emotional Screening System (BESS; Kamphaus & Reynolds, 2007). The BESS screens for externalizing, internalizing, school problem behaviors, and adaptive skills in children and adolescents (ages 3–18 years). More problem-specific measures that address the content of that group (e.g., the CDI-2 [Kovacs, 2011]) for Depression or the MASC-2 for childhood anxiety (March, Parker, Sullivan, Stallings, & Conners, 1997). For screening and regular progress monitoring we recommend measures like the Behavior Intervention Monitoring Assessment System (BIMAS; McDougal, Bardos, & Meier, 2011) or the Youth Outcomes Questionnaire (Dunn, Burlingame, Walbridge, Smith, & Crum, 2005).

An area of recent exploration with regards to children and adolescents is the concept of emotional intelligence (EQ), as children with high EQ are believed to be better able to regulate their emotional distress and handle adversity more effectively. This is a concept that we believe is key to RE-CBT work with children and adolescents and may be something that a clinician wishes to assess in an RE-CBT group. The Bar-On Emotional Quotient Inventory: Youth Version (EQ-I:YV; Bar-On & Parker, 2000) is a self-report measure for youth ages 7 through 18 and provides an overall EQ score which is subdivided into scores on four domains: Intrapersonal, Interpersonal, Stress Management, and Adaptability.

Finally, given that the focus of RE-CBT groups is on changing student thinking, we believe it is important to assess students' irrational thinking or automatic thoughts. In doing so, group leaders may be better served to examine how effective the RE-CBT component is within-group treatment as it relates to changing unhelpful thinking. With regard to irrational thinking in children and adolescents, we recommend the revised version of the Child and Adolescent Scale of Irrationality (CASI; Terjesen, Kassay, & Anderson, 2017). The CASI is a self-report measure of irrational beliefs of children and adolescents, which yields scores on six scales, including self-downing, dependence, conformity, demandingness, low frustration tolerance, and discomfort anxiety, in addition to a total irrationality score. Additionally, group leaders may also wish to consider using the Children's Automatic Thoughts Scale (CATS; Schniering & Rapee, 2002) which is a self-report of negative beliefs commonly seen to both internalizing and externalizing problems.

General Cognitive Behavioral Assessment Guidelines

As developmentally younger children may have difficulty in problem identification, emotional labeling, and introspection they may require a slower pace within the group and more experiential exercises and games to enhance assessment as well as treatment engagement. Further, asking students to recall prior events may be challenging as well. A relatively simple approach to collecting data about events occurred that has a greater likelihood of being accurate is to have students complete an "emotion and thought log" (see Appendix B). Conducting a functional analysis of behavior may be another important factor to consider in the assessment. This may help determine if the student engages in this behavior to change something in their environment (parent/teacher behavior), gain attention, avoid discomfort, or for sensory reasons. These logs (and the consequences received for behavior) may help in understanding this.

While not specific to RE-CBT, assessing for and then remediating problem-solving skill deficiencies is important given that the solutions often selected by children and adolescents are poor. The RE-CBT group therapist may want to determine whether the student knows effective ways of behaving but as a result of their style of thinking they do not behave appropriately, or have they not learned alternative problem-solving options. The direction you take clinically may vary depending upon whether or not you need to teach emotional along with practical problem skills.

As the RE-CBT group progresses, the group leader may utilize a number of group exercises (discussed below) to determine whether or not a group member has learned how to challenge unhealthy thoughts and develop more effective, healthy ways of thinking and behaving. This assessment can be through observation and may be accomplished through a rational role play exercise to assess both the students' overt behavior as well as to determine whether they are able to think and therefore behave more rationally in this role play.

Core Content in RE-CBT Groups with Children and Adolescents

While the focus of the RE-CBT group may vary as a function of the presenting problem and the developmental level of the group members there are some general areas that we have found are helpful for a group leader to consider when running groups as well as some group exercises and strategies that the group leader may wish to incorporate.

To begin, while the RE-CBT model is fairly straightforward conceptually, we believe that the group leader would benefit from having a strong conceptual understanding of RE-CBT and its techniques utilized as a mechanism of change. Having a group leader who is able to communicate differences between irrational evaluations and appraisals of misinterpretations (inferences, absolutes, evaluations) is helpful. Which thoughts (inferences or evaluations) group leaders target for change may vary depending upon the developmental level of the child. RE-CBT group leaders may work on challenging distorted interpretations of reality ("He doesn't like me"), the absolute ("I NEED him to like me all the time") or evaluative beliefs ("It's AWFUL that he doesn't like me"). Conceptually, these three cognitions are very different and the group process allows for the leader and the group members to target one or all types of belief systems but what to focus on may vary by group members age with more inference challenging occurring with younger group members.

These distorted interpretations of reality (incorrect conclusions/predictions) are an example of where group therapy may be more effective in treating these beliefs than individual treatment. Peers are often a great source of data collection and feedback and may help provide evidence that contradicts the belief. As an example, if a student says "Teacher X doesn't like me!" another group member may point out that she disagrees with that inference and offer evidence to the contrary. With regards to the challenging of absolutes and derivative evaluative assumptions (e.g., "It is awful that she doesn't like me!), group therapy can be very helpful in that group members who share common absolutes and irrational evaluations can be helped by their peers to see that they are not alone in this experience. Through hearing their peers discuss similar evaluative beliefs, group members may come to realize how faulty/unhelpful that way of thinking truly is. Further, the RE-CBT group therapy approach may offer models of peers who have successfully changed different types of cognitions and as such they may be able to apply them on their own or with the support of the group.

As part of emotive education, we encourage RE-CBT group leaders to present the idea that extreme negative emotions (such as high degrees of anger, anxiety, depression) interfere with overall healthy functioning. This can even lead the most reasonable students into saying or doing something that they wish they had not, that may cause problems at school, at home, or with friends. This may be facilitated by the group leader having group members recall the last time they made a bad decision. We then will ask them what they were thinking and feeling when they made that decision and whether they ever let what they felt, emotionally, make the decision for them. Students are often fairly good at recalling bad decisions and once one student is able to identify the role their affect played in this decision it may open the door for their peers to do so as well. Group leaders may wish to use video examples to help show how people may make bad decisions when they are extremely upset. We believe emphasizing that unhealthy emotions like stress, anxiety, anger, and depression interfere with their ability to make smart choices is key to promoting motivation for change.

Another part of emotive-education that we believe benefits from early and repeated exposure in RE-CBT groups is the distinction between non-hurtful and hurtful emotions. Non-hurtful emotions occur when students are dealing with difficult situations and they experience being annoyed, irritated, or aggravated. These non-hurtful emotions allow students to problem solve and manage things effectively in difficult situations. Hurtful emotions lead to escalating conflict, name calling, and a number of emotional (anger, depression, anxiety) and behavioral (avoidance, aggression) manifestations. We make sure to highlight that students will "feel" something when adversity occurs, and RE-CBT work focuses on helping them experience more of the healthy, appropriate negative emotions.

K. Doyle (personal communication, February 14, 2005, 2003) offers some suggested exercises for group settings that we think are excellent in general and that have specific applications to the REBT group therapy process with children and adolescents. We have highlighted a few below.

- Introduction Exercises: Have students finish the sentence, "One thing I'm hoping to gain from this group is …". We have found that this is helpful in terms of goal setting and it allows children and adolescents to hear what their peers are looking to work toward and may serve to further allow other group members to help them in the group process.
- Comprehensive Self-Inventory: Have each student use paper and pencil to assess their strengths and weaknesses; have them start on the weaknesses that they think might be remediable. With younger students you may have them draw pictures. This approach again helps with increasing insight into their problem as well as helping with goal selection.
- Expectations/Fears: Each student is asked to report his/her expectations and fears about participating in the group. We find this to be particularly helpful when working with children and adolescents, as it helps normalize cognitions they may be experiencing and may also allow for clarification of misconceptions of the group process that they may have. We also see this as a way of further clarifying specific rules of the group therapy process that are often concerns of students (e.g., confidentiality).
- Best and Worst Day: Here, group members are asked to draw a composite of their best and worst day in the past month or so and share these with the group. The group leader facilitates a conversation about what kinds of experiences make a "good" day and what are the common ingredients in a "bad" day. The group leader may help in looking for patterns of thinking that may differentiate between the two.
- Learning from Mistakes: Students are asked to think of a situation that they believe they did not handle particularly well. More specifically they are asked to close their eyes and try and recall the feelings and thoughts that they had at the time. They are then asked to write them down and share them with the group and allow the group to help them identify any thought distortions. The group leader may have them discuss what they would have liked to have happen and have the group develop a list of rational beliefs and coping statements that might have been helpful.
- Strongest Hour: This we usually try to do right after the Learning from Mistakes exercise. In this exercise, students are asked to recall a time when they relied primarily on themselves to deal with a difficult situation. We ask them to bring the situation clearly to mind by recalling the details (the setting, the people involved, the time and place, the things said, etc.). We help them experience

both satisfaction and pride about their successful handling of themselves in the situation. This may work particularly well for students with Low Frustration Tolerance, as they may see that they can handle adversity and things are not too difficult. We ask them to recall what they told themselves during that situation and discuss how they can increase the likelihood of thinking and behaving that way again in the future. This is a very powerful exercise for child and adolescent groups as peers hear of the success of their colleagues, which may serve to motivate them.

- Dear Dr. Rational: Each student writes a brief letter or email about one of their problems, as though they were writing to Oprah or Dr. Phil (the Dear Abby reference gets lost on the youth of today). These letters are then passed around the room and each person answers someone else's letter in writing. We encourage that they help each other come up with a practical solution as well as a solution that utilizes the rational thinking they have been developing.
- Evidence Against IBs: In this exercise for older students, on one side of an index card we have students write down their irrational beliefs, while on the other side, they write five negative things that have happened to them because they think this way. Students are then encouraged to read the card several times a week to remind them of how that belief is not working for them.
- Anonymous Disputing: This exercise occurs with students who possess a good understanding of the REBT framework, and most specifically of disputation. Students are asked to write down their irrational beliefs and pass them forward on a piece of paper to the group leader. The group leader reads them aloud and the group as a whole provides challenges or disputes for them. We have modified this at points to use a small ball as a "hot potato" exercise, in which group members throw the ball to their peers to try and involve all in the art of disputation.
- Shame-Attacking: This is one of the more well-known of the REBT techniques and involves having individuals do something or tell the group to do something which they would normally never do (typically for fear of others' negative reactions). We have found the group format to be an excellent forum for this in that peers support one another and also do not let each other "off the hook" for non-completion of the exercise.
- Round of Applause: Have students applaud something or someone they are grateful for. We have used this exercise at the beginning and the end of the group, around holidays (Thanksgiving or New Year's resolution) and have found this to be a very fun and enjoyable exercise. The group leader leads standing ovations, whistles, cheering for positive things/people, and helps refocus the group members on positive things in their lives, which is contrary to what the focus is of many therapy groups. We actively reinforce group participants.
- Positive Talk: Usually done in conjunction with the round of applause and it often serves the same purpose. Each student is asked to talk positively about themselves for a full 2 min. (If they qualify or modify what they say, they get a penalty of an additional 30 s.)

- Role-Play: Group members are asked to think of upcoming situations that they are apprehensive about (e.g., exam, social event) and act them out with other group members. Students can use this opportunity to provide feedback on the behavior of their peers as well as offer hypotheses as to what they are experiencing cognitively.
- Reverse Role-Play: This exercise is usually done after group members are familiar with one another. In this exercise, one group member takes another's irrational beliefs and holds onto them rigidly and forcefully. The student who presented the irrational belief has to try and talk the role-player out of the firmly held belief. This reinforces vigorous disputing for the individual and may further provide a model for their peers.
- Hotseat: One at a time, group members take the "seat" and as many participants as want to give feedback (both positive and negative), while the student remains silent. This helps students to learn to accept feedback from others and then as a group we process how the student felt and the validity of some of this feedback.

RE-CBT Group Research with Children and Adolescents

A complete review of all the research of Rational Emotive and Cognitive Behavioral group treatment approaches is beyond the scope of this chapter; however, we would like to highlight some recent findings. In her meta-analytic review, Esposito (2009) examined the effectiveness of both individual and group-based Rational Emotive Behavior Therapy (REBT) with children and adolescents. Of the studies reviewed, a significant majority (87.5%) were conducted within the school environment and delivered in a group-based format (77.8%). The effect size of 0.87 for those treatments done in a group-based format was equivalent to treatment provided on an individual basis (Esposito, 2009).

In addition, it has been demonstrated that REBT and CBT approaches are effective methods when used in non-clinical groups of children and adolescents. For example, Trip, Vernon, and McMahon (2007) conducted a meta-analytic review of Rational Emotive Education (REE) and reported that REE had a powerful effect on lessening irrational beliefs and dysfunctional behaviors.

Finally, Matta (2014) in her meta-analytic review of 98 articles on group-based psychotherapy in the school environment, found a medium to large overall within-group treatment effect size ($M = 0.67$, $SD = 0.65$), suggesting that school-based group therapy is effective in meeting the mental health needs of children and adolescents. She also reported that group treatment conditions showed significantly greater improvement than did individual treatment conditions. Finally, she reported that the modality of cognitive behavioral therapy produced one of the highest effect sizes, but it was not found to be significantly higher than other modalities.

Together these results provide significant evidence in support of the use of RE-CBT in group treatment of children and adolescents across multiple disorders and presenting problems. Further research is needed to allow group leaders to understand specifically what it is about the RE-CBT group therapy process that leads to change in working with children and adolescents. Clearly, written treatment manuals that lend themselves to research replicability and that have high practical utility with group leaders are further warranted. As a whole, RE-CBT as a therapeutic approach works well with children and adolescents, and it is hopeful that we will continue to see further applications of RE-CBT group therapy techniques with varied populations of children and adolescents.

Test Yourself Questions

1 What factors are important to consider when determining if a student would benefit from individual or group RE-CBT?
2 What challenges may exist in group therapy that may not exist during individual treatment and what are the best practices to address them?
3 Consider what the advantages are to having an open-ended group as opposed to a close-ended group and how do we best continue to promote efforts to change?

Appendix A: Pre-Group Contract for an REBT Group with Students

Group Contract

- I agree to attend all group sessions. If I will miss a group session, I will discuss this with the group leader in advance.
- I agree to actively participate in all group sessions and activities.
- I agree to actively work toward reaching my goals.
- I agree to complete all group assignments.
- I agree to be honest at all times in the group, both with myself and with other group members.
- I promise that I will not be physically or verbally abusive to either the group leader or other students in this group.
- *Confidentiality*: I agree to respect the privacy of all other students in this group. I promise not to discuss anything said or done in this group, except during group sessions. I understand that this applies even to talking to other group members when outside the group. The rules of confidentiality have been explained to me, and I understand and accept these rules.

I (Print Name) have carefully read all the above rules about joining this group. I understand these rules, including confidentiality; I promise to follow them, and I accept that there will be serious consequences if I break any of these rules.

____________ ____________
Signature Date

Appendix B: Emotion Log

Student Name: ______________________ Date: ________________________

Date	Time	Activating Event	Beliefs	Emotion	Intensity (1-10)	Duration	Action
10/10/20	11:00:00 AM	Parents said "no" to movie with friends	"It's Not fair"; "I should be allowed to go"	Angry	8	45 Min	After yelling, I watched TV, checked social media, and played with my little brother

References

American Psychiatric Association. (2013). *Diagnostic and statistical manual of mental disorders* (5th ed.). Arlington, VA: Author.

Bar-On, R., & Parker, J. D. A. (2000). *Emotional Quotient Inventory: Youth Version (EQ-i:YV): Technical manual*. Toronto, Canada: Multi-Health Systems.

Burlingame, G. M., Cox, J. C., Davies, D. R., Layne, C. M., & Gleave, R. (2011). The group selection questionnaire: Further refinements in group member selection. *Group Dynamics: Theory, Research, and Practice, 15*(1), 60–74. https://doi.org/10.1037/a0020220

Burlingame, G. M., Strauss, B., & Joyce, A. (2013). Change mechanisms and effectiveness of small group treatment. In M. J. Lambert (Ed.), *Bergin and Garfield's handbook of psychotherapy and behavior change* (6th ed., pp. 640–689). New York: Wiley.

Corey, G., Corey, M. S., Callanan, P., & Russell, J. M. (1992). *Group techniques: Second edition. Pacific grove*. California: Brooks/Cole Publishing Company.

Corey, M. S., & Corey, G. (1997). *Groups: Process and practice*. Pacific Grove, CA: Brooks/Cole Publishing Company.

Corey, M. S., & Corey, G. (2013). *Groups: Process and practice* (9th ed.). Pacific Grove, CA: Brooks/Cole Publishing Company.

David, D., Cotet, C., Matu, S., Mogoase, C., & Stefan, S. (2018). 50 years of rational-emotive and cognitive-behavioral therapy: A systematic review and meta-analysis. *Journal of Clinical Psychology, 74*(3), 304–318. https://doi.org/10.1002/jclp.22514

DiGiuseppe, R., Linscott, J., & Jilton, R. (1996). Developing the therapeutic alliance in child-adolescent psychotherapy. *Applied and Preventative Psychology, 5*, 85–100.

DiGiuseppe, R. A., Doyle, K. A., Dryden, W., & Backx, W. (2013). *A practitioner's guide to rational-emotive behavior therapy*. Oxford: Oxford University Press.

Dunn, T. W., Burlingame, G. M., Walbridge, M., Smith, J., & Crum, M. J. (2005). Outcome assessment for children and adolescents: Psychometric validation of the Youth Outcome Questionnaire 30.1 (Y-OQ®-30.1). *Clinical Psychology & Psychotherapy, 12*(5), 388–401. https://doi.org/10.1002/cpp.461

Elkin, A. (1983). Working with children in groups. In A. Ellis & M. E. Bernard (Eds.), *Rational-emotive approaches to the problems of childhood* (pp. 485–507). New York: Plenum Press.

Ellis, A. (1997). REBT and its application to group therapy. In J. Yankura & W. Dryden (Eds.), *Special applications of REBT: A therapist's casebook* (pp. 131–161). New York: Springer.

Ellis, A. (2002). REBT and its application to group therapy. In W. Dryden & M. Neenan (Eds.), *Rational-emotive behaviour group therapy* (pp. 30–54). Philadelphia: Whurr Publishers.

Esposito, M. (2009). *REBT with children and adolescents: A meta-analytic review of efficacy studies* (Unpublished doctoral dissertation). St. John's University, Jamaica, NY.

Flanagan, R., Povall, L., Dellino, M. J., & Byrne, L. (1998). A comparison of problem solving with and without rational-emotive behavior therapy to improve children's social skills. *Journal of Rational-Emotive and Cognitive-Behavior Therapy, 16*, 125–134.

Fuhriman, A., Burlingame, G. M., Seaman, S. W., & Barlow, S. H. (1999). Validating a behavioral measure of catharsis, cohesion, and insight, in group therapy. In *annual conference of the Society for Psychotherapy Research*. Braga, Portugal.

Garber, J., Frankel, S. A., & Herrington, C. G. (2016). Developmental demands of cognitive behavioral therapy for depression in children and adolescents: Cognitive, social, and emotional processes. *Annual Review of Clinical Psychology, 12*, 181–216. https://doi.org/10.1146/annurev-clinpsy-032814-112836

Grave, J., & Blissett, J. (2004). Is cognitive behavior therapy developmentally appropriate for young children? A critical review of the evidence. *Clinical Psychology Review, 24*, 399–420.

Hales, R. E. (2008). *The American Psychiatric Publishing textbook of psychiatry* (5th ed.). Arlington, VA: American Psychiatric Publishing.

Kamphaus, R. W., & Reynolds, C. R. (2007). *BESS behavioral and emotional screening system manual*. Bloomington: Pearson.

Kovacs, M. (2011). *Children's depression inventory: second edition (Manual)*. New York: MultiHealth Systems.

Lieberman, M. A., & Golant, M. (2002). Leader behaviors as perceived by cancer patients in professionally directed support groups and outcomes. *Group Dynamics: Theory, Research, and Practice, 6*(4), 267–276. https://doi.org/10.1037/1089-2699.6.4.267

March, J. S., Parker, J. D., Sullivan, K., Stallings, P., & Conners, C. K. (1997). The multidimensional anxiety scale for children (MASC): Factor structure, reliability, and validity. *Journal of the American Academy of Child and Adolescent Psychiatry, 36*, 554–565. https://doi.org/10.1097/00004583-199704000-00019

Matta, A. (2014). *Efficacy of school-based group therapy with children and adolescents: A meta-analytic review* (Unpublished doctoral dissertation). St. John's University, Jamaica, NY.

McDougal, J. L., Bardos, A. N., & Meier, S. T. (2011). *Behavior intervention monitoring assessment system technical manual*. Toronto: Multi-Health Systems.

Merikangas, K. R., He, J., Burstein, M., Swanson, S. A., Avenevoli, S., Cui, L., et al. (2010). Lifetime prevalence of mental disorders in U.S. adolescents: Results from the National Comorbidity Study – Adolescent Supplement (NCS-A). *Journal of the American Academy of Child and Adolescent Psychiatry, 49*(10), 980–989.

National Council for Community Behavioral Healthcare. (2009). *Children's mental health fact sheet*. Washington, DC: National Council for Community Behavioral Healthcare.

National Federation of Families for Children's Mental Health. (2008). *Children mental health prevalence, needs, & barriers*. Rockville, MD: National Federation of Families for Children's Mental Health.

Schniering, C. A., & Rapee, R. M. (2002). Development and validation of a measure of children's automatic thoughts: The children's automatic thoughts scale. *Behaviour Research and Therapy, 40*(9), 1091–1109.

Shechtman, Z., & Gluk, O. (2005). An investigation of therapeutic factors in children's groups. *Group Dynamics: Theory, Research, and Practice, 9*(2), 127–134. https://doi.org/10.1037/1089-2699.9.2.127

Smead, R. (1995). *Skills and techniques for group work with children and adolescents*. Champaign, IL: Research Press.

Terjesen, M. D., & Esposito, M. A. (2006). Rational-emotive behavior group therapy with children and adolescents. In A. Ellis & M. E. Bernard (Eds.), *Rational emotive behavioral approaches to childhood disorders: Theory, practice, and research* (pp. 385–414). New York: Springer.

Terjesen, M. D., Kassay, K. S., & Anderson, D. L. (2017). Evaluation of the psychometric properties of a measure of child irrationality. *Journal of Rational Emotive and Cognitive-Behavioral Therapy, 35*, 413–431. https://doi.org/10.1007/s10942-017-0269-z

The President's New Freedom Commission on Mental Health. (2003). *Achieving the promise: Transforming mental health care in America*. Rockville, MD: The President's New Freedom Commission on Mental Health.

Trip, S., Vernon, A., & McMahon, J. (2007). Effectiveness of rational-emotive education: A quantitative meta-analytical study. *Journal of Cognitive and Behavioral Psychotherapies, 7*, 81–93.

Yalom, I. D. (1995). *The theory and practice of group psychotherapy*. New York: Basic Books.

Yalom, I. D., & Leszcz, M. (2005). *The theory and practice of group psychotherapy*. New York: Basic Books.

Chapter 6
Rational Emotive and Cognitive Behavioral Therapy in Working with Parents

Robyn Kurasaki and Mark D. Terjesen

Parental Affect, Parenting Behaviors, and Impact on Children

At some point in their parenting journey, parents experience elevated levels of anger, anxiety, and depression. These heightened affective states have been linked to a number of child diagnoses and parenting practices. The interplay of parent affect, parent behavior, and child outcomes has been demonstrated in the parenting literature. While a complete review of the research in this area is beyond the scope of this chapter, it is important to discuss the relationship between parent affect and parent behavior, as clinicians need an understanding of these empirical links when developing a case conceptualization and treatment plan.

Anger

Parent anger is a common unhealthy negative emotion. Anger severity can range among parents and across situations; however, unhealthy anger has been associated with punitive, hostile, and inconsistent practices and child abuse (Ateah & Durrant, 2005; Del Vecchio, Jablonka, DiGiuseppe, Notti, & David, 2017; Leung & Slep, 2006; Stith et al., 2009). Experiencing extreme and/or chronic anger makes it difficult to implement positive and consistent parent practices and strategies (Ben-Porath, 2010), as those with increased levels of anger implement discipline inconsistently (Del Vecchio & O'Leary, 2008). These parents often engage in these

R. Kurasaki
New Hyde Park School District, New Hyde Park, NY, USA

M. D. Terjesen (✉)
Department of Psychology, St. John's University, Queens, NY, USA
e-mail: Terjesem@stjohns.edu

M. Bernard, M. D. Terjesen (eds.), *Rational-Emotive and Cognitive-Behavioral Approaches to Child and Adolescent Mental Health: Theory, Practice, Research, Applications*, https://doi.org/10.1007/978-3-030-53901-6_6

ineffective practices to quickly terminate their child's negative experience. The serious consequences that parent anger can have on the child and family have been well documented in studies highlighting the link between parenting and child outcomes. In their meta-analytic review of risk factors for child physical abuse, Stith and colleagues (2009) found that parent anger/hyperreactivity had one of the larger effect sizes as it related to child physical abuse. In the same review, anger was also strongly related to child neglect. Thus, parents experiencing unhealthy anger need assistance in coping with their child's behavior. By increasing their ability to tolerate their child's affective and behavioral experiences, parents may be in a more calm state to engage in effective parenting practices that include positive and consistent practices in response to their child's behavior.

Anxiety

Anxiety is a common unhealthy negative emotion experienced by parents. Parents often report worrying about their child's life success and physical well-being (Fisak, Holderfield, Douglas-Osborn, & Cartwright-Hatton, 2012). While concern can be normal and adaptive, anxiety usually develops when a parent believes that their situation will not improve. There have been numerous studies implicating parental anxiety in the etiology of child anxiety and depression (Biederman et al., 2006; Burstein & Ginsburg, 2010), however, not to externalizing symptoms (van der Bruggen, Stams, & Bögels, 2008). Although the exact transmission is unclear, anxious parents often model anxious behaviors and cognitions and engage in parent practices that exhibit higher levels of parental control that fosters child anxiety (Burstein & Ginsburg, 2010; Creswell & O'Connor, 2006; van der Bruggen et al., 2008). These parents can have perfectionist thoughts and worry about its impact on themselves and their child (Affrunti & Woodruff-Borden, 2015). Further, these parents can have worrisome beliefs related to their child's behavior or condition (Joyce, 1990). These cognitions were found to predict parenting behaviors with anxious parents described as being low in warmth, highly critical, overcontrolling, granting less autonomy in their children, and more reinforcing of avoidance to feared stimuli (Moore, Whaley, & Sigman, 2004; van der Bruggen et al., 2008; Walling, Mills, & Freeman, 2006). In addition, elevated levels of parental anxiety may impact their ability to develop and employ effective coping skills, which can reinforce anxiety among parents (Ginsburg & Schlossberg, 2002). In turn, ineffective coping skills may lead to avoidance of parenting situations perceived as threatening, which can model and reinforce avoidant behaviors of the child (van der Bruggen). Therefore, it is important for the clinician to consider to what degree their client's parental anxiety impacts their ability to implement for children who present with both internalizing and externalizing behaviors.

Depression

Understanding the interplay of parent and child variables may be even more important to consider when working with parents who experience depression. England and Sim (2009) reported that over 15 million children in the United States live in a home where at least one parent had one or more episodes of a major depressive disorder. Depressed mood in parents is characterized by irritable, hostile, and rejecting parenting styles. Parents with depressive symptoms engage in negative appraisals of their child, leading to more negative verbal and physical parent-child interactions (Dix & Meunier, 2009; Garber, Keiley, & Martin, 2002). Often these interactions have less positive monitoring/supervision, sensitivity, and involvement (Mustillo, Dorsey, Conover, & Burns, 2011). In addition, mothers with a history of depressive symptoms and maltreatment were more likely to use maladaptive parent strategies such as physical and psychological aggression (Wolford et al., 2019). Parent's depressed mood has been linked to child externalizing behavior (Barker et al., 2011), and children with parents who experience both anxiety and depressed mood are at higher risk for internalizing problems (Kuckertz, Mitchell, & Wiggins, 2018). Subsequently, these children are at risk for developing an emotional and behavioral disorder (Forehand et al., 2012). Recently, research has shown that the parent behaviors of mothers with depression can change with intervention, which may lead to more positive outcomes for their children (Compas et al., 2011).

Child Disabilities/Chronic Illness

Parents of children with disabilities (e.g., developmental disabilities) and/or chronic illness report higher levels of psychological distress than parents of children without disabilities (Baker et al., 2002; Benson & Karloff, 2009; Dabrowska & Pisula, 2010; McStay, Dissanayake, Scheeren, Koot, & Begeer, 2014). These parents are at increased risk for depression and other mental health problems (Abbeduto et al., 2004; Resch, Elliott, & Benz, 2012). Parents who experience stress and unhealthy negative emotions often utilize ineffective parent practices that create, maintain, or contribute to their child's social-emotional difficulties and family dysfunction. Parents with children with disabilities also endorsed elevated levels of irrational thinking and a higher degree of stress and viewed their child's symptoms as more stressful (Witt, 2005). In addition, these parents may have poorer treatment adherence as many struggle to implement strategies to manage their emotions and their child's behavior. Although levels of child impairment can vary, the relationship between child impairment and parent well-being is mediated by optimism and self-efficacy (Baker et al., 2005). Therefore, with higher risk and prolonged factors contributing to their distress, these parents' need for social support and tools to examine their belief system is critical. These parents may also need assistance in implementing appropriate parent practices tailored to the needs of their child (Kurasaki & Terjesen, 2012).

Clinicians would benefit from having an understanding about parenting practices as it relates to child outcomes. Knowing which parent practices are associated with parent symptomology or negative affect helps clinicians develop interventions that target changing these affective experiences to develop positive parent practices that can improve child outcomes and parent-child relationship satisfaction. It is also important for clinicians to transmit this knowledge through psychoeducation to parents. By understanding the factors that contribute to and maintain parent anger, anxiety, and depression, clinicians can design treatment protocols that target parenting beliefs that interfere with their parenting practices (Fukushima-Flores & Miller, 2011). Therefore, parents who experience anxiety and/or depressed mood would likely benefit from understanding how their own cognitive, affective, and behavioral symptomology as well as their child's behavior influences their parenting practices and child outcomes. RE-CBT can be a useful tool to help parents manage their emotions and improve their behavioral responses. RE-CBT can assist parents by addressing the faulty cognitions that underlie their emotional and behavioral experiences. With a more rational belief system and additional resources like psychoeducation and social support, parents will be better equipped to engage in more effective parent practices resulting in more positive parent, child, and family outcomes.

Theory of Rational Emotive and Cognitive Behavioral Therapy

Rational emotive behavioral therapy (REBT).is considered to be a present-oriented clinical intervention that works collaboratively with clients to change unhealthy thoughts/beliefs, dysfunctional emotions, and maladaptive behaviors (DiGiuseppe, Doyle, Dryden, & Backx, 2013). REBT is considered to be the first formal system under the cognitive behavioral therapy (CBT) spectrum (Hollon & DiGiuseppe, 2010; MacLaren, Doyle, & DiGiuseppe, 2015). The CBT umbrella attempts to group a number of therapies together that share common elements and clinical applications. REBT targets the client's unhealthy thoughts and beliefs associated with a specific trigger or activating event; clinicians can help clients challenge beliefs and replace them with healthy alternatives to prevent or change undesirable emotions and behaviors. REBT helps clients learn that these unhealthy emotions (e.g., anger, anxiety, depression, and guilt) are not *caused* by the actual events, but rather these beliefs develop from how the person perceives, interprets, and evaluates events (MacLaren et al., 2015). Some may view these stressors or events in an unhealthy manner ("I can't believe that just happened" or "This is the *worst* thing and *I can't stand it!*") and, as such, experience a number of unhealthy emotional states. Thus, the application of RE-CBT with parents is based on the premise that parent beliefs, emotions, and behaviors are interrelated and that clinically they are best considered together rather than in isolation.

This chapter will discuss the theory and practice of RE-CBT in clinical work with parents and, where appropriate, highlight the distinctive components of the model. For a thorough review of the distinctiveness of REBT, refer to Dryden (2015). Since its initial development, REBT has established empirical support as a clinical intervention for a number of populations and for various diagnoses (David et al., 2005, 2008; David, Cotet, Matu, Mogoase, & Stefan, 2018; Ford, 2008; Harris, Davies, & Dryden, 2006; Sava, Maricutoiu, Rusu, Macsinga, & Virgă, 2011; Szentagotai & Freeman, 2007).

The theory and practice of REBT are based on the ABC explanatory sequence of emotional disturbance. In the ABC model, the A stands for "activating event," B stands for an evaluative "belief" about A, and C stands for the consequences (emotional or behavioral) that one experiences (David et al., 2005). Clinicians provide psychoeducation of the ABC model to parents and help them to apply that knowledge to themselves as parents. By having parents understand the ABC model, they will learn that their negative emotional response (e.g., anger, stress, depression) derives from how they consider and evaluate these negative life events rather than by the events themselves (Ellis, Gordon, Neenan, & Palmer, 1997). The ABC connection is fundamental to eliciting therapeutic change. The ABC model of REBT with parents will be briefly explained through examples provided below.

Typically, parents may tend to believe that it is the situation that they are in (A) that causes their emotional responses or consequences (C). As an example, a parent may incorrectly make the causal link: "If my children would just listen to me, I wouldn't have to get angry at them and then yell at them." The parents are making a causal connection between their children's behaviors and their emotional and behavioral responses as parents. The model of REBT proposes that there is a middle step between the activating event (*A*, their children's behavior) and the consequences (*C*, anger and yelling), in which the A is evaluated by the parent, giving rise to these consequences. This middle evaluative component is the beliefs and is the *B* of the model. These are the beliefs, evaluations, or cognitions that the parent has about the activating events (Ellis et al., 1997). There can be considerable variability in how parents may evaluate and interpret these events. Some parents may have beliefs that would be considered to be healthy and flexible in nature (rational belief; rB), while others may have thoughts that are dysfunctional or inflexible (irrational belief; iB) (Ellis et al., 1997). These healthy rational beliefs lead to healthy or typical affective and behavioral functioning, while unhealthy irrational beliefs often lead to unhealthy affective and behavioral functioning (DiGiuseppe et al., 2013).

In the example provided above in response to their children's behavior, the parent who yells at and gets angry with their children may believe "She *should* listen to me." The *should* would be considered to be an iB as it is leading to negative and unhealthy emotional states and parenting strategies. It is also considered to be an iB, as it is inconsistent with reality (i.e., they aren't listening) and holding that belief is not useful for them. Alternatively, a parent who responds in a different manner, both affectively and behaviorally, may have a different interpretation of the same behavior (i.e., child not listening). These parents may still want to change their child's behavior but may have a rB such as "While I really *want* my child to listen to me, getting angry does not help her listen, makes me more upset, and just causes me more difficulties." Parents who engage in healthier affective states (e.g., annoyance as opposed to anger) may still try and change their child's behavior and will be in a better position to make better parenting decisions as opposed to the parents who endorse those illogical, unhealthy, dysfunctional ideas about their child's behavior.

The C within the ABC model represents the consequences that one experiences as a function of their beliefs (Bs) about the activating events (A) (MacLaren et al., 2015). Ellis argued that emotional or behavioral Cs that develop as a result from irrational beliefs are considered to be unhealthy, while those that develop from more flexible rational beliefs are more healthy for the individual (Ellis et al., 1997). In the same example, the parent who endorses irrational beliefs related to the child's behavior (i.e., not listening) may experience an unhealthy emotion (anger) and may then engage in poor parenting practices (e.g., yelling or corporal punishment) in an effort to change their child's behavior. Alternatively, the parent who had more healthy beliefs or rational ways of thinking may feel frustrated at their child's behavior instead of anger, and their choice of parenting strategies may be more effective both in their choice and implementation as they are not directly interfered with by their own unhealthy negative emotional state.

Upon helping clients recognize their irrational beliefs, the clinician works with them to actively challenge and dispute (D) these beliefs through a variety of cognitive, emotive, and behavioral techniques (DiGiuseppe et al., 2013). The process of disputation allows clients the opportunity to recognize that the way they were thinking about certain adversities was unhealthy, illogical, and not consistent with reality. Upon having the client recognize this, clinicians work with clients to replace these unhealthy iBs with more healthy rBs (Ellis et al., 1997) which in turn will lead to more appropriate and productive emotions and behaviors.

Research on RE-CBT with Parents

There are a number of evidence-based parenting programs that have resulted in improved child and parent outcomes. Many have followed a more traditional behavioral approach, while more contemporary programs have included a cognitive component or have also targeted stress reduction. There is considerable support for behavioral parent training (BPT; Evans, Owens, & Bunford, 2014) where clinicians offer direct training to parents on strategies to handle their children's behavior (Forgatch & Patterson, 2010; Raghibi, Fouladi, & Bakhshani, 2014). These programs often target effective communication, use of a reward and consequence system, establishing clear rules and expectations, use of time-out, etc. While these approaches are effective, it is important to consider that they do not work for all parents and that perhaps what makes it challenging for some is the fact that they may be experiencing any number of negative affective states, which may interfere with their performance of these parenting skills. As such, clinical work with parents may want to integrate direct work in teaching effective parenting skills while also teaching a rational emotive-cognitive behavioral approach to reduce stress and other negative emotions, increasing ability to execute these skills.

The research on cognitive behavioral therapy with parents is quite impressive as a whole, and over the last 15 years, we have seen the empirical support for REBT with parents grow. Both approaches have been repeatedly examined in terms of the impact of REBT and CBT on parenting affect, parenting practices, and child behavior.

Several recent studies have looked at the effectiveness of CBT approaches with several populations. A recent study by Wong and colleagues (2018) examined the impact of a group CBT-based program on parental cognitions, stress, and self-efficacy among Chinese parents of children with ADHD. The authors reported small to moderate effects on most of the outcome variables at two time points (posttreatment and follow-up) and recommend that group CBT be considered for parents with ADHD children. To look at if there is any additive component of a CBT-based approach, Sanders and McFarland (2000) contrasted a behavioral family intervention (BFI) with a cognitive behavioral family intervention (CBFI) in an effort to reduce the depression reported by mothers and disruptive behavior problems. While there were no differences between treatments in terms of reducing maternal depression and child behavior at post-intervention, a difference did emerge at a 6-month follow-up with 53% of the families in the CBFI condition showing reliable reductions in both areas compared to only 13% in the BFI (13%) condition. These results may highlight the additive value of integrating CBT in the treatment of parental depression and during parent training.

In what is probably the most comprehensive review of "cognitively enhanced" behavioral parent programs (EPT), Gavita and Joyce (2008) examined the effectiveness of group-based parenting interventions in reducing children's disruptive behavior and parental distress. The results gathered from a sample of 238 parents lend considerable support for the rationale to include rational emotive and cognitive behavioral strategies into more traditional parent training programs. The enhanced condition had a small effect ($d = 0.25$) in comparison with the more standard treatment program on child disruptive behavior, but (and perhaps more interesting) they reported that parents in the EPT condition were more improved in terms of parenting practices compared to the standard behavioral programs (at both post-intervention ($d = 0.25$) and follow-up ($d = 0.36$). These results offer support and encouragement for further research that examines specific cognitions as well as strategies to effectively change them to lead to behavioral and affective change in parents and ultimately their children.

In trying to understand the mechanism of change, Jiang and colleagues (2018) looked at whether parent cognitions are related to short- and long-term changes in parenting behaviors during treatment for children with ADHD-I. Among their findings they reported that positive and negative posttreatment parenting outcomes were related to improvements in parent cognitive errors and lend support for the possibility of the role of parent cognitions as mediators of treatment effects on parenting.

In sum, the current research supports the need to target cognitions in clinical work with parents, but additional research is needed to determine how these changes in thinking occur. In the next section, the mechanism of change will be discussed through an RE-CBT lens, with a focus on the specific approaches to challenging unhealthy beliefs and developing more adaptive ways of thinking, feeling, and behaving.

RE-CBT with Parents

The integration of parents in the clinical work with youth is not new, and many treatment programs recognize the important role that parents play in their child's development and seek to integrate them into treatment. Direct clinical treatment of the child alone is often limited if the context in which the behavior occurs does not change. Therefore, RE-CBT can be applied in a number of ways with parents to assist in positive affective and behavioral changes for them and their children. Prior to beginning any formal RE-CBT with parents, it is important that clinicians provide parents with psychoeducation about *why* children misbehave and how their role as parents is important in facilitating change. Working with parents to conduct an analysis of their child's behavior has led to positive treatment outcomes (Miller & Lee, 2013). Clinicians work with parents to help them recognize environmental variables that are maintaining their children's behavior. This will include their current and past parent practices. Clinicians can illustrate to parents the cyclical nature of how their child behaviors impact their behaviors and vice versa. Similarly, parents can gain insight into how their practices may maintain child behavior and impact their children's functioning. Then, offering psychoeducation as to what are effective behavioral strategies for their specific children can assist in discerning if the parents did not know effective parenting techniques or were aware of them but just had difficulty implementing them in a consistent and effective manner. Finally, it is important for clinicians to enhance the parent's knowledge and the model of RE-CBT as it applies to both parents and children. By helping parents understand how the beliefs that they may have about their role as parents or about their child are related to their emotional and behavioral responses, they may then be able to determine if they are prepared for clinical work targeting their affective and behavioral choices.

As stated earlier, parents who may be experiencing unhealthy negative emotions such as anger, anxiety, depression, or guilt may be challenged to effectively implement adaptive parenting practices which may result in the development of emotional and behavioral problems in childhood (Kurasaki & Terjesen, 2012). RE-CBT with parents recognizes that when parents experience unhealthy negative emotions, they can be more likely to engage in ineffective negative parenting practices, which may create, maintain, or contribute to children social-emotional difficulties (Kurasaki & Terjesen, 2012). The processes by which we work on changing these unhealthy negative emotions and behaviors to healthier ones involve the RE-CBT clinician working with parents to identify, challenge, and change these irrational beliefs sustaining unhealthy negative emotions and behaviors among parents. Further, clinicians may want to consider parent affect and cognitions as it relates not only to their ability to intervene with their children but also from their ability to benefit from clinical work. That is, in RE-CBT, clinicians would benefit from considering how the parent's irrational beliefs may not only impact their ability to implement change in their home but also prevent their participation in the treatment plan (i.e., "It's too difficult to do this").

In the next section, specific irrational beliefs parents experience will be broken down through the RE-CBT model, and additional information on how clinicians can differentiate how to work with parental inferences as opposed to parental evaluations will be provided.

Parent Irrational Beliefs

There are a number of parent irrational beliefs that are consistent with the REBT model and have been linked to parent emotional responses (Bernard, 1990; Kurasaki, 2009). Within the REBT framework, there are four core categories of irrational beliefs: demandingnesss, awfulizing, frustration intolerance, and global evaluations of human worth (DiGiuseppe et al., 2013). Each of these beliefs will be discussed below with clinical strategies on how to assist parents in challenging these beliefs and develop newer healthier ones.

Demandingness

In regard to parenting, parent demands may be seen to be rigid, unrealistic, and absolute expectations of themselves as parents, of their children, or of others (e.g., partners or extended family members). Bernard (1990) offered examples of parent irrational demands: "My child *should* behave well and do what I say" or "My child *must* do well in everything" (Bernard, 1990, p. 300). Parents who strongly hold on to these irrational demands may often experience anger and as a result may make ineffective parenting decisions. Each type of demand endorsed by a parent may lead to different emotional experiences and behavioral outcomes. As an example, when parents hold demands about their children (e.g., "They should listen to me!"), they may experience anger as a result and then engage in ineffective parenting strategies like corporal punishment. Alternatively, parents who have demands about their roles as parents (e.g., "I should be a better parent!") may experience guilt or depression.

Awfulizing

Awfulizing beliefs are considered to be exaggerations of negative consequences that individuals may not consider to be "terrible" and "awful" in nature. These beliefs may be a precursor to parents having unhealthy negative emotions, and an example of such a belief for parents may be "It's awful that my child has a problem" (Bernard, 1990, p. 300).

Some parents may consider their child's behavior as well as their own inability to effectively manage the behavior as "awful." These catastrophic-type thoughts may lead to parents experiencing anxiety, depression, and even guilt. As an example, parents of children diagnosed with autism spectrum disorder (ASD) may have irrational catastrophic beliefs regarding the diagnosis, the child, and themselves as parents. Upon hearing of their child's diagnosis, parents may blame themselves and believe "This is *awful* and it is all my fault" and experience depression. When considering some of the learning challenges that their child may experience going forward, parents may catastrophize and awfulize about the implications of the diagnosis. "This is the *worst* thing that could ever happen to a child. This is horrible" are common irrational beliefs of many parents.

Frustration intolerance

The REBT model consists of another type of irrational belief that is called frustration intolerance (FI; DiGiuseppe et al., 2013). Earlier, FI was referred to as low frustration tolerance (LFT) and was characterized as an intolerance for discomfort. Parents with FI often would have irrational beliefs such as "It is *too hard* to solve my child's problems" (Bernard, 1990) or "I *cannot stand* my child's behaviors" which may lead to a number of unhealthy emotional experiences. FI may present itself in extreme forms in regard to their child's behavior as well as their own. They may also have beliefs about implementing behavioral strategies to manage their child's behavior ("This is too hard! I can't stand this!") as well as the effort required to manage their children's behavior and have more of an FI philosophy as it relates to parenting (e.g., "Parenting shouldn't be so hard. I can't stand all that I have to do."). Finally, we have found that some parenting choices are driven by FI for the judgment of others. That is, when a child is tantruming in front of others, parents may think that they cannot stand others judging them and may give in to the child's behavior, which further reinforces the negative behavior of the child or use more harsh parenting strategies to attempt to immediately terminate the child's tantrum.

Ratings of Worth

The last category of irrational beliefs involves global ratings of worth and can be directed at their children or at themselves as parents. These irrational beliefs exist on the premise that a parent or others can be given a single rating of value or worth. An example of this would be "I am worthless because my child has so many problems" (Grieger & Boyd, 1983). When considering their child's behavior, parents may compare themselves to other parents and think "I'm not a good parent. I'm such an idiot. I cannot do anything right as a parent and I am no good." As a consequence, they may experience signs of depression and develop a learned helplessness mindset and stop engaging with their child as no matter what they do, they think it will be ineffective.

In addition to ratings of self, parents may rate or evaluate their partner (e.g., "They're stupid") or their child ("they are bad!"), which may lead to extreme negative feelings that may further impact their relationship and familial functioning. In both cases it is important when working with parents to discuss the concept of rating oneself as opposed to rating one's behavior. This is particularly important with parents, as they may in fact have made some poor parental decisions that were ineffective. By rating themselves as *totally stupid*, as opposed to their behavior being rated as ineffective, it may lead to unhealthy emotions and behavioral decisions.

Disputing/challenging

After collaboratively working to identify the automatic thoughts and irrational beliefs of parents, clinicians may want to challenge these beliefs to develop newer, more logical, functional ways of thinking. Within the REBT framework, these challenges are referred to as disputation (DiGiuseppe et al., 2013). The different types of disputing described in the REBT literature (i.e., empirical, logical, semantic, heuristic/functional; see Bernard, 2004) can be used to identify, challenge, and change the iBs to rBs. Below we offer examples as to how clinicians may wish to challenge each of the aforementioned irrational beliefs when working with parents.

Disputing frustration intolerance can be challenging in working with parents as some of their children's behaviors can be VERY challenging. When disputing iBs, it is important to validate a lower level of their affective experience (e.g., annoyance as opposed to anger) while also pointing out the differences between something being difficult to handle and something being TOO difficult to deal with. It is recommended that the clinician acknowledge that certain aspects of parenting are more difficult than others, while reminding them that believing it is *too* difficult only sets up another emotional barrier to applying effective parenting strategies. Through questioning, parents may report other times that they have perceived their child's behavior as "too difficult and unbearable." The clinician may use an evidence-based (empirical) approach toward challenging their FI beliefs. That is, they may say: "While I see that you thought it was too difficult to deal with in the past, you did handle it, albeit with frustration." This dispute may be combined with a functional challenge of the belief with the clinician asking: "Is thinking this is TOO hard helping you deal with this? Does thinking this way lead to more difficulties for you?" Having parents understand that while their child's behavior may in fact be difficult and they don't like it, they can stand it, may assist in reducing negative affect in the moment and increasing implementation of positive parenting practices in response to their child's behavior.

Having parents work to identify and dispute "catastrophic" thinking begins by first having parents recognize that through telling themselves a number of awfulizing thoughts (e.g., "This is the WORST thing ever"), it will lead to both unhealthy affect (i.e., anxiety, depression) and ineffective parenting. Having parents empirically evaluate just how *bad* the situation would be and challenge these irrational beliefs from a functional (i.e., "Does thinking this way help me deal with this problem?) and semantic (i.e., "How do I define awful?; What are the things that are truly bad and does this meet that standard?") approach may likely reduce their level of negative affect.

In disputing the demands of parents, a combination of functional disputes (i.e., "How does thinking he should listen and getting angry help me deal with my children?") can be especially helpful when combined with an empirical dispute (i.e., "I am saying he *should* listen, but what do I know is true….he doesn't!") and logical one (i.e., "Does my demand they listen make sense?").

Disputing global self-ratings (i.e., "My worth as a parent depends on my child's behavior") is critical in working with parents. Having parents consider if thinking this way is valid (empirical) and does it help them reach their goals (functional) may lead to more adaptive affective and parent behavioral experiences. Working toward accepting that their worth is independent from both their child's behavior and their own will lead to more healthy negative emotions and more effective parenting decisions. Having parents recognize that we are complex and that everyone has good and bad traits/behaviors can help toward changing these beliefs.

Development of Rational Beliefs

Finally, after working with parents to catch and challenge their iBs, the RE-CBT model seeks to replace these faulty patterns of thinking with healthier rational self-statements. These rBs are theoretically and empirically a variation of the unhealthy irrational beliefs. That is, if clients change the belief of "It's terrible my children don't listen to me" to "Hopefully they listen next time," that does not directly replace the evaluation (awfulizing) of their child's behavior. As an example if a parent believes that "My children *should* listen to me," the clinician would help the parent challenge/dispute that thought (e.g., "Why should they? What is their history of listening? Does thinking that they should and getting angry when they don't helping you to think that way? Do they listen?); the clinician would work with the parent to develop a healthier, empirically sound, logical, rational alternative. An example of this may be "While I really would like my children to listen to me, I know that they do not always, and getting angry doesn't help them or me. I don't like it but can deal with it and try and handle it better going forward." When working with parents on developing a rational alternative, it is important to acknowledge what negative affect would also be healthy (i.e., frustration as opposed to anger) and validate what their goals are. It is important to also model having the rB be stronger in tone and conviction over the initial iB.

Special Considerations

When using RE-CBT with parents, there are a number of factors that warrant consideration. First, the age of child and the nature of the problem may impact parents differently. Before providing RE-CBT or any psychological services, practitioners would benefit from considering the challenges of parenting at their child's respective stage of development. Thus, RE-CBT practitioners may wish to gain an understanding of the mental and physical state of their clients' parent and consider unique activating events, specific irrational beliefs, and common maladaptive emotions parents commonly experience. For example, infancy and toddlerhood require high levels of parent attention and involvement. At these stages, children are significantly dependent on parents to address their basic physical and psychological needs. Parents often describe this joyful period as one with fatigue, worry, and stress. For example, as new mothers experience biological changes as a result of pregnancy and birth, they may also experience the realization that many maternal activities do not go as planned. By being cognizant of postpartum depression and parents with little environmental resources, clinicians may want to address these factors. New parents may hold irrational beliefs or unrealistic expectations about their performance as parents and the impact on their child. For example, mothers may experience guilt or shame around difficulties with breastfeeding. Parents may also experience high levels of anxiety for their child's well-being and less relationship satisfaction as they can be frustrated when they are unable to help soothe their crying child. Often times, these parents place unhealthy demands on themselves and hold self-downing, awfulizing, or low frustration tolerance beliefs such as "I must be able to breastfeed," "My baby should not be crying this much," or "I am a bad mother/father because my baby won't sleep or eat" and "I can't take the crying." This coupled with lack of sleep and less time to care for ones self can make this time period extremely difficult. Toddlerhood can be an equally stressful period for parents. This period is characterized by many changes in cognitive, linguistic, physical, and emotional functioning within the child (Lieberman, 1995). At this young age, it can feel like an emotional rollercoaster, with the word "no" frequently heard in the household (Lieberman). As toddlers are constantly exploring their environment, this stage continues to involve high levels of vigilance, keeping the child stimulated and safe, while teaching them new skills like toileting. These requirements can coincide with many healthy and unhealthy emotions of varying intensity. Parents may experience anger toward their child's behavior, which is accompanied by unhealthy demands and frustration intolerance. Further, when a child has delays in their developmental milestones, parents can experience heighted levels of distress. They may blame themselves for their child's difficulties, hold unhealthy demands about their child's functioning, and ultimately experience anger, depression, anxiety, shame, or guilt.

The school-aged years of development span childhood and adolescence. Children face the demands of compulsory education and increase their social networks. Parent involvement expands beyond caring for basic needs, to assisting their child to be contributing members of society. During these years, supervision of their child's behavior becomes progressively more challenging as the child spends less time in the home. Parents can often feel unhealthy negative emotions around their child's increased autonomy, school performance, or with significant changes like going off to college. These years can also be difficult when a child experiences learning difficulties and engages in high risk or self-harm behaviors. Parents may hold irrational beliefs toward themselves or their child's behavior, some of which could include "My child should respect my house rules," "They should be doing better in school," and "I can't stand it when he/she does that." RE-CBT practitioners want to be mindful of secondary negative emotions. For example, parents may experience guilt or shame about their own negative reactions to their child's behavior.

RE-CBT practitioners can assist parents in handling the challenges of parenting by considering the unique experiences they face across their child's development. These diverse activating events can often be marked with unhealthy negative emotions and dysfunctional parenting behaviors that can impact parent-child interactions and overall family functioning. Therefore, clinical work may improve when RE-CBT practitioners familiarize themselves with these stage-specific situations to understand what the parent is experiencing. This will allow for the challenge of specific irrational beliefs and replacement of more healthy ways of thinking. Not only will this reduce unhealthy negative emotions, but also it can make parents more apt to engage in positive parenting practices, seek additional resources, and make effective parenting decisions.

RE-CBT therapists may also want to consider parental expectations about their child's behavior and examine if their expectations are developmentally appropriate.

In addition to helping the parents learn adaptive strategies to manage affect and behavior, RE-CBT may also help parents manage their emotions more effectively beyond the role of parenting. That is, the principles in place and clinical skills learned during RE-CBT with parents may generalize to other areas of the parent's life (e.g., work, finances, friendships) and may then lead to adaptive response in those areas which may in turn help them in their role as parents.

Summary

Given the high rates of negative affective states among parents, the RE-CBT approach appears to be a useful tool to promote healthier emotional functioning in parents, which can increase implementation of child behavioral interventions. The RE-CBT model may help parents become more in control of their emotions by identifying and subsequently changing their unhealthy beliefs and increasing their ability to implement effective behavioral strategies. Further, they will be modeling effective ways of thinking, feeling, and behaving for their children.

Test Yourself Questions

1. Clinically, what would be some important areas to consider before introducing a behavioral strategy for parents in working with their child's behavior?
2. What variables may impact on the effectiveness of RE-CBT with parents?
3. How would you dispute the belief that a parent may have about? "My children NEVER listen to me and I *can't* stand it!"

References

Abbeduto, L., Seltzer, M. M., Shattuck, P., Krauss, M. W., Orsmond, G., & Murphy, M. M. (2004). Psychological well-being and coping in mothers of youths with autism, Down syndrome, or fragile X syndrome. *American Journal of Mental Retardation, 109*(3), 237–254.

Affrunti, N. W., & Woodruff-Borden, J. (2015). Parental perfectionism and overcontrol: Examining mechanisms in the development of child anxiety. *Journal of Abnormal Child Psychology, 43*, 517–529. https://doi.org/10.1007/s10802-014-9914-5

Ateah, C., & Durrant, J. (2005). Maternal use of physical punishment in response to child misbehavior: Implications for child abuse prevention. *Child Abuse & Neglect, 29*, 169–185. https://doi.org/10.1016/j.chiabu.2004.10.010

Baker, B. L., Blacher, J., Crnic, K. A., & Edelbrock, C. (2002). Behavior problems and parenting stress in families of three-year-old children with and without developmental delays. *American Journal on Mental Retardation, 107*(6), 433–444.

Baker, B.L., Blacher, J. and Olsson, M.B. (2005), Preschool children with and without developmental delay: behaviour problems, parents' optimism and well-being. *Journal of Intellectual Disability Research, 49*, 575–590. https://doi.org/10.1111/j.1365-2788.2005.00691.x.

Barker, E. T., Hartley, S. L., Seltzer, M. M., Floyd, F. J., Greenberg, J. S., & Orsmond, G. I. (2011). Trajectories of emotional well-being in mothers of adolescents and adults with autism. *Developmental psychology, 47*(2), 551–561. https://doi.org/10.1037/a0021268

Ben-Porath, D. D. (2010). Dialectical behavior therapy applied to parent skills training: Adjunctive treatment for parents with difficulties in affect regulation. *Cognitive and Behavioral Practice, 17*(4), 458–465.

Benson, P. R., & Karlof, K. L. (2009). Anger, stress proliferation, and depressed mood among parents of children with ASD: A longitudinal replication. *Journal of Autism and Developmental Disorders, 39*(2), 350–362. https://doi.org/10.1007/s10803-008-0632-0.

Bernard, M. E. (1990). Rational-emotive therapy with children and adolescents: Treatment strategies. *School Psychology Review, 19*, 294–304.

Bernard, M.E. (2004). *The REBT therapist's pocket companion for working with children and adolescents* (pp. 245). New York: Albert Ellis Institute.

Biederman, J., Petty, C., Faraone, S. V., Henin, A., Hirshfeld-Becker, D., Pollack, M., et al. (2006). Effects of parental anxiety disorders in children at high risk for panic disorder: A controlled study. *Journal of Affective Disorders, 94*, 191–197.

Burstein, M., & Ginsburg, G. S. (2010). The effect of parental modeling of anxious behaviors and cognitions in school-aged children: An experimental pilot study. *Behaviour Research and Therapy, 48*(6), 506–515.

Compas, B. E., Forehand, R., Thigpen, J. C., Keller, G., Hardcastle, E. J., Cole, D. A., et al. (2011). Family group cognitive-behavioral preventive intervention for families of depressed parents: 18- and 24-month outcomes. *Journal of Consulting and Clinical Psychology, 79*, 488–499.

Creswell, C., & O'Connor, T. G. (2006). Anxious cognitions in children: An exploration of associations and mediators. *British Journal of Developmental Psychology, 24*, 761–766. https://doi.org/10.1348/026151005X70418

Dabrowska, A., & Pisula, E. (2010). Parenting stress and coping styles in mothers and fathers of pre-school children with autism and Down syndrome. *Journal of Intellectual Disabilities, 54*(3), 266–280.

David, D., Szentagotai, A., Eva, K., & Macavei, B. (2005). A synopsis of rational-emotive behavior therapy (REBT): Fundamental and applied research. *Journal of Rational-Emotive & Cognitive-Behavior Therapy, 23*(3), 175–221. https://doi.org/10.1007/s10942-005-0011-0

David, D., Szentagotai, A., Lupu, V. and Cosman, D. (2008). Rational emotive behavior therapy, cognitive therapy, and medication in the treatment of major depressive disorder: A randomized clinical trial, posttreatment outcomes, and six-month follow-up. *Journal of Clinical Psychology, 64*, 728–746. https://doi.org/10.1002/jclp.20487

David, D., Cotet, C., Matu, S., Mogoase, C., & Stefan, S. (2018). 50 years of rational- emotive and cognitive-behavioral therapy: A systematic review and meta-analysis. *Journal of Clinical Psychology, 74*(3), 304–318. https://doi.org/10.1002/jclp.22514

Del Vecchio, T., Jablonka, O., DiGiuseppe, R., Notti, J., & David, O. (2017). Psychometric evaluation of the parent anger scale. *Journal of Child and Family Studies, 26*, 3013–3025. https://doi.org/10.1007/s10826-017-0824-3

Del Vecchio, T., & O'Leary, S. G. (2008). Predicting maternal discipline responses to early child aggression: The role of cognitions and affect. *Parenting: Science and Practice, 8*(3), 240–256. https://doi.org/10.1080/15295190802204827

DiGiuseppe, R. A., Doyle, K. A., Dryden, W., & Backx, W. (2013). *A practitioner's guide to rational-emotive behavior therapy*. Oxford: Oxford University Press.

Dix, T., & Meunier, L. N. (2009). Depressive symptoms and parenting competence: An analysis of 13 regulatory processes. *Developmental Review, 29*(1), 45–68.

Dryden, W. (2015). *Rational emotive behaviour therapy*. London: Routledge. https://doi.org/10.4324/9781315749433

Ellis, A., Gordon, J., Neenan, M., & Palmer, S. (1997). *Stress counseling: A rational emotive behavior approach*. New York: Springer Publishing Company.

England, M. J., & Sim, L. J. (Eds.). (2009). *Depression in parents, parenting, and children: Opportunities to improve identification, treatment, and prevention*. Washington, DC: National Academies Press.

Evans, S. W., Owens, J. S., & Bunford, N. (2014). Evidence-based psychosocial treatments for children and adolescents with attention-deficit/hyperactivity disorder. *Journal of Clinical Child & Adolescent Psychology, 43*, 527–551. https://doi.org/10.1080/15374416.2017.1390757

Fisak, B., Holderfield, K., Douglas-Osborn, E., & Cartwright-Hatton, S. (2012). What do parents worry about? Examination of the construct of parent worry and the relation to parent and child anxiety. *Behavioural and Cognitive Psychotherapy, 40*(5), 542–557. https://doi.org/10.1017/S1352465812000410

Ford, P. W. (2008). *Effect of methodological improvements and study quality on REBT treatment outcome research since 1990: A meta-analysis* (Unpublished Doctoral dissertation). St. John's University, New York.

Forehand, R., Thigpen, J. C., Parent, J., Hardcastle, E. J., Bettis, A., & Compas, B. E. (2012). The role of parent depressive symptoms in positive and negative parenting in a preventive intervention. *Journal of Family Psychology, 26*(4), 532–541. https://doi.org/10.1037/a0028406

Forgatch, M. S., & Patterson, G. R. (2010). Parent Management Training—Oregon Model: An intervention for antisocial behavior in children and adolescents. In J. R. Weisz & A. E. Kazdin (Eds.), *Evidence-based psychotherapies for children and adolescents* (pp. 159–177). New York: The Guilford Press.

Fukushima-Flores, M., & Miller, L. (2011). FRIENDS Parent Project: Effectiveness of parent training in reducing parent anxiety in a universal prevention program for anxiety symptoms in school children. *Behaviour Change, 28*(2), 57–74. https://doi.org/10.1375/bech.28.2.57

Garber, J., Keiley, M. K., & Martin, N. C. (2002). Developmental trajectories of adolescents' depressive symptoms: Predictors of change. *Journal of Consulting and Clinical Psychology, 70*(1), 79–95. https://doi.org/10.1037/0022-006X.70.1.79

Gavita, O. A., & Joyce, M. R. (2008). A review of the effectiveness of group cognitively enhanced behavioral based parent programs designed for reducing disruptive behavior in children. *Journal of Cognitive and Behavioral Psychotherapies, 8*(2), 185–199.

Ginsburg, G. S., & Schlossberg, M. C. (2002). Family-based treatment of childhood anxiety disorders. *International Review of Psychiatry, 14*(2), 143–154. https://doi.org/10.1080/09540260220132662

Grieger, R. M., & Boyd, J. D. (1983). Childhood anxieties, fears, and phobias. In A. Ellis & M. E. Bernard (Eds.), *Rational-emotive approaches to the problems of childhood* (pp. 211–237). New York: Plenum Press.

Hardcastle, E. J., Bettis, A., & Compas, B. E. (2012). The role of parent depressive symptoms in positive and negative parenting in a preventive intervention. *Journal of Family Psychology, 26*(4), 532–541. https://doi.org/10.1037/a0028406

Harris, S., Davies, M. F., & Dryden, W. (2006). An experimental test of a core REBT hypothesis: Evidence that irrational beliefs lead to physiological as well as psychological arousal. *Journal of Rational-Emotive and Cognitive-Behavioral Therapy, 24*, 101–111. https://doi.org/10.1007/s10942-005-0019-5

Hollon, S. D., & DiGiuseppe, R. (2010). Cognitive psychotherapies. In J. C. Norcross & G. VandenBos (Eds.), *History of psychotherapy: Continuity and change* (2nd ed.). Washington, DC: American Psychological Association.

Jiang, Y., Haack, L. M., Delucchi, K., Rooney, M., Hinshaw, S. P., McBurnett, K., et al. (2018). Improved parent cognitions relate to immediate and follow-up treatment outcomes for children with ADHD-predominantly inattentive presentation. *Behavior Therapy, 49*(4), 567–579.

Joyce, M. R. (1990). Rational-emotive parent consultation. *School Psychology Review, 19*, 304–315.

Kuckertz, J. M., Mitchell, C., & Wiggins, J. L. (2018). Parenting mediates the impact of maternal depression on child internalizing symptoms. *Depression & Anxiety, 35*, 89–97. https://doi.org/10.1002/da.22688

Kurasaki, R. E. (2009). *The role of parental cognition, negative affect, and behavior on predicting child academic achievement and social-emotional well-being*. ProQuest.

Kurasaki, R. E., & Terjesen, M. D. (2012). Helping couples deal with chronic medical or mental illness of a partner or child. In A. Vernon (Ed.), *Cognitive and rational-emotive behavior therapy with couples*. New York: Springer.

Leung, D. W., & Slep, A. M. S. (2006). Predicting inept discipline: The role of parental depressive symptoms, anger, and attributions. *Journal of Consulting and Clinical Psychology, 74*(3), 524–534. https://doi.org/10.1037/0022-006X.74.3.524

Lieberman, A. F. (1995). *The emotional life of a toddler*. New York: Free Press.

MacLaren, C., Doyle, K. A., & DiGiuseppe, R. (2015). Rational emotive behavior therapy: theory and practice. In H. Tinsley, S. H. Lease, & N. S. Giffin-Wiersma (Eds.), *Contemporary theory and practice in counseling and psychotherapy* (pp. 233–263). Los Angeles, CA: Sage.

McStay, R. L., Dissanayake, C., Scheeren, A., Koot, H. M., & Begeer, S. (2014). Parenting stress and autism: The role of age, autism severity, quality of life and problem behavior of children and adolescents with autism. *Autism, 18*(5), 502–510.

Miller, F. G., & Lee, D. L. (2013). Do functional behavioral assessments improve intervention effectiveness for students diagnosed with ADHD? A single-subject meta-analysis. *Journal of Behavior Education, 22*, 253–282. https://doi.org/10.1007/s10864-013-9174-4

Moore, P. S., Whaley, S. E., & Sigman, M. (2004). Interactions between mothers and children: Impacts of maternal and child anxiety. *Journal of Abnormal Psychology, 113*(3), 471–476. https://doi.org/10.1037/0021-843X.113.3.471

Mustillo, S., Dorsey, S., Conover, K., & Burns, B. (2011). Parental depression and child outcomes: The mediating effects of abuse and neglect. *Journal of Marriage and Family, 73*, 164–180. https://doi.org/10.2307/29789565

Raghibi, M., Fouladi, S., & Bakhshani, N. M. (2014). Parent training and behavior therapy on behaviors of children with attention deficit-hyperactivity disorder. *Health Scope, 3*. https://doi.org/10.17795/jhealthscope-15418

Resch, J., Elliott, T., & Benz, M. (2012). Depression among parents of children with disabilities. *Families, Systems & Health, 30*, 291–301. https://doi.org/10.1037/a0030366

Sanders, M. R., & McFarland, M. (2000). Treatment of depressed mothers with disruptive children: A controlled evaluation of cognitive behavioral family intervention. *Behavior Therapy, 31*(1), 89–112. https://doi.org/10.1016/S0005-7894(00)80006-4

Sava, F. A., Maricutoiu, L. P., Rusu, S., Macsinga, I., & Virgă, D. (2011). Implicit and explicit self-esteem and irrational beliefs. *Journal of Cognitive and Behavioral Psychotherapies, 11*, 97–111.

Stith, S., Liu, T., Davies, L., Boykin, E., Alder, M., Harris, J., et al. (2009). Risk factors in child maltreatment: A meta-analytic review of the literature. *Aggression and Violent Behavior, 14*, 13–29. https://doi.org/10.1016/j.avb.2006.03.006

Szentagotai, A., & Freeman, A. (2007). An analysis of the relationship between irrational beliefs and automatic thought in predicting distress. *Journal of Cognitive and Behavioral Psychotherapies, 7*(1), 1–9.

van der Bruggen, C., Stams, G., & Bögels, S. (2008). Research review: The relation between child and parent anxiety and parental control: A meta-analytic review. *Journal of Child Psychology and Psychiatry, & Allied Disciplines, 49*, 1257–1269. https://doi.org/10.1111/j.1469-7610.2008.01898.x

Walling, B., Mills, R., & Freeman, W. (2006). Parenting cognitions associated with the use of psychological control. *Journal of Child and Family Studies, 16*, 642–659. https://doi.org/10.1007/s10826-006-9113-2

Witt, K. (2005). *The role of parental irrationality and child autism characteristics on parental stress level* (Unpublished Doctoral dissertation). St. John's University, New York.

Wolford, S. N., Cooper, A. N., & McWey, L. M. (2019). Maternal depression, maltreatment history, and child outcomes: The role of harsh parenting. *American Journal of Orthopsychiatry, 89*(2), 181–191. https://doi.org/10.1037/ort0000365

Wong, D. F. K., Ng, T. K., Ip, P. S. Y., Chung, M. L., & Choi, J. (2018). Evaluating the effectiveness of a GroupCBT for parents of ADHD children. *Journal of Child and Family Studies, 27*, 227–239. https://doi.org/10.1007/s10826-017-0868-4

Chapter 7
The Rational Emotive Behavior Therapy Approach to Working with Families

Olga Gulyayeva Fuller, Brooke Edelman, and Tamara Del Vecchio

Treatments that include family members, such as parents, grandparents, and siblings, are often considered the treatment of choice for childhood disorders (Carr, 2019). Family-based treatments are shown to be beneficial in reducing child distress and maladaptive behavior beyond outcomes from individual child therapy alone (e.g., Dowell & Ogles, 2010). Further, therapy incorporating other family members is considered the first line of treatment for youth conduct disorder, substance abuse, and eating disorders, producing better outcomes than individual therapy for each of these concerns (Borduin, Curtis, & Ronan, 2004; Eisler et al., 1997; McCart, Priester, Davies, & Azen, 2006; Stanton & Shadish, 1997). Family-based therapy may also be indicated for mood and anxiety disorders. Psychoeducational family treatment has been found to increase knowledge about childhood mood symptoms, improve family relationships, and decrease symptoms of depression and mania for children with mood disorders (Fristad, Goldberg-Arnold, & Gavazzi, 2002, 2003; Miklowitz et al., 2004; Pavuluri et al., 2004). Family therapy is as effective as individual therapy in the treatment of major depression among youth, leading to remission in two-thirds to three-quarters of cases at 6-month follow-up, and is more effective than individual therapy in maintaining posttreatment improvement (Stark, Banneyer, Wang, & Arora, 2012). Moreover, some reviews suggest that the effectiveness of family-based treatment for childhood anxiety disorders is more effective than individual therapy when parents also present with anxiety disorders (e.g., Barmish & Kendall, 2005).

In this chapter, we will describe the rational emotive behavior therapy (REBT) approach to families and review its effectiveness.

O. G. Fuller · B. Edelman · T. Del Vecchio (✉)
St. John's University, Queens, NY, USA
e-mail: delvecct@stjohns.edu

M. Bernard, M. D. Terjesen (eds.), *Rational-Emotive and Cognitive-Behavioral Approaches to Child and Adolescent Mental Health: Theory, Practice, Research, Applications*, https://doi.org/10.1007/978-3-030-53901-6_7

Overview of the Rational Emotive Behavioral Approach to Family Therapy

REBT was developed by Albert Ellis in 1955 and is rooted in Stoic philosophy and the idea that one's attitudes about life, rather than the events and experiences that a person has, are responsible for one's disturbance (Ellis, 1982). In a description of REBT philosophy, Dryden (2002, p. 349) quotes the philosopher Epictetus, "Men are disturbed not by things, but by the views which they take of them." Thus, REBT encourages a philosophic transformation in terms of the beliefs that individuals hold true and their related behaviors and emotions as the means for change (Ellis & Dryden, 1997). As with all cognitive behavioral therapies, REBT conceptualizes psychological distress in terms of the interplay between cognitions, emotions, and behaviors. REBT's approach to therapy places cognitions, or beliefs, at the core of all disturbance. REBT's A-B-C model (Fig. 7.1) suggests that beliefs (B) about an activating event (A) result in behavioral and emotional consequences (C).

Although REBT was initially developed and used with individuals, it can and has been readily applied to work with families (Ellis & Dryden, 1997). The rational emotive behavioral approach to working with families (REBT-F) emphasizes each individual's perception and interpretation of events within the family environment and the extent to which these individual beliefs penetrate the family system (Hutcheson, 2019). When working with families, the content of the As, Bs, and Cs focuses on activating events within the family context (Fig. 7.2), beliefs that each family member has about those events, and the emotional and behavioral consequences that they experience and exhibit as a result of those beliefs. If these beliefs

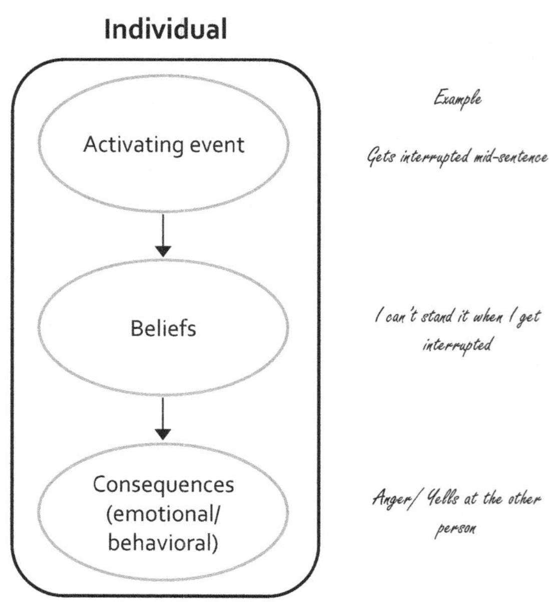

Fig. 7.1 The A-B-Cs of REBT

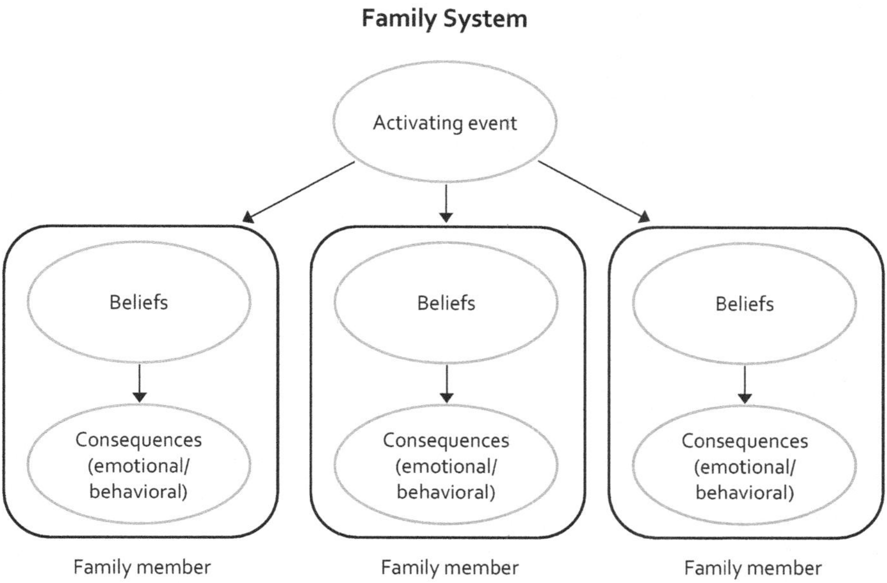

Fig. 7.2 The A-B-Cs of REBT-F

are rational (e.g., flexible, logical, nondogmatic, and grounded in evidence), then the Cs that follow will be adaptive, healthy, and functional (DiGiuseppe, Doyle, Dryden, & Backx, 2014). If the beliefs are irrational (e.g., rigid, inflexible, and dogmatic), then the consequences are likely to be dysfunctional, unhealthy, and maladaptive. While irrational beliefs may lead to family members experiencing anger, anxiety, or guilt, the endorsement of more flexible, rational ways of thinking will lead to healthy negative affective experiences like frustration, concern, or regret. Thus, the goal of therapy is to help family members recognize their irrational beliefs and replace them with flexible, logical beliefs. For example, a teenage son arrives home after curfew (A). The son thinks that he is generally a good kid and that one late arrival is not a big deal. However, his mother believes that her son's coming home late indicates the start of a trend toward risky behavior and starts having some "worst case scenario" thoughts and *catastrophizes* (B), and as a result, she feels worried and persistently questions her son about his whereabouts (C). On the other hand, his father believes that his son has disregarded his rules out of disrespect and he *shouldn't* do this (B), and as a result, he feels angry and argues with his son when he arrives home (C).

REBT-F groups irrational beliefs into four categories: demandingness, awfulizing, frustration intolerance, and global evaluations of worth (DiGiuseppe et al., 2014). Demandingness refers to the belief that things (events, actions, people, self) must be a certain way. Awfulizing refers to the belief, or pattern of beliefs, that an event or situation will have catastrophic, awful, horrible outcomes. Frustration intolerance (formerly called low frustration tolerance) refers to the belief that one cannot stand or tolerate a given event or situation. Global evaluations of

Table 7.1 Examples of irrational beliefs

Irrational belief	Example
Demandingness	*My parents should be fair* *My son must not disrespect me*
Awfulizing	*My daughter will end up homeless and destitute after failing all her classes because she does not study enough*
Frustration intolerance	*I can't work on our family's budget because it's too hard*
Global evaluations of worth	*My husband is a totally worthless, terrible person because he never comes home on time*

worth refer to the belief that the worth of oneself or others is contingent on a quality or aspect of that person (e.g., see Table 7.1).

In REBT-F, meta-emotional disturbance, or disturbance about one's disturbed emotions, often results in a secondary set of A-B-Cs (DiGiuseppe et al., 2014). For instance, a mother's guilt about how angry she was at her child yesterday may lead her to think "I'm a terrible mother," and then this irrational thought interferes with her ability to effectively set limits for her child. In these cases, a C (e.g., anger) serves as the A for another B (e.g., I'm a terrible mother) and a new C (e.g., guilt and ineffective limit setting). When working with families, it is important to also identify and understand how one family member's C may serve as the A for another member of the family. For instance, when a child argues with her brother (A), thinks "he shouldn't bother me all the time" (B), gets angry, and screams (C), her being angry and screaming (A) leads her mother to think "I can't deal with this" (B) and respond with anger (C). It is important for the clinician to work on identifying these patterns and interactions of As, Bs, and Cs not just within one person's experience but also between the various family members in the room (Fig. 7.3).

REBT-F in Practice

Assessment in REBT-F is emphasized both at the beginning of treatment as well as throughout therapy. To evaluate the functioning of family members, we would recommend that clinicians consider measures for the individual family members that reflect their personal areas of difficulty. That is, if one family member is experiencing considerable distress/anxiety within the context of the family, clinicians may want to assess this and monitor changes during the course of treatment. While there are no specific measures to evaluate the functioning of the family that were derived from REBT-F, clinicians may wish to consider other family functioning measures developed through other theoretical orientations. While a complete review of all family assessment measures is beyond the scope of the present chapter, the reader is referred to Hamilton and Carr (2016) to increase familiarity with the psychometrics of varied measures of family functioning.

Establishing and agreeing upon both individual and shared realistic goals for treatment is of utmost importance, as they act as motivating factors to encourage

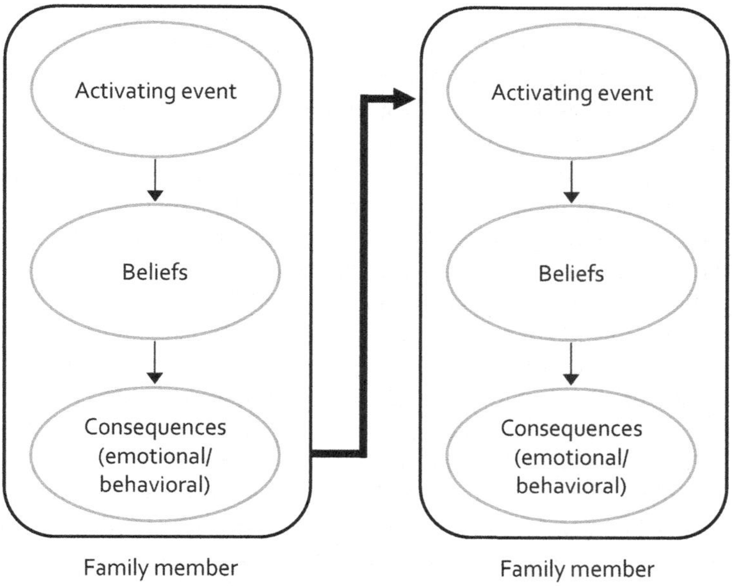

Fig. 7.3 A-B-C interactions between family members

change in each member of the family. REBT-F sessions are structured with agendas agreed upon and tailored to the goals of the family. For each session, if multiple goals are identified, one is selected as the target, and other goals are deferred. The therapist works to balance competing or opposing agendas of family members present in the session by noticing reactions of the individual family members and identifying the beliefs that are unique to individual family members as well as beliefs that are shared among the family (Friedberg, 2006). Ultimately, family members, with the therapist's assistance and guidance, come to a consensus about which goals to address first, with the understanding that some compromise and turn-taking may be necessary. The therapist emphasizes the need to address goals related to changing the beliefs of one or more members of the family rather than changing the activating event related to the family member's distress (Wachtler, 2019).

Once the A, B, and C of a specific situation that have led to conflict within the family have been identified, therapeutic focus is placed on establishing the B-C connection. The B-C connection is the concept that no one and nothing can *make* a person feel or act something (DiGiuseppe et al., 2014). It is common in colloquial conversation to say "he made me so angry" or "that movie made me depressed" – the A-C connection. However, letting go of the A-C connection belief is critical to REBT-F. At the core of REBT's view on disturbance is that one's thoughts and beliefs (B) about an activating event are responsible for that person's emotional and behavioral reaction to that event (C). If an individual holds on to the belief that factors outside himself are responsible for his emotions and the B-C connection is not established, then he does not accept responsibility for his own emotions and does not yet have the fundamental rationale for disputing irrational beliefs (that the only person who can make him feel a certain way is himself). The B-C connection is important in individual REBT therapy and perhaps even more so when working with families. Given how frequently family conflict involves blame of another family member (Alexander, 1973; Patterson, 1982), in REBT-F, the emphasis is placed on one's own emotional and behavioral responsibility.

Critical to its effectiveness is REBT-F's teaching of techniques to identify, dispute, and change irrational beliefs to more rational beliefs, thereby changing the behavioral and emotional consequences an individual has about a given situation or event. The role of the therapist is to guide the family members to identify and challenge dysfunctional beliefs about the family. Furthermore, the therapist demonstrates the mutuality of cognitions, behaviors, emotions, and family relationships.

REBT-F uses cognitive, emotive, and behavioral techniques to achieve the goal of helping the family dispute these beliefs, and thus, as with other forms of CBT, this process is collaborative, active, and directive. The therapist uses both Socratic and didactic approaches to present session content and to dispute and challenge irrational beliefs. Specifically, the therapist challenges irrational beliefs using strategies such as functional disputes, empirical disputes, psychoeducation, rational coping statements, role playing, inference chaining, Socratic questioning, and humor (Cluxton-Keller, 2011; DiGiuseppe et al., 2014). Examples are listed in Table 7.2.

REBT-F does not emphasize the absolute factual truth about an activating event or belief. That is, the clinician does not spend time trying to determine who is "correct" in their reporting as to what occurred but rather focuses on the beliefs and behavioral and emotional consequences associated with the perceived activating event. Clinicians work to reframe what the client reports ("They should leave me alone and when they don't it really angers me") to a healthier cognitive ("I understand that you really don't like when your parents get on you about completing

Table 7.2 Examples of disputations and challenges to irrational beliefs

Strategy	Example
Functional dispute	*How is this emotion/belief/behavior helping you?*
Empirical dispute	*What evidence/which facts support your belief?*
Psychoeducation	*Teach new rational beliefs/provide facts and information to facilitate formation of rational beliefs*
Rational coping statements	*Teach/ask family members to rehearse a succinct, rational statement to be used in place of the current irrational belief*
Role playing	*Asking a married couple to have the conversation as the other person and then provide feedback*
Inference chaining	*Asking a client who is anxious to suppose that the feared outcome they are imagining will come true, asking them to explain what that would mean for them, and repeating the process until irrational beliefs are identified and can be disputed*
Socratic questioning	*Asking leading questions to better understand client's beliefs and to then help client understand why the belief is irrational*
Humor	*Using irreverence, humor, and sarcasm to emphasize inconsistencies within irrational beliefs, while strengthening the therapeutic relationship*

your school work") and affective ("and when you think that way, I would imagine that would be frustrating") state that validates the clients experience and also promotes the B-C connection within the REBT framework as to ownership of emotions.

An empirical solution (Ellis's view on Beck's Cognitive Therapy; Beck, 1976) addresses the inferences and perceptions about the A (If a father is worried that his son will hate him and never speak to him again for enforcing rules and has awfulizing, catastrophic beliefs, the therapist would ask what evidence he has for this worry and how likely this is to happen). However, the philosophical, elegant solution that Ellis favored instead encourages the client to assume the worst. Here, the therapist accepts the premise or inference that the client puts forth and tells the client to "suppose this is true." In this situation, rather than working with hypothetical probabilities and likelihoods, the therapist is able to get to the core of the disturbance more efficiently, or *elegantly*, by exploring what this event would mean to the client and the effect that this irrational belief is having on the client's life. In a similar example, if a mother is hurt and angry about her teenage son's behavior and suggests that he does not care about his parents anymore, that he missed his father's birthday surprise party on purpose, the REBT-F therapist would not focus on whether the mother's ideas about her son are true or false. Instead, the mother would be asked to suppose that this is true and that her son did miss the party on purpose and to instead address the beliefs she has about what this might mean. What beliefs about her son are leading her to feel anger and hurt? Is the mother demanding that he act a certain way? Does his behavior in this instance mean that he is a worthless, terrible human being? REBT-F makes a distinction between the elegant and inelegant empirical solutions, favoring the use of the elegant solution to help individuals cope with the reality they are perceiving (DiGiuseppe et al., 2014).

To review, reinforce, consolidate, and generalize the session content, a key component of every REBT-F session is negotiating a homework assignment that every member of the family can practice between sessions. The homework is conceptualized as a collaborative process between clinician and family members in order to increase the motivation and commitment of the client to complete. Homework assignments can take various forms and may include rehearsal of rational statements, behavioral exercises, and emotive exercises (imagery, etc.), each tailored to the content covered in the session (e.g., an adolescent is asked to rehearse the statement "I would prefer it if my parents stopped nagging me about my grades, but there is no reason why they must," while his mother is asked to picture the catastrophic "worst case scenario" of her son failing high school and then visualize herself and her family coping with the situation by signing him up for a trade school). The negotiation of homework assignments conveys the importance of practice and underscores the idea that change takes effort and time. REBT-F teaches clients to identify and dispute their irrational beliefs, many of which are deep-seated and have been present for a long time. Rather than suggesting a quick fix for a problem within the family, REBT-F presents the opportunity for a change in a family member's philosophy and view of their family. REBT-F aims to help family members *get* better rather than just *feel* better, which requires commitment and motivation on the part of each family member. It is often necessary to remind clients that happiness and positive emotions are not the goal of REBT-F and that the aim of changing one's beliefs to be rational rather than irrational will likely result in healthy negative emotions (e.g., concern, frustration, regret) and adaptive coping behaviors (e.g., more effective communication and problem-solving), rather than happiness, which is usually not realistic given an unpleasant A.

REBT-F holds several principles to be true, and sessions are conducted with these principles in mind (Ellis, 1993). At the core are the concepts of unconditional acceptance of oneself, of others, and of life, unconditional human worth, and the idea of personal responsibility for one's emotions and behaviors. REBT-F holds that all humans have equal worth and that the worth of a person is unconditional; it does not increase or decrease based on their actions or characteristics (Dryden, 2019). REBT-F holds true the idea that pain is a part of life and that by accepting this as reality, one can cope with and adapt to that reality, whereas denying this fact and struggling against it will result in unnecessary suffering. The definition of acceptance in REBT-F is more akin to acknowledgement rather than that of approval – a point that frequently needs to be clarified with clients. Rather than striving to be happy about or approving of an event or a person, the goal is to acknowledge the circumstances and reality of the situation with some appropriate, healthy negative affect without it resulting in disturbance or suffering.

REBT-F and Other Family-Based Therapies

REBT-F Versus Family Systems Therapy REBT-F is in agreement with some aspects of family systems therapy in that treatment of the family can be an effective way to help individuals within the family system (Ellis, 1982). Similar to family systems therapy, REBT-F uses an active-directive, problem-solving approach and goal-oriented strategies. However, REBT-F emphasizes the importance of treatment of family members for their individual disturbances in addition to working with the family as a system. REBT-F suggests that disturbed relationships stem from the attitudes and views family members have about family situations. In Ellis's (1978) writings on REBT-F, he suggested that family systems therapy tends to "neglect" the individual family members within the system and thus leaves the self-disturbing aspects of the individuals unaddressed. Furthermore, while family systems therapy focuses on understanding and changing the A (past events, experiences, and situations that occur), REBT-F emphasizes the B (beliefs and attitudes about those events). Ellis's REBT-F maintains that changes made to a family system are likely to be superficial and short-lived, with individual family members' problems needing to be addressed for meaningful change to occur in the family (Ellis, 1982, 2001). Family systems therapy accepts clients' worldviews and tries to reframe them, whereas REBT-F challenges these beliefs directly and helps to show individuals how they are responsible for creating their emotional disturbance as well as the problems within the family (Ellis, 2001; Guterman, 1991).

Further, REBT-F tends to focus more on cognitions than traditional family therapy (Ellis, 1978). Ellis (1962) described REBT-F as a cognitive theory, viewing symptoms and disturbance as a product of intrapsychic processes within individuals at the individual level. However, for family systems therapists, the goal of therapy is to address emotional disturbance by changing patterns of interactions between family members (Fisch, Weakland, & Segal, 1982). Although the assessment differs between REBT-F and family systems therapy, with REBT-F seeking to identify the irrational beliefs that are causing disturbance in the family, and family systems therapists seeking to diagnose the maladaptive patterns in the functioning and interactions between family members, the techniques used in therapy are often more similar than different. The use of role play, behavioral homework assignments, and learning and practicing problem-solving skills is present in both REBT-F and family systems therapy (Russell & Morrill, 1989). Russell and Morrill (1989) propose a hybrid model that combines elements of REBT-F and family systems therapy, suggesting that the family therapist may consider both the independent problems and disturbance of the individuals as well as the interdependence of family members.

REBT-F Versus Psychoanalytic Family Therapy Although Ellis is considered to be the grandfather of CBT (DiGiuseppe et al., 2014) and is known for his legacy of developing and disseminating REBT, a cognitive behavioral therapy, Ellis actually began his career by training in psychoanalysis. In his clinical practice early on in his career, Ellis found that psychoanalysis was less efficient in helping his clients, particularly those with relationship and sex problems, than a more direct, active approach (Ellis, 1975). Although the theoretical framework and techniques that Ellis used in REBT-F were a substantial departure from his psychoanalytic training, Ellis did not reject the importance and value of the relationship between the therapist and the client (therapeutic alliance). In contrast to the psychoanalytic view of families, Ellis believed that a present-centered, direct approach to therapy was more effective and that while REBT-F may reveal the unconscious thoughts and demands of a family member, these demands are rarely repressed and usually just outside of conscious awareness (Ellis, 2001). Though REBT-F rejects psychoanalytic personality formation theories, REBT-F agrees with the idea that the individual's emotional disturbance is at the core of family difficulties.

REBT-F Versus Behavioral Family Therapy REBT-F is considered a form of CBT (Ellis, 1982). It incorporates techniques like operant conditioning, in vivo desensitization, and exposure. As with many other behavioral therapies, REBT-F also teaches effective relationship skills and problem-solving in addition to using cognitive, behavioral, and emotional interventions. REBT-F, along with most other forms of CBT, takes an active and directive approach with clients, empowering and requiring individuals to take responsibility for their problems rather than viewing themselves as the passive victims or recipients of misfortune and negative life events. Ellis viewed REBT-F as a humanistic and pragmatic framework of therapy (Ellis, 1978). REBT-F favors self-control over conditioning, as excessive reinforcement from the therapist may result in family members becoming overly dependent on this form of conditioning.

Evidence for REBT-F

While rational emotive behavior therapy is established as an effective approach to family counseling (e.g., David, Cotet, Matu, Mogoase, & Stefan, 2017; Ellis, 1982, 1993, 2001; Ellis & Dryden, 1997; Wachtler, 2019), empirical work is limited. To our knowledge, no author has systematically reviewed the efficacy or effectiveness of REBT-F.

Despite the dearth of outcome research for REBT-F specifically, the research on rational emotive behavior therapy as a psychological intervention for individuals is sound. Hundreds of studies provide support for REBT's basic theory and efficacy (David, 2015). REBT is effective for a range of psychological concerns in adults, children, and adolescents, including disruptive behavior (Gaviţa, David, Bujoreanu, Tiba, & Ionuţiu, 2012), parent stress (Joyce, 1995), obsessive-compulsive disorder (Emmelkamp & Beens, 1991), depression (David, Szentagotai, Lupu, & Cosman, 2008), and psychosis (Meaden, Keen, Aston, Barton, & Bucci, 2013), among others (David, Szentagotai, Eva, & Macavei, 2005). Research also demonstrates the effectiveness of REBT compared to other treatments. For example, one review found REBT to be equally effective to alternative treatments, including systematic desensitization and combination treatments, for the treatment of anxiety symptoms (Engels, Garnefski, & Diekstra, 1993). More recently, REBT has been found to be moderately more effective when compared to other interventions for both irrational beliefs and psychological outcomes more generally (David et al., 2017).

Research on the impact of REBT for specific family conditions is also scant. One case study found REBT may be effective in helping couples adapt to the loss of a child. In the case, the therapist used the A-B-C model to emphasize the couple's dysfunctional, distressing beliefs using techniques like legitimizing and normalizing (Malkinson & Brask-Rustad, 2013). While the treatment was effective in promoting rational cognitions surrounding death, the study did not measure changes in emotional disturbances, and thus, the impact on psychological functioning is unclear. Other studies more clearly demonstrate the impact of REBT on emotional outcomes. For example, rational emotive group therapy may be effective in reducing symptoms of depression among teenagers of divorced parents (Bistamann et al., 2015). A rational emotive protocol was also found to be effective for caregivers in alleviating death anxiety and psychological distress, defined by self-reported levels of depression and anxiety (Onyechi et al., 2016). Further, improvements in caregivers were maintained at follow-up in the experimental group compared to a treatment-as-usual group. However, the unique effects of protocol cannot be determined, as the participants also received other therapeutic techniques including relaxation, imagery, and Gestalt.

However, there is substantial research supporting the use of cognitive behavioral therapy for families. Cognitive behavioral family therapy (CBFT) produces equal or better results than individual therapy across a range of disorders, including depression (Stark et al., 2012), adolescent eating disorders (Bulik, Baucom, Kirby, & Pisetsky, 2011), child conduct disorders (Kaminski & Claussen, 2017), comorbid anxiety and ADHD (Maric, van Steensel, & Bögels, 2018), obsessive-compulsive disorder (O'Leary, Barrett, & Fjermestad, 2009), and psychosomatic disorders (Khodayarifard & Zardkhaneh, 2012). Further, improvements from CBFT are long-lasting (e.g., O'Leary et al., 2009). There is some evidence to suggest that CBFT is most effective for younger children, when parents are more likely to participate as co-therapists and carry out the intervention at home (Cottrell, 2003).

The efficacy of REBT, together with support for the use of cognitive behavioral interventions for families, suggests the effectiveness of REBT-F. Clearly, though, more scholarly work is needed to consider REBT-F an evidence-based intervention. Outcomes from controlled experiments demonstrating superior results from REBT-F (defined by improved emotional outcomes) over other schools of family therapy, alternative therapies, and placebo therapies would support the efficacy of REBT for families. Beyond supporting its efficacy, there are many additional questions to explore in subsequent research. For example, what are the most critical aspects of REBT-F? What measures can be developed to better evaluate outcome? Is REBT-F indicated in some situations and more generalized CBFT in others?

When to Use Family-Based Therapy

Ellis believed that families whose members are young, active, verbal, intelligent, and sensitive would benefit most from REBT-F (Ellis, 2005). However, unlike other family therapies, REBT-F is also effective for "difficult customers" (e.g., psychotic, borderline, etc.), as it helps clients work toward accepting themselves as they are and helps family members to accept their relatives as they are, including the disturbances and mental illnesses they may have (Ellis, 1973, 1982). For instance, REBT-F may teach children to accept their parents who suffer from psychosis, substance abuse, etc. or teach parents to accept their disabled children rather than holding demands that they must be or act a certain way or that they cannot deal with the reality of their family member's illness (Ellis, 1982).

From early work in the area, there are some contraindications for therapy with families (Ackerman, 1966). For example, family-based therapy can be problematic in the treatment of psychotic young adults. Guttman (1973) reports on several cases in which family therapy precipitated or aggravated a psychotic breakdown of the patient. Further, open communication and confrontation may worsen the condition of the psychotic patient (McDermott Jr, 1981). It is also reasonable to assume that the limited cognitive awareness of even pre-psychotic patients would preclude effective cognitive behavioral work. Wolska (2011) suggests avoiding family or couple therapy whenever one member has a severe mental illness. Other contradictions include dishonesty of family members (e.g., due to a valid family secret), addiction problems, extremely rigid defenses, and preoccupation with disengagement from the family, all of which prevent meaningful interpersonal work (Ackerman, 1966; Wolska, 2011).

Summary and Conclusion

The REBT framework of examining and changing the beliefs one has about an activating event in order to change one's emotions from disturbed to healthy negative emotions has been shown to be effective for many different disorders, symptom presentations, and client types. This approach has also been applied clinically to family-based work. REBT-F shares many similarities with other forms of family-based therapy; however it also maintains some unique attributes that make REBT-F a sound clinical choice when working with families whose members are "difficult customers" for therapy. Despite its widespread clinical use and long-standing theoretical and philosophical foundations, empirical research about REBT-F is still relatively limited. We recommend that additional research about REBT-F be conducted with the intent to better understand and further legitimize REBT-F as an effective, evidence-based treatment for families.

Test Yourself

1. Why is establishing the B-C connection particularly important at the outset of therapy with families? What may happen if this is unsuccessful?
2. Which of the REBT principles is most important for working with families?
3. What are some key differences/distinguishing features between REBT-F and other family therapies? For whom is REBT-F most effective?
4. What is the purpose of homework in REBT-F? How is homework addressed in REBT-F sessions? What are some types of possible homework activities?
5. Who is the ideal candidate for REBT-F? For which condition(s) is REBT-F most indicated?

References

Ackerman, N. W. (1966). *Treating the troubled family*. New York: Basic Books. https://doi.org/10.1093/sw/13.3.114

Alexander, J. F. (1973). Defensive and supportive communication in normal and deviant families. *Journal of Consulting and Clinical Psychology, 40*, 223–231. https://doi.org/10.1037/h0034514

Barmish, A. J., & Kendall, P. C. (2005). Should parents be co-clients in cognitive-behavioral therapy for anxious youth? *Journal of Clinical Child and Adolescent Psychology, 34*, 569–581. https://doi.org/10.1207/s15374424jccp3403_12

Beck, A. T. (1976). *Cognitive therapy and the emotional disorders*. New York: International Universities Press.

Bistamann, M. N., Jais, S. M., Jusoh, A. J., Rahman, A. M. A., Arif, M. A. S. M., & Razali, M. M. S. (2015). The effect of REBT structured counseling group towards the grief and depression among teenagers of divorced parent. *International Journal of Education and Research, 3*, 113–122.

Borduin, C., Curtis, N., & Ronan, K. (2004). Multisystemic treatment: A meta-analysis of outcome studies. *Journal of Family Psychology, 18*, 411–419. https://doi.org/10.1037/0893-3200.18.3.411

Bulik, C. M., Baucom, D. H., Kirby, J. S., & Pisetsky, E. (2011). Uniting couples (in the treatment of) anorexia nervosa (UCAN). *International Journal of Eating Disorders, 44*, 19–28. https://doi.org/10.1002/eat.20790

Carr, A. (2019). Family therapy and systemic interventions for child-focused problems: The current evidence base. *Journal of Family Therapy, 41*, 153–213. https://doi.org/10.1111/1467-6427.12226

Cluxton-Keller, F. (2011). Rational emotive behavior therapy. In L. Metcalf (Ed.), *Marriage and family therapy* (pp. 129–146). New York: Springer. https://doi.org/10.1891/9780826106827.0006

Cottrell, D. (2003). Outcome studies of family therapy in child and adolescent depression. *Journal of Family Therapy, 25*, 406–416. https://doi.org/10.1111/1467-6427.00258

David, D. (2015). Rational emotive behavior therapy (REBT). In R. L. Cautin & S. O. Lilienfeld (Eds.), *Encyclopedia of clinical psychology*. Wiley-Blackwell: Hoboken, NJ.

David, D., Cotet, C., Matu, S., Mogoase, C., & Stefan, S. (2017). 50 years of rational-emotive and cognitive-behavioral therapy: A systematic review and meta-analysis. *Journal of Clinical Psychology, 74*, 304–318. https://doi.org/10.1002/jclp.22514

David, D., Szentagotai, A., Eva, K., & Macavei, B. (2005). A synopsis of rational-emotive behavior therapy (REBT): Fundamental and applied research. *Journal of Rational-Emotive & Cognitive-Behavior Therapy, 23*(3), 175–221. https://doi.org/10.1007/s10942-005-0011-0

David, D., Szentagotai, A., Lupu, V., & Cosman, D. (2008). Rational emotive behavior therapy, cognitive therapy, and medication in the treatment of major depressive disorder: A randomized clinical trial, posttreatment outcomes, and six-month follow-up. *Journal of Clinical Psychology, 64*, 728–746. https://doi.org/10.1002/jclp.20487

DiGiuseppe, R., Doyle, K. A., Dryden, W., & Backx, W. (2014). *A practitioner's guide to rational-emotive behavior therapy*. New York: Oxford University Press. https://doi.org/10.1093/med:psych/9780199743049.003.0017

Dowell, K. A., & Ogles, B. M. (2010). The effects of parent participation on child psychotherapy outcome: A meta-analytic review. *Journal of Clinical Child & Adolescent Psychology, 39*, 151–162. https://doi.org/10.1080/15374410903532585

Dryden, W. (2002). Rational emotive behaviour therapy. In W. Dryden (Ed.), *Handbook of individual therapy* (4th ed., pp. 347–372). London, UK: Sage.

Dryden, W. (2019). The distinctive features of rational emotive behavior therapy. In *Advances in REBT* (pp. 23–46). Cham, Switzerland: Springer.

Eisler, I., Dare, C., Russell, G. F. M., Szmukler, G., le Grange, D., & Dodge, E. (1997). Family and individual therapy in anorexia nervosa: A 5-year follow-up. *Archives of General Psychiatry, 54*, 1025–1030. https://doi.org/10.1001/archpsyc.1997.01830230063008

Ellis, A. (1962). *On theory and practice of RET*. New York: Albert Ellis Institute.

Ellis, A. (1973). *Humanistic psychotherapy: The rational-emotive approach*. New York: McGraw-Hill.

Ellis, A. (1975). The rational-emotive approach to sex therapy. *The Counseling Psychologist, 5*(1), 14–22. https://doi.org/10.1177/001100007500500106

Ellis, A. (1978). A rational-emotive approach to family therapy. Part I: Cognitive therapy. *Rational Living, 13*, 15–19.

Ellis, A. (1982). Rational-emotive family therapy. In A. M. Horne & M. M. Ohlsen (Eds.), *Family counseling and therapy* (pp. 302–328). Itasca, IL: F.E. Peacock Publishers.

Ellis, A. (1993). The rational-emotive therapy (RET) approach to marriage and family therapy. *The Family Journal, 1*, 292–307. https://doi.org/10.1177/1066480793014002

Ellis, A. (2001). *How to stop destroying your relationships*. New York: Citadel.

Ellis, A. (2005). Rational emotive behavior therapy. In R. J. Corsini & D. Wedding (Eds.), *Current psychotherapies* (pp. 166–201). Thomson Brooks/Cole Publishing Co.

Ellis, A., & Dryden, W. (1997). *The practice of rational-emotive therapy* (2nd ed.). New York: Springer.
Emmelkamp, P. M., & Beens, H. (1991). Cognitive therapy with obsessive-compulsive disorder: A comparative evaluation. *Behaviour Research and Therapy, 29*, 293–300. https://doi.org/10.1016/0005-7967(91)90120-R
Engels, G. I., Garnefski, N., & Diekstra, R. F. (1993). Efficacy of rational-emotive therapy: A quantitative analysis. *Journal of Consulting and Clinical Psychology, 61*, 1083–1090. https://doi.org/10.1037/0022-006x.61.6.1083
Fisch, R. T., Weakland, J. H., & Segal, L. (1982). *The tactics of change*. San Francisco: Jossey-Bass.
Friedberg, R. D. (2006). A cognitive-behavioral approach to family therapy. *Journal of Contemporary Psychotherapy, 36*, 159–165. https://doi.org/10.1007/s10879-006-9020-2
Fristad, M., Goldberg-Arnold, J., & Gavazzi, S. (2002). Multifamily psychoeducation groups (MFPG) for families of children with bipolar disorder. *Bipolar Disorder, 4*, 254–262. https://doi.org/10.1034/j.1399-5618.2002.09073.x
Fristad, M., Goldberg-Arnold, J., & Gavazzi, S. (2003). Multifamily psychoeducation groups in the treatment of children with mood disorders. *Journal of Marital and Family Therapy, 29*, 491–504. https://doi.org/10.1111/j.1752-0606.2003.tb01691.x
Gaviţa, O. A., David, D., Bujoreanu, S., Tiba, A., & Ionuţiu, D. R. (2012). The efficacy of a short cognitive-behavioral parent program in the treatment of externalizing behavior disorders in Romanian foster care children: Building parental emotion-regulation through unconditional self- and child-acceptance strategies. *Children and Youth Services Review, 34*, 1290–1297. https://doi.org/10.1016/j.childyouth.2012.03.001
Guterman, J. T. (1991). Developing a hybrid model of rational-emotive therapy and systemic family therapy: A response to Russell and Morrill. *Journal of Mental Health Counseling, 13*, 410–413.
Guttman, H. A. (1973). A contraindication for family therapy. *Archives of General Psychiatry, 29*, 352–355. https://doi.org/10.1001/archpsyc.1973.04200030050007
Hamilton, E., & Carr, A. (2016). Systematic review of self-report family assessment measures. *Family Process, 55*, 16–30. https://doi.org/10.1111/famp.12200
Hutcheson, C. L. (2019). Cognitive behavioral family therapy. In L. Metcalf (Ed.), *Marriage and family therapy: A practice-oriented approach* (p. 95–118). Springer Publishing Company.
Joyce, M. R. (1995). Emotional relief for parents: Is rational-emotive parent education effective? *Journal of Rational-Emotive & Cognitive-Behavior Therapy, 13*, 55–76. https://doi.org/10.1007/bf02354557
Kaminski, J. W., & Claussen, A. H. (2017). Evidence base update for psychosocial treatments for disruptive behaviors in children. *Journal of Clinical Child & Adolescent Psychology, 46*, 477–499. https://doi.org/10.1080/15374416.2017.1310044
Khodayarifard, M., & Zardkhaneh, S. A. (2012). Cognitive behavior family therapy of psychosomatic disorders with an emphasis on positive psychotherapy. *Psychology, 3*, 1104–1109. https://doi.org/10.4236/psych.2012.312a163
Malkinson, R., & Brask-Rustad, T. (2013). Cognitive behavior couple therapy-REBT model for traumatic bereavement. *Journal of Rational-Emotive & Cognitive-Behavior Therapy, 31*, 114–125. https://doi.org/10.1007/s10942-013-0164-1
Maric, M., van Steensel, F. J. A., & Bögels, S. M. (2018). Parental involvement in CBT for anxiety-disordered youth revisited: Family CBT outperforms child CBT in the long term for children with comorbid ADHD symptoms. *Journal of Attention Disorders, 22*, 506–514. https://doi.org/10.1177/1087054715573991
McCart, M. R., Priester, P., Davies, W. H., & Azen, R. (2006). Differential effectiveness of cognitive-behavioral therapy and behavioral parent-training for antisocial youth: A meta-analysis. *Journal of Abnormal Child Psychology, 34*, 527–543. https://doi.org/10.1007/s10802-006-9031-1

McDermott Jr., J. F. (1981). Indications for family therapy: Question or non-question? *Journal of the American Academy of Child Psychiatry, 20*, 409–419. https://doi.org/10.1016/s0002-7138(09)60998-5

Meaden, A., Keen, N., Aston, R., Barton, K., & Bucci, S. (2013). *Cognitive therapy for command hallucinations: An advanced practical companion*. New York: Routledge. https://doi.org/10.4324/9780203086544

Miklowitz, D., George, E., Axelson, D., Kim, E., Birmaher, B., Schneck, C., et al. (2004). Family-focused treatment for adolescents with bipolar disorder. *Journal of Affective Disorders, 82*, 113–128. https://doi.org/10.1016/j.jad.2004.05.020

O'Leary, E. M. M., Barrett, P., & Fjermestad, K. W. (2009). Cognitive-behavioral family treatment for childhood obsessive-compulsive disorder: A 7-year follow-up study. *Journal of Anxiety Disorders, 23*, 973–978. https://doi.org/10.1016/j.janxdis.2009.06.009

Onyechi, K., Onuigbo, L., Eseadi, C., Ikechukwu-Ilomuanya, A., Nwaubani, O., Umoke, P., et al. (2016). Effects of rational-emotive hospice care therapy on problematic assumptions, death anxiety, and psychological distress in a sample of cancer patients and their family caregivers in Nigeria. *International Journal of Environmental Research and Public Health, 13*, 929. https://doi.org/10.3390/ijerph13090929

Patterson, G. R. (1982). *Coercive family process*. Eugene, OR: Castalia Publishing Company.

Pavuluri, M., Grazyk, P., Henry, D., Carbray, J., Heidenreich, J., & Miklowitz, D. (2004). Child- and family-focused cognitive behavioural therapy for pediatric bipolar disorder: Development and preliminary results. *Journal of the American Academy of Child and Adolescent Psychiatry, 43*, 528–537. https://doi.org/10.1097/00004583-200405000-00006

Russell, T. T., & Morrill, C. M. (1989). Adding a systemic touch to rational-emotive therapy for families. *Journal of Mental Health Counseling, 11*, 184–192.

Shadish, W. R., Montgomery, L. M., Wilson, P., Wilson, M. R., Bright, I., & Okwumabua, T. (1993). Effects of family and marital psychotherapies: A meta-analysis. *Journal of Consulting and Clinical Psychology, 61*, 992–1002. https://doi.org/10.1037/0022-006x.61.6.992

Stanton, M. D., & Shadish, W. R. (1997). Outcome, attrition, and family-couples treatment for drug abuse: A meta-analysis and review of the controlled, comparative studies. *Psychological Bulletin, 122*, 170–191. https://doi.org/10.1037//0033-2909.122.2.170

Stark, K., Banneyer, K., Wang, L., & Arora, P. (2012). Child and adolescent depression in the family. *Couple and Family Psychology: Research and Practice, 1*, 161–184.

Wachtler, B. E. (2019). REBT with families. In W. Dryden & M. Bernard (Eds.), *REBT with diverse client problems and populations*. Cham, Switzerland: Springer. https://doi.org/10.1007/978-3-030-02723-0_14

Wolska, M. (2011). Marital therapy/ couples therapy: Indications and contraindications. *Archives of Psychiatry and Psychotherapy, 13*, 57–64.

Part II
Childhood Disorders, Difficulties and Different Populations

Chapter 8
RE-CBT in the Treatment of Anxiety, Fears, and Phobias Among Youth

Michael Hickey and Stephanie Schwartz

Chapter Overview

This chapter provides a comprehensive overview of anxiety, fear, and phobias in children and adolescents and clinical treatment of these problems using rational emotive and cognitive behavioral therapy (RE-CBT) approaches. As there are several anxiety disorders often diagnosed during childhood and adolescence, they may each present with some unique characteristics that warrant clinical attention. While some differences among the disorders will be periodically addressed, the content of this chapter is primarily focused on the clinical similarities/underlying mechanisms among these disorders and how RE-CBT treatment strategies can be applied in a transdiagnostic manner across the various anxiety disorders.

The first sections of this chapter cover etiology, assessment, and research. Subsequent sections provide information on developmental considerations, best practice guidelines, and specific interventions utilized in RE-CBT treatment of anxiety disorders, fears, and phobias. Concluding sections include a case study and discussion of treatment in the school setting. The information in this chapter reflects advances in theory and research to provide an evidence-oriented resource for mental health professionals working with anxiety disorders.

M. Hickey (✉)
Center for Psychological Evaluation and the Center for Treatment and Research of Obsessive-Compulsive & Related Disorders, Albert Ellis Institute, New York, NY, USA

S. Schwartz
Anxiety Disorders Center, Child Mind Institute, New York, NY, USA

M. Bernard, M. D. Terjesen (eds.), *Rational-Emotive and Cognitive-Behavioral Approaches to Child and Adolescent Mental Health: Theory, Practice, Research, Applications*, https://doi.org/10.1007/978-3-030-53901-6_8

Overview of Anxiety, Fears, and Phobias in Children and Adolescents

Anxiety involves emotional, cognitive, behavioral, and physiological components. Fears are typical in children and adolescents, and subclinical symptoms of anxiety are common in the general pediatric population (Muris, Meesters, Merckelbach, Sermon, & Zwakhalen, 1998). When symptoms of anxiety are persistent and severe and result in significant distress or impaired functioning, they are indicative of an anxiety disorder (Muris, Merckelbach, Mayer, & Prins, 2000). Anxiety disorders are characterized by excessive fear and anxiety, behavioral disturbances, faulty cognitions, and somatic symptoms. Furthermore, for an anxiety disorder to be present, symptoms must persist for a specified period, to ensure that the anxiety or fear is not transient or developmentally appropriate. The various anxiety disorders differ in the objects or situations that lead to the fear and anxiety, but the disorders share many common features including intense anxiety that is unrealistic or out of proportion to the situation, intrusive thoughts that are unwanted and uncontrollable, and behavioral avoidance of situations that are not inherently dangerous. Furthermore, somatic complaints, such as restlessness and stomach aches, are very common in youth with anxiety disorders (Ginsburg, Riddle, & Davies, 2006). While the cause of anxiety disorders isn't fully understood, these disorders are thought to be triggered and maintained by a combination of genetic and environmental factors.

Anxiety disorders impact a significant number of children and adolescents, and in recent years, there has been an increase in anxiety disorder diagnoses among youth (Bitsko et al., 2018). The worldwide prevalence of anxiety disorders among youth is estimated to be 6.5%, which is higher than the prevalence of depressive disorders, attention-deficit hyperactivity disorders, and disruptive disorders in children and adolescents (Polanczyk, Salum, Sugaya, Caye, & Rohde, 2015). In a parent survey of children's health, among parents who reported youth with anxiety disorders, anxiety was rated as mild for 48%, moderate for 36.8%, and severe for 15.2% (Bitsko et al., 2018). Having anxiety as a child is associated with being diagnosed with an anxiety disorder in adolescence, and gender and heredity are both factors associated with the development of anxiety disorders (Bittner et al., 2007). Beginning at puberty, females are more likely than males to have an anxiety disorder, and anxiety disorders are more likely in youth who have parents with anxiety (Beidel & Turner, 2007; Merikangas et al., 2010).

The *Diagnostic and Statistical Manual of Mental Disorders* (DSM-5) distinguishes anxiety disorders and includes selective mutism, separation anxiety disorder, specific phobia, social anxiety disorder, generalized anxiety disorder, agoraphobia, and panic disorder (American Psychiatric Association (APA), 2013). Anxiety disorders are also highly comorbid with one another and often co-occur with affective disorders, including major depressive disorder; externalizing disorders, including attention-deficit/hyperactivity disorder; eating disorders; and substance abuse disorders (Garber & Weersing, 2010; Predescu, Asztalos, & Sipos, 2018; Russo & Beidel, 1994; Seligman & Ollendick, 2011). Anxious children and adolescents are at risk for a number of negative outcomes, including poor academic performance and impaired social functioning (Mychailyszyn, Mendez, & Kendall, 2010; Scharfstein & Beidel, 2014). Furthermore, untreated anxiety disorders pose the threat of long-term consequences such as additional psychiatric disorders and occupational difficulties (Bittner et al., 2007; Woodward & Fergusson, 2001).

Among the anxiety disorders, the earliest incidence occurs with selective mutism, separation anxiety disorder, and some types of specific phobias (Becker et al., 2007; Kessler et al., 2005; Wittchen, Stein, & Kessler, 1999). Selective mutism involves an inability to speak in certain situations where speech is expected, despite being able to verbalize fluently in other situations. Prevalence rates of selective mutism based on clinic and school samples range between 0.03% and 1% (Carbone et al., 2010; Viana, Beidel, & Rabian, 2009). Children with selective mutism are often talkative at home with immediate family members but have restricted speech with certain people, in certain settings, or while engaging in certain activities. These children often do not verbally participate in school or the community, and many also do not verbalize with peers (APA, 2013). In addition, children with selective mutism frequently do not communicate their needs, such as letting an adult know that they need to go to the bathroom or that they are injured.

Separation anxiety disorder involves excessive and persistent fear about separating from caregivers. The prevalence is estimated to be approximately 4% in children and 1.6% in adolescents (Cartwright-Hatton, McNicol, & Doubleday, 2006; Kessler, Petukhova, Sampson, Zaslavsky, & Wittchen, 2012; Thapar et al., 2015). Youth with separation anxiety disorder may refuse to go to school, playdates, or other activities where they experience separation from a major attachment figure. This can lead to problems with academic functioning and peer relationships (APA, 2013). Some youth also have difficulty being apart from parents in the home setting and may not engage in play or activities of daily living (e.g., bathing, sleeping) without a caregiver nearby. Children with separation anxiety commonly engage in catastrophic thinking that if separated from their parents or caregiver something bad will happen to them.

Specific phobias among youth involve excessive and intense fear of a situation or object. Prevalence rates are estimated to be 5% in children and 16% in adolescents (Kessler et al., 2012; Ollendick, King, & Muris, 2002). Specific phobias are categorized into types including animal type, such as dogs; natural environment type, such as thunderstorms; blood-injection or injury type, such as getting shots; situation type, such as elevators; and other type, such as vomiting. Youth with a specific phobia may become tearful, act aggressive or oppositional, or engage in clingy behavior with caregivers when they encounter the situation or object they fear (APA, 2013). Youth with specific phobia often do not recognize that the intensity of their fear is irrational. They commonly hold distorted beliefs about how likely the situation is to occur and their level of distress if they were to face the object or situation they fear.

Social anxiety disorder typically has a first onset in late childhood or adolescence, while panic disorder, agoraphobia, and generalized anxiety disorder generally have initial incidence in late adolescence or early adulthood (Beesdo et al., 2007; Kessler et al., 2005; Wittchen & Fehm, 2003). Prevalence rates of social anxiety disorder, panic disorder, and agoraphobia have been found to be less than 1% in children (Almqvist et al., 1999; Costello, Mustillo, Erkanli, Keeler, & Angold, 2003; Ford, Goodman, & Meltzer, 2003; Sugawara et al., 1999). Social anxiety disorder involves fear of being embarrassed, laughed at, or negatively evaluated. Youth with social anxiety disorder often expect worst-case scenarios, such as that they will be made fun of, or believe they know what others are thinking about them, such as that they are stupid. The prevalence of social anxiety disorder in adolescents is approximately 9% (Merikangas et al., 2010). Children and adolescents with social anxiety disorder often restrict their participation at school, prefer engaging in solitary activities, and avoid activities where attention is on them, such as having their picture taken or eating in front of others. Generalized anxiety disorder involves excessive worry about a variety of events or activities, such as school, performance, social relationships, and health. Similar to social anxiety disorder, prevalence rates have been found to be less than 1% in children (Almqvist et al., 1999; Costello et al., 2003; Ford et al., 2003). For adolescents, the prevalence rate is approximately 2% (Merikangas et al., 2010). Youth with generalized anxiety disorder may be perfectionistic, may get stuck on "little things," and generally engage in worst-case scenario thinking patterns. Panic disorder involves recurrent unexpected panic attacks that involve various physiological symptoms and at least 1 month of persistent worry about additional panic attacks or a change in behavior related to the attacks (APA, 2013). The prevalence of panic disorder in adolescents is approximately 2% (Merikangas et al., 2010). Youth with panic disorder often avoid situations that could be triggering, such as crowded places or engaging in physical activity, and may make frequent trips to the doctor or school nurse. Lastly, agoraphobia involves marked anxiety and subsequent avoidance of two of the following: using public transportation, being in open spaces, being in enclosed spaces, standing in line or being in a crowd, or being outside of the home alone. The prevalence of agoraphobia in adolescents is approximately 2% (Merikangas et al., 2010). Children and adolescents with agoraphobia may refuse to go to school or other activities outside of the home and may exhibit clingy behavior and reassurance seeking from caregivers. Those with panic disorder or agoraphobia commonly hold distorted beliefs that their feared situations are likely to occur in the future and engage in awfulized thinking about how distressing they would be.

Assessment and Diagnosis of Anxiety, Fears, and Phobias in Children and Adolescents

As with the assessment of all psychiatric disorders, it is important in the initial diagnostic evaluation for the clinician to ask questions about the child's behavior, diagnostic symptoms, developmental history, and family history. A thorough assessment allows the clinician to formulate a case conceptualization and treatment plan. Assessment should be multifaceted and include both the objective and subjective assessment of symptoms. A comprehensive assessment involves clinical interviews with the child, parents, teachers, and other individuals with knowledge of the child, as appropriate, child self-report measures, parent report measures, teacher report measures, and clinical observations.

The use of a structured interview that includes specific questions about a child's behavior based on the criteria for each psychiatric disorder in the *Diagnostic and Statistical Manual* is a useful tool. The Anxiety Disorders Interview Schedule, Parent/Child Version (ADIS-IV), is a comprehensive semi-structured clinical interview that assesses for the DSM-4 diagnostic criteria for anxiety disorders, as well as additional psychiatric disorders. While a revised version of this instrument reflecting DSM-5 updates is not yet available, the ADIS is still useful in assessing anxiety disorders in children as DSM-5 core features of anxiety disorders are highly consistent with DSM-4.

Rating scales involve sets of questions about a child's behaviors and emotions and are also helpful tools to aid in diagnosis. Many rating scales offer self, parent, and teacher report versions, which allow for reports from multiple perspectives. Some of the commonly used rating scales for anxiety in clinical practice are the Multidimensional Anxiety Scale for Children, Second Edition (MASC-2; March, 2012); Screen for Child Anxiety Related Emotional Disorders (SCARED; Birmaher et al., 1999); Spence Children's Anxiety Scale (SCAS; Spence, 1997); State-Trait Anxiety Inventory for Children (STAIC; Spielberger, 1971); Revised Children's Manifest Anxiety Scale (RCMAS; Reynolds & Richmond, 2008); and the Fear Survey Schedule for Children-Revised (FSSC-R; Ollendick 1983). While rating scales should not be used solely as a diagnostic tool, they do provide information about whether a certain area (e.g., anxiety) is elevated compared to same-aged peers. In addition, as thoughts are key in the development of anxiety, as well as a target for clinical change, measures that evaluate specific unhealthy thoughts or beliefs may be helpful. An example is the Child and Adolescent Scale of Irrationality (CASI; Terjesen, Kassay, & Anderson, 2017), which is a rational emotive behavior therapy (REBT)-specific measure that assesses for irrational beliefs.

Anxiety is conceptualized as being triggered and maintained by a combination of biological predisposition and environmental factors (Gross & Hen, 2004). A major component of cognitive behavioral therapy (CBT) with children is to change what is maintaining the anxiety.

Children with anxiety disorders try hard to not experience anxiety or to get rid of the negative feeling if it happens. The most common way to ensure that anxiety is not experienced is to avoid or stay away from anxiety-activating situations (Arnaudova, Kindt, Fanselow, & Beckers, 2017). This maintains the anxiety as the child learns that avoiding objects or situations feels much better than approaching them, which in turn leads to more avoidance. When assessing for anxiety disorders, it is important for the clinician to get a thorough understanding of the various objects or situations that elicit the anxiety and prompt the anxiety-driven behavior of avoidance. Furthermore, anxious youth often rely on their parents help to avoid their anxiety, which is commonly referred to as accommodation (Lebowitz & Omer,

2013). Accommodation involves changes in parents' behavior with the intent to prevent or reduce the child's distress. This may involve family members participating in a child's rituals, modifying personal or family routines, or answering reassurance-seeking questions. Speaking in place of a child with selective mutism, sleeping in bed with a child with separation anxiety disorder, or repeatedly answering a reassurance-seeking question of a child with emetophobia (i.e., "is this going to make me sick?") are all examples of parent accommodation. Notably, accommodation should be distinguished from healthy protection, or assisting a child to stay away from things that are truly dangerous, and reassurance seeking should be distinguished from giving information, or answering once to a question that the child does not know the answer (Lebowitz et al., 2013). An accommodation checklist created by Lebowitz and Omer (2013) may be helpful when assessing for accommodations with parents.

Research on RE-CBT with Child and Adolescent Anxiety, Fears, and Phobias

The American Academy of Child and Adolescent Psychiatry identifies CBT as the most empirically supported approach for treating anxious youth based on several randomized controlled trials conducted in multiple settings (Sawyer & Nunez, 2014). One of the largest randomized controlled trials (RCTs) to date that examined the efficacy of CBT for children and adolescents with anxiety disorder diagnoses is the Child/Adolescent Anxiety Multimodal Study (CAMS) (Compton et al., 2010). This study included participants with diagnoses of generalized anxiety disorder, social anxiety disorder, and separation anxiety disorder and found that both CBT and pharmacological treatment were efficacious in reducing anxiety symptoms and associated disability. Other RCTs have also demonstrated that CBT is effective in treating anxiety among youth (Seligman & Ollendick, 2011), and positive effects have been shown for diagnostic recovery (Sawyer & Nunez, 2014), academic functioning (Nail et al., 2015), and social competence (Wood, 2006). Comparatively, the literature has been scarce when it comes to research specifically on clinical work utilizing REBT with anxious children, although studies to date have shown that REBT with children and adolescents has resulted in decreased anxiety (DiGiuseppe & Kassinove, 1976; Warren, Deffenbach, & Broding, 1976; Wessel & Mersch, 1994). More recently, a meta-analysis of REBT with children and adolescents found a moderately positive effect of REBT on anxiety (Gonzalez et al., 2004). Research on specific REBT interventions for child and adolescent mental health problems has increased in recent years. For example, a newly developed rational emotive education program (SELF kit) was found to provide reductions in internalizing and externalizing symptoms in preschool children (Opre, Buzgar, & Dumulescu, 2018). In addition, the short Rational Parenting Program (sRPP) and the RETMAN rational stories intervention (RETMAN), which both stem from the REBT approach, have been shown to have a positive impact on child emotional and behavioral problems, including reductions in anxiety problems (Gavita & Calin, 2013). Furthermore, a recent pilot study found that children and adolescents who were provided a brief presentation on REBT principles followed by engaging in the *Feeling Better* mini video game, part of the *REThink* therapeutic online platform, showed a significant increase in their ability to correctly identify functional emotions (David, Predatu, & Cardos, 2018).

RE-CBT treatment for anxiety disorders aims to target the somatic, cognitive, and behavioral aspects of anxiety. The common components of RE-CBT for children with anxiety are psychoeducation, relaxation training, cognitive restructuring, exposure to feared situations, and homework. Cognitive restructuring and exposure have been identified as critical ingredients of CBT that significantly accelerate symptom reduction (Peris et al., 2015). Homework has been discussed as an integral part of treatment as it allows an individual to practice the skills or material covered in the session. Homework has been demonstrated to be related to treatment outcome in adult studies of CBT, although there has been less research on whether homework is an essential component in CBT with children (Hudson & Kendall, 2002). One study that was correlational in nature failed to find a significant relationship between homework compliance and outcome (Hudson & Kendall, 2002). However, it is thought that youth should practice skills outside of the session in order to increase the likelihood of mastery. Homework tasks vary and may involve having the child practice relaxation techniques, rehearse cognitive coping statements, or engage in exposures.

Given that parental factors contribute to the onset and maintenance of anxiety, parent involvement in treatment is often crucial (Lebowitz et al., 2013). Parent involvement in therapy may include parent psychoeducation, improving parent-child interactions, reducing accommodation, and contingency management. It has been shown that children whose parents actively participate in treatment show significantly more remission in long-term follow-up than those with limited parent participation (Walczak, Esbjørn, Breinholst, & Reinholdt-Dunne, 2017). Parent involvement may be particularly beneficial with younger children or when there is at least one parent who has anxiety (Aydin, 2014). In addition, school personnel may also be involved in the treatment process, particularly if the child's anxiety manifests in the educational setting, as is often the case for children with anxiety disorders, particularly selective mutism and separation anxiety disorder. In many cases, transparency with the school about the child's presentation and treatment plan is beneficial so that school personnel are equipped with the knowledge of what they can do to best support the child. School involvement can vary in scope from consultation with the clinician about helpful accommodations for the child to having school personnel involved in exposure tasks (Kingery et al., 2006). The application of RE-CBT in school settings is discussed in greater detail later in this chapter.

Developmental Considerations

It is essential to consider a child's age and developmental level when using RE-CBT, as young children may not benefit from the central cognitive elements of the approach. Piagetian developmental theory places children between the ages of 2 and 7 in the preoperational stage of cognitive development, which highlights a time of significant language development as well as an inability to use cognitive operations, such as logic (Piaget, 1964). While children in this age group have the verbal ability to orally engage with a therapist, their lack of sophistication in cognitive functioning may limit their ability to participate in the cognitive therapeutic process (Grave & Blissett, 2004). CBT is based on a rationalist paradigm, as it involves logically analyzing one's thoughts, disputing irrational thoughts, and thinking abstractly (Grave & Blissett, 2004). Most children under age 8 do not have the cognitive capabilities to understand and participate in these aspects of CBT. Furthermore, a core principle of CBT is that thoughts, feelings, and behaviors are interrelated. Causal reasoning allows an individual to comprehend that one's thoughts impact how one feels and behaves, which is essential in understanding the rationale for cognitive restructuring, which involves identifying, challenging/disputing, and replacing maladaptive cognitions. Disputation can be empirical (gathering data and evidence to refute the irrational belief), logical (using reason and logical thinking to refute the irrational belief), and pragmatic/functional (questioning how holding onto an irrational belief is helping the individual achieve their goals) (DiGiuseppe, Doyle, Dryden, & Backx, 2014).

Younger children can benefit from less complex techniques to modify cognitions. Rather than engaging the child in the steps to identify and challenge maladaptive cognitions, such as "I think something really bad is going to happen," the therapist can assist a young anxious child with generating simple coping statements (i.e., "I can get through this;" "I'm strong and can do hard things;" "It's okay to feel worried sometimes;" "I'm not in danger right now"). Given the cognitive limitations of children under age 8, the behavioral component of exposure is the core of treatment with young children. As young children don't have the capacity for causal reasoning, they cannot understand the cycle of negative reinforcement that occurs from avoiding feared objects or situations. A solid understanding of this pattern is the rationale for exposure, and thus young children may not be internally motivated to engage in facing their fears. As a result, external reinforcement, such as tangible rewards, is often used to motivate children to engage in exposure work. Some young children are able to participate in simple cognitive work, such as reflecting on past exposures that went well and then using this information to manage anticipatory anxiety for subsequent exposures (Grover, Hughes, Bergman, & Kingery, 2006).

Best Practice Guidelines

Currently the American Psychological Association (APA) has established clinical practice guidelines for depression and obesity in children and adolescents, but it has yet to publish guidelines specific to children and adolescents experiencing anxiety disorders (American Psychological Association, 2019). However, the APA emphasizes the necessity of evidence-based practice in psychology (EBPP), which includes the application of empirically supported interventions (American Psychological Association, 2005). As discussed earlier in this chapter, the cognitive behavioral therapies are the most empirically supported approaches for treating anxious youth (Sawyer & Nunez, 2014), and therefore RE-CBT is the gold standard in treating anxiety, fears, and phobia.

The most recently published practice parameter for the assessment and treatment of children and adolescents with anxiety disorders published by the American Academy of Child and Adolescent Psychiatry (AACAP; Connolly & Bernstein, 2007) offers a variety of practice guidelines for clinicians working with children and adolescents with anxiety disorders. First, it is imperative that clinicians are familiar with normal age-appropriate worries and fears and to be able to distinguish them from anxiety disorders. For example, there is a difference between a shy child and one that experiences debilitating social anxiety. Therefore, when assessing children and adolescents, best practice involves carefully examining the impact on the child or adolescents functioning. In order to provide a comprehensive assessment, the AACAP recommends a formal evaluation to determine the severity of anxiety symptoms and differential diagnosis to rule out other physical conditions that may be mimicking anxiety. Assessment and treatment should also involve a multimodal, multi-informant approach and can include parent and child clinical interviews, parent and teacher rating scales, child self-report measures, and behavioral observations (Mychailyszyn et al., 2011).

As discussed earlier in this chapter, RE-CBT interventions should be tailored to a child's developmental level and presentation of symptoms to ensure best practice. For example, a 6-year-old child with a phobia of dogs will likely respond much better to a graded exposure protocol rather than spending significant amounts of time with cognitive restructuring. Similarly, a child who has not reached a developmental level of abstract thinking will likely not benefit from traditional disputation methods and would better respond to the development and rehearsal of coping statements to manage anxiety.

Best practice in the treatment of anxiety fears and phobia also involves appropriate involvement of family and parents. It is important to have all parties be made aware of confidentiality policies, and this is particularly important in establishing a trusting relationship when working with adolescents. While confidentiality is important, research shows that involving parents in aspects of treatment can maximize its effectiveness (Walczak et al., 2017). Parents and family members can support the process of therapy by not accommodating the child's anxiety (e.g., opting to not provide reassurance, allowing the child to stay home from school when anxious) and by implementing behavioral contingencies to reinforce target behaviors that are inconsistent with escape and/or avoidance.

RE-CBT in the Treatment of Anxiety, Fears, and Phobias in Children and Adolescents

As previously outlined earlier in this chapter, the common components of RE-CBT for children and adolescents with anxiety, fears, and phobia are comprised of psychoeducation, relaxation training/somatic management, cognitive restructuring, and exposure. Behavioral contingencies are also often put into place to support treatment. These methods are adapted to a child's age and developmental level and may be modified based on symptom presentation. Given the number of anxiety disorders that are diagnosed in children and adolescents, this section will primarily emphasize on the clinical similarities among the disorders and how RE-CBT can be applied across the spectrum of childhood anxiety disorders.

Establishing rapport is a critical component in therapy and especially when working with anxious youth and their parents. When working with anxious youth, a strong therapeutic alliance is particularly important as the therapist will eventually be working with them to systematically confront their anxiety triggers, irrational beliefs, and feared stimuli, which will likely be uncomfortable. It is therefore crucial that the child or adolescent trusts the therapist and that realistic goals and expectations are agreed upon. Providing good psychoeducation (discussed in detail below) including a clear rationale for treatment can help facilitate this process. It is also beneficial to foster autonomy particularly with older children and adolescent clients. They can be assured that they are going to be an active part of the treatment, which could be in opposition to an authoritarian relationship that they may be used to with other adult figures in their lives. In our experience, getting to know the client by inquiring about their interests, social life, family relationships, etc. is often time well spent in that it shows the adolescent you are genuinely interested in getting to know them and it may also reveal clinically useful information.

Parents of children with anxiety, fears, and phobias are often very anxious themselves (Casline et al., 2018). Assisting parents with their own fears can help build a trusting relationship between parent(s) and the therapist. Parents may hold several irrational beliefs such as "My child should not have to experience so much anxiety." "I can't stand seeing my child so distressed…It is terrible!" They may also experience self-blame and self-downing. "I should've been less over-protective. I gave my child anxiety and I am such a bad parent." RE-CBT therapists can address these anxiety-provoking irrational beliefs in a supportive and educational manner so that parents can effectively be involved in the therapy process. If parental disturbance is significant, they may require individual or family therapy as an adjunct to their child's therapy.

Psychoeducation

Before a child or adolescent can be effectively treated with RE-CBT, it is critical that parents and children be educated as to the key theoretical and treatment components as well as a basic level of understanding of the etiology and maintenance of anxiety. There are common elements of psychoeducation that are important for both parents and children. For example, understanding the ABC model of RE-CBT and the importance of the interplay between thinking, emotion, and behavior is important for both parents and children alike. REBT theory holds that it is irrational beliefs (B), rather than activating events (A), that lead to consequences (C), such as emotions or behaviors. Children and adolescents can learn through the use of rational stories, metaphors, games, and modeling (Cristea, Stefan, David, Mogoase, & Dobrean, 2016; Vernon, 2019). This can be done in a creative manner that will engage the child or adolescent. For example, preliminary evidence has shown positive results for teaching children and adolescents to distinguish functional and dysfunctional negative emotions through the use of a mini video game, which can be played on a smartphone or tablet (David et al., 2018).

Information regarding the nature of anxiety and resulting escape/avoidance behaviors that are maintained by negative reinforcement can be tailored for the child or adolescent to comprehend (Abramowitz, Deacon, & Whiteside, 2019; Cristea et al., 2016). For example, the fight or flight response can be discussed in an age-appropriate manner. Children and adolescents are often familiar with the expression "What goes up, must come down," and this can be used to describe the sympathetic and parasympathetic nervous system response when a panic attack occurs. Another illustrative metaphor can be used to explain the negative reinforcement cycle and rationale for exposure therapy. The therapist may present a pool party scenario where one child jumps into a pool and jumps right out because he is thinking that he can't stand being in the cold water and his friend jumps in, stays in the pool, gets used to the water, and ultimately has fun with his friends. Socratic questions about the differences in thinking between the two children can help teach and reinforce the B-C connection. In addition, the process of getting "used to" the temperature of the water can be an effective way of teaching the concept of habituation.

Relaxation Training

Relaxation training has been an important component in managing anxiety in RE-CBT since its inception (Ellis, 1998). Over 95% of youth with anxiety disorders experience at least one somatic symptom, and this is pronounced in those with generalized anxiety disorder and separation anxiety disorder (Crawley et al., 2014). Somatic complaints in anxious children and adolescents include but are not limited to stomach aches, headaches, muscle tension, increased respiration and heart rate, shaking, and blushing. These sensations can be quite scary for children and may elicit secondary emotional disturbance (e.g., anxiety about their somatic symptoms originally triggered by anxiety). Therefore, it is important for practitioners to incorporate relaxation strategies, particularly when the child or adolescent is so physiologically aroused that it may be difficult for them to attend to cognitive and behavioral interventions.

Children and adolescents can be taught to identify their unique physiological/somatic sensations when feeling anxious and use them as cues to employ relaxation strategies (Mychailyszyn et al., 2011). Specific relaxation strategies that can be incorporated into the treatment of children and adolescents with anxiety include diaphragmatic breathing, progressive muscle relaxation, and relaxing imagery (Cristea et al., 2016; Kendall & Hedke, 2006). When working with younger children, diaphragmatic breathing can be introduced as belly breathing, and children often find it enjoyable to place a pillow on their stomach and watch it move up and down as they learn to effectively inhale and exhale through their diaphragm. Creating relaxation imagery can also be a collaborative and enjoyable exercise where the therapist can work with the child to put together a story and scene that they find to be peaceful, enjoyable, and relaxing.

Cognitive Restructuring

Children and adolescents who experience anxiety hold at least one irrational belief, if not several. Irrational beliefs are characterized as rigid, illogical, and inconsistent with reality and interfere with goal attainment. According to contemporary REBT theory, there are four irrational beliefs: demandingness, awfulizing/catastrophizing, frustration intolerance, and global evaluations of human worth (DiGiuseppe et al., 2014). Helping the child or adolescent to effectively identify and replace their irrational beliefs with rational beliefs, which are flexible, logical, and consistent with reality, will serve to change their anxiety to a healthier negative emotion of concern. As previously indicated, a child's developmental level will determine the method in which an RE-CBT practitioner conducts cognitive restructuring. Children younger than 11 years of age frequently have not developed abstract reasoning skills, and therefore the RE-CBT therapist should align cognitive restructuring to the child's developmental level and may pose ways to think when encountering feared stimuli as opposed to a Socratic disputation style (Bernard, Ellis, & Terjesen, 2006).

Many children and adolescents with anxiety engage in awfulizing or catastrophic thinking (e.g., "It will be terrible if I do poorly on this test") and frustration intolerance (e.g., "I can't stand the idea of getting a bad grade) in addition to demandingness (e.g., "I absolutely have to do well on this test") and global evaluations of worth (e.g., "I am a failure because I got a bad grade"). Consider an adolescent experiencing social anxiety. She may believe that she must always know what to say when asked a question and it would be terrible if she didn't. It is important to help this adolescent change her demands to preferences and to decatastrophize the situation. This can be done through a variety of disputation strategies. Vernon (2019) emphasizes the utility of reverse role play in helping younger children in addition to encouraging them to be "fact detectives" as a way to identify evidence contrary to their irrational beliefs. A catastrophe scale may also be used, sometimes in the form of a thermometer, where a child or adolescent thinks of the worst thing possible and, in the aforementioned case, then places their difficulty answering the question on the scale to show that,while bad, it is not the end of the world. For children and adolescents who believe they can't stand a certain situation or the resulting sensations of anxiety, it is important to help them see that they have in fact tolerated discomfort in the past and, while uncomfortable, they were able to get through it. This also helps to foster self-efficacy and will be useful when conducting exposure exercises.

Many anxious children and adolescents also hold irrational beliefs in the form of global evaluations of worth. For example, children with performance anxiety at school or other forms of social anxiety may believe that they must get a good grade and, if not, they are a failure. Helping children and adolescents to separate their behavior from their worth and foster self-acceptance is critical. This can be done through a variety of strategies. Anxious students may benefit from creating a self-acceptance circle that lists their positive and negative traits and behaviors, strengths, weaknesses, etc. so they can see that it is not helpful nor logical to entirely rate themselves based on a success or failure. A friend dispute can also be helpful for some children and adolescents with anxiety. That is, the clinician may ask: "What would they tell a friend who believed they were stupid because they answered a question incorrectly in front of the class?"

While various disputation strategies can be helpful in generating rational beliefs, it is important that therapists encourage children and adolescents to rehearse them on a regular basis. Coping statements for anxiety can be written on index cards and reviewed on a regular basis for younger children. Adolescents may choose to write their rational beliefs and coping statements in their smartphones and set reminders to review them. Parents can also play a role in supporting this process by ignoring irrational statements and reinforcing the use of rational coping statements.

Exposure to Feared Situations

Exposure to feared situations and reduction of safety behaviors is a critical component of RE-CBT treatment of anxiety, fears, and phobias. Consistent with the cognitive restructuring approaches, the purpose of exposure therapy is to disconfirm fear-based expectations and/or the belief that feelings of anxiety are intolerable (Abramowitz et al., 2019). Exposure therapy is particularly effective for children and adolescents with separation anxiety, social anxiety, panic disorder, and phobias. A traditional fear hierarchy is constructed with the child or adolescent. For younger children, the clinician may choose to refer to the hierarchy as a fear ladder, and clinicians can use illustrated images of a ladder and work together with the child/adolescent and/or their parents to create a list of about 10–15 anxiety-activating items or situations that are avoided due to the fear or anxiety. The items are then ranked in the order of least to most distressing via subjective units of distress (SUDs) scale.

Traditionally, exposure has been conducted in a graded fashion (Abramowitz et al., 2019) which involves moving up the ladder from exposure to stimuli with lower to higher SUDs and that the child or adolescent stays in the situation until habituation has occurred (e.g., 50% reduction in SUDs). However, emphasis is now shifting from an emotional processing model to an inhibitory learning model where safety-based associations compete with fear-based danger associations. Therefore, when conducting exposures with children and adolescents, it is important to emphasize that their extreme fear-based associations in fact did not occur and that they were able to tolerate the discomfort of the anxiety (Abramowitz et al., 2019). Thus, habituation does not necessarily have to occur for the exposure to be successful, and there may be some utility to selecting exposure exercises at random as opposed to the traditional graded method, which can also facilitate self-efficacy in managing anxiety and confronting fears.

Case Study: The Case of Isabella

Isabella is a 15-year-old high school sophomore who was referred for rational emotive and cognitive behavioral therapy (RE-CBT) by her school psychologist due to recent problems related to anxiety and panic. Isabella was born in a Western European country but was raised in the United States since she was 5 years old. Much of her extended family still resides in Europe, though her parents live and work in the United States. During the initial session, Isabella's mother revealed that her father has a history of depression but was reluctant to seek treatment, highly due to cultural stigma. While both Isabella and her mother described Isabella as a perfectionist and high achiever, Isabella had never experienced significant anxiety until recently when she had her first panic attack. Furthermore, Isabella had no prior experience with psychotherapy or mental health treatment other than a couple of meetings with her school psychologist.

At the time of Isabella's first session, it was clear that her anxiety and panic were having a significant impact on her functioning. Isabella reported that her first panic attack occurred about a month prior to seeking treatment after watching a television show where one of the characters had a psychotic break. An intellectually curious adolescent, Isabella did some Internet research on psychosis and schizophrenia. She reported that as she was engaging in this research, she began to have the thought "What if I have a psychotic break?" Isabella then described experiencing symptoms typical of a panic attack. She experienced accelerated heart rate, light-headedness, numbness in her fingers, feelings of unreality (derealization), and accompanying thoughts that she was going crazy and even possibly dying. She immediately found her mother who tried to reassure her that she was okay and that she was not dying or going crazy and her panic soon subsided. Two days after the initial panic attack, Isabella was taking an exam at school, and she began to experience some numbness in her fingers which quickly led to another panic attack. She told her teacher who excused her from the exam and sent her to the school psychologist, who called her mother to pick her up. Isabella subsequently had an appointment with her medical doctor who concluded that there was no apparent medical cause for her panic symptoms and that it was likely anxiety.

During the initial session, the preceding background information was gathered, and this therapist began to establish a therapeutic alliance by validating the difficult nature of Isabella's symptoms and engaging in brief casual conversation about her interests as well as her perceived strengths and weaknesses. Goals for therapy were identified, and Isabella wanted to learn how to tolerate and eventually decrease her panic attacks and how to avoid making herself unnecessarily anxious in anticipation of having a panic attack. A thorough functional assessment also revealed that Isabella often sought reassurance from her mother regarding her mental well-being, avoided situations that may draw attention to physiological sensations and fears (e.g., exercise, being alone with her thoughts, watching tv shows/movies with individuals with mental illness), and frequently researched symptoms of schizophrenia on the Internet.

Psychoeducation was a critical component in commencing Isabella's treatment. This therapist explained the fight or flight response to Isabella and had her reflect on her own experiences with her panic attacks in that they became very intense but then eventually passed in about a 10-minute time period. In the psychoeducation phase, Isabella was educated about panic attacks in that they do not involve passing out, dying, or going crazy. However, in subsequent sessions, the therapist did not provide reassurance to Isabella. The therapist explained that this was necessary because it was important for her to tolerate uncertainty and utilize her own coping skills. Psychoeducation was also provided to Isabella's mother in a joint session early in therapy. She agreed that she would not accommodate Isabella and specifically would refrain from providing reassurance that she was not psychotic. Isabella's mother also agreed that she would not take her out of school if she was experiencing heightened anxiety.

Relaxation training and management of somatic symptoms involved teaching Isabella diaphragmatic breathing and implementing grounding exercises when she was experiencing symptoms of derealization and depersonalization. For the first 2 weeks of therapy, Isabella practiced diaphragmatic breathing twice a day for about 5–10 minutes. Her grounding exercises involved noticing five things she could see, hear, feel, taste, or smell, and she also found it useful to focus on the sensation of her feet touching the floor as she walked.

A major component of Isabella's treatment involved cognitive restructuring. Isabella held many irrational beliefs regarding her ability to tolerate her panic symptoms. She *demanded* that she not have panic attacks and that her symptoms were *terrible* and *unbearable*. Isabella also spent a lot of time ruminating about the possibility of impending panic attacks. She *catastrophized* that if she were to experience panic symptoms she would go crazy and that would be the *worst thing* in the world. As a result, Isabella paid excessive attention to bodily sensations and *demanded* that she not feel any physical discomfort that in any way resembled her panic symptoms. The majority of cognitive restructuring centered on Isabella's demand for control and presumed inability to tolerate her panic symptoms. Through structured disputing, Isabella was able to see that, paradoxically, the more she demanded that she not experience her symptoms, the more likely she was to notice otherwise harmless sensations. Pragmatic disputes were particularly helpful for Isabella as she was able to notice this phenomenon and soon began to relinquish control. She changed her thinking from "I absolutely must not experience panic symptoms" to "I don't like my panic symptoms and wish I didn't have to deal with this, but I have strategies to cope when they happen." In addition, by drawing Isabella's attention to the fact that she experienced panic attacks and nothing horrible happened as a result, she was able to logically and empirically dispute beliefs that they were awful and unbearable. Through her previous experiences, she had evidence to the contrary that, while very uncomfortable, she was able to tolerate the discomfort. Finally, Isabella also benefited from labeling her panic symptoms as her brain responding to a false alarm. She was able to remind herself that she was not truly in danger, which allowed her to remind herself that panic symptoms were not consistent with having a psychotic break.

Behavioral interventions were introduced to augment and support cognitive restructuring. While Isabella learned relaxation strategies, it was important that she reinforce the effective new belief that she could tolerate the discomfort. Interoceptive exposure exercises (e.g., running in place to increase heart rate, breathing through a straw to simulate difficulty breathing, and spinning in an office chair to bring on dizziness) were completed in session for several sessions and were assigned as homework. Eventually, Isabella no longer avoided these sensations and began to return to her exercise routine that she has been avoiding. Her safety-seeking behaviors were also addressed and eliminated. When Isabella had the urge to do research on schizophrenia or "google" her symptoms, she was instructed to utilize one of her coping skills instead and to remind herself that she did not need to know the answers and that she could tolerate the uncertainty.

Isabella was quite motivated and spent a lot of time practicing her relaxation strategies, cognitive restructuring techniques, exposure exercises, and elimination of safety behaviors for homework. As a result, Isabella's frequency of panic attacks decreased. By accepting them for what they were, decatastrophizing, and showing herself that she could tolerate the discomfort, Isabella also spent much less time ruminating, and her anticipatory anxiety changed to a healthy concern. Over the course of 10 weeks of therapy, Isabella reached most of her treatment goals and presently only attends therapy once a month for maintenance and relapse prevention.

Adaptation of RE-CBT in the Schools for Anxiety, Fears, and Phobias

Given the short-term and directive nature of RE-CBT, it has been applied effectively in schools, and numerous studies have investigated its effectiveness in school settings (Bernard, 2008; Ginsberg et al., 2012; Mychailyszyn et al., 2011). Moreover, RE-CBT interventions targeted at addressing anxiety, fears, and phobia are particularly beneficial given that these emotional problems are often activated in school settings (Mychailyszyn et al., 2011). Younger children, for example, often experience separation anxiety from their caregivers, and older children and adolescents are confronted with a range of anxiety-activating triggers from developing social relationships and fitting in to demands for high achievement, test anxiety, and even fears of violence in the schools.

Mychailyszyn et al. (2011) have shown the efficacy of modifying the Coping Cat (Kendall & Hedke, 2006) program into schools for delivery by school psychologists, school social workers, and guidance counselors. For accessibility reasons in the school environment, they suggest decreasing the traditional 50-minute session to 30 minutes and increasing the amount of sessions per week. Mychailyszyn and colleagues also emphasize the importance of parental involvement to reinforce principles learned and to assist with homework compliance. Other practical considerations include the delivery of exposure-based components of the Coping Cat program in school. While several feared stimuli may be present in the school setting, which can facilitate the process, it may be difficult to reintegrate children into the classroom environment if their fear response has not adequately habituated. The authors suggest allocating extra time at the end of the session to include a pleasant activity to help decrease distress and also to schedule exposure tasks for after school.

The You Can Do It! Education (YCDI) cognitive behavioral intervention program on emotional resilience has also been shown to be effectively implemented in primary school settings (grades 4–6) with promising results (Bernard, 2008). This program is based on cognitive behavioral and social-emotional learning principles and assists children in learning how to identify, challenge, and replace irrational thinking in a systematic eight-session protocol. This program allows for effective use in schools because it can be presented in a once-a-week format during small group counseling sessions. Findings particularly relevant for students experiencing anxiety included increased ability to cope with distressful events and ability to calm themselves when experiencing anxious feelings (Bernard, 2008).

Similarly, Saelid and Nordahl (2017) examined the effects of educating adolescent students with subclinical anxiety and depression about REBT's ABC model and compared the REBT condition to an individual attention placebo (ATP) condition and a no treatment control condition. In a three-session protocol, the students were taught the ABC model and utilized the REBT self-help form to identify and dispute irrational beliefs. Both the REBT and ATP conditions resulted in significant reduction in anxious and depressed symptoms, but only the REBT significantly reduced dysfunctional thinking and maintained symptom reduction at 6-month follow-up. This study provides promising support that teaching the ABC model and utilizing brief, structured intervention can fit well in a school setting and can have clinical utility for students experiencing anxiety.

Another advantage of the adaptation of RE-CBT in schools is that services may be available to anxious children and adolescents who may otherwise not have the means to obtain evidence-based services in a clinical setting. For example, Ginsburg, Becker, Drazdowski, and Tein (2012) conducted a pilot study comparing the effectiveness of CBT vs. usual care in an urban public school setting of primarily African American youth and found significant and clinically meaningful improvements in symptoms of anxiety and functioning in a 7–9-week session protocol delivered by novice CBT school-based clinicians.

There are important limitations to consider when adapting RE-CBT in the schools for this population. Depending on the setting, there may be limited resources and/or qualified professionals to provide the services needed to effectively treat children and adolescents with anxiety, fears, and phobia. For example, Miller, Short, Garland, and Clark (2010) evaluated a CBT intervention program (Taming Worry Dragons) administered by teachers in a public elementary school setting. The intervention did not yield significant reduction in anxiety symptoms on either self- or parent-report measures. However, observations from teachers indicated benefits in normalizing anxiety, increased empathy for other students, and provision of a common language to talk about worries.

In conclusion, rational emotive and cognitive behavioral therapy (RE-CBT) is an evidence-based form of psychotherapy used to successfully treat anxiety, fears, and phobias in children and adolescents. This has been supported by a wealth of published studies including numerous randomized control trials. As a result, RE-CBT therapists have a variety of effective assessment and intervention strategies that have been outlined in this chapter to successfully treat a range of anxiety disorders that present in children and adolescents. While several of the interventions (e.g., relaxation training, cognitive restructuring, exposure) are also used in RE-CBT treatment of anxious adults, it is imperative to tailor these treatment methods to be consistent with the child/adolescent's developmental level. In addition to traditional clinical settings, RE-CBT has been utilized in a variety of prevention and intervention programs in school settings, thus maximizing the availability of short-term effective treatment for anxious youth in need of mental health services.

Questions

1. Anxiety disorders are often maintained by a cycle of negative reinforcement. Describe this cycle and give an example.
2. It is important for parents to provide their children with healthy protection, whereas accommodation can maintain and worsen anxiety. Describe the difference between healthy protection and accommodation.

3. Sarah is a 14-year-old ninth grade student who is skipping school because she fears negative judgments regarding her school performance from her teachers and peers. What irrational beliefs may Sarah be holding? What type of exposure exercises would be appropriate to get Sarah back to regularly attending school?

References

Abramowitz, J. S., Deacon, B. J., & Whiteside, S. P. H. (2019). *Exposure therapy for anxiety: Principles and practice* (2nd ed.). New York: The Guilford Press.

Almqvist, F., Puura, K., Kumpulainen, K., Tuompo-Johansson, E., Henttonen, I., Huikko, E., et al. (1999). Psychiatric disorders in 8–9-year-old children based on a diagnostic interview with the parents. *European Child & Adolescent Psychiatry, 8*(S4), IV17–IV28.

American Psychiatric Association. (2013). *Diagnostic and statistical manual of mental disorders* (5th ed.). Washington, DC: Author.

American Psychological Association. (2005). *Policy statement on evidence-based practice in psychology*. Retrieved from https://www.apa.org/practice/guidelines/evidence-based-statement

American Psychological Association. (2019). *APA clinical practice guideline development*. Retrieved from https://www.apa.org/about/offices/directorates/guidelines/clinical-practice

Arnaudova, I., Kindt, M., Fanselow, M., & Beckers, T. (2017). Pathways towards the proliferation of avoidance in anxiety and implications for treatment. *Behaviour Research and Therapy, 96*, 3–13.

Aydin, A. (2014). Parental involvement in cognitive-behavioral therapy for children with anxiety disorders. *Turkish Journal of Psychiatry, 25*(3), 181–189.

Becker, E. S., Rinck, M., Türke, V., Kause, P., Goodwin, R., Neumer, S., et al. (2007). Epidemiology of specific phobia subtypes: Findings from the Dresden Mental Health Study. *European Psychiatry, 22*(2), 69–74.

Beesdo, K., Bittner, A., Pine, D. S., Stein, M. B., Höfler, M., Lieb, R., et al. (2007). Incidence of social anxiety disorder and the consistent risk for secondary depression in the first three decades of life. *Archives of General Psychiatry, 64*(8), 903–912.

Beidel, D. C., & Turner, S. M. (2007). Clinical presentation of social anxiety disorder in children and adolescents. In *Shy children, phobic adults: Nature and treatment of social anxiety disorders* (pp. 47–80). Washington, DC: American Psychological Association.

Bernard, M. E. (2008). The effect of You Can Do It! Education on the emotional resilience of primary school students with social, emotional, behavioural and achievement challenges. *Proceedings of the Australian Psychological Society Annual Conference, 43*, 36–40.

Bernard, M. E., Ellis, A., & Terjesen, M. (2006). Rational-emotive behavioral approaches to childhood disorders: History, theory, practice and research. In A. Ellis & M. E. Bernard (Eds.), *Rational-emotive behavioral approaches to childhood disorders: History, theory, practice, and research* (pp. 3–84). New York: Springer Science + Business Media, Inc.

Birmaher, B., Brent, D. A., Chiappetta, L., Bridge, J., Monga, S., & Baugher, M. (1999). Psychometric properties of the Screen for Child Anxiety Related Emotional Disorders (SCARED): A replication study. *Journal of the American Academy of Child and Adolescent Psychiatry, 38*(10), 1230–1236.

Bitsko, R. H., Holbrook, J. R., Ghandour, R. M., Blumberg, S. J., Visser, S. N., Perou, R., et al. (2018). Epidemiology and impact of health care provider-diagnosed anxiety and depression among US children. *Journal of Developmental & Behavioral Pediatrics, 39*(5), 395–403.

Bittner, A., Egger, H. L., Erkanli, A., Costello, E. J., Foley, D. L., & Angold, A. (2007). What do childhood anxiety disorders predict? *Journal of Child Psychology and Psychiatry, 48*(12), 1174–1183.

Carbone, D., Schmidt, L. A., Cunningham, C. C., McHolm, A. E., Edison, S., St. Pierre, J., et al. (2010). Behavioral and socio-emotional functioning in children with selective mutism: A comparison with anxious and typically developing children across multiple informants. *Journal of Abnormal Child Psychology, 38*(8), 1057–1067.

Cartwright-Hatton, S., McNicol, K., & Doubleday, E. (2006). Anxiety in a neglected population: Prevalence of anxiety disorders in pre-adolescent children. *Clinical Psychology Review, 26*(7), 817–833.

Casline, E. P., Pella, J., Zheng, D., Harel, O., Drake, K. L., & Ginsburg, G. (2018). Parental responses to children's avoidance in fear-provoking situations: Relation to child anxiety and mediators of intervention response. *Child & Youth Care Forum, 47*, 443–462.

Compton, S. N., Walkup, J. T., Albano, A. M., Piacentini, J. C., Birmaher, B., Sherrill, J. T., et al. (2010). Child/Adolescent Anxiety Multimodal Study (CAMS): Rationale, design, and methods. *Child and Adolescent Psychiatry and Mental Health, 4*(1), 1.

Connolly, S. D., & Bernstein, G. A. (2007). Practice parameter for the assessment and treatment of child and adolescents with anxiety disorders. *Journal of the American Academy of Child and Adolescent Psychiatry, 46*(2), 267–283.

Costello, E. J., Mustillo, S., Erkanli, A., Keeler, G., & Angold, A. (2003). Prevalence and development of psychiatric disorders in childhood and adolescence. *Archives of General Psychiatry, 60*(8), 837–844.

Crawley, C. A., Caporino, N. E., Birmaher, B., Ginsburg, G., Piacentini, J., Albano, A. M., et al. (2014). Somatic complaints in anxious youth. *Child Psychiatry & Human Development, 45*, 398–407.

Cristea, I. A., Stefan, S., David, O., Mogoase, C., & Dobrean, A. (2016). *REBT in the treatment of anxiety disorders in children and adults* (Springer briefs in psychology). Cham, Switzerland: Springer International Publishing.

David, O. A., Predatu, R. M., & Cardos, R. A. (2018). A pilot study of the Rethink online video game applied for coaching emotional understanding in children adolescents in the therapeutic video game environment: The feeling better resource game. *Journal of Evidence-Based Psychotherapies, 18*(1), 57–67.

DiGiuseppe, R., & Kassinove, H. (1976). Effects of a rational-emotive school mental health program on children's emotional adjustment. *Journal of Community Psychology, 4*(4), 382–387.

DiGiuseppe, R. A., Doyle, K. A., Dryden, W., & Backx, W. (2014). *A practitioner's guide to rational emotive behavior therapy* (3rd ed.). New York: Oxford University Press.

Ellis, A. (1998). *How to control your anxiety before it controls you*. Secaucus, NJ: Carol Publishing.

Ford, T., Goodman, R., & Meltzer, H. (2003). The British child and adolescent mental health survey 1999: The prevalence of DSM-IV disorders. *Journal of the American Academy of Child & Adolescent Psychiatry, 42*(10), 1203–1211.

Garber, J., & Weersing, V. R. (2010). Comorbidity of anxiety and depression in youth: Implications for treatment and prevention. *Clinical Psychology: Science and Practice, 17*(4), 293–306.

Gavita, O. A., & Calin, A. (2013). Retman rational stories versus rational parenting program for the treatment of child psychopathology: Efficacy of two formats of rational-emotive behavior therapy. *Journal of Cognitive and Behavioral Psychotherapies, 13*(1), 33–56.

Ginsburg, G. S., Becker, K. D., Drazdowski, T. K., & Tein, J. Y. (2012). Treating anxiety disorders in inner city schools: Results from a pilot randomized controlled trial comparing CBT and usual care. *Child & Youth Care Forum, 41*, 1–19.

Ginsburg, G. S., Riddle, M. A., & Davies, M. (2006). Somatic symptoms in children and adolescents with anxiety disorders. *Journal of the American Academy of Child & Adolescent Psychiatry, 45*(10), 1179–1187.

Gonzalez, J. E., Nelson, J. R., Gutkin, T. B., Saunders, A., Galloway, A., & Shwery, C. S. (2004). Rational emotive therapy with children and adolescents. *Journal of Emotional and Behavioral Disorders, 12*(4), 222–235.

Grave, J., & Blissett, J. (2004). Is cognitive behavior therapy developmentally appropriate for young children? A critical review of the evidence. *Clinical Psychology Review, 24*(4), 399–420.

Gross, C., & Hen, R. (2004). Genetic and environmental factors interact to influence anxiety. *Neurotoxicity Research, 6*(6), 493–501.

Grover, R. L., Hughes, A. A., Bergman, R. L., & Kingery, J. N. (2006). Treatment modifications based on childhood anxiety diagnosis: Demonstrating the flexibility in manualized treatment. *Journal of Cognitive Psychotherapy, 20*(3), 275–286.

Hudson, J. L., & Kendall, P. C. (2002). Showing you can do it: Homework in therapy for children and adolescents with anxiety disorders. *Journal of Clinical Psychology, 58*(5), 525–534.

Kendall, P. C., & Hedke, K. A. (2006). *Coping cat workbook* (2nd ed.). Ardmore, PA: Workbook Publishing.

Kessler, R. C., Berglund, P., Demler, O., Jin, R., Merikangas, K. R., & Walters, E. E. (2005). Lifetime prevalence and age-of-onset distributions of DSM-IV disorders in the national comorbidity survey replication. *Archives of General Psychiatry, 62*(6), 593–602.

Kessler, R. C., Petukhova, M., Sampson, N. A., Zaslavsky, A. M., & Wittchen, H.-U. (2012). Twelve-month and lifetime prevalence and lifetime morbid risk of anxiety and mood disorders in the United States. *International Journal of Methods in Psychiatric Research, 21*(3), 169–184.

Kingery, J. N., Roblek, T. L., Suveg, C., Grover, R. L., Sherrill, J. T., & Bergman, R. L. (2006). They're not just "little adults": Developmental considerations for implementing cognitive-behavioral therapy with anxious youth. *Journal of Cognitive Psychotherapy, 20*(3), 263–273.

Lebowitz, E., & Omer, H. (2013). *Treating childhood and adolescent anxiety: A guide for caregivers*. Hoboken, NJ: Wiley.

March, J. S. (2012). *Multidimensional anxiety scale for children* (2nd ed.). North Tonawanda, NY: Multi-Health Systems.

Merikangas, K. R., He, J., Burstein, M., Swanson, S. A., Avenevoli, S., Cui, L., et al. (2010). Lifetime prevalence of mental disorders in U.S. adolescents: Results from the national comorbidity survey replication–adolescent supplement (NCS-A). *Journal of the American Academy of Child & Adolescent Psychiatry, 49*(10), 980–989.

Miller, L. D., Short, C., Garland, E. J., & Clark, S. (2010). The ABCs of CBT: Evidence-based approaches to child anxiety in public school settings. *Journal of Counseling & Development, 88*, 432–438.

Muris, P., Meesters, C., Merckelbach, H., Sermon, A., & Zwakhalen, S. (1998). Worry in normal children. *Journal of the American Academy of Child & Adolescent Psychiatry, 37*(7), 703–710.

Muris, P., Merckelbach, H., Mayer, B., & Prins, E. (2000). How serious are common childhood fears? *Behaviour Research and Therapy, 38*(3), 217–228.

Mychailyszyn, M. P., Mendez, J. L., & Kendall, P. C. (2010). School functioning in youth with and without anxiety disorders: Comparisons by diagnosis and comorbidity. *School Psychology Review, 39*(1), 106–121.

Mychailyszyn, W. P., Beidas, R. S., Benjamin, C. L., Edmunds, J. M., Podell, J. L., Cohen, J. S., et al. (2011). Assessing and treating child anxiety in schools. *Psychology in the Schools, 48*(3), 223–232.

Nail, J. E., Christofferson, J., Ginsburg, G. S., Drake, K., Kendall, P. C., McCracken, J. T., et al. (2015). *Child & Youth Care Forum, 44*, 327–342.

Ollendick, T. H. (1983). Reliability and validity of the Revised Fear Survey Schedule for Children (FSSC-R). *Behaviour Research and Therapy, 21*(6), 685–692.

Ollendick, T. H., King, N. J., & Muris, P. (2002). Fears and phobias in children: Phenomenology, epidemiology, and aetiology. *Child and Adolescent Mental Health, 7*(3), 98–106.

Opre, A., Buzgar, R., & Dumulescu, D. (2018). Empirical support for self kit: A rational emotive education program. *Journal of Cognitive and Behavioral Psychotherapies, 13*(2a), 557–573.

Peris, T. S., Compton, S. N., Kendall, P. C., Birmaher, B., Sherrill, J., March, J., et al. (2015). Trajectories of change in youth anxiety during cognitive—behavior therapy. *Journal of Consulting and Clinical Psychology, 83*(2), 239–252.

Piaget, J. (1964). Part I: Cognitive development in children: Piaget development and learning. *Journal of Research in Science Teaching, 2*(3), 176–186.

Polanczyk, G. V., Salum, G. A., Sugaya, L. S., Caye, A., & Rohde, L. A. (2015). Annual research review: A meta-analysis of the worldwide prevalence of mental health disorders in children and adolescents. *Journal of Child Psychology and Psychiatry, 56*(3), 345–365.

Predescu, E., Asztalos, A. B., & Sipos, R. (2018). *Prevalence and treatment of anxiety disorders comorbidities in a clinical Romanian sample of children and adolescents with psychiatric disorders*. Retrieved from https://www.intechopen.com/online-first/prevalence-and-treatment-of-anxiety-disorders-comorbidities-in-a-clinical-romanian-sample-of-children

Reynolds, C. R., & Richmond, B. O. (2008). *Revised children's manifest anxiety scale: Second edition (RCMAS-2)*. Los Angeles: Western Psychological Services.

Russo, M. F., & Beidel, D. C. (1994). Comorbidity of childhood anxiety and externalizing disorders: Prevalence, associated characteristics, and validation issues. *Clinical Psychology Review, 14*(3), 199–221.

Saelid, G. A., & Nordahl, H. M. (2017). Rational emotive behaviour therapy in high schools to educate in mental health and empower youth health. A randomized controlled study of a brief intervention. *Cognitive Behaviour Therapy, 46*(3), 196–210.

Sawyer, M. C., & Nunez, D. E. (2014). Cognitive-behavioral therapy for anxious children: From evidence to practice. *Worldviews on Evidence-Based Nursing, 11*(1), 65–71.

Scharfstein, L. A., & Beidel, D. C. (2014). Social skills and social acceptance in children with anxiety disorders. *Journal of Clinical Child & Adolescent Psychology, 44*(5), 826–838.

Seligman, L. D., & Ollendick, T. H. (2011). Cognitive-behavioral therapy for anxiety disorders in youth. *Child and Adolescent Psychiatric Clinics of North America, 20*(2), 217–238.

Spence, S. H. (1997). Structure of anxiety symptoms among children: A confirmatory factor-analytic study. *Journal of Abnormal Psychology, 106*(2), 280–297.

Spielberger, C. D. (1971). Anxiety as an emotional state. In C. D. Spielberger (Ed.), *Anxiety: Current trends in theory and research*. New York: Academic Press.

Sugawara, M., Mukai, T., Kitamura, T., Toda, M. A., Shima, S., Tomoda, A., et al. (1999). Psychiatric disorders among Japanese children. *Journal of the American Academy of Child & Adolescent Psychiatry, 38*(4), 444–452.

Terjesen, M. D., Kassay, K. S., & Anderson, D. L. (2017). Evaluation of the psychometric properties of a measure of child irrationality. *Journal of Rational-Emotive and Cognitive-Behavioral Therapies, 35*, 413–431. https://doi.org/10.1007/s10942-017-0269-z

Thapar, A., Pine, D. S., Leckman, J. F., Scott, S., Snowling, M. J., & Taylor, E. (Eds.). (2015). *Rutter's child and adolescent psychiatry* (6th ed.). West Sussex, UK: Wiley.

Vernon, A. (2019). REBT with children and adolescents. In W. Dryden & M. E. Bernard (Eds.), *REBT with diverse client problems and populations* (pp. 243–263). Cham, Switzerland: Springer Nature Switzerland.

Viana, A. G., Beidel, D. C., & Rabian, B. (2009). Selective mutism: A review and integration of the last 15 years. *Clinical Psychology Review, 29*(1), 57–67.

Walczak, M., Esbjørn, B. H., Breinholst, S., & Reinholdt-Dunne, M. L. (2017). Parental involvement in cognitive behavior therapy for children with anxiety disorders: 3-year follow-up. *Child Psychiatry & Human Development, 48*(3), 444–454.

Warren, R., Deffenbach, J., & Broding, P. (1976). Rational-emotive therapy and the reduction of test anxiety in elementary school students. *Rational Living, 11*, 28–29.

Wessel, I., & Mersch, P. P. A. (1994). A cognitive-behavioural group treatment for test-anxious adolescents. *Anxiety, Stress & Coping: An International Journal, 7*(2), 149–160.

Wittchen, H.-U., & Fehm, L. (2003). Epidemiology and natural course of social fears and social phobia. *Acta Psychiatrica Scandinavica, 108*(s417), 4–18.

Wittchen, H.-U., Stein, M. B., & Kessler, R. C. (1999). Social fears and social phobia in a community sample of adolescents and young adults: Prevalence, risk factors and co-morbidity. *Psychological Medicine, 29*(2), 309–323.

Wood, J. (2006). Effect of anxiety reduction on children's school performance and social adjustment. *Developmental Psychology, 42*(2), 345–349.

Woodward, L. J., & Fergusson, D. M. (2001). Life course outcomes of young people with anxiety disorders in adolescence. *Journal of the American Academy of Child & Adolescent Psychiatry, 40*(9), 1086–1093.

Chapter 9
REBT-CBT in the Treatment of Trauma Among Children and Adolescents

Jaco Rossouw

PTSD develops in response to exposure to actual or threatened death, serious injury or sexual violence (American Psychiatric Association, 2013). Symptoms can develop in response to directly experiencing the traumatic event, such as being sexually or physically assaulted and being exposed to a natural disasters, accidents or injuries. Symptoms may also manifest itself as a result of witnessing the event as it occurs to others or learning that the traumatic event occurred to a close family member or close friend (American Psychiatric Association, 2013). PTSD is characterised by intrusive memories of the traumatic event, avoidance of reminders to the trauma (internal and external) and hyperarousal symptoms. If left untreated, PTSD often develops into a chronically debilitating condition with substantial functional impairment. Further, PTSD has a high co-morbidity with other psychiatric disorders such as other anxiety disorders, substance abuse disorders and mood disorders, with depression being the most common (McLaughlin et al., 2013).

The rates of trauma exposure reported internationally in studies vary considerably (Finkelhor, Omrod, Turner, & Hamby, 2005; McLaughlin et al., 2013). In a national epidemiological study in the United State (USA), three out of five adolescents reported experiencing at least one traumatic stressor (McLaughlin et al., 2013). Earlier studies from the United States examined the prevalence of trauma exposure in school samples and reported rates of exposure to trauma ranging from 40% to 70% (Giaconia et al., 1995; Jenkins & Bell, 1994). In their review of 2000 children aged 10–16, Finkelhor and Dziuba-Leatherman (1994) reported that 24% of their sample stated they had been victims of physical assault, sexual assault or kidnapping.

J. Rossouw (✉)
Centre for Cognitive-Behaviour Therapy, Cape Town, South Africa

Department of Psychiatry, Faculty of Medicine and Health Science, Stellenbosch University, Stellenbosch, South Africa

M. Bernard, M. D. Terjesen (eds.), *Rational-Emotive and Cognitive-Behavioral Approaches to Child and Adolescent Mental Health: Theory, Practice, Research, Applications*, https://doi.org/10.1007/978-3-030-53901-6_9

According to Alisic et al. (2014) in a review of studies from North America, Europe, Australia and Asia, 16% of children and adolescents exposed to potentially traumatic events will develop PTSD. There is a scarcity of epidemiological studies reporting on the prevalence rates of trauma exposure and PTSD of children and adolescents in low- and middle-income countries (LIMICs). The PTSD prevalence rate in low- and middle-income countries (LIMICs) is higher than in high-income countries (HICs). One reason is that the majority of children and adolescents living in war-torn areas is from LIMICs. Children in LIMICs that are war torn or embroiled in armed conflict settings have a high risk of trauma exposure (World Health Organization, 2013). It is estimated that 230 million children live in countries suffering with armed conflict (UNICEF, 2014). These children are exposed to displacement, becoming a refugee, torture, kidnapping, rape or recruitment as a child soldier (UNICEF, 2014). A meta-analysis of children affected by war suggests a PTSD prevalence rate of 47% (Attanayake et al., 2009). The PTSD prevalence rate among child soldiers is estimated to be between 35% and 97% (Bayer, Klasen, & Adam, 2007; Derluyn, Broekaert, Schuyten, & De Temmerman, 2004). The rate of gender-based violence and domestic violence is also higher in LMICs (WHO, 2013). The exposure to domestic and gender-based violence has a profound effect on the mental health of the children and adolescents witnessing or experiencing these events and can include developing PTSD. The estimated PTSD rates for adolescents (Hiller et al., 2016) show a rate of 21% in the first month after a trauma; this spontaneously declines to 15% at 3 months, 12% at 6 months and 11% at 1 year after a trauma. Spontaneous recovery after 6 month therefore seems unlikely.

Exposure to trauma is associated with multiple negative outcomes, including most mental disorders, academic underperformance, poor social and interpersonal functioning and physical health problems. Logically, a major consequence of exposure to trauma is PTSD. PTSD has a high co-morbidity with other mental health disorders among youth and specifically depressive conditions, ranging from a low mood to major depression (Brent et al., 1995; Das-Munshi et al., 2016; Yule, 1994). Kilpatrick et al. (2003) reported that 41% of adolescents with PTSD met criteria for major depression by age 18 compared to 8% among their peers. PTSD is also associated with a significantly increased risk for social anxiety (33%), specific phobia (29%), alcohol dependence (46%), drug dependence (25%) and suicidal ideation and attempts (Kilpatrick et al., 2003; Rojas et al., 2017).

Assessment and Diagnosis of PTSD

PTSD is characterised by the presence of intrusion symptoms. These symptoms present as distressing involuntary memories of the traumatic event, flashbacks or nightmares. In younger children, the distressing memories may not appear distressing and can be expressed as play re-enactment. Younger children may also have dreams with content that seem unrelated to the trauma (APA, 2013). Individuals struggling with PTSD secondary to exposure to the traumatic event often present with persistent avoidance of internal and external reminders to the event. This avoidance of internal reminders is an attempt to avoid distressing memories, thoughts and feelings related to the traumatic event (APA, 2013). Further, individuals with PTSD individuals may present with changes in cognition and mood. Cognitive changes can include difficulty remembering important aspects of the traumatic event and the presence of unhelpful thoughts about themselves, others or the world. Individuals with PTSD could present with thoughts such as "I am incompetent to prevent these dangers" and "The world is a dangerous place". They present with an enduring negative emotional state that can include fear, anger, guilt, shame and horror. They also can experience themselves as detached or estranged from others and struggle to experience positive emotions such as happiness, satisfaction and love. Significant changes in arousal and reactivity associated with the traumatic event occur and can present as irritable behaviour and angry outbursts expressed as verbal or physical aggression, reckless or self-destructive behaviour, hypervigilance, exaggerated startle response, problems of concentration and/or sleep disturbance (APA, 2013).

When considering a diagnosis of PTSD, the trauma symptoms need to be present for at least 1 month prior to assessment. If symptoms are present for less than 1 month, clinicians may wish to consider an acute stress disorder diagnosis. In cases where trauma events occurred over an extended period of time (e.g., repeated sexual victimisation among youth), the presentation may be different. As a consequence, the presentation of long-standing complex PTSD is now covered as a separate diagnosis in ICD-11.

A number of commonly used self-report checklists or structured interviews are available to assist in the diagnosis of PTSD in children and adolescents. The Clinician-Administered PTSD Scale for Children and Adolescents (CAPS-CA) is a structured interview used for diagnostic assessment of PTSD in 8–15 year olds. The UCLA PTSD Reaction Index (UCLA PTSD-RI; Steinberg, Brymer, Decker, & Pynoos, 2004) is an interview schedule used with 6–18 year olds. Self-report and clinician-administered scales commonly used are the Child PTSD Symptom Scale (CPSS5) (Foa, Asnaami, Zang, Capaldi, & Yeh, 2018). The self-report scale (CPSS5) is also helpful to measure progress during treatment. The Child Post-traumatic Cognitions Inventory measures negative trauma-related beliefs among 7–17 year olds (Meiser-Stedman et al., 2009). Self-report measures to measure associated symptoms such as depression and substance abuse disorders can also be helpful to gauge treatment response.

Research on RE-CBT with Children and Adolescents with PTSD

PTSD is a diagnosis with a very strong evidence base for trauma-focussed psychological treatment in adults. A review reporting on treatment of adult PTSD found trauma-focussed interventions to be effective in the treatment of PTSD (Bisson et al., 2007). Bisson et al. (2007) concluded that specifically trauma-focussed CBT and eye movement desensitisation and reprocessing (EMDR) therapy were more effective in reducing PTSD symptoms than other non-trauma-focussed psychological therapies in adults.

While comparatively there are not as many studies examining the treatment of trauma among youth, the evidence base for the psychological treatment of PTSD in children and adolescents is expanding with ongoing studies. A Cochrane meta-analytic study (Gillies, Taylor, Gray, O'Brien, & D'Abrew, 2013) identified 14 studies (totalling 758 participants; aged 3–18 years) on the treatment of PTSD in children and adolescents. The types of trauma the participants had been exposed to included sexual abuse, interpersonal violence, natural disasters and motor vehicle accidents. The psychological interventions used in these studies were cognitive behavioural therapy (CBT), exposure-based interventions, supportive counselling, EMDR, narrative therapy and psychodynamic therapy. The majority of studies compared a psychosocial treatment to a control group. The authors concluded that there is evidence for the effectiveness of psychosocial therapies for the treatment of PTSD in children and adolescents. Specifically, CBT was identified as the most effective therapy for treating PTSD in children and adolescents – with maintained gains of up to a month following treatment.

A more recent meta-analysis of interventions for children and adolescents with PTSD (Morina, Koerssen, & Pollet, 2016) identified 41 randomised control trials (RCTs) – of which 39 were psychological interventions and 2 psychopharmacological interventions. The researchers concluded that psychological interventions are effective in treating PTSD in children and adolescents. Trauma-focussed CBT was found to be the most studied form of intervention and resulted in medium to large effect sizes, when compared to waitlist and active control conditions at post- and follow-up assessment. Interventions were also effective in reducing co-morbid depression symptoms. The authors concluded that psychological interventions can effectively reduce PTSD symptoms in children and adolescents.

A recent review of TF-CBT studies (De Arellano et al., 2014) identified ten RCT studies and concluded that TF-CBT is a viable treatment for reducing trauma-related symptoms among children and adolescents. TF-CBT has also been shown to be effective in LIMIC settings utilising both experienced clinicians and task-shifted care to community mental health workers with varying degrees of experience and qualification, including lay counsellors with a limited formal education (Holtzhausen, Ross, & Perry, 2015). Cohen, Mannarino, Kliethermes, and Murray (2012) also found TF-CBT to be helpful in treating children and adolescents with complex PTSD and provide practical strategies for applying TF-CBT to this population.

More recently, four RCT studies of adolescents (Foa, McLean, Capaldi, & Rosenfield, 2013; Gilboa-Schechtman et al., 2010; Rossouw et al., 2016; Rossouw, Yadin, Alexander, & Seedat, 2018) investigated a trauma-focussed CBT intervention prolonged exposure therapy for adolescents (PE-A) and reported significant improvement in PTSD symptom severity compared with a non-trauma-focussed intervention. The Foa et al. (2013) study added a dissemination component, by training community-based rape crisis centre counsellors to provide PE-A. The study demonstrated that PE-A can be implemented at a community level. Rossouw et al. (2016, 2018) demonstrated similar results in a LIMIC community-based (schools) environment in a task-shifted (psychotherapy naive nurses) RCT.

Ellis (1994) expanded on the REBT theories of Moore (1992) and Warren and Zgourides (1991) who argued individuals who experience trauma will present with one or more irrational beliefs such as "they should be invulnerable and not overreact to traumatic events", that "they should have behaved better during the event", "that a 'just' world should exist" and that "they should act well in practically all situations to allow them to accept themselves as a 'good' person". These unhelpful demands (rigid demands rather than preferences, wishes, desires or hopes) are often experienced at two levels, primary and secondary. At a primary level, this would lead to demands about the situation and the role of the traumatised person, such as "the rape should not have occurred" (the world is a safe place) and that as someone who was raped "I should have managed the situation better" (and therefore I am not competent or capable). However, at the secondary level (secondary disturbance) the focus is on demands about symptoms experienced such as "I should absolutely not be fearful, or have any intrusions (nightmares, flashbacks)". Within the treatment of PTSD, the contribution from REBT of a secondary disturbance is recognised as an important factor that interferes with emotional processing (Foa & Kozak, 1986). It is often misperceived that the focus of REBT is only on the cognitive components within CBT. However, exposure therapy as part of the treatment of PTSD from a REBT perspective is well documented (Ellis, 1994).

Hyland, Shevlin, Adamson, and Boduszek (2014) offer empirical evidence for REBT conceptualisation of PTSD. It was found that "demandingness" predicted symptoms of intrusion, hyperarousal, avoidance and dysphoria through derivative irrational beliefs of worth rating, frustration intolerance and awfulising. Hyland et al. (2014) concluded that targeting demands and derivatives thereof is important in the amelioration of PTSD symptoms.

The advantage of REBT is that it aims for philosophical change of core beliefs. In other CBT approaches, the targeted level of cognitive distortions does not always address these core beliefs. Proponents of REBT argue that processing of an event can be addressed at three levels of cognition: (1) inferential cognitions, (2) schematic/imperative cognitions and (3) evaluative cognitions (DiGuiseppe, Doyle, Dryden, & Backx, 2013). Inferential cognitions refer to our perceptions of reality and the conclusions we make from these perceptions and are similar to automatic thoughts. An example for trauma among youth may be a student recalling that these events/context or individuals are dangerous: going out alone is putting me in harms way. REBT argues that targeting only this level, although helpful, does not address change of one's philosophical core beliefs. Evaluative cognitions refer to irrational beliefs that are derived from the more central imperative demands. Imperative demands are thoughts about the way reality should be. These imperative demands are more akin to schemas and may include beliefs such as I should not have these thoughts, and if I do, it shows that I am weak and have no control over these dangerous thoughts.

The benefit of including REBT into the already existing evidence-based trauma-focussed interventions is discussed below with similarities between techniques used in REBT and TF-CBT and PE-A clarified.

Developmental Considerations in Treating PTSD

With younger children (children with language ability, from 3 to 12 years of age, depending on the individual child), the imaginal exposure or trauma narrative can include a trauma recounting that consists of a direct telling of the trauma event. The child can also be assisted to access the memories via storytelling, drawing or co-storytelling. The processing of the trauma memories does not utilise a directive cognitive restructuring format in very young children. They would rather be helped to address inferential cognitions with a discussion about probability and severity regarding core beliefs. As an example, if a student had been exposed to a traumatic event such as a robbery, the clinician may help them look at the data. That is, they may ask: "how many times you have walked into a shop and a robbery occurred? Let's also ask your family and your friends". The use of an effective alternative philosophy or rational belief (RB) for the unhelpful belief can be helpful in how they consider/evaluate the situation. Working on changing an unhealthy thought of "the world must not be an extremely dangerous place" to a RB of "The world can sometimes be a dangerous place, but mostly tends to not be; as much as I would like it to not be dangerous, it sometimes will be and that insisting that it should not be a dangerous place will not make it so at least some, even though not a lot, of the time" can offer a realistic, healthy view to promote healthier functioning.

Best Practice Guidelines for Treating PTSD in Children and Adolescents

The International Society for Traumatic Stress Studies (ISTSS) provides comprehensive information on treating trauma, training and assessment tools (www.istss.org) (International Society for Traumatic Stress Studies, n.d.). ISTSS developed a publication, *Effective Treatments for PTSD* (second edition), and the United Kingdom's National Institute for Health and Clinical Excellence (NICE) published *PTSD: The management of PTSD in adults and children in primary and secondary care* (www.nice.org.uk/guidance/ng116) (NICE, n.d.). The NICE publication offers guidance on the treatment of PTSD in children and adolescents. NICE recommends an individual trauma-focussed CBT intervention for children 5–6 years of age who present more than 1 month after a traumatic event as well as for children 7–17 years who present more than 1 month after a traumatic event. NICE recommends that treatment should be based on a validated manual, typically be provided over 6–12 sessions, be presented by trained providers with ongoing supervision, be adapted to the child's age and development and involve caregivers of the child. The treatment should include the following aspects: psychoeducation about reactions to trauma, safety planning and strategies for managing arousal and flashbacks, processing of trauma memories, processing of trauma-related emotions, restructuring of trauma-related meanings for the individual, address avoidance, preparation for ending treatment and booster sessions if needed in relation to significant dates.

RE-CBT in the Treatment of PTSD

The two evidence-based trauma-focussed approaches developed for children and adolescent PTSD described here are the TF-CBT approach of Drs. Tony Mannarino, Esther Deblinger and Judith Cohen (www.tfcbt.org) and the adolescent-specific PE-A protocol (Foa, Chrestman, & Gilboa-Schechtman, 2008).

TF-CBT was designed as an outpatient program for children and adolescents 3–18 years of age and their parents or caregivers and is delivered in 8–25 sessions. TF-CBT has eight components (the first of which has two pieces) that include psychoeducation and parenting skills, relaxation, affect modulation, cognitive coping and processing, a trauma narrative, in vivo mastery of trauma reminders, conjoint child-caregiver sessions and enhancing safety and development (de Arellano et al., 2014).

PE-A was designed as a program for adolescents 13–18 years of age and can be provided as a stand-alone treatment or combined with consultations with primary caregivers and consists of 7–14 weekly, 60- to 90-minute sessions. Treatment comprises of eight modules and cover psychoeducation on treatment rationale, gathering information on the trauma, identifying the index trauma and conducting a breathing retraining exercise, a discussion of common reactions to trauma, in vivo exposure (confronting trauma reminders in real life), imaginal exposure (remembering and recounting the traumatic memory), generalisation of skills learned in treatment and relapse prevention.

The need for an adolescent-specific protocol is secondary to adolescents being in a unique developmental stage, and, accordingly, the CBT manuals developed to treat PTSD in adults or younger children may not be directly applicable to this age group. Treatment protocols that include preadolescent children have multiple components that also include parent sessions that would not be directly relevant to an adolescent population. The symptom presentation of PTSD in adolescents is deemed to be closer to the presentation in adults than in children (Pine & Cohen, 2002).

Foa et al. (2008) adapted the PE treatment manual for adults to be suitable as a treatment manual for adolescents (PE-A). Notably, the four studies discussed earlier (Foa et al., 2013; Gilboa-Schechtman et al., 2010; Rossouw et al., 2016, 2018) provide evidence for the utilisation of the adapted adult protocol (PE) for use with adolescents (PE-A).

Theories of PE-A and TF-CBT

PE-A and the Emotional Processing Theory of Fear

PE is based on the emotional processing theory (EPT) of fear (Foa & Kozak, 1986). In brief, EPT proposes that memory structures made up of associated stimulus, response and meaning elements are organised as a program to avoid or escape danger and form a representation of fear. When something in the environment matches an element of a fear structure, it activates the fear structure, and it spreads through the fear network. Foa and Rothbaum (1998) in applying EPT to PTSD proposed that the fear structure of PTSD includes excessive stimulus and response elements and pathological meaning elements. Thus, a child that was sexually assaulted in an open field on her way to school would associate walking alone on a walk way bordering on open fields as dangerous. The problematic meaning elements associated with this fear structure may include "I should have prevented this from happening" or "I am always in danger".

In PTSD (Foa & Riggs, 1993; Foa & Rothbaum, 1998), emotional processing theory posits that two core unhelpful cognitions underlie the development and maintenance of PTSD, namely, the world is completely dangerous and one is totally incompetent to control this. As a result, an effective psychological treatment for trauma would require changing the pathological elements of a fear structure. In PTSD, after a traumatic event, the trauma survivor incorporate the view of the world as extremely dangerous and themselves as incompetent to deal with the consequences of the trauma, in fear structures. With a diagnosis of PTSD, individuals systematically avoid trauma-related memories and activities that serve as reminders off the trauma and thus maintain these pathological elements, with the consequence being chronic PTSD. PE-A treatment involves allowing the trauma survivor the opportunity to be in the presence of the trauma reminders, both trauma memories (imaginal exposure) and external triggers in the environment (in vivo exposure), repeatedly. The repeated prolonged exposure provides disconfirming information that allow the pathological elements of the fear structure to be challenged and a corrective learning experience to occur. Rauch and Foa (2006) found that changes in beliefs about incompetence and dangerousness of the world are associated with greater reduction in PTSD symptoms.

TF-CBT Theoretical Framework

TF-CBT is a CBT-based intervention. It is however a hybrid intervention that includes elements of attachment theory, neurobiology, family therapy and humanistic theory (Cohen, Mannarino, & Deblinger, 2006). The model is based in stress management models such as stress inoculation therapy (SIT) with the goal of preparing children by providing psychoeducation, relaxation and emotion regulation.

This is followed with gradual exposure (Cohen et al., 2006) that involves exposing the child gradually to trauma reminders and trauma memories. Caregivers are critical models for coping with trauma and are included in the treatment.

Treatment Protocols

TF-CBT Protocol

TF-CBT sessions are structured to allow the therapist to meet individually with the child as well as in sessions with the child and the caregivers together. Caregivers also meet with the therapist individually to receive training in effective parenting skills. The model is designed to be trauma focussed and have exposure-based elements to every session. At the completion of every component of treatment, a conjoint session with the child and caregiver serves to review the content covered in that component. About one-third of therapy time is spent on stabilisation (emotion regulation) skills, another third on trauma narration and processing and the last third for conjoint work, in vivo mastery and safety. This distribution of time might vary according to the trauma exposure of the child, such as in the case of complex long-term childhood trauma, when the time spent on emotion regulation might be longer.

Overview of the Components of Treatment of TF-CBT

Psychoeducation is focussed on building a relationship, reducing stigma and modelling to not avoid trauma-related content. This entails providing information on the trauma, such as prevalence rates, common myths, common reactions to trauma, emotional and behavioural difficulties and different feelings (fear, guilt, shame and anger).

Parenting training also begins at the start of treatment and continues throughout the treatment. Within this model parental support and effective parenting are seen as a strong predictor of therapy outcome (Cohen & Mannarino, 2000). Parental skills taught to caregivers include time out, praise, selective attention, contingency reinforcement and effective instructions and consequences.

Relaxation strategies taught include focussed breathing, mindfulness, meditation and progressive relaxation. The children are exposed to multiple types of relaxation, and the ones that are a best fit for the child are then implemented. Other techniques such as yoga, exercise, art and listening to music might also be used.

Affective expression and modulation intends to help the child to identify feelings. The therapist helps the child to recognise, name and express feelings, while confirming that these feelings are appropriate and normal. The therapist helps the child to link these emotions with trauma reminders. Children are taught strategies to regulate their emotions more effectively.

Cognitive coping helps the child to identify thoughts and to understand the link between a trigger, thoughts, feelings and behaviour. The idea that it is possible to change feelings and behaviour by changing thoughts is emphasised. These skills are used to change trauma-related cognitions that are unhelpful.

Trauma narration and processing is the gradual exposure component that focus on the memories of the specific trauma(s) experienced by the child. Trauma narration takes many forms and includes writing, drawing in a storybook, writing a poem or performing a skit. The aim is to allow the child to recount the memory of the trauma while in the safety and supportive environment of a therapeutic relationship. The therapist assists the child to identify and change trauma-related cognitions that are unhelpful. The caregiver is also engaged in clinical work to discuss the trauma in sessions with the therapist. The therapist also, if appropriate, discusses the trauma recounting of the child with the caregiver. At the end of this component, the child typically shares their trauma story in a conjoint session with the child and caregiver.

In vivo mastery centres around helping the child to face safe trauma-related triggers and to decrease unhelpful avoidant behaviours. This is presented as an exposure plan with a gradual increase in discomfort levels. The caregiver plays an important role as exposure to these triggers is practised outside of the office.

Enhancing future safety and development are covered towards the end of treatment and provide the child and caregiver with skills to cope with future stressors. This includes teaching personal safety skills that aims to reduce risk for re-victimisation.

PE-A Protocol

PE-A (Foa et al., 2008) consist of 7–14 weekly, 60- to 90-minute sessions. Sessions with caregivers and conjoint sessions with caregivers and the adolescent are part of the protocol and will take place during the treatment process, if required or possible. Treatment consists of eight modules with a varying number of sessions per module dependent on the adolescent's presentation. These modules are outlined in Table 9.1. Homework exercises are provided at every session to practise skills taught after each session. This includes listening to audio recordings of sessions and to recorded imaginal exposure sessions.

REBT Integrated Into Trauma-Focussed Interventions

Treatment effectiveness for both TF-CBT and PE-A is established. However, some patients do not respond to treatment, and research is ongoing on how to improve treatment response rates and on lowering the treatment dropout rate. In both TF-CBT and in PE-A, cognitive restructuring is covered. In TF-CBT, cognitive disputing is covered in the cognitive coping component. In PE-A cognitive changes is

Table 9.1 Prolonged exposure for adolescents module

Module	Focus
Module 1	Provides information on the treatment rationale of PE-A
Module 2	Gather information on the trauma, identify the index trauma and conduct a relaxation and emotion regulation skill by teaching breathing retraining
Module 3	Focus on discussing common reactions to trauma
Module 4	Expose to external triggers, and include a discussion of the rationale for in vivo exposure (confronting trauma reminders in real life), construction of an in vivo hierarchy and assignment of in vivo homework
Module 5	Focus on internal triggers, namely, the trauma memories, that consist of the presentation of the rationale for imaginal exposure (recounting the traumatic memory), conducting imaginal exposure for 15–45 minutes and cognitively processing this remembering experience
Module 6	Imaginal exposure focussing on the worst moments of the trauma memory
Module 7	Focussed on generalisation of skills learned in treatment and on relapse prevention
Module 8	Comprises a final project, such as making a collage detailing the trauma and the gains made in treatment

implemented in the psychoeducation and common reactions to trauma module by providing information about PTSD, the maintenance of symptoms and treatment through information sharing and a Socratic dialogue interviewing style. During the imaginal exposure module, cognitive changes occur during imaginal exposure and during the processing discussion after recounting the trauma memory as the corrective learning experience secondary to being in the presence of the trauma memory allows for new information on the dangerousness of remembering the trauma. This corrective learning experience is solidified during the Socratic dialogue-oriented processing discussion. During in vivo exposure homework (both while setting the homework task, practising the in vivo homework and discussing the homework task at the next session), a similar corrective learning process is facilitated by a Socratic dialogue-oriented discussion of the experience and the changes in distress as well as in cognition. The addition of a more direct core cognitive restructuring component, central to REBT, allows for a more elegant change of core beliefs.

REBT can help to highlight the core beliefs of demands and the derivatives from these demands of catastrophising, global worth rating (self, other and world) and frustration intolerance that contribute to unhealthy, unhelpful negative emotions and behaviours. The irrational, unhelpful beliefs are discovered using the ABC model. When the patient is able to identify the irrational beliefs, the helpfulness and validity of the belief are evaluated through disputation. This is followed by establishing an effective alternative philosophy.

Rigid demands regarding your inability to avert danger (self-blaming), demanding that the world should not be a dangerous place as well as that you should be able to control your PTSD symptoms (not experience intrusions such as nightmares or flashbacks), have been shown to be related to chronic PTSD (Foa, Hembree, & Rothbaum, 2007). The use of functional, empirical and logical/pragmatic disputes to address these core beliefs is helpful to establish a new effective response.

PTSD Case Study of PE-A Treatment of Adolescent

Kuhle (a fictional case based on cases treated) is a 15-year-old female adolescent who was repeatedly sexually assaulted while being held captive by an older man within a rural setting. As the perpetrator was a prominent man in her community, she had to leave the rural community where she was raised to live with her father, with who she had limited contact during her childhood. She was referred for counselling by a teacher at her school in who she confided regarding her traumatic sexual assault.

After the completion of her intake interview (MINI-Kid) and completing a self-report version of the CPSS5 and the Children's Depression Inventory (Kovacs, 1985), the diagnosis of PTSD and depression was discussed and clarified as the best way to describe the symptoms that she was experiencing. Kuhle was introduced to PE-A as a possible treatment for her symptoms. The rationale of PE-A was discussed. The importance of understanding that PTSD is a reaction to being reminded of her traumatic experience was discussed. Further, it was pointed out that by trying to avoid being reminded of or remembering the traumatic experience it is creating a situation in which she is inadvertently blocking effective emotional processing of the emotions associated with remembering. An explanation of the techniques used in PE-A, namely, imaginal exposure (recounting the trauma memory to address internal triggers of emotion associated with the trauma event), in vivo exposure (real-life experiments to address external triggers of memories that are associated with the trauma event) and addressing the trauma-related beliefs, was provided to her. Initial reservations around the intervention that included concern around remembering and discussing the memories of the trauma were addressed by identifying the inferences and associated irrational beliefs around how distressing it would be for her to do so and her concern about her ability to tolerate the discomfort associated with doing so. Breathing retraining, an abdominal breathing technique, was demonstrated and practised as a skill to be used for general stress management and for emotion regulation. Homework was to listen to the recording of the first session, practise the breathing retraining technique daily and read a summary of the main points of the session that was provided. As her mother was not living with her and her father was not able to attend any sessions due to work commitments, she was provided with a summary of what the treatment entailed and what was discussed at the first session to give to her father.

Module 2 also started with the completion of the self-report measures and checking on her homework assignment. An initial discussion that served to open the discussion around being sexually assaulted was initiated with clear instructions to merely focus on the context and broad details of the traumatic events. This was achieved by asking questions and directing Kuhle to not describe the details of her experience to prevent too much emotional engagement at this stage of treatment. Kuhle described that she was invited by the older man to the next village, over a weekend. With limited availability of public transport and an opportunity to go visit a friend in the next village, she was excited to drive with him. While driving he proceeded to tell her how attractive he finds her and proceeded to touch her leg. She told him she was not comfortable with this, and he stopped. When they arrived at the village, he took her to a house and then locked her in a room. He proceeded to sexually assault her repeatedly over the course of the weekend. When he returned on the Sunday, she waited for him next to the door and as he opened the door surprised him and managed to escape. She described that the first attempt to rape her was the worst and led to the most intrusive recollections and emotion. This was identified as the index trauma. This was followed by a discussion on how it can be difficult to talk about things that make you upset and that it gets easier with practice. Her homework was to listen to the recording of the session, review the secret weapons form she filled in, practise the breathing and provide the "How can I help?" handout to her father to provide him with guidance on how he can help her during the treatment process.

Module 3 was spent on discussing the common reactions people with PTSD experience in response to trauma and normalising Kuhle's symptoms. This module in concert with the data gathering module mapped out Kuhle's specific symptoms and was used as the basis for the imaginal and real-life exposure hierarchies. This module also educated Kuhle about the symptoms of PTSD and helped her view her own symptoms as common reactions to trauma rather than as a personal failure or a sign of irreparable damage. The topics covered included discussing fear and anxiety as a common reaction to trauma, feeling on edge, re-experiencing, flashbacks, nightmares, avoidance, emotional numbness, anger, guilt and shame, a sense of losing control, change of perception of self and the world and a perception of hopelessness as common reactions to trauma. In discussing these symptoms with Kuhle, she agreed that she experienced several of the symptoms.

Adolescents will often hide their reactions because they think they are the only ones experiencing these symptoms and this is a sign of weakness, extreme pathology or moral failure. They imagine most other people would have coped far better than them. Emphasising the fact that their reaction is a common reaction will help them to feel less lonely and less ashamed. From an REBT perspective, identifying and discussing secondary disturbance can be helpful to facilitate acceptance of the symptoms. The unrealistic expectations around not experiencing the emotions or not having such severe emotions are helpful to address at this point. The acceptance of emotions will help with emotion tolerance that will facilitate engaging with the emotion later in treatment (imaginal and in vivo exposure).

After covering the list of common reactions, Kuhle summarised her own common reactions. As homework she was asked to look out for the presence of more common reactions and asked to write new ones down to discuss at the next session. She had to practise breathing retraining and listen to a recording of the session.

Module 4 introduced in vivo exposure and reviewed the rationale for in vivo exposure and taught Kuhle how to rate her anxiety with the help of the stress thermometer (SUD scale). Kuhle created a hierarchy of external triggers that included activities that are perceived as more dangerous than they are in reality. Exposure of this type may be trauma specific, such as talking to men or boys in safe settings. Situations that are reminders of the traumatic event are people, places and activities that trigger memories of the event and are avoided because the memories are associated with uncomfortable feelings such as fear, shame, guilt, anger or a sense of helplessness. These include trauma reminders such as wearing similar clothing as on the day of the trauma, smelling odours or hearing music that were present during the trauma. Being in the presence of people that were present or remind of people present at the trauma event (even though they were not involved in causing the trauma) is also avoided.

In adolescents with co-morbid depression as was the case with Kuhle, situations or activities that increase pleasure or demonstrate competence can be assigned, not because they are related to the trauma but the patient avoids them due to a loss of interest. This activity is called behavioural activation and is helpful with participants that withdrew after the trauma. These activities include re-engaging in sport, friendships, chores or other enjoyable or important events. These items might not lead to excessive anxiety and might be very low on the hierarchy but are important from numbing symptoms and avoidance perspective. They can typically be attempted early on in the exposure.

Kuhle initiated the first real-life experiment during her session and completed others for homework. This module remains active until the end of treatment. Kuhle tackled the items on the hierarchy in a stepwise fashion for homework. Kuhle identified a friend and adult in her community to help her to implement the in vivo exposure homework.

Module 5 focussed on practising the second exposure technique, recounting the memory. Recounting the memory can be done in several ways; however, the preferred method is imaginal exposure. If the patient is unable to verbally recount the memory, other methods such as writing down the memory, drawing the memory through different pictures or recounting it through stories can be suggested. After each exposure session, time is spent emotionally processing the memory, and challenging unhelpful thoughts as necessary. Kuhle chose to recount her trauma memory. This is done by retelling the trauma repeatedly during a 15- to 45-minute period and by rating your discomfort every 5 minutes on a SUD scale during the imaginal exposure. Typically, the first and second telling are the hardest and proper processing is very important. During processing, time was spent to address what Kuhle learnt from the imaginal exposure exercise.

With an REBT-enhanced approach, Kuhle evaluated her beliefs that "all men and boys are dangerous and will sexually abuse her if she allows them close to her and that staying away from all men is the best way to prevent getting hurt". She was helped to develop an effective response (E), "I am mostly safe in the presence of others, including men, some men might be dangerous and exploring relationships with boys mostly will be pleasant and fun, even though some risk of getting hurt might be present". The module is repeated at least for two additional sessions as long as the patient is advancing well. During imaginal exposure Kuhle's worst moments of her trauma memory were identified. Once Kuhle felt less anxious with retelling the entire memory, she advanced to Module 6, the worst moments module. Module 6 focussed on recounting the worst moments of the trauma memory. Kuhle started with recounting the worst moment of her trauma event based on her own report and also the therapist's observations.

Module 7 and 8 focussed on consolidating the skills learned during the previous sessions and ended with a final project such as a collage.

Adaptation of RE-CBT in Schools for PTSD

Within LIMIC environments and even in high-income countries, the lack of access to mental health services is increasingly being recognised (Weinmann & Koesters, 2016). The requirement of access to centralised treatment and the lack of mental healthcare specialists (MHS) available at most community-level clinics often lead to treatment delays and perceptions within the community that treatments for mental disorders do not exist or are inaccessible (Weinmann & Koesters, 2016). Stigma associated with seeking help for mental disorders, combined with the lack of availability of evidence-based treatments for mental disorders in the community, often results in patients only using mental health services as an absolute last resort (van de Water, Rossouw, van der Watt, Yadin, & Seedat, 2018).

Therefore, a current research priority is for more implementation-level evidence-based treatment trials that would demonstrate the effectiveness of task-shifted, community-based, psychosocial treatments in LMIC settings (Tomlinson et al., 2009). In order to provide both accessible and effective treatments, common mental disorders like PTSD, depression, other anxiety disorders and also substance use disorders could be addressed within the community by non-specialist health workers (NSHW) (Kilpatrick et al., 2003). Services offered should include protocol-driven psychosocial treatments tailored for these mental health disorders – especially in the most vulnerable populations (Cohen, 2010).

A study in South Africa (Rossouw et al., 2018) demonstrated the implementation of the PE-A protocol in a task-shifted (previously psychotherapy naive nurses) RCT at high schools in low-income areas around Cape Town, South Africa. The study demonstrates that with appropriate supervision NSHWs can effectively treat adolescents at their schools for interpersonal traumas that include sexual assault, physical assault and witnessing murder or physical assault of others. No adaption of the original PE-A protocol was required. In qualitative interviews with the providers, treatment coordinators at the schools and the adolescents, the only comment around improvement of the protocol was suggestions to use local metaphors in explaining treatment components (van de Water et al., 2018).

Test Yourself

1. Describe some of the key factors to consider in the assessment of PTSD to guide case conceptualisation and treatment planning.
2. Consider the role of parents in TF-CBT and PE-A and how as a clinician you would work to promote their participation in clinical treatment where appropriate.
3. How might REBT be effectively used to support exposure-based approaches and modify beliefs related to the trauma?

References

Alisic, E., Zalta, A. K., Van Wessel, F., Larsen, S. E., Hafstad, G. S., Hassanpour, K., et al. (2014). Rates of post-traumatic stress disorder in trauma-exposed children and adolescents: Meta-analysis. *British Journal of Psychiatry, 204*(5), 335–340.

American Psychiatric Association. (2013). *Diagnostic and statistical manual of mental disorders* (5th ed.). Washington, DC: American Psychiatric Association.

Attanayake, V., McKay, R., Joffres, M., Singh, S., Burkle Jr., F., & Mills, E. (2009). Prevalence of mental disorders among children exposed to war: A systematic review of 7920 children. *Medicine, Conflict and Survival, 25*, 4–19.

Bayer, C. P., Klasen, F., & Adam, H. (2007). Association of trauma and PTSD symptoms with openness to reconciliation and feelings of revenge among former Ugandan and Congolese child soldiers. *Journal of the American Medical Association, 298*, 555.

Bisson, J. I., Ehlers, A., Matthews, R., Pilling, S., Richards, D., & Turner, S. (2007). Psychological treatments for chronic post-traumatic stress disorder. *The British Journal of Psychiatry, 190*(2), 97–104. https://doi.org/10.1192/bjp.bp.106.021402

Brent, D. A., Perper, J. A., Moritz, G., Liotus, L., Richardson, D., Canobbio, R., et al. (1995). Posttraumatic stress disorder in peers of adolescent suicide victims: Predisposing factors and phenomenology. *Journal of the American Academy of Child and Adolescent Psychiatry, 34*, 209–215. https://doi.org/10.1097/00004583-199502000-00016

Cohen, A. C. (primary author), The Work Group on Quality Issues & the AACAP Work Group on Quality Issues (WGQI). (2010). Practice parameters for the assessment and treatment of children and adolescents with posttraumatic stress disorder. *Journal of the American Academy of Child and Adolescent Psychiatry, 49*, 414–430.

Cohen, J. A., & Mannarino, A. P. (2000). Predictors of treatment outcome in sexually abused children. *Child Abuse and Neglect, 24*(7), 983–391.

Cohen, J. A., Mannarino, A. P., & Deblinger, E. (2006). *Treating trauma and traumatic grief in children and adolescents*. New York: Guilford Press.

Cohen, J. A., Mannarino, A. P., Kliethermes, M., & Murray, L. A. (2012). Trauma-focused CBT for youth with complex trauma. *Child Abuse Neglect, 36*(6), 528–541. https://doi.org/10.1016/j.chiabu.2012.03.007

Das-Munshi, J., Lund, C., Mathews, C., Clark, C., Rothon, C., & Stansfeld, S. (2016). Mental health inequalities in adolescents growing up in post-apartheid South Africa: Cross-sectional survey, SHaW study. *PLoS One, 11*, e0154478. https://doi.org/10.1371/journal.pone.0154478

de Arellano, M. A., Lyman, D. R., Jobe-Shields, L., George, P., Dougherty, R. H., Daniels, A. S., et al. (2014). Trauma-focused cognitive-behavioral therapy for children and adolescents: Assessing the evidence. *Psychiatric Services, 65*(5), 591–602. https://doi.org/10.1176/appi.ps.201300255

Derluyn, I., Broekaert, E., Schuyten, G., & De Temmerman, E. (2004). Post-traumatic stress in former Ugandan child soldiers. *Lancet, 363*, 861.

DiGuiseppe, R. A., Doyle, K. A., Dryden, W., & Backx, W. (2013). *A Practitioner's guide to rational emotive behavior therapy* (3rd ed.). New York: Oxford University Press.

Ellis, A. (1994). *Reason and emotion in psychotherapy: A comprehensive method to treating human disturbance. Revised and updated.* New York: Birch Lane Press.

Finkelhor, D., & Dziuba-Leatherman, J. (1994). Children as victims of violence: A national survey. *Pediatrics, 94*(4 Pt 1), 413–420.

Finkelhor, D., Omrod, R., Turner, H., & Hamby, S. L. (2005). The victimization of children and youth: A comprehensive, national survey. *Child Maltreatment, 10*, 5–25.

Foa, E. B., Asnaami, A., Zang, Y., Capaldi, S., & Yeh, R. (2018). Psychometrics of the child PTSD symptom scale for DSM-5 for trauma exposed children and adolescents. *Journal of Clinical Child & Adolescent Psychology, 47*(1), 38–46.

Foa, E. B., Chrestman, K., & Gilboa-Schechtman, E. (2008). *Prolonged exposure manual for children and adolescents suffering from PTSD*. New York: Oxford University Press.

Foa, E. B., Hembree, S. P., & Rothbaum, B. O. (2007). Treatments that work. In *Prolonged exposure therapy for PTSD: Emotional processing of traumatic experiences: Therapist guide*. Oxford, UK/New York: Oxford University Press.

Foa, E. B., & Kozak, M. J. (1986). Emotional processing of fear: Exposure to corrective information. *Psychological Bulletin, 99*, 2–35.

Foa, E. B., McLean, C. P., Capaldi, S., & Rosenfield, D. (2013). Prolonged exposure vs supportive counselling for sexual abuse-related PTSD in adolescent girls: A randomized clinical trial. *JAMA, 310*(24), 2650–2657. https://doi.org/10.1001/jama.2013.282829

Foa, E. B., & Riggs, D. S. (1993). Posttraumatic stress disorder in rape victims. In J. Oldham, M. B. Riba, & A. Tasman (Eds.), *Annual review of psychiatry* (Vol. 12, pp. 273–303). Washington, DC: American Psychiatric Association.

Foa, E. B., & Rothbaum, B. O. (1998). *Treating the trauma of rape: Cognitive-behavioral therapy for PTSD*. New York: The Guilford Press.

Giaconia, R. M., Reinherz, H. Z., Silverman, A. B., Pakiz, B., Frost, A. K., & Cohen, E. (1995). Traumas and posttraumatic stress disorder in a community population of older adolescents. *Journal of the American Academy of Child and Adolescent Psychiatry, 3*, 1369–1380. https://doi.org/10.1097/00004583-199510000-00023

Gilboa-Schechtman, E., Foa, E., Shafran, N., Aderka, I. M., Powers, M. B., Rachamim, L., et al. (2010). Prolonged exposure vs dynamic therapy for adolescent PTSD: A pilot randomized controlled trial. *Journal of the American Academy of Child and Adolescent Psychiatry, 49*(10), 1034–1042. https://doi.org/10.1016/j.jaac.2010.07.014

Gillies, D., Taylor, F., Gray, C., O'Brien, L., & D'Abrew, N. (2013). Psychological therapies for the treatment of post-traumatic stress disorder in children and adolescents (review). *Evidence-Based Child Health: A Cochrane Review Journal, 8*(3), 1004–1116. https://doi.org/10.1002/ebch.1916

Hiller, R. M., Meiser-Stedman, R., Fearon, P., Lobo, S., McKinnon, A., Fraser, A., et al. (2016). Research review: Changes in the prevalence and symptom severity of child posttraumatic stress disorder in the year following trauma – a meta-analytic study. *Journal of Child Psychology and Psychiatry, 57*, 884–898.

Holtzhausen, L., Ross, A., & Perry, R. (2015). Working on trauma: A systematic review of TF-CBT work with child survivors of sexual abuse. *Social Work, 52*(4). https://doi.org/10.15270/52-2-528

Hyland, P., Shevlin, M., Adamson, G., & Boduszek, D. (2014). The organization of irrational beliefs in posttraumatic stress symptomology: Testing the predictions of REBT theory using structural equation modelling. *Journal of Clinical Psychology, 70*(1), 48–59.

International Society for Traumatic Stress Studies. (n.d.). Retrieved from http://www.istss.org/

Jenkins, E. J., & Bell, C. C. (1994). Violence among inner city high school students and post-traumatic stress disorder. In S. Friedman (Ed.), *Anxiety disorders in African Americans* (pp. 76–88). New York: Springer Publishing Co..

Kilpatrick, D. G., Ruggiero, K. J., Acierno, R., Saunders, B. E., Resnick, H. S., & Best, C. L. (2003). Violence and risk of PTSD, major depression, substance abuse/dependence, and comorbidity: Results from the National Survey of Adolescents. *Journal of Consulting Clinical Psychology, 71*, 692–700.

Kovacs, M. (1985). The children's depression, inventory (CDI). *Psychopharmacology Bulletin, 21*(4), 995–998.

McLaughlin, K. A., Koenen, K. C., Hill, E. D., Petukhova, M., Sampson, N. A., Zaslavsky, A. M., et al. (2013). Trauma exposure and posttraumatic stress disorder in a national sample of adolescents. *Journal of the American Academy of Child & Adolescent Psychiatry, 52*(8), 815–830. e14. https://doi.org/10.1016/j.jaac.2013.05.011

Meiser-Stedman, R., Shepperd, A., Bryant, R., Samon, K., Yule, W., Dagleish, T., et al. (2009). Development and validation of the child post-traumatic cognitions inventory. *Journal of Child Psychology and Psychiatry and Allied Disciplines, 24*, 47–51.

Moore, R. H. (1992). *Traumatic incident reduction: A cognitive-emotive resolution of the post-traumatic stress disorder (PTSD).* Clearwater, FL: Institute for Rational-Emotive Therapy.

Morina, N., Koerssen, R., & Pollet, T. V. (2016). Interventions for children and adolescents with posttraumatic stress disorder: A meta-analysis of comparative outcome studies. *Clinical Psychology Review, 47*, 41–54. https://doi.org/10.1016/j.cpr.2016.05.006

NICE. (n.d.). *Overview: Post-traumatic stress disorder: Guidance.* http://www.nice.org.uk/guidance/ng116

Pine, D. S., & Cohen, J. A. (2002). Trauma in children and adolescents: Risk and treatment of psychiatric sequelae. *Biological Psychiatry, 51*(7), 519–531. https://doi.org/10.1016/s0006-3223(01)01352-x

Rauch, S., & Foa, E. (2006). Emotional processing theory (EPT) and exposure therapy for PTSD. *Journal of Contemporary Psychotherapy, 36*, 61–65. https://doi.org/10.1007/s10879-006-9008-y

Rojas, S. M., Bilsky, S. A., Dutton, C., Badour, C. L., Feldner, M. T., & Leen-Feldner, E. W. (2017). Lifetime histories of PTSD, suicidal ideation, and suicide attempts in a nationally representative sample of adolescents: Examining indirect effects via the roles of family and peer social support. *Journal of Anxiety Disorders, 49*, 95–103.

Rossouw, J., Yadin, E., Alexander, D., Mbanga, I., Jacobs, T., & Seedat, S. (2016). A pilot and feasibility randomised controlled study of Prolonged Exposure Treatment and supportive counselling for post-traumatic stress disorder in adolescents: A third world, task-shifting, community-based sample. *Trials, 17*(1), 548.

Rossouw, J., Yadin, E., Alexander, D., & Seedat, S. (2018). Prolonged exposure therapy and supportive counselling for posttraumatic stress disorder in adolescents: Task-shifting randomised controlled trial. *The British Journal of Psychiatry, 213*(4), 587–594. https://doi.org/10.1192/bjp.2018.130

Steinberg, A. M., Brymer, M. J., Decker, K. B., & Pynoos, R. S. (2004). The University of California at Los Angeles post traumatic stress disorder reaction index. *Current Psychiatry Reports, 6*(2), 96–100.

Tomlinson, M., Rudan, I., Saxena, S., Swartz, L., Tsai, A. C., & Patel, V. (2009). Setting priorities for global mental health research. *Bulletin of the World Health Organization, 87*(6), 438–446. https://doi.org/10.1590/S0042-96862009000600012

UNICEF. (2014). *Press release: 2014 a devastating year for children.* https://www.unicef.org/media/media_78058.html. Accessed 8 March 2020.

van de Water, T., Rossouw, J., van der Watt, A. S. J., Yadin, E., & Seedat, S. (2018). Adolescents' experience of stigma when accessing school-based PTSD interventions. *Qualitative Health Research, 28*(7), 1088–1098.

Warren, R., & Zgourides, G. (1991). *Anxiety disorders; a rational-emotive perspective.* New York: Pergamon Press.

Weinmann, S., & Koesters, M. (2016). Mental health service provision in low and middle-income countries: Recent developments. *Current Opinion in Psychiatry, 29*(4), 270–275. https://doi.org/10.1097/YCO.0000000000000256

World Health Organization. (2013). *Guidelines for the management of conditions specifically related to stress.* Geneva, Switzerland: WHO.

Yule W. (1994). *Posttraumatic stress disorder* (pp. 223–240). New York: Plenum Pres.

Chapter 10
Depression in Children and Adolescents: RE-CBT Approaches to Assessment and Treatment

Ann Vernon

> It comes out of the blue, this insidious cloud that descends on me, envelops me, scares me, and changes me from an outgoing, upbeat teenager to a sullen, withdrawn stranger who fleetingly thinks of suicide as an escape. It's so overwhelming; it's like something crawls into my brain and literally takes over and I can't think straight. –16-year-old female

These words describe how many depressed young clients feel as they struggle with depression, which has become increasingly prevalent, especially among adolescents (Beevers, 2011; Monroe, 2018; Towery, 2016). In fact, since the 1940s, the rate of depression among youth has increased every decade, according to Paterson (2011). If left untreated, the negative ramifications are significant and profound, impacting future healthcare needs as children and adolescents grow into adulthood (Monroe, 2018). Without a doubt, effective diagnosis and early intervention are imperative, but in a report published by Mental Health America (Adams, 2018), 63% of youth with major depression receive no mental health treatment, which puts them more at risk for suicide and other serious problems.

Prevalence, Symptoms, and Related Disorders

Recent statistics indicate that in 2017, 2.3 million adolescents between the ages of 12 and 17 (approximately 9.4% of the population) experienced at least one major depressive episode (NIMH, 2017). Over the last 30 years, the proportion of

A. Vernon (✉)
University of Northern Iowa, Tucson, AZ, USA

M. Bernard, M. D. Terjesen (eds.), *Rational-Emotive and Cognitive-Behavioral Approaches to Child and Adolescent Mental Health: Theory, Practice, Research, Applications*, https://doi.org/10.1007/978-3-030-53901-6_10

15–16-year-olds who report feeling depressed has doubled, from 1 in 30 to 2 in 30 for boys and 1 in 10 to 2 in 10 for girls (Nuffield Foundation, 2012). A Newport Academy report (Monroe, 2018) cites statistics that lead to what they label as an epidemic of teen depression: since 2013, a 47% increase in depression among adolescent males and a 65% increase in adolescent females ages 12–17. According to Maughan, Collishaw, and Stingaris (2013), depression is still relatively low before puberty. However, the prevalence progressively increases until early adolescence, when the rate rapidly escalates and continues through late adolescence (Weir, 2019). It is significant to note that "Once adolescent girls reach puberty, their risk of depression is double that of their male classmates" (Paterson, 2011, p. 32). As Evans, Van Velsor, and Schumacher (2002) note, "Depression may be one of the most overlooked and under-treated psychological disorders of adolescence" (p. 211).

Although currently there is general agreement that childhood depression exits, until the late 1960s, there was considerable controversy regarding its existence prior to late adolescence or early adulthood because children were thought to be too developmentally immature to experience depression (Evans et al., 2002; Maughan et al., 2013). In fact, Merrell (2001) pointed out that there was "widespread denial that certain types of internalizing disorders, such as depression, could even exist in children" (p. 1). A common belief was that children and adolescents were basically immune from depression because childhood is a happy, carefree time, so they have nothing to be depressed about. Another typical belief was that mood swings are normal during adolescence; they are just part of growing up. These beliefs reflect three major misconceptions: first, that depression is caused by something, so if there are no disturbing events in children's lives, they won't be depressed; second, that disturbing events themselves cause depression; and third, that adolescent depression is just normal moodiness. In response to the first two misconceptions, it is true that situations, especially various kinds of loss, can be trigger events for depression. In addition, social media addiction, bullying, and school pressure can also lead to depression, according to a report by the Newport Academy (2018). However, there are also biological, genetic, and environmental factors (Woo & Keatinge, 2016), as well as early childhood traumatic events that contribute to depression (Powell & Logan, 2019). In addition, there are cognitive components to depression that cannot be ignored. In fact, "cognitive theory suggests that negative thinking plays a pivotal role in the development and/or maintenance of depression" (Rush & Nowels, 1994, p. 3).

With regard to the third misconception, there is a significant difference between "normal" adolescent moodiness and depression, which is more severe, atypical, and must be taken seriously (Koplewicz, 2002). Depression is the most common mental illness among teenagers (Towery, 2016) and is more than "just teenagers with 'growing pains' or in a moody stage" (Evans et al., 2002, p. 211).

Symptoms of Depression

Children and adolescents experiencing depression exhibit various symptoms, including the following: affective symptoms (sad or depressed mood, also expressed as irritability in children and adolescents); negative cognitive styles and attributions (pessimism, overgeneralization, and prediction of negative outcomes); decreased interest and pleasure in usual activities, which may result in apathy and social isolation; poor concentration, as well as difficulty making decisions; major change in eating and/or sleeping patterns; somatic complaints (unfounded headaches, stomachaches, muscle aches); behavioral problems such as acting out, temper tantrums, or aggressive behavior; restlessness, psychomotor agitation, listlessness, or lethargy; diminished self-esteem or feelings of worthlessness or guilt; fixation on past failures and exaggerated self-criticism; increased anger, hostility, and irritability; tearfulness; hopelessness and helplessness; and suicide ideation, recurrent thoughts or preoccupation with death, or suicide attempts (Curry & Hersh, 2014; Monroe, 2018; Morrison & Flegel, 2016).

A key indicator of depression is a marked drop in grades, and a hallmark characteristic is loss of interest in usual activities (Paterson, 2011). It is important to note that depression in children and youth may be differentiated from adult depression by hypersomnia, boredom, irritability, physical complaints, and lack of achieving expected weight gains (Clark, Jansen, & Cloy, 2012; Merrell, 2001). Evans et al. (2002) pointed out that as compared with adults, adolescents exhibit more interpersonal/peer difficulties, are more prone to demonstrate suicide ideation, and may exhibit anxiety or irritability rather than depressed mood. Common co-occurring problems include academic underachievement, school attendance problems, and school failure (Powell & Logan, 2019). Substance abuse disorders are also linked to depression, and depressed youth are twice as likely as other adolescents to have a substance abuse problem than other adolescents (Paterson, 2011).

Types of Depression

Depression is a broad term that includes several types of disorders (Morrison & Flegel, 2016; Woo & Keatinge, 2016). The first is *major depressive disorder* (MDD), which is an intense form of depression that consists of one or more major depressive episodes that last 2 or more weeks, with a typical episode duration lasting 2–9 months (Curry & Hersh, 2014). Symptoms include those listed previously, most notably sadness or irritable mood, sleep and appetite disturbance, decreased concentration, loss of pleasure in activities, and repetitive thoughts of death or suicide (Morrison & Flegel, 2016). This type of depression is much more common in adolescents than in children, and even after treatment and full recovery, MDD is likely to reoccur (Curry et al., 2011).

Persistent depressive disorder, or *dysthymia*, can be best described as "low-grade depression," according to Woo and Keatinge (2016, p. 242). This disorder combines dysthymic disorder and chronic MDD. The symptoms are usually less severe than in episodes of MDD, and it usually lasts 2 or more years. Clients with dysthymia are usually melancholic, have little energy, experience few positive feelings, and have a bleak outlook on life. They have trouble concentrating and experience problems with sleep and appetite. According to Stark, Sander, Yancy, Bronik, and Hoke (2000), dysthymia "may be more insidious than major depression relative to its long-term impact on the psychosocial adjustment of youth, and it appears to be more resistant to treatment" (p. 174). Young clients who have briefer and milder depressive episodes that are in response to a stressor may be diagnosed with adjustment disorder (Curry & Hersh, 2014).

A new type of depressive disorder described in the DSM-5 (Morrison & Flegel, 2016) is *disruptive mood dysregulation disorder* (DMDD), characterized by severe tantrums that can result in verbal or physical attacks on others. These temper outbursts often occur with slight or no provocation and are not consistent with the child's developmental age. Between outbursts, the child is typically angry and irritable. This disorder is more common in boys and is comorbid with other disorders such as ADHD.

Bipolar I and bipolar II disorders, which may be referred to as *pediatric bipolar disorder* (Rizvi, Ong, & Youngstrom, 2014), are complicated to diagnose in youth (Powell & Logan, 2019). Bipolar disorders are characterized by extreme mood and energy shifts and can look like other disorders such as attention-deficit/hyperactivity disorder (ADHD), post-traumatic stress disorder (PTSD), or other developmental variations and complications of mood during and after puberty (American Psychiatric Association, 2013). According to Morrison and Flegel (2016), late adolescence is the most common time for the onset of this disorder which affects approximately 1–3% of adolescents. There is very little information about how bipolar disorders are manifested in young children, and a diagnosis for children younger than age 6 is not recommended.

Who Is Most Vulnerable?

There are several factors that contribute to the development of depression. First, genetics must be considered because depression is more common when a parent or grandparent has also suffered from depression (Maughan et al., 2013; Mayo Clinic, 2018). Children of depressed parents are three times more likely to become depressed as compared with children who do not have a family history of depression (Maughan et al., 2013). However, Koplewicz (2002) warned that because adolescent depression is so common, most teenagers who have it do not have an immediate relative who is depressed. In addition to genetics, other family influences such as strained relationships, extensive conflict, ineffective communication and conflict resolution skills, and maladaptive parenting styles increase the risk of depression in youth (Woo & Keatinge, 2016).

Gender also predicts vulnerability. As previously noted, the prevalence rate for depression is similar in girls and boys prior to puberty, but particularly around age 13 and on into adulthood, about twice as many girls as boys experience depressive symptoms (Paterson, 2011). Although there is no comprehensive model to explain these sex differences, the fact is that girls have more cognitive, biological, and interpersonal vulnerability factors prior to adolescence, and they are more affected than boys during the transition to adolescence (Choate & Anderson, 2008). There are several other factors that make girls more vulnerable to depression than their male counterparts. First, they are more social and place greater value on relationships. Therefore, when things go wrong in a relationship, they are more vulnerable. Also, they are inclined to measure their self-worth on how successful they are in their relationships, so they are more likely to become depressed if they are rejected by their peers, according to Choate and Anderson. They tend to view themselves more negatively than boys, and this predicts a higher risk for depression. In addition, they are more likely than boys to blame themselves when things go wrong, which increases their vulnerability (Koplewicz, 2002). Biological factors also play a role in that the female sex hormones that kick in at puberty may have a special effect on the mood regulators in the brain (Waslick, Kandel, & Kakouros, 2002).

It is also important to know that anxiety is a strong predictor of vulnerability for depression. In fact, nearly half of depressed adolescents also have generalized anxiety disorder that almost always precedes depression (Berlinger, 2005).

The REBT/CBT Perspective on the Etiology of Depression

RE-CBT practitioners acknowledge the biological, neurochemical, and genetic predisposition to depression but maintain that distorted thinking and irrational beliefs play a pivotal role in the development, progression, and alleviation of depression (David, Cardea, Cardos, Oltean, & Stefan, 2019). REBT is "based on the assumption that many emotional problems such as depression and anxiety are caused by irrational thinking and mistaken assumptions, which in turn lead to low self-esteem, unnecessary guilt and shame, psychological stress, and maladaptive problem solving" (Merrell, 2001, p. 103). According to DiGiuseppe, Doyle, and Rose (2002), clinical depression results when individuals have one or more of the following beliefs: a negative view of self, a negative view of their environment, a bleak view of the future, the prediction that negative things will happen to them and that they can do little to improve them, the belief that they must do better and receive approval from significant others, and the notion that they should be treated better in life and it is horrible when this doesn't happen. "These negative thoughts about oneself, one's environment, and one's future result in feelings of sadness and disappointment. However...only when absolutistic demands that bad traits, an unpleasant environment, and a negative future *must not* exist will clinical depression ensue" (DiGiuseppe et al., 2002, p. 223).

According to this theory, depression is related to a belief about one's personal inadequacy, how awful and hopeless things are and how terrible it is not to have what one needs. Depressed clients believe that they are defective, unworthy, and inadequate and attribute unpleasant experiences to their own defects. Not only do they interpret events negatively, but they also have a bleak view of the future (Evans et al., 2002).

A basic premise of cognitive models is that depressive symptoms can be moderated by changing the cognitions that in depressed clients are marked by distortions in attributions, self-evaluations, and information processing such as catastrophizing, predicting negative outcomes, and selectively attending to the negative as opposed to positive aspects of events (Evans et al., 2002). If children are successful in changing their distorted thinking, they will experience behavioral and emotional improvement.

Years ago, Seligman (1995) cautioned that depression was at epidemic proportions among children and adolescents, and that, unfortunately, has not changed (Newport Academy, 2018). Seligman cited pessimistic thinking as a major contributor to this problem. He identified the following three cognitive errors associated with depression: permanence, pervasiveness, and personalization. He explained that children and adolescents who are most at risk for depression believe that the causes of bad events that happen to them are *permanent* as opposed to temporary. Therefore, they are more likely to think about their failures, rejections, or challenges as always being this way or *never* getting better. Depressed children also incorrectly assume that the cause of something negative is generalizable across all situations, or *pervasive*, as opposed to situationally specific. For example, if two students are in a contest and work hard, but neither is selected as the winner, the pervasive thinker would consider him or herself a total loser, whereas the non-pervasive thinker would understand that although he or she did not win the contest, it has nothing to do with being a failure or never doing anything right again. *Personalizing* refers to the idea that when bad things happen, children must blame themselves or others. Consequently, they feel depressed, ashamed, and guilty, in contrast to children who realistically evaluate each situation and do not internalize blame consistently because they are able to separate themselves from their performance.

Merrell (2001) also agreed that the way in which children think has a strong influence in the development of depression. He identified three models: attributions children make about their world, cognitive distortions, and the self-control model. According to Merrell, if children believe that they are helpless to influence or change events in their life, they may become depressed. Since they feel as if they have no power to make any changes, they see no use in trying. Second, children who have a negative view of themselves, the world, and the future and interpret their experiences in dysfunctional ways tend to become depressed. Third, the self-control model relates to the idea that depressed children have a dysfunctional way of monitoring events in their lives. They pay more attention to immediate as opposed to future consequences of behavior, they evaluate themselves unrealistically, they pay more attention to negative events than to positive events, and they criticize rather than reward themselves. All of these thinking patterns contribute to a young person's susceptibility to depression (Merrell, 2001).

Cognitive models of depression focus on changing distorted, irrational thinking in order to achieve emotional and behavioral change. The goal is to help depressed youth understand that if they change the way they think, they don't have to be paralyzed by their depression.

Developmental Considerations

From a developmental standpoint, children's ability to identify and verbalize how they are thinking, feeling, and behaving has a significant impact on the way therapy can be conducted. For example, young children often express their emotions behaviorally rather than verbally, in part because they have a limited feeling vocabulary (Morrison & Flegel, 2016; Vernon & Chen, 2019). However, since RE-CBT emphasizes the importance of psychoeducation, RE-CBT practitioners can readily adapt their approach to the age of the client, making concepts understandable. For instance, instead of asking a 6-year-old how being sad is affecting her at home or at school, the therapist could ask her to draw a picture of what it's like when she is sad and through discussion about the picture and identify the feelings expressed in order to build a feeling vocabulary. It can also be effective to read a book about a child with similar feelings and discuss it using content questions (What did the child in the story do when she felt sad?) and personalization questions (When you are sad, what do you do?)

Developmentally, children and preteens are more predisposed to irrational thinking because formal operational thinking does not begin to develop until early adolescence (Scott & Saginak, 2016; Vernon & Chen, 2019). As formal operational thinkers, adolescents are better able to hypothesize, think logically, identify consequences, and solve problems. However, as many scholars note (Newman & Newman, 2017; Scott & Saginak, 2016; Vernon & Chen, 2019), this shift to formal operational thinking is very gradual and inconsistent, so even during mid-adolescence (ages 15–18), teens still have difficulty thinking logically, distinguishing between facts and assumptions, and connecting cause and effect, all of which can result in multiple errors in judgment. Consequently, the RE-CBT therapist needs to employ a more concrete therapeutic approach with children and teens. Take the example of a young adolescent who was depressed because he failed a test but admitted that he hadn't prepared for it because studying was boring and he just didn't feel like doing it. As his therapist, I took some slips of paper and formed them into a paper chain. On the first link of the chain, I wrote "had a test to study for but didn't do it." Then on subsequent links we identified the consequences: he failed the test and had to retake it, his parents grounded him, he missed a party, and so forth. Then I took another chain, and we identified the same event, but this time he studied and passed the text, and there were no negative consequences. A visual, concrete approach such as this, which epitomizes RE-CBT treatment with young clients, takes into account their developmental limitations and helps them understand cause and effect, decisions, and consequences.

Another developmental factor to take into consideration is that children's sense of time is more immediate (Vernon & Chen, 2019). And since adolescents in particular have a tendency to react inappropriately or impulsively because the part of the brain that controls self-regulation is not fully developed (Newport Academy, 2018), they often make bad decisions in the moment. For example, young clients may not understand that they probably will not be depressed forever but their need for an immediate "fix" can result in a variety of self-defeating behaviors such as substance abuse, eating disorders, self-harm, and suicide as a way to end their pain (Vernon, 2009). Thus it is important for RE-CBT therapists to adapt techniques to the client's developmental level so that they clearly understand the negative consequences that can ensue as a result of thinking that they can't stand being depressed or that it will last forever.

One of my extremely depressed adolescent clients was seriously contemplating suicide, so I asked her if she would participate in an experiment. I filled a glass with water and asked her to squeeze drops of blue food coloring into the glass (the more drops, the greater the depression). Then I asked her to put an Alka-Seltzer tablet in the water and observe what happens. I explained that the foam from the tablet represents her depression bubbling up and increasing in intensity. I asked her to observe how long the foaming lasts (seconds). I used this analogy to help her understand that the intense depression doesn't last forever and that there were specific things that we could work on that would help lessen her depression, as if she were pouring some of that blue (depression) water down the drain. I then handed her a tube of toothpaste and asked her to squeeze some out and then squeeze it back in, which she learned was not possible. I compared that to suicide—if she attempts and succeeds, her life is over. RE-CBT therapists routinely use techniques like this to compensate for young clients' limited cognitive, emotive, or behavioral maturity.

Research on RE-CBT with Depressed Children and Adolescents

According to Curry and Hersh (2014), studies began examining the effect of CBT on young clients with depression as early as the 1980s, but the early studies focused more on school-based group interventions for those with mild to moderate depressive symptoms. While CBT was better than no treatment, it was not superior to other treatment approaches such as modeling or relaxation training. Curry and Hersh (2014) also noted that in the several studies focused on the link between thoughts, feelings, and behaviors, there was an emphasis on teaching cognitive and behavioral skills to increase knowledge about how to cope with depression by learning to restructure automatic negative thoughts and assumptions. These studies showed that cognitive interventions were effective in reducing depressive symptoms, but for those who were more severely depressed, CBT was not always sufficient as a stand-alone treatment.

In the later 1990s, with greater awareness about the prevalence and need for effective treatment for adolescent depression, the National Institute of Mental Health (NIMH) requested a study comparing CBT and fluoxetine (Prosac) for the short- and long-term treatment of adolescent MDD. This study, the Treatment for Adolescents with Depression Study (TADS), randomly assigned 439 adolescents to receive CBT, fluoxetine, a combination of both, or a pill placebo. Results indicated that the combination of CBT and medication was most effective, but not necessarily with severely depressed adolescents (Curry & Hersh, 2014).

More recent meta-analyses of CBT studies (Spielmans, Pasek, & McFall, 2007) compared CBT to other therapies and found that CBT was much more effective than other treatments if the outcomes were assessed with directly relevant measures. Curry and Hersh (2014) concluded that it is an effective treatment for adolescents with mild to moderate depression, "adds to the efficacy of medication for moderately depressed youths" (p. 27), and may add a protective layer for suicidal teens.

Best Practice Guidelines

In working with depressed children and adolescents, it is important that treatment correspond to the developmental level of the client (Clark et al., 2012). The American Academy of Pediatrics (AAP) (2018), updated guidelines of the American Psychological Association (Weir, 2019), and the National Institute for Health and Clinical Excellence guidelines (2005) recommend that treatment should include not only the young client but parents and/or other family members as well. The AAP guidelines also suggest developing a treatment plan with specific goals for functioning at home, with peers, and in school settings. In addition, for the first time, the AAP guidelines endorse a universal depression screening for adolescents age 12 and over as part of their regular wellness visit to a physician that also includes parental input on any observations or concerns related to their child's depression. Because suicide is also a risk factor for depressed youth, the National Institute for Health and Clinical Excellence (2005) guidelines stress the importance of routine suicide assessment by physicians who are often responsible for detecting and treating childhood and adolescent depression due to a shortage of mental health professionals.

The American Academy of Pediatrics (2018) recommends that psychotherapy should be a component when treating depression in youth, with a combination of medication and psychotherapy for adolescents with moderate to severe depression. The APA guidelines (Weir, 2019) recommend the use of cognitive behavioral therapy or interpersonal therapy in treating adolescents, but the guideline development panel of experts was unable to recommend any specific treatment for children. According to the AAP, a combination of CBT and medication is more effective than medication alone. Although medication may be a necessary part of treatment, the neural pathways in children and adolescents may not be fully developed, so extrapolating adult data on antidepressant medication may not be accurate. If medication is needed, selective serotonin reuptake inhibitors (SSRIs) such as Prozac, Zoloft, Lexapro, or Luvox are recommended, but tricyclic antidepressants should not be used because they are not beneficial.

Assessment and Diagnosis

Diagnosing depression is not as clear-cut as it is for other disorders, especially for children and adolescents. There are several reasons for this. First, many teenagers are normally moody, so adults might ignore the moodiness. Also, children and adolescents may not be able to clearly express their feelings or may not be aware of the symptoms and ask for help. Furthermore, unlike depressed adults who may be more consistently depressed and feel sad, depression in adolescents in particular is unstable. According to Koplewicz (2002), teenagers often have the ability to "snap out of it, even if it's just for a few hours" (p. 17). Furthermore, depressed adults usually lose their appetites and their sex drive and have trouble sleeping, whereas adolescents sleep and eat more and still have interest in sex. It is also important to note that young clients are more likely to be angry and irritable or to act out more, in part because they have difficulty verbalizing emotions. This may result in a misdiagnosis of conduct problems.

Young clients' verbal skills and their cognitive and emotional development will impact the degree to which they can express feelings and concerns (Morrison & Flegel, 2016). Therefore, when assessing depression in younger children, it is usually necessary to involve the parents. It is also advisable to obtain parental input with adolescents, in addition to their self-report.

The first step in assessment involves identifying the frequency, intensity, and duration of the symptoms and asking open-ended questions such as "What is it like when you are feeling depressed?" (Woo & Keatinge, 2016, p. 433). Practitioners can use a standardized self-report scale such as the *Reynolds Child Depression Scale* or the *Reynolds Adolescent Depression Scale* (cited in Merrell, 2001), the *Children's Depression Inventory* (Kovacs, 2011), or the *Beck Depression Inventory* for adolescents age 14 and older (Clark et al., 2012). For a less formal assessment, they can develop a checklist based on the *DSM5* symptoms or the characteristics identified previously in this chapter.

Other techniques that may prove useful in assessing the intensity, severity, and frequency of the depression include the following:

Mood chart (Vernon, 2002, p. 133). Young clients are given a chart listing the days of the week across the top and times of the day down the side. They are asked to rate each time period numerically—1 being very depressed or sad and 5 being happy, not depressed. This measure helps the practitioner as well as the client understand more about the frequency and intensity of the depressed feelings.

Emotional pie (Merrell, 2001, pp. 86–87). This is a pictorial way of helping clients evaluate their moods. The assessment is like a pie chart graph, and the child is asked to indicate for a specific period of time (day or week) how his or her mood states were divided, like pieces of a pie with different sizes. The child divides the pie and colors the feelings (i.e., blue/sad, yellow/happy, or labels them: H = happy, S = sad, etc.).

In REBT, the presumption is that how one thinks affects how one feels, so a critical aspect of the assessment process is the cognitive component. A measure that assesses cognitive variables is the *Automatic Thoughts Questionnaire for Children* (ATQ-C; Stark, Humphrey, Livingston, Laurent, & Christopher, 1993, as cited in Stark et al., 2000). This scale consists of 30 self-statements that the child rates according to how frequently each thought occurs. The *Cognitive Triad Inventory for Children* (CTI-C) (Kaslow, Stark, Printz, Livingston, & Tsai, 1992, as cited in Stark et al., 2000) assesses the child's sense of self, the world, and the future. The *Child and Adolescent Scale of Irrationality* (Bernard & Cronan, 1999) contains a distinct sub-scale assessing self-downing tendencies.

Other cognitive assessment strategies for identifying distorted thinking include the following:

The down arrow technique (Merrell, 2001, p. 90). This technique is adapted from Burns' vertical arrow technique and is more suitable for older children and adolescents because this assessment technique requires that clients have more abstract thinking skills. The intent is to identify underlying beliefs that contribute to the depressed mood. The practitioner will ask questions such as "So what?" and "What does that mean?" to help the client identify irrational beliefs that lead to depression.

Identifying cognitive distortions or thinking errors (Merrell, 2001, p. 92). This technique would also be more appropriate with older children or adolescents who are more cognitively mature. For this assessment, the client is given a handout with examples of distorted cognitions such as the following and is asked to put a check mark next to those that contribute to his or her depression. (Readers are encouraged to consult Merrell for more distortions that are not listed due to space constrictions.)

Binocular vision: looking at things so that they seem bigger or smaller than they really are.

Black and white thinking: looking at things as extreme opposites—for example, things are either all good or all bad.

Making it personal: blaming yourself for something that happened when you can't control it or are not responsible for it.

Overgeneralizing: drawing a conclusion based on a single event, assuming that you will always fail a test just because you failed once, for example.

Labeling: putting a negative label on yourself or someone else, such as "I'm a loser; he's stupid."

A thorough assessment includes emotions, cognitions, and behaviors. This is particularly important with depression because of the correlation between depression and suicide (Powell & Logan, 2019). Although the majority of depressed adolescents do not attempt or commit suicide, depressed adolescents are at an increased risk (Capuzzi & Gross, 2019). There is also a relationship between depression and self-mutilation (Leppma & Schimmel, 2019) and other self-defeating behaviors such as substance abuse (Powell & Logan, 2019) and eating disorders (Merrell, 2001), so these must be assessed as well. Depressed adolescents often journal or write poetry, so if they are willing to share, their writings often provide valuable insights. Other suggestions include the following.

S-T-E-B (Vernon, unpublished; adapted from Knaus, 1974). This technique involves giving the client a sheet of paper with S-T-E-B written across the top in four columns. S stands for a situation; what the client perceived as upsetting or depressing; T stands for thoughts (beliefs about the situation); E stands for emotions such as depression or other feelings; and B stands for behaviors—what did the client do when he or she had these emotions and thoughts. This technique generally elicits good information.

Checklist. Because it is often difficult or embarrassing for young depressed clients to identify what they do when they feel depressed, a checklist such as the following can be developed (with more items) and adapted for different-aged clients.

When I Feel Depressed or Very Sad, I:

1. Sleep a lot	Yes___No___Sometimes___
2. Isolate myself/withdraw from others	Yes___No___Sometimes___
3. Use drugs or alcohol	Yes___No___Sometimes___
4. Hurt myself (cuts, burns)	Yes___No___Sometimes___
5. Don't eat—or eat too much	Yes___No___Sometimes___
6. Cry a lot	Yes___No___Sometimes___

Assessing depression is an ongoing process, and multiple approaches should be used throughout the course of therapy.

Assessing Secondary Emotions

When assessing depression, it is important to look for secondary emotions, such as feeling angry, anxious, ashamed, guilty, or depressed about being depressed. This is very difficult to do with younger children because their feeling vocabulary is limited as it is, so asking them how they feel about feeling depressed is generally not very successful. However, adolescents are much better able to identify secondary emotions associated with their depression, although the therapist may have to be more directive in eliciting these emotions. One technique is to ask them to write a letter to their depression, which in my experience is an excellent way to help them identify the secondary emotions which the therapist deals with first before moving to the primary emotion.

Treatment

RE-CBT treatment of depression in young clients primarily involves the child or adolescent, but it is also important to include the parents, family, and school personnel to help them understand the nature of the depression and how it is manifested in young clients (Stone & Brott, 2019). In addition, these significant adults need to know the basic principles of RE-CBT so they can help the child or adolescent develop new strategies for managing their depressed feelings, challenging their distorted thinking, and changing self-defeating behaviors.

RE-CBT Therapeutic Interventions

In working with depressed youth who may be unable or unwilling to talk about their feelings, it is important at the first meeting to do some rapport building, which should include psychoeducation to help young clients understand what depression is and where it comes from. This is very important because depression can be very confusing and frightening, and a simple explanation about how the changes in brain restructuring contribute to emotional ups and downs is very helpful because they learn that they are not "crazy," that others their age also struggle with depression, and that there are many ways to help them deal with their depressed mood. Next, the RE-CBT therapist asks the client if there is a particular activating event associated with the depression or if the depression in itself is the activating event. Younger children often present with something that they think "makes them sad," so the therapist discusses this event and helps them identify and describe the feelings related to this incident. Adolescents may or may not identify a specific event because their depression is often more pervasive and not linked to anything specific. If this is the case, the therapist treats the depression as the activating event and elicits the secondary emotions about being depressed.

After the As and the Cs have been identified and discussed, the next step is to identify the Bs. For example, many depressed youth think they will never get better, that life isn't worth living, and that they are the only ones who are depressed, which makes them weird and unlikeable. The RE-CBT therapist looks for irrational beliefs related to self-downing, awfulizing and catastrophizing, frustration intolerance, and demandingness. Bernard (2004) identified irrational beliefs related to a typical activating event such as being rejected by peers, being teased, or not being included. Children and adolescents who are depressed about social rejection might infer that everyone is against them, that nobody likes them, that they will never be included or have any friends, and therefore they will never be happy. The think that they *must* be loved and approved of and that it is awful and unbearable to be rejected or teased; it proves they are worthless.

Once the beliefs are identified, the next step is to help clients learn to challenge their irrational beliefs using empirical, functional, and logical disputes such as

"Where's the evidence that you will always be depressed?" "How does it help you to think that you will always be depressed?" "Is it really logical to think that because you are depressed that you are also crazy?" "Just because your boyfriend rejected you, where is the proof that you are a loser or that nobody will ever want anything to do with you because he broke up with you?" "How is thinking that you are worthless because you were rejected helping you?" "Is it really logical to think that you will never get over this or that life is not worth living if this person isn't in your life?" The "best friend" dispute is also effective: "Would you tell your friend she is a total loser because her boyfriend broke up with her?" After your client says she would never say that, ask "So does it make sense to put yourself down and think you are a failure because your boyfriend broke up with you?"

Based on my own clinical experience in working with depressed children and adolescents, I find that it is often more effective to dispute inferences first because if they are not thinking clearly, this compounds their depression and they become overwhelmed, discouraged, and depressed about being depressed. As a result, they may act impulsively to alleviate their misery, like my client who took an overdose of drugs "just to put herself out of her misery for the night." Of course it never occurred to her that this could have been lethal. It depends on the nature of the problem and the degree of depression, but I think RE-CBT therapists have to be cautious about asking for the "worst-case scenario" right off the bat when working with children and young adolescents because they often don't think logically or have the ability to put things into perspective. Because they lack life experience, it may not be easy for them to see that even if the worst happens, they can eventually bounce back. Therefore, I have found that being empathic is extremely important: "I am sure you are in a difficult place now since your boyfriend broke up with you to date your girlfriend, and you probably wish that there was a law against it, but unfortunately there isn't. I know you are really depressed about this and think that nobody will ever consider you good enough to be their girlfriend, but does thinking that way help you feel less depressed? Would you like to work on your thoughts so that you can feel better?" I think of it as "coming in the back door…," eventually I will get to the demands and evaluations, but more slowly than if I were working with an adult.

I have also found that the most difficult irrational belief to dispute in young people is the demand that things or people should or shouldn't be the way they are. In the previous example, if I had asked "Is there any law that says your boyfriend shouldn't have broken up with you to date your best friend?," my client may have agreed that there wasn't a law, but she probably wouldn't really believe it, so that would not have been a very effective dispute. I find it best to use more "round about" ways to dispute this, such as "I know there is a school rule about not teasing others." But has someone ever teased you? And so even if there is a rule, does everyone always follow the rules? Does it make sense to get upset by thinking that this rule *should never* get broken?

The following interventions can also be used to help depressed children and adolescents (original ideas unless noted; these can be adapted depending on the age and developmental level of the client):

Doom and gloom glasses. Have two pair of glasses available, one with dark colored lenses and the other with clear lenses. Explain to clients that when they are depressed, they tend to look at things with the doom and gloom (dark) glasses. Give examples, using a situation they identify as depressing for them, such as getting a bad grade on a test. Have them put on the doom and gloom (dark) glasses and verbalize their thoughts about this event: that they are stupid and worthless, will never pass the class, they will be made fun of by others (and that would be horrible), and so forth. Explain concepts such as awfulizing, overgeneralizing, and equating self-worth with performance. Then have them put on the clear glasses and verbalize what they might be thinking if they had these on as opposed to the doom and gloom glasses.

When you need a helping hand (adapted from Vernon, 2002, p. 131). Invite the client to draw around his or her hand. At the base of the hand, have the client identify an event that is depressing for him or her, such as not receiving a prestigious scholarship. Then, between each of the fingers, have the client identify his or her irrational beliefs, such as this is awful, it's not fair, and this just proves I'm an unworthy big loser. Help the client dispute these thoughts, and have him or her write rational beliefs on each of the fingers to serve as a reminder of how to change thinking about a negative event.

Act as if. When young clients are depressed, they often feel powerless and give in to their depression. It is sometimes helpful to have them act as if they aren't depressed for a designated period of time each day, keeping a log of what they do so they can repeat these behaviors in the future.

Away with the blues (adapted from Vernon, 2002, pp. 126–127). This is an intervention that helps a young client learn how to deal with depressed feelings. First, have the client verbalize what it is that is depressing, such as parents getting a divorce. After some discussion about this, give the client a small glass pitcher of water and a bottle of blue food coloring. Ask the client to pour an amount of food coloring into the pitcher that depicts how depressing this is. Next, help the client identify the irrational beliefs (This is the worst thing that could ever happen to me; I will never be happy again). Then help the client identify less depressing thoughts: "There are worse things that could happen, like my parents could die; I'm sad now, but I probably won't be sad forever." As the client verbalizes each thought, ask him or her to pour some of the blue water down the drain (sink) as a visual reminder of how to decrease depressing feelings.

Depression toolbox (Vernon, 2009, pp. 127–128). When they are very depressed, it is often difficult for clients to remember happier times or think that they could ever be happy again. This simple technique involves having them identify artifacts that remind them of important people or events in their lives, rational coping self-statements, inspirational sayings or songs that "give them hope," books with a moral or rational message, etc. They can decorate a box with cheerful sayings or cartoons to make them laugh and put their artifacts inside the depression toolbox. When they are depressed, they can refer to the contents of their tool box to remind them of ways to cope.

Story time. Have clients write a story in which they pretend that they aren't depressed; what would they be thinking, feeling, and doing? Then help them establish a plan to make the story come true.

Fortune-telling. Oftentimes depressed clients think they can predict the future, thinking that they will always be depressed, which in turn does not motivate them to work on overcoming the depression. To help them address this, make a "crystal ball" by covering a ball with foil and glitter. Urge clients to look into this crystal ball and predict what is going to happen with a specific issue that is troubling them. Usually they say they can't, but the therapist can challenge this by giving examples of when they have in the past—such as "knowing they would fail a test" (but didn't) and so forth. Discuss the disadvantages of predicting the future if there isn't good evidence to support it.

Concrete objects. Use concrete objects as metaphors: a sponge, which signifies not "soaking" up negative, irrational thoughts; binoculars, as a reminder not to magnify things and make them bigger than they really are; and a kaleidoscope to remind them that there are always multiple, less depressing ways of looking at things.

An essential part of RE-CBT includes homework assignments as a way of reinforcing concepts learned during therapy. For example, clients can keep a mood chart, they can record their dysfunctional thoughts and write challenges, or they can watch humorous movies to make them laugh. Other homework assignments include getting physical exercise because it is a good way to combat depression, listening to upbeat music, or journaling about positive aspects of their day.

Case Study

Sixteen-year-old Larissa presented in therapy with depression, sharing that she had been depressed off and on for the past year but that lately it had become much worse. When asked if anything in particular triggered it, she replied that she used to get depressed when she had issues with her friends or boyfriend but that lately she felt depressed most of the time and it didn't relate to anything specific. During this first session, she clearly articulated that she felt overwhelmed, hopeless, and confused, and her responses to a short checklist (Hutt, 2019) revealed that she also had withdrawn from friends and family, had lost interest in most activities, had trouble sleeping, and had difficulty concentrating. She denied any suicidal attempts or other self-injurious behaviors but admitted that occasionally suicide fleetingly crossed her mind.

During this first session, I asked Larissa to complete the emotional pie assessment (previously described) so that I could more accurately determine how much of the time Larissa had been depressed during the past week. The visual representation indicated a significant amount of depression, as well as some anxiety and anger/frustration. We discussed her thoughts and feelings in more detail and, based on what she shared, collaborated on several goals for therapy: to elevate her depressed mood, to increase her tolerance to deal with the frustration of being depressed, and to address relationship issues. I told Larissa that while there is no "quick fix," there were things we could work on during therapy that would help her gain better control over her emotions. At the end of the first session, I asked Larissa to complete the *Beck Depression Inventory* (which confirmed a diagnosis of MDD) and to keep track of her moods on a daily basis using the mood chart.

After reviewing her mood chart at the beginning of the second session, I used a psychoeducational approach to explain how depression is common in teenagers and why and then oriented her to RE-CBT by explaining that depression can also result from dysfunctional negative thoughts such as "I can't stand being depressed—it's too hard to fight it, I will never get over this or be happy again, I must be a loser since I have problems in relationships," and so forth. I also helped her understand that it is not an event itself that creates the negative feelings—it is how she thinks about it—so if she can learn to change her negative thoughts, she can reduce the intensity of her depression. I gave Larissa a handout, *Identifying Cognitive Distortions and Thinking Errors* (Merrell, 2001), and together we discussed how these types of thoughts can lead to depression. Her homework assignment was to keep a record of her thoughts.

During the third session, Larissa shared her dysfunctional thought record. I then explained more about the connection between thoughts, feelings, and behaviors. I asked Larissa if she could share a recent event that contributed to her depression. Larissa said that her boyfriend hadn't returned her phone calls twice last week and he had ignored her on a several occasions. She was able to identify some irrational beliefs: he shouldn't treat me like this; because he is ignoring me, he must not love my anymore; it would be horrible if he broke up with me—and it would prove that I am a loser.

I used the analogy of a robot, asking Larissa if her boyfriend was like a robot that she could just wind up and he would do exactly what she wanted. She acknowledged that she couldn't make him do what she wanted, and I stressed that although she could not control him, she could control her thoughts about his behavior. I helped her understand that when she thought she couldn't stand to be ignored, predicted that he didn't love her anymore, and assumed that they would break up (which would prove that she was a loser) she became more depressed. I asked Larissa to check off thoughts on the *Identifying Cognitive Distortions and Thinking Errors* handout (Merrell, 2001) that corresponded to her irrational beliefs, and I introduced the concept of challenging her thoughts, asking her questions such as the following: "Has your boyfriend ever ignored you before, and if so, did he break up with you?" "How does it help you to assume that he doesn't care about you? Do you have evidence to support that assumption?" "If your best friend came to you and said she was a loser because her boyfriend broke up with her, would you agree with her? Is it really logical to think *you* are a loser if your boyfriend breaks up with you?" "Obviously you don't want him to break off the relationship, but do you know others who have survived break ups? Is it helpful for you to think you could never get over this if he broke up with you?"

At the end of this session, Larissa understood more about how her negative thoughts were contributing to her depression, but she still struggled with the actual disputation process, so I taught her how to use an REBT self-help form and requested that she complete one after each emotionally upsetting event. I also gave her the book *Feeling Better: CBT Workbook for Teens* (Hutt, 2019) and asked her to read it.

During the next several sessions, Larissa and I worked through the REBT self-help homework sheets, which were beneficial. However, she continued to struggle with the belief that her depression was unbearable, so I had her read *The Little Engine that Could* (Piper, 1986) and suggested that she read this simple book every day and make a list of things she could do and had already done to prove to herself that she could stand this, even if it was hard. I also had her implement a self-reward system so that each day she managed to stand the depression she could do something nice for herself.

Over the course of therapy, I also used bibliotherapy—*Conquer Negative Thinking for Teens* (Alvord & McGrath, 2017)—behavioral activation, and expressive writing, where Larissa pretended she was an advice columnist offering help about overcoming depression. In addition, because she still tended to think about a bleak future, I asked her to think about what she wanted out of life, take photos of these things, and make a collage to remind her to stay focused on the future and not predict doom and gloom. Larissa was a motivated client, and the various interventions I used helped her work through her depression as she changed her thinking.

Conclusion

Depression is a very serious disorder which is often under-identified and under-treated in children and adolescents, in part because they don't ask for help or because they present with different symptoms than adults. Given the increasing prevalence of depression in the child and adolescent population (Bennett, Jones, & Smith, 2014; Mayo Clinic, 2018), it is imperative that practitioners employ the most efficacious treatment strategies. While further research needs to be conducted, CBT has been shown to be an effective form of therapy in treating depression. The purpose of this chapter has been to highlight the various ways RE-CBT can be an effective component of a comprehensive treatment plan for depressed youth.

Test Yourself

1. What factors may contribute to the development and maintenance of depression among youth?
2. How are rational emotive and cognitive behavioral approaches modified for diagnosis and treatment of depression as a function of child developmental level?

3. What are common beliefs endorsed by children with depression and how might you apply disputation strategies to help challenge these beliefs and develop more effective/helpful ways of thinking?

References

Adams, J. U. (2018). *Regular screening can find teen depression, but getting treatment isn't easy.* Retrieved from https://www.washingtonpost.com/national/health-science/regular%2D%2Dscreening

Alvord, M. K., & McGrath, A. (2017). *Conquer negative thinking for teens: A workbook to break the nine thought habit that are holding you back.* Oakland, CA: Instant Help Books.

American Academy of Pediatrics. (2018). *American Academy of Pediatrics publishes teen depression guidelines that equip physicians to tackle mental health issues.* Retrieved from https://www.aap.org/en-us/about-the-aap/aap-press-room/Pages/AAP-Publishes-Teen-Depression-Guidelines-aspx

American Psychiatric Association. (2013). *Diagnostic and statistical manual of mental disorders* (5th ed.). Arlington, VA: Author.

Beevers, C. G. (2011). Introduction: Evidence-based practice for major depressive disorder. In D. W. Springer, A. Rubin, & C. G. Beevers (Eds.), *Treatment of depression in adolescents and adults* (pp. 1–20). Hoboken, NJ: Wiley.

Bennett, C., Jones, R. B., & Smith, D. (2014). Prevention strategies for adolescent depression. *Advances in Psychiatric Treatment, 20*(2), 116–124.

Berlinger, N. T. (2005). *Rescuing your teenager from depression.* New York: Harper Collins.

Bernard, M. E. (2004). *The REBT therapist's pocket companion for working with children and adolescents.* New York: Albert Ellis Institute.

Bernard, M. E., & Cronan, F. (1999). The child and adolescent scale of irrationality: Validation data and mental health correlates. *Journal of Cognitive Psychotherapy: An International Quarterly, 13*, 121–132.

Capuzzi, D., & Gross, D. R. (2019). "I don't want to live:" The adolescent at risk for suicidal behavior. In D. Capuzzi & D. R. Gross (Eds.), *Youth at risk: A prevention resource for counselors, teachers, and parents* (7th ed., pp. 219–254). Alexandria, VA: American Counseling Association.

Choate, L., & Anderson, K. (2008). *Girls and women's wellness: Contemporary counseling issues and interventions.* Alexandria, VA: American Counseling Association.

Clark, M. S., Jansen, K. L., & Cloy, J. A. (2012). *Treatment of childhood and adolescent depression.* Retrieved from https://www.aafp.org/afp/2012/0901/p442.html

Curry, J. F., & Hersh, J. (2014). Development and evolution of cognitive behavior therapy for depressed adolescents. *Journal of Rational-Emotive and Cognitive Behavior Therapy, 32*(1), 15–30.

Curry, J. F., Silva, S., Rohde, P., Ginsberg, G., Kratochvil, C., Simmons, A., et al. (2011). Recovery and recurrence following treatment for adolescent major depression. *Archives of General Psychiatry, 68*, 263–270.

David, D., Cardea, D., Cardos, R., Oltean, H., & Stefan, S. (2019). REBT and depressive disorders. In W. Dryden & M. E. Bernard (Eds.), *REBT with diverse client problems and populations* (pp. 23–44). Cham, Switzerland: Springer.

DiGiuseppe, R., Doyle, K. A., & Rose, R. D. (2002). Rational emotive behavior therapy for depression: Achieving unconditional self-acceptance. In M. A. Reinecke & M. R. Davison (Eds.), *Comparative treatments of depression* (pp. 220–248). New York: Springer.

Evans, J. R., Van Velsor, P., & Schumacher, J. E. (2002). Addressing adolescent depression: A role for school counselors. *Professional School Counseling, 5*, 211–218.

Hutt, R. L. (2019). *Feeling better: CBT workbook for teens*. Emeryville, CA: Althea Press.

Knaus, W. J. (1974). *Rational emotive education: A manual for elementary school teachers*. New York: Institute for Rational Living.

Koplewicz, H. S. (2002). *More than moody: Recognizing and treating adolescent depression*. New York: Berkley Publishing.

Kovacs, M. (2011). *Children's depression inventory 2*. North Tonawanda, NY: Multi-Health Systems, Inc.

Leppma, M., & Schimmel, C. J. (2019). Children and challenges: Counseling from a growth mindset perspective. In A. Vernon & C. J. Schimmel (Eds.), *Counseling children and adolescents* (5th ed., pp. 338–379). San Diego, CA: Cognella.

Maughan, B., Collishaw, D. P., & Stingaris, A. (2013). Depression in childhood and adolescence. *Canadian Academy of Child and Adolescent Psychiatry, 22*(1), 35–40.

Mayo Clinic. (2018). *Teen depression*. Retrieved from www.mayoclinic.org/diseases-conditions/teen-depression/symptoms-causes/syc-20350985

Merrell, K. W. (2001). *Helping students overcome depression and anxiety: A practical guide*. New York: Guilford Press.

Monroe, J. (2018). *Teenage depression rates rising*. Retrieved from https://www.newportacademy.com/resources/mental-health/teen-depression-study

Morrison, J., & Flegel, K. (2016). *Interviewing children and adolescents: Skills and strategies for effective DSM-5 diagnosis* (2nd ed.). New York: Guilford Press.

National Institute for Health and Clinical Excellence. (2005). *Depression in children and young people: Identification and management in primary, community and secondary care (Clinical Guideline CG28)*. Leicester, UK: British Psychological Society.

Newman, B. M., & Newman, P. R. (2017). *Development through life: A psychosocial approach*. Boston: Cengage.

Newport Academy. (2018). *Adolescent depression in schools*. Retrieved from https://www.newportacademy.com/

NIMH. (2017). *Prevalence of major depressive episode among adolescents*. Retrieved from https://www.nimh.nih.gov/health/statistics/major-depression.shtml

Nuffield Foundation. (2012). *Increased levels of anxiety and depression as teenage experience changes over time*. Retrieved from http://www.nuffieldfoundation.org/news/increased-levels-anxeity-and-depression

Paterson, J. (2011). Young and depressed. *Counseling Today, 54*(1), 32–35.

Piper, W. (1986). *The little engine that could*. New York: Platt and Munk.

Powell, M. J., & Logan, C. R. (2019). Identifying and preventing mood disorders in children and adolescents. In D. Capuzzi & D. R. Gross (Eds.), *Youth at risk: A prevention resource for counselors, teachers, and parents* (7th ed., pp. 117–133).

Rizvi, S. H., Ong, M. L., & Youngstrom, E. A. (2014). Bipolar disorder in children and adolescents: An update on diagnosis. *Clinical Practice, 11*, 665–676.

Rush, A. J., & Nowels, A. (1994). Adaptation of cognitive therapy for depressed adolescents. In T. C. R. Wilkes, G. Belsher, A. J. Rush, & E. Frank (Eds.), *Cognitive therapy for depressed adolescents* (pp. 3–21). New York: Guildford Press.

Scott, S. K., & Saginak, K. A. (2016). Adolescence: Emotional and social development. In D. Capuzzi & M. D. Stauffer (Eds.), *Human growth and development across the lifespan: Applications for counselors* (pp. 347–386). Hoboken, NJ: Wiley.

Seligman, M. E. P. (1995). *The optimistic child: A proven program to safeguard children against depression and build lifelong resilience*. New York: Harper.

Spielmans, G. I., Pasek, L. F., & McFall, J. P. (2007). What are the active ingredients in cognitive and behavioral psychotherapy for anxious and depressed children? A meta-analytic review. *Clinical Psychology Review, 27*, 642–654.

Stark, K. D., Sander, J. B., Yancy, M. G., Bronik, M. D., & Hoke, J. A. (2000). Treatment of depression in childhood and adolescence: Cognitive-behavioral procedures for the individual and family. In P. C. Kendall (Ed.), *Child and adolescent therapy* (pp. 173–234). New York: Guilford Press.

Stone, T., & Brott, P. E. (2019). Counseling children and adolescents with exceptionalities. In A. Vernon & C. J. Schimmel (Eds.), *Counseling children and adolescents* (5th ed., pp. 258–293). San Diego, CA: Cognella.

Towery, J. (2016). *The anti-depressant book: A practical guide for teens and young adults to overcome depression and stay healthy*. Palo Alto, CA: Jacob Towery.

Vernon, A. (2002). *What works when with children and adolescents: A handbook of individual counseling techniques*. Champaign, IL: Research Press.

Vernon, A. (2009). *More what works when with children and adolescents: A handbook of individual counseling techniques*. Champaign, IL: Research Press.

Vernon, A., & Chen, P. C. (2019). Working with children, adolescents, and their parents: Practical applications of developmental theory. In A. Vernon & C. J. Schimmel (Eds.), *Counseling children and adolescents* (5th ed., pp. 1–36). San Diego, CA: Cognella.

Waslick, B. D., Kandel, R., & Kakouros, A. (2002). Depression in children and adolescents: An overview. In D. Shaffer & B. D. Waslick (Eds.), *The many faces of depression in children and adolescents* (pp. 1–36). Washington, DC: American Psychiatric Publishing.

Weir, K. (2019). *APA offers new guidance for treating depression*. Retrieved from https://www.apa.org/monitor/2019/09/ce-corner-depression

Woo, S. M., & Keatinge, C. (2016). *Diagnosis and treatment of mental disorders across the lifespan*. Hoboken, NJ: Wiley.

Chapter 11
Self-Acceptance: REBT as the Psychological Armor that Protects Children and Adolescents

Michael Bernard

Historically, *self-acceptance* has long been a stimulus for personal change and development in Eastern and Western religion and culture, as well as in psychological literature (see Bernard's edited book, 2013, *The Strength of Self-Acceptance*). Different theologies (e.g., Christianity, Buddhism), psychological theories (e.g., Humanism), and therapies (e.g., REBT; ACT) view *self-acceptance* as a catalyst for the alleviation of emotional misery as well as an energizer, supporting growth toward happiness and fulfillment. Research continues to show that *self-acceptance* is strongly related to mental health and well-being in people of all ages.

Self-acceptance means acknowledging that one is a complex, imperfect human being capable of making mistakes as well as significant accomplishments. One possesses a realistic awareness of one's strengths and weaknesses. One accepts oneself in spite of one's imperfections and because of one's uniqueness. One refrains from self-criticism, avoiding rating one's self-worth based on other people thinking negatively of what one does, the way one looks, or when one perceives not living up to one's expectations.

Self-acceptance is not an excuse for accepting one's bad or inappropriate behavior. In fact, with strong self-acceptance, it is much easier to realistically evaluate what one does and to work on changing behavior that is inappropriate or self-defeating.

Self-acceptance is not self-esteem (Barrish, 1997; Ellis, 2005). Self-esteem refers to our judgments about how much we like or value ourselves and is based on comparisons with others and on the extent to which we achieve personal goals. Not taking things personally gives people the resilience, confidence, and wisdom to change those things about yourself that need changing and the calmness to accept those things that you cannot change.

M. Bernard (✉)
Melbourne Graduate School of Education, University of Melbourne, Parkville, VIC, Australia
e-mail: m.bernard@unimelb.edu.au

M. Bernard, M. D. Terjesen (eds.), *Rational-Emotive and Cognitive-Behavioral Approaches to Child and Adolescent Mental Health: Theory, Practice, Research, Applications*, https://doi.org/10.1007/978-3-030-53901-6_11

Albert Ellis and his colleagues (e.g., Ellis, Wolfe, & Moseley, 1968) have written about the pernicious effects of self-depreciation on the mental health of children and the need for adults to not only combat young people's tendencies to negatively self-rate but also explicitly teach self-acceptance.

> Teach children to never rate themselves in terms of their behavior and to separate judgments of their actions from judgments of self-worth. Encourage them to acknowledge and accept responsibility for their *traits* and *behaviors* –both good and bad- without evaluating *themselves* as good or bad. Help combat children's tendencies towards self-downing by reminding them they are made up of many good qualities (and some that are not so helpful) and that they do not lose their good qualities when bad things happen. Explain to children that all human beings are capable and likeable in their unique ways and, therefore, it is good for children to accept themselves unconditionally without having to prove themselves. (Ellis, Wolfe, & Moseley, 1968, *How to Raise an Emotionally Healthy, Happy Child*)

In 1968, Albert Ellis founded *The Living School* for elementary-age students at what was then called the Institute for Rational Living (New York City). There, children were not only taught the standard academic curriculum but also *Rational Emotive Education* (Knaus, 1974) – a curriculum of lessons designed to teach emotional literacy including the role of thinking in emotions and behavior and a variety of rational beliefs including high frustration tolerance, acceptance of others, and self-acceptance.

Why Self-Acceptance in Young People Must Be Addressed

Chronic depression and high anxiety result from the attitude of *self-depreciation* and a *lack* of strong self-acceptance. Due to social and developmental factors, many young people feel badly about themselves.

To combat young people's tendencies to self-depreciate, parents and teachers can help young people to not rate their self-worth based on their achievements, what others think of them, or their body image but rather to display "self-acceptance" – regardless of external factors.

Self-Acceptance in Young People: What It Looks Like

> Two girls receive the same cyber message on several occasions saying that each looks FAT and UGLY. Carmen is quite devastated, feeling extremely anxious and depressed about the impact of the message on her popularity, while Alex pays little attention to the message, reminds herself that she is a worthwhile person, and returns an SMS saying that the sender should have paid more attention in their recent health class on celebrating differences and not judging people by their appearance, culture, or behavior.

The emotional impact of this cyberbullying event is dramatically different for the two girls because of the different attitude or mindset of each girl. As a consequence of her attitude of *self-depreciation*, Carmen takes being cyberbullied quite personally thinking "Because I am being picked on for my physical appearance, there must be something wrong with me. I now think less of myself and I must be a real loser."

In contrast, Alex's attitude of *self-acceptance* literally protects her. She refuses to rate her self-worth and value based on another's opinion of her, instead thinking "I accept myself no matter what" and "I am me and that's OK."

The Pressure Is on Kids

The research indicates that 50% of young people today say they feel very stressed compared with 30% in 2003 (Bernard & Stephanou, 2017).

Social media isn't helping, with young people constantly being shown what it means to be successful, physically attractive, and cool. A myriad of mobile devices makes it that much easier to tease and bully – and get away with it. Young people feel they are constantly being judged, requiring "likes" and other people's approval just to feel worthwhile. Our kids are doing all they can to live up to and meet their peer's expectations. Plus, there is a ton of pressure on young people, from parents and teachers, to perform well in school.

Many parents today are very anxious about their children. Consequently, many parents are overprotecting their children, with the result being that many young people feel very vulnerable and lack resilience, partly because they do not possess strong self-acceptance.

Research Facts

- 58% of young people worry excessively about what others think of them.
- 35% say that when they do badly in their schoolwork, they think "I'm a failure."
- In primary and secondary schools, student self-acceptance is associated with positive emotions and high levels of life satisfaction.
- In primary and secondary schools, student self-depreciation is associated with negative emotions and low levels of life satisfaction.
- Student self-depreciation, anxiety, and anger are often seen alongside behavior problems and teacher ratings of students' low effort in school.

Child Developmental Considerations

Fortunately, many very young children (3–6 years) tend to perceive themselves in a very favorable light (Harter, 2012). However, those that experience a high incidence of negative encounters with other people and with their learning can be heard thinking aloud: "I'm a loser," "I'm hopeless," and "I'm a bad kid." By the age of 8, these negative self-evaluations can become internalized, automatic, and pervasive.

Children in middle to late childhood (8–10 years) are more at risk for developing negative self-evaluations than younger children (Harter, 2012). Due to their increasing abilities to see themselves through the eyes of others as well as be concerned by the discrepancy between the way they would like to be (ideal self) and the way they really are (real self), they demonstrate great vulnerability to self-depreciation and low self-esteem.

Adolescents bring additional challenges with adolescent egocentrism emerging in 11–13 year olds (e.g., Elkind, 1967). The way they view themselves may be very unrealistic. Their construction of an *imaginary audience* reflects the false assumption that others, particularly peers, are as preoccupied with their behavior and appearance as they are and that peers are constantly submitting them to scrutiny and critical evaluation. While academic achievements are also important to self-evaluations, perceptions of physical appearance top the list in terms of the correlation with feelings of overall self-worth. During this stage, because of an increase in negative self-evaluations, physical development, hormones, timing of puberty, and stressful life events, depression rates rise from 2–5% to 8%.

Self-Acceptance Versus Self-Depreciation

In some ways, it is easier to illustrate the meaning of self-acceptance by its converse, self-depreciation (also referred to as self-downing or negative self-rating). Semantically, self-depreciation involves the mislabeling of one's overall value as a person as worthless, hopeless, or failure. Logically, self-depreciation is seen as a non sequitur where a conclusion is reached that because one (or more) aspect of one's behavior or traits is bad, therefore, all aspects of oneself are bad. Empirically, self-depreciation results from selective abstraction of one or more aspects of one's negative behavior or traits to arrive at the false conclusion that all aspects of oneself are bad.

The significant role self-depreciation plays in a young person's low self-esteem, hopelessness, and depression is illustrated below using the ABC model of emotions (Ellis, 1994). The bolded type reflects self-rating (from Bernard, 2004b).

Example 1

Activating events: loss of parental love through desertion/abandonment/neglect or death

Beliefs:

> Inferences (conclusions, predictions): My parent doesn't love me. It's my fault my parent never wants to see me. I cannot do anything to get his/her to love me. I cannot be happy without his/her love. Life is not worth living if I cannot have his/her love.

Absolutes (shoulds, oughts, musts, needs): I need my parent's love.
Evaluations: I cannot bear to live without her love. *This proves how unlovable and hopeless I am.* This is terrible.

Consequence (emotional, behavioral): down, crying, periods of inactivity, avoidance of people and tasks, tiredness, irritability

Example 2

Activating events: poor school performance
Beliefs:

Inferences (conclusions, predictions): I'm not good at any of my schoolwork and never will be. I am hopeless in everything I do.
Absolutes (shoulds, oughts, musts, needs): I should/must achieve in my schoolwork.
Evaluations: It is awful to make mistakes and do so poorly; I really can't stand it. *This proves I am really a total failure.*

Consequence (emotional, behavioral): down, crying, periods of inactivity, avoidance of people and tasks, tiredness, irritability

Example 3

Activating events: social rejection, teasing, no one to play with, not being invited, loss of boyfriend/girlfriend
Beliefs:

Inferences (conclusions, predictions): Everyone is against me. Everyone is teasing me. No one likes me. I'll never have any friends.
I can't be happy without his/her love or attention.

Absolutes (shoulds, oughts, musts, needs): I need people to like and approve of me.
Evaluations: It is awful to be criticized, laughed at, and alone. I can't stand it. *This proves that I really am a hopeless person.*

Consequence (emotional, behavioral): down, crying, periods of inactivity, avoidance of people and tasks, tiredness, irritability

Research on Self-Acceptance

One of the problems we see in understanding the concept of self-acceptance is that it is often defined inconsistently. Further, self-acceptance is also used interchangeably with the concepts of self-worth and self-esteem, making it difficult to truly understand self-acceptance, its relationship to mental health, and ultimately the strategies that may be used to promote this concept.

Research reveals the relationship of low self-acceptance as indicated by a high degree of self-depreciation and childhood disorders (e.g., Ellis & Bernard, 2006). For example, using the *Child and Adolescent Scale of Irrationality* to measure self-depreciation, Bernard and Cronan (1999) found significant positive relationships between self-depreciation, trait anxiety, trait anger, and teacher ratings of student low effort in school and behavior problems. Pannes (1963) found significant associations between low dogmatism in adolescents and low degrees of self-acceptance. Self-acceptance has been shown to be related to both internalizing and externalizing behaviors (Kassay, Terjesen, & Smidt, 2010) as well as academics (Brooks, 1999) among both clinical samples and typically developing youth.

I designed a scale that contains items reflecting dimensions of positive self-regard as well as negative self-evaluation. In its original form, 12 items were written tapping each dimension and were edited and agreed to by three different experts in rational emotive behavior therapy. The survey was administered to 254 students (169 in grades 5/6; 85 in grades 7/8) in 4 different schools in Victoria, Australia. An exploratory factor analysis revealed a two-factor solution with eight items being dropped due to item-factor loadings lower than 0.50. The factors were negatively correlated (0.49).

Items loading on factor 1 "positive self-regard" but not factor 2 reflect self-awareness of positive attributes especially when faced with negative events.

- When I think about what I cannot do very well, I still accept who I am.
- When I get a lower grade than I want, I am good at reminding myself I am capable.
- When I look in the mirror and see something I don't like (e.g., my skin, my hair, my nose), I know I still have good things about me.
- I know a lot about my good qualities.

Factor 2 "negative self-evaluation" consists of items that reflect global self-rating as well as the importance of other people's opinions and school performance as a basis for determining one's value as a person.

- When my friends don't ask me to do things with them, I think I'm a loser.
- People would like me a lot more if I wasn't such a loser.
- When things are boring, I think I'm a dull and uninteresting person.
- I am someone who needs my friends to like me to feel important and to be worthwhile.
- When I don't succeed in a subject that is important to me, I am likely to think I'm a complete failure.

To examine the relationship of positive self-regard and negative self-evaluation to the emotional life and life satisfaction of young people, the revised 16-item *Child and Adolescent Survey of Positive Self-Regard and Self-Acceptance*, Huebner's (2001) *Students' Life Satisfaction Scale* (6-item short form), and the 20-item *Positive and Negative Affect Scale for Children* (Laurent et al., 1999) were administered to 175 students (90 in grades 5/6; 85 in grades 7/8) in 4 different schools in Victoria, Australia. Significant relationships are reported in Table 11.1.

Table 11.1 Relationship between self-regard and negative self-evaluation with positive/negative emotions and life satisfaction

	Positive affect	Negative affect	Life satisfaction
Positive self-regard	0.55	−0.22	0.63
Negative self-evaluation	−0.37	0.38	−0.51
Total	0.52	−0.34	0.64

Positive affect correlated 0.58 with life satisfaction, whereas negative affect correlated −0.53. No gender differences were found, and there was some evidence that older students score lower in factor 1 (positive self-regard) than younger students.

Both dimensions, positive self-regard and negative self-evaluation, were associated with life satisfaction. As might be expected, positive self-regard was most strongly correlated with the experience of positive emotions, while negative self-evaluation was most strongly correlated with the experience of negative emotions. Overall, these preliminary findings suggest that education programs for young people should include learning experiences that promote the development of positive self-regard and the elimination of negative self-evaluation.

The buffering impact of self-acceptance may also be seen in research that looked at the development of body dissatisfaction and psychopathology (Maxwell & Cole, 2012). The authors reported that adolescents' use of self-acceptance strategies appeared to attenuate the relation between body dissatisfaction and psychopathology. Now the scales that measured self-acceptance may not be exactly in line with the conceptualization of self-acceptance for this chapter (e.g., "I would say to myself that I am perfect the way I am," "I would tell myself that I like the way I look"); these results may provide insights into healthy and unhealthy strategies that adolescents may use to manage negative affective states and body dissatisfaction, may warrant further investigation, and further support the importance of this concept as a buffer to pathology.

In sum, self-acceptance has been demonstrated to be related to healthy affective states and behavior among youth and also has been used as a component of varied clinical interventions and educational programs that have resulted in positive outcomes. The combination of the continued efficacy of cognitive behavioral interventions for youth with the desire for more preventative programming and efficiency of clinical work may in fact spur further investigation into examining the science of self-acceptance among youth.

Working 1:1

In teaching a young person's self-acceptance (e.g., Bernard & Joyce, 1984), a prerequisite step often involves the disputing of self-depreciation. You can explain that disputing involves asking three questions about one's thinking:

1. Is what I am thinking true? Is there evidence to support what I am thinking?
2. Is my thinking logical? Does it make sense to think this way?
3. Does it help me to think this way? Does my thought help me to achieve my goals and manage my emotions?

When a young person answers "no" to any one of these questions, they should, with your help, try to change the thought to one that is true, sensible, and helpful.

To dispute self-downing, you will want to show young clients how their thinking "I'm hopeless, a loser" does not make sense and is not true. You can begin by having the young person identify a range of positive and negative traits using a self-concept circle divided into segments with pluses and minuses in each segment. Once completed, ask the young client "Does it make sense to think because something bad happened (e.g., poor grade, teased, rejection) that you are totally bad?" "Do you lose all your positive qualities when you make something bad happen?" You can also discuss the concept of human fallibility. Indicate that everyone is born as a mistake maker and, as such, it never makes sense to think "I must not make mistakes" as mistakes are inevitable.

An example of semantic disputation of self-depreciation is seen in the following exchange between a therapist and young client.

T: So, let me get this straight. When you were not invited to the party at Mary's house and your friend was, you thought of yourself as a "loser." Is that what you thought?
C: Yeah, I mean like Dina and Stephanie were invited.
T: Well, I would upset myself about what happened, too. But, if you don't want to get so down, let's examine what you were telling yourself and see if it is rational.
C: OK.
T: When you think of yourself as a loser, the word "loser" means more than "I am not popular enough with Mary to get invited to her party."

The word "loser" means loser in everything you have done, are doing, and will be doing. It means your total essence is one of being a loser. Now, is your use of the word "loser" really true to this meaning?

During individual counseling sessions, specific interventions can target self-acceptance in developmentally and culturally appropriate ways that facilitate healthy development in young clients (Bernard, Vernon, Terjesen, & Kurasaki, 2013). As with classroom guidance activities, it is more effective if a variety of interventions employing different creative arts techniques are employed because there is a greater likelihood that younger clients will retain the concepts.

Ann Vernon has indicated the following (from Bernard et al., 2013):

> Young children respond well to concrete techniques, such as using a balloon and a hard rubber ball to emphasize "bouncing back" after being put down, for example. For a child struggling with this issue, give him a balloon to blow up and tie, then give him a straight pin and ask him to prick the balloon with it until it pops. Then have him prick the rubber ball with the pin, discussing the difference between the balloon that pops and a rubber ball…the ball is still intact but the balloon isn't. Use this method to help the child see that if he per-

> sonalizes everything and thinks he is what others say he is when they put him down, he "deflates," whereas if he thinks about his strengths and weaknesses and doesn't personalize every bad thing others say about him, he will be much more likely to "bounce back" like a rubber ball….
>
> Teenagers are notorious for "soaking up the negative" when peers call them names or put them down, so a concrete strategy that works well with this age group is to use a large sponge and a bucket of water. First have them hold the sponge when it is dry and light, then dip it in the bucket of water and hold it again. They readily realize that it is much heavier when it is wet. Draw the analogy that if they "soak up" everything others say about them without "wringing out" the sponge and differentiating between who they are and what others say they are, their self-acceptance is negatively impacted.

During individual counseling sessions, it is also important to help clients learn that they are complex human beings with multiple characteristics. Mental health practitioners and school counselors can use an intervention called The Whole Picture (Vernon, 2009, pp. 279–280) to convey this concept to clients struggling with this issue. Use a child's puzzle, a sheet of construction paper that is cut into ten shapes that fit together like a puzzle, transparent tape, and a pen. First have the client put the puzzle together, discussing what happens if there are missing pieces and that all pieces are needed to see the whole picture. Then give her the construction paper puzzle pieces, and explain that this is a personal puzzle. She needs to think about different "pieces" of herself and write them on the individual pieces and then put her puzzle together and tape it. Again, discuss how all parts are needed for the "whole picture."

Another technique that can be used to enhance self-acceptance and teach clients to avoid equating their self-worth with how they describe themselves is called Who, Me? Yes, You (Vernon, 2009, p. 281). This intervention requires a short checklist with characteristics such as intelligent, fun to be with, responsible, dependable, loyal, trustworthy, outgoing, popular, good looking, musically talented, and so forth. The client completes the checklist, and you discuss which characteristics were like or unlike him, asking if he is "better" if he has more check marks. Then ask the client to read the characteristics out loud, saying "I am only a good person if I am _______ (intelligent, responsible, and so forth)." Tape recording this and playing it back help clients really hear what they are saying: I am only a good person if…, and have proven to be an effective way of helping them understand that they are good regardless of specific characteristics.

Another intervention appropriate for adolescents is to engage them in an activity called IAWAC (Vernon, 2002, pp. 74–76). This strategy helps teenage clients understand that they don't have to take every criticism or comment personally and put themselves down as a result, helping them accept themselves and build emotional resiliency. First, give the client a sheet of paper with the letters IAWAC written across it, informing her that this paper represents her self-worth. Next, tell her a story about a girl who gets up late for school and is yelled at by her parents for being irresponsible, which sets off her whole day. She is almost late for the bus, so she can't sit with her friends who ignore her; she misses most of the problems on the algebra board drill and considers herself stupid, and she forgets to go to play practice, so her parents cite this as yet another example of her irresponsible behavior. As you read the story, instruct the client to tear off a part of her IAWAC sign each time she or someone else is critical of her. By the end of the story, there won't be much left of her worth. Then give her another IAWAC sign, and tell the story again, but this time instead of tearing off part of the sign when she misses problems and calls herself stupid, the girl in the story thinks to herself, "I'm not a stupid person…I just missed problems," and tears off a smaller part of the sign. Or, instead of tearing off a large piece of her sign when her parents called her irresponsible, she could tear off a small piece while thinking to herself, "I may not be the most responsible kid, but that doesn't make me a bad person." At the end of the story, discuss the rational self-talk that helped the girl in the story be more accepting of herself and how the client might use these concepts to deal with her own lack of self-acceptance.

Strategies for Disputing "Self-Downing"

1. To dispute self-downing, you will want to show young clients how their thinking "I'm hopeless, a loser" does not make sense and is not true. You can begin by having your young client come up with a range of positive and negative traits using a self-concept circle divided into segments with pluses and minuses in each segment. Once completed, ask the young client "Does it make sense to think because something bad happened (e.g., poor grade, teased, rejection) that you are totally bad?" "Do you lose all your positive qualities when you make something bad happen?"
2. Discuss the concept of *human fallibility*. Indicate that everyone is born as a mistake maker and, as such, it never makes sense to think "I must not make mistakes" as mistakes are inevitable.
3. Teach the following ideas to help engender both *self-acceptance* and *other-acceptance*:

   (a) Every person is complex, not simple.
   (b) I am complex, not simple.
   (c) Every person is made up of many positive and negative qualities.
   (d) I am made up of many positive and negative qualities.
   (e) A person is not all good or all bad because of some of his or her characteristics.
   (f) I am not all good or all bad.
   (g) When I only focus on the negative characteristics of a person, I feel worse about the person.
   (h) When I only focus on my negative qualities, I feel worse about myself.
   (i) Focusing only on the negative qualities of someone else and thinking he is totally bad are irrational. People who do the wrong thing also have other positive qualities.

(j) Only focusing on my negative qualities and concluding "I am hopeless" are irrational. Even when I do the wrong thing, I still retain my positive qualities.

4. Ask a young client: "Would you put a friend of yours down because she didn't do well in a subject or wasn't invited to a party? Would it make sense to think that she was a total loser?" Once young client agrees, ask: "Well then, why are you putting yourself down because of what happened. If you would not put your friend down, does it make sense to put yourself down?"
5. Explain that a person's worth cannot be calculated from a person's performance.
   Use an analogy. Ask: "Would you junk a car if it had a flat tire?" When the young client can see that it would not make sense to do so, you can help him begin to see that junking himself when something bad happens does not make sense.
6. For children who are depressed due to perceived loss of love from a parent through divorce, abuse, or abandonment, gather evidence (instances of loving behavior) to prove or disprove the automatic thoughts "My parent doesn't love me." If it appears that there is no evidence of loving behavior on the part of the child's parent, be prepared to dispute the child's irrational belief that he needs his parents' love, that he will not be able to be happy without it, and that he is unlovable.

Case study (from Bernard et al., 2013). The following case study illustrates further application of self-acceptance principles in individual counseling. The client is a 15-year-old female, referred to counseling by her parents who are concerned about her depression which they feel directly relates to low self-esteem and the pressure she puts on herself because she thinks she has to be perfect.

During the first session with Amanda, she admitted that she was very self-critical and that it contributed in a major way to her depression. When asked to talk more about feeling depressed, she stated that it was because she was ugly, fat, stupid, and unpopular. In fact, she was an attractive young woman who was not at all overweight and who was obviously not stupid based on the fact that her grades were all As and Bs. According to her parents, she did have friends and even a boyfriend, but as is typical with adolescents, those relationships would be on again and off again, which caused Amanda to think that she wasn't popular or worthy of having a boyfriend when the relationships were rocky. Unbeknownst to her parents, when she went through periods where she was rejected by friends or fighting with her boyfriend, she admitted to drinking rather heavily and also toyed with the idea of becoming anorexic because she thought that might make her more attractive.

It was so apparent that this young client had an unrealistic picture of herself and for some time had only seen herself in a negative light, which resulted in a lot of insecurity and anxiety, as well as depression. During an initial session, I gave her an envelope and asked her to write words describing the "public" Amanda on the outside – words that others would use to describe her. Although most of them were negative, there were a few positives. Then I invited her to write words that she used to describe herself – characteristics that others may not even know about her – and put those on slips of paper inside the envelope. When we discussed what she had written, it was once again very evident that she basically didn't see her strengths, only her weaknesses. Even challenging her perception that she was stupid with the fact that she got As and Bs was difficult because she stubbornly held onto the notion that she was stupid because she didn't get all As and because she didn't, she wasn't a good person. In challenging this, I asked her if she would consider her best friend a bad person because she didn't get all As, and Amanda said she wouldn't. "So if you wouldn't think your friend was a bad person, why would you think you are? Does that make sense?" She admitted that it didn't make much sense, but I could tell we needed to continue to work on letting go of this irrational belief.

It also appeared that Amanda was like Velcro; everything that was implied or directly stated or even misinterpreted by her would automatically "stick" to her. For example, when her best friend was sitting by someone else, Amanda assumed she didn't like her and that she wasn't worthy of her friendship. Or, when her boyfriend didn't call her at the exact time he had said he would, she assumed he was out with another girl because she wasn't good enough for him. Incidents like this depressed her even more to the point where she didn't concentrate well at school and resulted in some bad grades on tests. Of course, this further confirmed her perception that she was stupid.

Several different interventions were employed over the course of many months to address self-acceptance issues, which seemed to be the root of Amanda's problems and were spiraling out of control. First, I shared the concept of unconditional self-acceptance – USA – with her, emphasizing that humans are fallible people who make mistakes, that they are not their behavior, and that one doesn't have to be perfect to be worthwhile. To get these points across, I used an intervention entitled USA (Vernon, 2002, p. 78), which involved giving her a paper bag labeled USA. Inside the bag were five strips of paper with the following phrases, one per card: school performance; peer relationships; sports, music, or drama; jobs or chores; and daughter. I then explained that it is not good to globally rate herself as a good or a bad person, but rather, she should remember that she is comprised of many different traits and that it is preferable to rate those to give her a more accurate picture of herself. I encouraged her to think about her performance in each area and rate herself on a 1–5 scale, as objectively and factually as possible. True to form, she did not rate herself high in any category, so I challenged her perception that she was average in music with the fact that she had recently been asked to try out for an honor choir. "But I know I won't make the final cut," she said. "You have a crystal ball?" I asked. "And even if you don't make it, doesn't the fact that you were asked to try out mean that you have better than average musical ability?" She reluctantly agreed. "But even if you actually had average or below average talent, does that make you a bad person?" I asked. "I guess not" was her response. I continued to work with her on each of the areas listed on the cards, helping her see that she did have strengths as well as weaknesses but that her worth as a person wasn't related to her performance or her behavior.

Another intervention was used to help her accept herself more unconditionally. Because she had a tendency to jump to conclusions that she wasn't good enough, I asked her to write down every single negative thought she had ever had about herself. Then one by one, we went through the list, and I asked her to prove to me that she in fact was that "bad." For example, one of the things on her list was that she was inconsiderate. I asked for an example, and she provided one. "Well," I said, "surely there must be lots of other examples; name a few more." She really couldn't think of any at the moment, so I asked her if it was in fact accurate to label herself as inconsiderate when she could only recall one incident. After doing some of this sort of challenging, I then asked her to select ten labels that she could let go of because they were one-time occurrences or overgeneralizations. She selected these and then wrote them on individual slips of paper and stuffed them into balloons that she then blew up and tied. We went outside and she let them go. We continued to do this for the next two sessions until we got to the point where she had a more realistic concept of herself and was able to accept the labels that were left as part of her, but not defining her as a good or a bad person.

Another intervention used to help Amanda address her perfectionism was Too Perfect? (Vernon, 2009, pp. 283–285). This intervention utilized a short checklist with items such as I must be perfect because if I'm not, I'm not worthwhile, I must be perfect so that I am better than others, I must be perfect because others will like me better, and so forth. After she checked off the items that applied to her, we discussed the reasons why she thought she had to be perfect and talked about where her "should be perfect" ideas were coming from. Then she filled out a worksheet with three columns: why must I be perfect? advantages of being perfect, and disadvantages of being perfect. There were multiple lines under each category so that she could thoroughly explore this issue. Together we discussed her irrational idea that she had to be perfect to be accepted and worthwhile and weighed the advantages and disadvantages of demanding that she always be perfect. This took repeated work, but she gradually relaxed her self-imposed standards and found out that others still accepted her even if she wasn't perfect.

Helping children and adolescents understand and internalize the concept of self-acceptance isn't easy, but as this case illustrated, there are various ways to help them learn the concepts, and the end result benefits clients in numerous ways. If they can begin to think that they are worthwhile individuals regardless of their performance and to accept themselves with strengths as well as weaknesses, they will be better able to face.

School-Home Practices for Strengthening Self-Acceptance in Young People

For younger children (less than 8 years), the path to strong self-acceptance is paved by parents, teachers, and significant others through:

- Encouraging them to make positive, realistic judgments of how smart they are, their physical abilities, and how they look and behave
- Being proud of their achievements

- Providing evidence and discussion about when they learn new things that are hard, through their effort and trying new ways to do things, they become smarter and better learners
- Not judging them by their behavior and what they have or have not accomplished
- Encouraging them to *not* compare their achievements with others
- When faced with difficulty and challenges, modeling self-acceptance self-talk by thinking out loud "I am me and that's ok. I am still proud of who I am."
- Teaching self-talk that adults can rehearse with younger children when they are faced with difficulty in learning new skills or being treated badly by a peer:
  - "Just because those kids don't want me to play doesn't mean I'm a total loser"
  - "Some kids take longer than others to learn to read. I just need to keep practicing and I know I'll get there."
  - "Just because they called me a loser doesn't mean it's true. I know I'm not a total loser and that's the most important thing."

As children mature, the following practices can be employed by teachers and parents to promote self-acceptance.

Practice 1. Introduce Young People to Self-Acceptance
Say that self-acceptance can help you to think and feel positive, confident, and resilient when faced with tough situations like being teased or not achieving a result you hoped for. Explain the meaning of self-acceptance: "Accepting yourself as a worthwhile person no matter what, and being proud of who you are." Explain that self-downing or self-depreciation means thinking untrue, unhelpful things, such as that you are totally hopeless or a failure when you haven't been successful, someone is behaving poorly toward you, or you do not like aspects of your body image.

Practice 2. Communicate Unconditional Positive Regard
When disciplining or critiquing, do so without negative attitude or hostility. Focus on the young person's behavior, and try not to make him/her feel bad about him/herself as a person because of lack of achievement or poor behavior.

Practice 3. Illustrate How Self-Acceptance Can Help Young People Deal with Difficulty
If a child makes an error on an art project and begins to cry, the teacher or parent could help the child cope with the situation of making a mistake and rehearse statements such as "We all make mistakes, but just because we made a mistake does not mean that we are bad." If a child becomes upset due to a physical impairment, rehearsing self-acceptance statements could include "I don't like that I need hearing aids, but it doesn't make me any less awesome, and it's not going to stop me from coming to school."

Practice 4. Challenge and Change the Young Person's Self-Downing Thinking
For example, if a young person is down in the dumps, say: "One good way to think when you've had a bit of a setback is to remind yourself of your good points and not to put yourself down." Use an analogy. Ask: "Would you trash an entire car if it had just one flat tire?" When young people can see that it would not make sense to do

so, you can help them begin to see that trashing him or herself when one bad thing happens does not make sense either.

Practice 5. Help Young People Become Aware of and Appreciate Their Positive Qualities
To develop young people's sense of positive self-regard, have them take stock of their individual positive skills, strengths, and personality traits, including, and aside from, school performance.

Practice 6. Review with Young People Examples of Self-Accepting Thinking (Self-Talk)
Here are examples of self-accepting self-talk that can be discussed with young people for dealing with difficult situations and events:

Happening: You get a C- in English.
Self-talk: "Let's try and get more out of the next exam and do more practice. My value as a person is not decided by a test/exam score."
Happening: Being excluded from a game.
Self-talk: "I can cope with being excluded; it doesn't mean I am a loser. I am who I am, I'm still proud of whom I am. I don't need to be included in a game to feel good about myself, to be a worthwhile people."

Conclusion

Self-acceptance is vital to the emotional well-being and productivity of all members of a school community – students, teachers, support staff, administrators, and parents. Self-acceptance should be explicitly incorporated as a core value of a school and incorporated within school culture. All members of a school community will benefit. It is clear that more research needs to be conducted to determine the relationship of self-acceptance to character strengths and social-emotional skills as well as to isolate its influence in effecting positive change in young people. It would be good to learn more about the relationship of self-acceptance and self-regard in terms of their relative contributions to positive emotions and life satisfaction of young people.

Test Yourself

1. In your communication with students, parents, and teachers, how would you differentiate self-acceptance from self-esteem?
2. What factors exist that may make overcoming the myth of self-esteem and promoting self-acceptance more challenging?
3. What role does self-depreciation play in self-acceptance, and how can clinicians and educators work to overcome this?

Appendix 1

Child and Adolescent Survey of Self-Acceptance (Bernard, 2012)

Gender: (circle one): boy girl School: ________________
Grade/Class: ________

When you are ready to begin, please reach each sentence below and pick your answer by circling a number from "1" to "5." The five possible answers for each sentence are:

1 = strongly disagree 2 = disagree 3 = not sure 4 = agree 5 = strongly agree

For example, if you were given the sentence "I like to read comic books," you would circle a "1" if you strongly disagree. If you were given the sentence "I like to keep my room neat and tidy," you would circle a "5" if you strongly agree. Please be sure to answer all of the questions.

	Strongly disagree	Disagree	Not sure	Agree	Strongly agree
1. When I think about me, I am proud of whom I am	1	2	3	4	5
2. Saying something stupid in front of others shows I am an idiot	1	2	3	4	5
3. When my father or mother criticizes me for doing the wrong thing, I know that I still have my good points	1	2	3	4	5
4. I am someone who needs my friends to like me to feel important and to be worthwhile	1	2	3	4	5
5. When a classmate treats me unfairly, I think I must be a hopeless person	1	2	3	4	5
6. When a classmate teases me about the way I look or talk or what I say, I think it is okay to be different	1	2	3	4	5
7. When my friends don't ask me to do things with them, I think I'm a loser	1	2	3	4	5
8. When I get a lower grade than I want, I am good at reminding myself that I am capable	1	2	3	4	5
9. When I think about what I cannot do very well, I still proud of who I am	1	2	3	4	5
10. People would like me more if I wasn't such a loser	1	2	3	4	5
11. When I don't succeed in school in a subject that is important to me, I am likely to think I'm a complete failure	1	2	3	4	5
12. I know a lot about my positive qualities	1	2	3	4	5
13. When things are boring, I think I'm a dull and uninteresting person	1	2	3	4	5

	Strongly disagree	Disagree	Not sure	Agree	Strongly agree
14. When I look in the mirror and see something I don't like (e.g., my hair, my skin, my nose), I know I still have good things about me	1	2	3	4	5
15. When I make mistakes in my schoolwork, I can think of things I am good at	1	2	3	4	5
16. I am someone who needs to get good grades to feel important and worthwhile	1	2	3	4	5

Positive self-regard: ___ + ___ + ___ + ___ + ___ + ___ + ___ + ___
1 3 6 8 9 12 14 15

Negative self-evaluation: ___ + ___ + ___ + ___ + ___ + ___ + ___ + ___
2 4 5 7 10 11 13 16

References

Barrish, I. J. (1997). Teaching children how to feel good without rating themselves. *Journal of Rational-Emotive & Cognitive-Behavior Therapy, 15*(1), 71–79.

Bernard, M. E. (2004b). *The REBT therapist's pocket companion for working with children and adolescents*. New York: Albert Ellis Institute.

Bernard, M. E. (2012). *The character strength of self-acceptance: I accept myself no matter what.* East Melbourne, VIC: The Bernard Group.

Bernard, M. E. (Ed.). (2013). *The strength of self-acceptance* (p. 288). New York: Springer.

Bernard, M.E., & Stephanou, (2017). A. Ecological levels of social and emotional wellbeing of young people. *Child Indicators Research, 11*, 661–679. DOI 10.1007/s12187-017-9466-7.

Bernard, M. E., & Cronan, F. (1999). The child and adolescent scale of irrationality: Validation data and mental health correlates. *Journal of Cognitive Psychotherapy: An International Quarterly, 13*, 121–132.

Bernard, M. E., & Joyce, M. R. (1984). *Rational-emotive therapy with children and adolescents: Theory, treatment strategies, preventative methods*. New York: Wiley.

Bernard, M. E., Vernon, A., Terjesen, M., & Kurasaki, R. (2013). Self-acceptance in the educational and counseling of young people. In M. E. Bernard (Ed.), *The strength of self-acceptance. Theory, research and application* (pp. 155–192). New York: Springer Press.

Brooks, M. (1999). *Achievers and underachievers in regular and special education: An examination of their mindset for achievement and foundations for learning.* Unpublished master's thesis, California State University, Long Beach.

Elkind, D. (1967). Egocentrism in adolescence. *Child Development, 38*, 1025–1034.

Ellis, A., Wolfe, J., & Moseley, S. (1968). *How to raise an emotionally healthy, happy child.* New York: Albert Ellis Institute.

Ellis, A. (1962; 1994 rev ed.). *Reason and emotion in psychotherapy.* Secaucus, NJ: Lyle Stuart and Citadel Press.

Ellis, A. (2005). *The myth of self-esteem*. Amherst, NY: Prometheus.

Ellis, A., & Bernard, M. E. (Eds.). (2006). *Rational emotive behavioral approaches to childhood disorders*. New York: Springer.

Harter, S. (2012). *The construction of the self. Developmental and Sociocultural Foundations* (2nd ed.). New York: Guilford Press.

Kassay, K., Terjesen, M., & Smidt, D. (2010). *Measuring irrationality in children: Re-standardization and validation of the CASI.* Poster presented at the American Psychological Association 118th Annual Convention (Division 12), San Diego, CA, August 2010.
Knaus, W.J. (1974). *Rational emotive education: A manual for elementary school teachers.* New York: Albert Ellis Institute.
Laurent, J., Catanzaro, S. J., Joiner, T. E., Rudolph, K. D., Potter, K. I., Lambert, S., et al. (1999). A measure of positive and negative affect for children: Scale development and preliminary validation. *Psychological Assessment, 11*, 326–338.
Maxwell, M. A., & Cole, D. A. (2012). Development and initial validation of the adolescent responses to body dissatisfaction measure. *Psychological Assessment, 24*(3), 721–737. https://doi.org/10.1037/a0026785
Pannes, E. (1963). The relationship between self-acceptance and dogmatism in junior-senior high school students. *Journal of Educational Sociology, 36*, 419–426.
Vernon, A. (2002). *What works when with children and adolescents: A handbook of individual counseling techniques.* Champaign, IL: Research Press.
Vernon, A. (2009). *More what works when with children and adolescents: A handbook of individual counseling techniques.* Champaign, IL: Research Press.

Chapter 12
A Rational Emotive, Cognitive Behavioral Approach in Clinical Work with Suicidal and Non-suicidal Self-Injurious Behaviors Among Children and Adolescents

Nora Gerardi and Ennio Ammendola

Overview of Suicide and Self-Harm Behaviors

Suicide can be defined as an intentional and self-directed behavior which results in one's own death (Maris, 2019). Suicide is a leading cause of death worldwide, with an estimated 793,000 suicide death in 2016. These numbers indicate an annual global age-standardized rate of 10.5 individuals for every 100,000 people (World Health Organization [WHO], 2016). In 2017, suicide was the second leading cause of death for persons aged 10–14, 15–19, and 20–24. After a stable period from 2000 to 2007, suicide rates for persons aged 10–24 increased 56% from 2007 to 2017 (Centers for Disease Control and Prevention [CDC], 2017).

Non-suicidal self-injury (NSSI) is understood as being directly linked with suicide (Hollander, 2017). While they are distinct and separate behaviors, NSSI has been shown to elevate risk for suicide (Miller, Rathus, & Linehan, 2007). Throughout this chapter, we discuss NSSI and use the definition provided by the International Society for the Study of Self-Injury (ISSS). The ISSS defines NSSI as the "deliberate destruction of body tissue without suicidal intent and for the purposes not socially or culturally sanctioned" (ISSS, 2018). While NSSI is a separate and distinct behavior from a suicide attempt as it is done without intent to die, NSSI is one of the best predictors of eventual suicide (Miller et al., 2007); that is, risk of suicide increases 50–100 times within the first 12 months after an episode of NSSI, compared to the general population risk (Cooper et al., 2005).

N. Gerardi (✉)
Psychologist at Cognitive & Behavioral Consultants, New York, NY, USA

Queens College, New York, NY, USA

E. Ammendola
Fordham University, New York, NY, USA

M. Bernard, M. D. Terjesen (eds.), *Rational-Emotive and Cognitive-Behavioral Approaches to Child and Adolescent Mental Health: Theory, Practice, Research, Applications*, https://doi.org/10.1007/978-3-030-53901-6_12

NSSI is a term that captures a complex set of human behaviors associated with a wide variety of externalizing and internalizing conditions. There are several models and theories related to NSSI: the medical model, the self-verification theory, the biosocial theory, the addiction model, the experiential avoidance model, and the more recently developed stage model of NSSI (Houston, 2017), which are reviewed in Table 12.1. These theories are essential in clinical practice because they assist in clinical decision-making by considering if the NSSI is a separate diagnostic entity or if it is present also in other clinical conditions.

The prevalence of completed suicides is easier to identify and quantify in objective data as compared to NSSI; that is, NSSI represents a range of behaviors (e.g., cutting, burning, punching oneself) which are more diverse and broad, thus harder to capture accurately and completely. In a recent meta-analysis (Swannell, Martin, Page, Hasking, & St. John, 2014), the estimated prevalence for NSSI among adolescents was 17.2%, 13.4% among young adults 18–25 years old, and 5.5% among adults.

Suicidal behaviors (e.g., suicidal ideation and suicide attempts) and NSSI are associated with a wide range of severe clinical psychiatric diagnoses and other dysfunctional behavioral problems (Vaughn, Salas-Wright, Underwood, & Gochez-Kerr,

Table 12.1 Models and theories related to NSSI

The self-verification theory by Swann (1981)	The author posits that adolescents have a strong desire to confirm and stabilize their firmly held self-views. For example, adolescents who see themselves as unworthy will look for evidence from others that perceive them as unworthy
The biosocial theory by Linehan (1993)	It suggests that borderline personality disorder (BPD) is a disorder of self-regulation and particularly of emotional regulation, which results from biological irregularities combined with specific dysfunctional environments, as well as from their interaction and transaction over time. Adolescents with chronic negative emotions and invalidating environments may engage in NSSI in response to intense negative emotions
The addiction model by Faye (1995)	The author conceptualizes NSSI as an addictive behavior suggesting that the increase in negative emotions before NSSI is analogous to the aversive withdrawal symptoms experienced by drug users. The experiential avoidance model posits that the primary mechanism that maintains the NSSI is the negative reinforcement in the form of escape from or avoidance of unwanted emotional experiences
The stage model of NSSI by Williams and Hasking (2010)	The authors propose that clients experience several stages in their episodes of NSSI, which parallel the development of other addictive behaviors (e.g., development of substance abuse). Stage 0: No self-harm behavior (no NSSI) Stage 1: Experimental NSSI (initial act of NSSI) Stage 2: Exploration (discover physical and mental responses to the NSSI) Stage 3: Encapsulation (NSSI as primary coping) Stage 4: Pervasive dysfunction (persistent NSSI) These stages aim to examine whether coping skills and emotion regulation moderate the relationship between psychological distress and NSSI and how NSSI may be maintained overtime if it effectively regulates emotions, thus becoming addictive in theory

2015). For example, chronic suicidal and NSSI behaviors are a diagnostic criterion for borderline personality disorder (Selby, Bender, Gordon, Nock, & Joiner, 2012). In addition to borderline personality disorder, these behaviors are also comorbid with anxiety and depressive disorders, substance abuse, eating disorders, and post-traumatic stress disorder (Vaughn et al., 2015).

Assessment of Suicide and Self-Harm Behaviors

As suicidality and NSSI exist across a spectrum of symptoms (including thoughts and behaviors), a comprehensive assessment is essential. Given the broad range of disorders with which suicidal behaviors co-occur, mental health practitioners should assess for history or current suicidal behaviors regardless of the reason for referral. There are many behaviors across the suicide spectrum that warrant assessment, including passive and active suicidal ideation, suicide preparation or planning, suicide attempt history, and reasons for living. Research has demonstrated that several variables get in the way of comprehensive risk assessment, including clinician emotions such as fear (Linehan, Comtois, & Ward-Ciesielski, 2012) and skills deficits in conducting an assessment. As such, several structured measures have been developed that provide clear, direct questions to assess a range of suicidal behaviors. Two of these evidence-based structured measures for risk assessment that can be utilized with students are the Columbia Suicide Severity Rating Scale (C-SSRS; Posner et al., 2008) and the Linehan Risk Assessment and Management Protocol (L-RAMP; Linehan, 2009). An overview of these assessment measures is provided below.

Assessment of Suicide

Columbia Suicide Severity Rating Scale (C-SSRS)

The questionnaire provides specific instructions to the assessor, including a series of simple and direct questions. These questions assess three domains of suicidality: (1) suicide ideation, (2) suicide preparatory behaviors, and (3) suicide attempts (Columbia Lighthouse Project, 2016). The C-SSRS is appropriate for use with all ages. Several studies have validated the relevance and effectiveness of the questions used to assess suicide risk, including the how the questions assess the likelihood that someone will make a suicide attempt (Columbia Lighthouse Project, 2016). The measure has also been found to reliably identify who is most at risk for engaging in suicidal behaviors (Columbia Lighthouse Project, 2016). The reader is referred to a summary of the research on the C-SSRS put forth by the Columbia Lighthouse Project, which can be accessed with the following link: http://cssrs.columbia.edu/documents/c-ssrs-supporting-evidence/.

The C-SSRS has many benefits to practitioners, namely, its simple, efficient, and evidence-supported nature. Available in 103 different languages, the scale has been successfully implemented across many settings, including schools, college campuses, military, fire departments, the justice system, primary care, and scientific research. In addition, the C-SSRS is free to use and easily accessible online at https://cssrs.columbia.edu/wp-content/uploads/C-SSRS_Pediatric-SLC_11.14.16.pdf. Practitioners who wish to utilize the C-SSRS are expected to complete a brief training on the utilization of this measure, which is also available free of charge via an online interactive training model.

Linehan Risk Assessment and Management Protocol (L-RAMP)

The L-RAMP (Linehan, 2009; Linehan, 2014) is a structured formal assessment of current suicide risk designed as a treatment form for clinicians to fill out during sessions (Linehan et al., 2012). This form was created for use with adults (Linehan et al., 2012), though may still be a helpful tool for clinicians as the L-RAMP documents both the clinician's risk assessment and interventions provided, those not provided, and the rationale for intervention choices (Linehan et al., 2012).

The L-RAMP outlines acute risk factors and protective factors, based on the literature and research for suicidal behaviors. Following the risk assessment section, the L-RAMP directs the clinician through a series of clinical interventions. If certain options were not chosen or utilized, the protocol prompts clinicians to document their thinking process as related to selection of intervention and procedures. Finally, steps for receiving consultation on the case and follow-up with the client are documented. This structure provides many benefits to the clinician, as it prompts for both assessment and documentation of factors pertinent to suicide risk, as well as a range of intervention options (e.g., conducting a behavioral or chain analysis of the suicidal behavior, using problem-solving strategies, developing a crisis plan).

To use the L-RAMP, training is not required for clinicians who already have formalized

training in risk assessment although Linehan (2009) recommend that clinicians obtain formalized training in suicide risk assessment (e.g., attending a 2-day workshop).The protocol is available for free online and can be accessed with the following link: http://depts.washington.edu/uwbrtc/wp-content/uploads/LSSN-LRAMP-v1.0.pdf.

Assessment of NSSI

Assessment of suicidal behaviors should also include an assessment of NSSI, a behavior which is both separate from suicidality (inherent in its name, there is no suicidal intent) and, at the same time, a potent risk factor for suicidal behaviors (Chesin et al., 2017; Grandclerc, De Labrouhe, Spodenkiewicz, Lachal, & Moro,

2016). When assessing NSSI, practitioners will want to consider assessing the methods, function(s), and severity. Structured and semi-structured measures also exist for the assessment of NSSI; the International Society for the Study of Self-Injury provides a repository of validated and reliable measures of NSSI on its website (the reader is referred to https://itriples.org/category/measures/). One such measure is the Non-Suicidal Self-Injury Assessment Tool (NSSI-AT; Whitlock, Exner-Cortens, & Purington, 2013). This measure was developed and validated with a college-age population (Whitlock et al., 2013), though can be used with youth. The NSSI-AT guides practitioners through a series of questions that assess NSSI characteristics, functions, frequency, age of onset, severity, and practice patterns (Whitlock et al., 2013). The structured nature of this measure allows practitioners to comprehensively assess this complex behavior.

In sum, when working with youth, it is important that practitioners assess suicidality across the spectrum of life-threatening behaviors, including suicidal thinking, preparation or planning, NSSI, and suicide attempts. Structured measures and questionnaires are recommended for the assessment of suicide and NSSI, as both behaviors warrant a careful and comprehensive understanding.

Best Practice Guidelines in Suicide Risk Assessment in School Settings

The National Association of School Psychologists (NASP) offers several resources for school psychologists regarding best practices and guidelines for suicide prevention and intervention. NASP (2015) states that school personnel have both a legal and ethical responsibility to both recognize and respond to student suicidality. NASP (2015) recommends that schools assemble a crisis team comprised of trained staff who can effectively intervene with students at risk for suicidal behavior; members of the team should receive regular (annual) training on the warning signs associated with suicide as well as referral procedures for students who display suicidal thinking and actions. The crisis response team is recommended to develop clear suicide risk assessment, intervention, and postvention (responses after a suicide has occurred) policies and procedures (NASP, 2015). Lieberman, Poland, and Kornfeld (2014) also highlight the importance of assessing for both risk and protective factors (e.g., risk factors including psychological disorders, history/current bullying, history/current NSSI). Further, Lieberman et al. (2014) also stress the importance of actively seeking out and identifying youth at risk for suicide, for example, administering screening tools to students and training school staff to notice imminent warning signs of suicide risk (e.g., suicide threats, plan/method/access to means, sudden changes to mood and behavior). In sum, themes in recommendations for best practices include school staff training, preventive measures to identify students at risk, conducting comprehensive suicide risk assessments, and intervening by notifying parents and referring the student to appropriate and evidence-based treatment (Lieberman et al., 2014; NASP, 2015).

Treatment and Intervention for Suicidal and Self-Harm Behaviors

RE-CBT Treatment and Intervention

The traditional framework of REBT has, since its inception, emphasized the three main psychological aspects of human functioning: thoughts, emotions, and behaviors, with the understanding that these three processes are almost always intertwined and interrelated and that changes in one will often produce changes in the others (DiGiuseppe, Doyle, Dryden, & Backx, 2014). I (EA) propose an integration of REBT with a continual behavioral analysis of suicidal thoughts/behaviors and NSSI present in all phases of the treatment and will provide an overview of the model below in clinical work with youth. Comprehensive outpatient REBT for suicidality and NSSI consists of three modalities of treatment: (1) assessment, (2) intervention, and (3) family sessions.

Assessment

The assessment phase is one of the most critical steps in working with youth who present with NSSI and suicidal behaviors as it promotes the process of making sure to identify the functions and maintaining factors of behaviors across the suicide spectrum. Some of the most commonly cited functions of NSSI include affect regulation, self-punishment, and communication of distress (Klonsky, 2009). Clinicians may wish to consider some of the measures highlighted earlier like the Non-Suicidal Self-Injury Assessment Tool (NSSI-AT).

As the function of behaviors strongly connects to intervention, understanding these are critical and therefore a main goal of assessment. During this phase, the concept expressed by Dryden (1998) of "understanding the person in the context of his problems" (UPCP) is important to consider. This concept states that the strategic assessment and planning process requires not just defining and understanding the problem but also a description of the broader context of the client and his/her problem behaviors (e.g., situations in which the person is more likely to engage in NSSI). In applying this concept to working with clients who engage in NSSI, I refer to it as the "understanding the person in the context of his/her NSSI" (UPCN). Table 12.2 presents the application of the UPCN with a student who engages in NSSI; clinicians may use this as a guide to assist in case conceptualization and treatment planning.

Table 12.2 Important considerations in assessment of NSSI within the UPCN model

Assessment step	Description	Sample questions
Type(s) of NSSI client reports	Gathering specific information about the NSSI	What do you use when you self-harm? Describe what this behavior looks like for you. *The clinician is encouraged to evaluate if the client engages in common forms of NSSI such as cutting and burning. The clinician should ask for specific methods utilized (e.g., NSSI using a shaving razor). The clinician should evaluate all historical NSSI methods, as well as the most commonly used current method*
NSSI history	Recalling the client's initial event, frequency, and intensity of NSSI	When was the first time you engaged in NSSI? What do you remember about this first time? How often do you currently engage in NSSI?
NSSI relationship	Evaluating how the client perceives their relationship to the NSSI.	How does NSSI work for you or help you? What do you feel after you engage in NSSI?
NSSI risk factors	Evaluating personal affective, behavioral, and contextual variables that put the client at greater risk for NSSI	What triggers make you engage in NSSI? What are the times you are at greater risk? What emotions do you typically feel before you engage in NSSI? Are there specific places where you are more likely to engage in NSSI (e.g., at home and in your room)?
NSSI premonitory urges	Discussing awareness of warning signs prior to engaging in NSSI	What happens/what do you experience right up until the point that you cannot resist the urge to NSSI? What do you notice in your body before you engage in NSSI?
NSSI protective factors	Evaluating personal affective, behavioral, and contextual variables that reduce risk for NSSI	When do you feel content, without thoughts or urges related to NSSI?
NSSI coping skills	Recalling strategies that the client has used to manage/deal with the urge to engage in NSSI	What have you done so far to help yourself manage the urge to engage in NSSI? Do you engage in any other activities instead? Can you recall a time when you had the urge to engage in NSSI and did not act on the urge? What do you remember about this time?
NSSI contextual A	Evaluating contextual triggers prior to NSSI that the client may perceive activated them to engage in NSSI behavior	If being alone in your room is a risk factor for you, what is stopping you from leaving your room?
NSSI past A	Reviewing past activating events from previous NSSI episodes	What did trigger you in the past to engage in these behaviors?

(continued)

Table 12.2 (continued)

Assessment step	Description	Sample questions
NSSI recent A	Reviewing activating events that are not imminent NSSI risk factors but are still freshly remembered by the client	Can you recall a recent incident/trigger that you then ended up doing the behavior? What has lately triggered you that you still remember?
NSSI present A	Discussing the activating event at the center of the client's attention in our current session	What was it about that incident that you were most upset/disturbed about?
NSSI immediate A	Discussing the A that puts the client at high risk of a new episode of NSSI	What has to happen for you to go immediately to NSSI?
NSSI contextual C	Evaluating affective state the client feels *after* engaging in NSSI behavior	How does your body feel when you engage in NSSI?
NSSI contextual IB	Identifying irrational beliefs (IBs) that may lead to the client engaging in NSSI behavior	What thoughts do you have/what are you telling yourself when you engage in NSSI?
NSSI contextual RB	Identifying rational beliefs (RBs) that may lead to the client managing their urge to engage in NSSI behavior	When you feel the urge to engage in NSSI, but you do not, what are you telling yourself to stop from harming yourself?

While Table 12.2 offers guidance for gathering the contextual history as well as affective states associated with NSSI, I think it is important to briefly elaborate on the role of beliefs and why they also are integral to client history of NSSI. As discussed elsewhere in this edited volume, irrational beliefs (IBs) are thoughts that are rigidly held and may often present themselves in terms of "musts/shoulds." They tend to be inflexible, inconsistent with reality, and illogical and interfere with the adolescent's psychological well-being (e.g., "I can't stand feeling this way! I have to control my emotions"). As an alternative, rational beliefs (RBs) are considered to be more flexible in nature and often present themselves in the form of preferences. These thoughts tend to be consistent with reality and logical and promote the adolescent's psychological well-being (Dryden, 1996). An example would be thinking "This is uncomfortable and I do not like feeling this way and *want* this discomfort to go away, but I do not have to cut myself to feel better." Ellis (1994) argued that the irrational, dogmatic musts are at the very core of emotional disturbances, while nondogmatic preferences are at the very core of psychological health. As such, clinicians will want to assess for the presence of both of these types of beliefs and use the assessment phase to understand if either IBs or RBs are key links preceding NSSI urges or behaviors.

Lastly, a crucial step in completing the assessment is identifying any activating events or triggers related to NSSI. This is the antecedent or "A" in the REBT ABC model (DiGiuseppe et al., 2014), and there may be several antecedents related to NSSI. In adapting Shea's (2002) work on suicide assessment, I (EA) have reframed the A in the ABC proposed by REBT with respect to four major components of the client's suicidality, which are described in Table 12.2: the past A (activating event from previous NSSI), the recent A (activating events that are not imminent risk factors but are still freshly remembered by the client), the present A (activating event at the center of the client's attention in our current session), and finally, the immediate A (the A that puts the client at high risk of NSSI).

Discussion of application of these assessment steps will be presented in further detail in the case study.

Intervention

A nine-step REBT treatment sequence in conducting clinical work using the information gained during the UPCN phase is presented in Table 12.3. This model incorporates that information with some modifications to the REBT model. A few noteworthy clinical considerations are outlined below.

In step 2 (orientation to REBT Model as it relates the NSSI), the clinician may consider whether to use a B-C or A-C model. In the B-C language, which is more consistent with the traditional REBT model, clients understand that it is their beliefs/thoughts that are responsible for how they feel; alternatively, in the A-C language, clients believe that the event or stressor that they have experienced is what is responsible for how they feel. In a proposed modification of the REBT model, clients who engage in NSSI may not have awareness of their thoughts and beliefs and as such may benefit initially from an A-C model. That is, the A-C model may be more effective when clients are unable to identify an explicit irrational belief (IB) that is related to their engagement in NSSI. For example, a client might communicate to the clinician: "This happened to me...and I *felt/did* this" (A-C), instead of "Something happened to me...I was *thinking*...then I felt/did this" (B-C). When there is an absence of such statements related to thoughts, the A-C model may be a better fit. Clients who engage in NSSI tend to provide initial narratives in A-C terms (without thoughts) because they think that the critical A leads them to directly engage in NSSI. That is, some clients are mostly event-driven ("It is about what happened to me") and not thought-driven ("I keep telling myself I cannot stand my life"). Therefore, B's role may be underemphasized at the beginning, while A is overengaged. The emphasis on A is why initially it may be more productive to focus on the A-C connection to stabilize the NSSI episodes and then introduce the B-C connection later in the treatment.

Table 12.3 The nine-step REBT treatment sequence during the UPCN

Step 1 Problem identification	Completing the FBA; identifying the NSSI as the main presenting problem; educating the client about the nature of the NSSI (e.g., hypothesized function[s] of NSSI such as emotion regulation). *Do you want to work on reducing NSSI?*
Step 2 Orientation to REBT model as it relates the NSSI	Educating the client to the ABC (activating event-belief-consequence) model or the ABBC model (activating event/bypassing the beliefs/emotional and behavioral consequences) of NSSI. ABC: *Over the next few sessions, you will learn how to identify an activating event in the presence of the NSSI that characterizes your environment, how you feel about that activating event, and what thoughts you hold in the face of the NSSI. You will also learn to generate a functional equivalent to those thoughts.* ABBC: *Over the next few sessions, you will learn how to identify an activating event in the presence of the NSSI that characterizes your environment and how you feel about that activating event. Later in therapy, you will learn a new way to help yourself, called the B-C connection, which will help you to identify what thoughts you hold in the face of the NSSI make you feel in a certain way. You will also learn to generate a functional equivalent to those thoughts*
Step 3 Assessment of functional impairment	Identifying the emotional and behavioral consequences and evaluating them in terms of their degree of functional impairment. *Tell me about what happens after you engage in NSSI. What do you feel? What happens afterward?*
Step 4 Clarifying beliefs related to NSSI behaviors	Assessment of client's IBs (demandingness, awfulizing, frustration intolerance, self-condemnation, and other condemnation) that may lead to NSSI. Clarifying questions at this point of the treatment are "were you aware of any thoughts in your mind about NSSI?" "are you aware now, with me, of what you thought when you wanted to engage in NSSI?"
Step 5 Making the belief-consequence connection	Reinforcing to clients the connection between their IBs and emotional and behavioral consequences (C). Clarifying questions may be "What are you telling yourself at B to feel depressed and thus engage in NSSI?"
Step 6 Challenging and disputing the client IBs	Work with client to examine and challenge the IBs from a logical ("does thinking this way make sense?"), functional ("how does thinking this way help you?"), empirical ("what do we know about this thought?"), and semantic perspective ("you say this is *terrible*, let's look at the literal meaning of the word")
Step 7 Strengthening the rational beliefs (RBs)	Clinician works with clients to practice and strengthen their RBs as the healthy/adaptive alternative to their IBs. An example would be *This is tough; I have stood this before but clearly don't like it. It won't be easy but I don't have to cut myself. I can deal with the discomfort*
Step 8 Putting it all together	Clinician works with clients on implementing concepts/skills learned into practice. Involves generating a crisis response plan (identify emotional crisis, list of problem-solving tools, identify social support) with specific instructions for what to do during periods of crisis *When you feel depressed, remember to evaluate your thought, take a break, and reach out to a friend*

(continued)

Table 12.3 (continued)

Step 9 Long-term planning	Emphasizing to clients that the new learning will lead to profound affective, behavioral, and philosophical changes in their lives by adapting this healthier belief system. *When your conviction in the healthier belief system is high enough, you will start acting in ways aligned with those beliefs. You will tolerate feeling depressed, even though it is hard, without engaging in NSSI*

Second, to promote the difference between the B-C and the A-C language, I propose that an ABBC model in certain clinical cases may be more effective. In the ABBC model, A stands for an activating event, BB stands for bypassing the belief (still implicit) about that event, and C stands for the consequences (emotional or behavioral) of holding the implicit belief B. It is suggested that when clients are at a highly aroused affective state and at considerable risk for NSSI, clinicians may wish to initially bypass any resistance at the B level by prioritizing the A-C connection in session and, only later, go back to the B-C connection when the clients become able to focus on their cognitive patterns. For example, the clinician could say, "I am interested in what you were thinking and telling yourself when you made yourself feel so angry, but I can see that you are so emotionally upset that we are going to come back to your thoughts at a later point. For now, I would like to understand what happened to you that made you feel like this."

A common error that we have seen beginning clinicians make in the application of REBT is that they think that clients will "feel better" simply by challenging/disputing their irrational beliefs. We argue that it is just as important to strengthen the rational belief that is a direct alternative to the irrational one. That is, instead of thinking "I can't stand this. It is too much to handle and the only way my stress will go away is to engage in NSSI!," we would work with clients to believe more healthy, adaptive beliefs that are the alternative to the irrational type of belief such as "This is tough; I have stood this before but clearly don't like it. It won't be easy but I don't have to do cut myself. I can deal with the discomfort." At times, clients may fail to distinguish between the more flexible rational belief and the rigid irrational one. As stressed by DiGiuseppe, Leaf, Exner, and Robin (1988), it is important to highlight the importance of building up rational preferences, while also challenging/weakening the irrational belief that is causing emotional disturbance and having the client engage in NSSI.

Family Sessions

Family support is crucial during the REBT treatment course for youth engaging in NSSI, as well as with maintaining treatment gains. Tatnell, Kelada, Hasking, and Martin (2014) found that the level of perceived family support was significantly associated with stopping NSSI. Within an REBT framework, the clients' perception of family support is likely to promote positive interactions, feelings of security, and a sense of connectedness that enhance adaptive functioning and more competencies in becoming aware of their ABCs or ABBCs when at risk of NSSI.

Family members are crucial in the process of the functional behavior assessment because the function of the NSSI is defined by the context, and family members become instrumental in identifying areas to work on in session such as communication, behavioral, and emotional reactions to the NSSI behaviors. Parents learn to identify their child's perceived alienation, criticism, and disconnectedness from others or themselves as playing a major role in perpetuating NSSI.

Lastly, REBT provides parents, caregivers, or other family members with an educational framework to address the adolescents' emotions related to the NSSI and then assist them with problem-solving and skill building to target the dysfunctional interactions. Parents learn that NSSI is only the tip of the iceberg, and so they learn to understand NSSI as a way of coping with stressful thoughts and emotions. Consequently, parents model strategies for expressing and managing strong emotions.

DBT Treatment and Intervention for Suicidality Among Youth

DBT was initially developed by Marsha Linehan for the treatment of high-risk, chronically suicidal adult women diagnosed with borderline personality disorder (BPD; Linehan, 1993; Linehan, Armstrong, Suarez, Allmon, & Heard, 1991). DBT is an evidence-based treatment that blends standard cognitive behavioral approaches with Eastern philosophy and meditation-based practices (Heard & Linehan, 1994).

Comprehensive outpatient DBT includes four modes of treatment: (1) individual therapy, (2) skills training, (3) phone coaching, and (4) consultation team. An overview of these modes is provided below as it relates to working with youth who engage in comprehensive DBT.

Individual Therapy In DBT, therapists and clients agree to work on goals together as a team, both putting forth their best efforts to make treatment as effective as possible. Targets in individual therapy are organized within a target hierarchy that includes life-threatening behaviors, therapy-interfering behaviors, and quality-of-life interfering behaviors (Linehan, 1993). Targets are attended to in this order, such that the therapy goals are first to reduce suicide and self-harm behaviors, keeping the client safe, alive, and committed to building a life worth living. Individual therapy typically occurs once a week. As clinically indicated, the individual therapist may conduct family sessions with the client.

Skills Training DBT skills training is conducted in a group format, typically for 2–2.5 hours once a week. The standard length of skills training is approximately 7 months. Groups are led by both a leader and co-leader, who teach skills in the domains of mindfulness, distress tolerance, emotion regulation, and interpersonal effectiveness (Linehan, 1993; Rathus & Miller, 2014). Each skills group begins with a mindfulness exercise, followed by review of skills practice/assigned homework for the first half. The second half of the group is didactic in nature, teaching the new skills content.

Phone Coaching All clients in DBT are provided with phone coaching, meaning that the client's individual therapist is on call 24/7 to help manage crisis behaviors, skills generalization, and repairs to the therapeutic relationship. While 24/7 phone coaching was developed as part of the initial comprehensive DBT protocol, this modality may be modified in settings such as schools. The school setting inherently provides an opportunity for in-the-moment coaching for students in distress. School-based DBT practitioners may "coach" students to use their DBT skills in situations that arise during the school day and are not available to be reached 24/7 by phone.

Consultation Team All DBT therapists sit on a consultation team that meets weekly. This mode of treatment is sometimes thought of as "therapy for the therapists." DBT therapists add themselves to the consultation team agenda to request help with applying DBT principles and strategies.

DBT-A (Rathus & Miller, 2014) modifies skills training such that both adolescents and their parents attend a multifamily skills group (MFSG) together. A fifth module (see Developmental Considerations section) titled "walking the middle path" is added to DBT-A skills training. Parents who participate in the MFSG also receive a coach, available for coaching for skills generalization 24/7. The parent coach is one of the group skills trainers. Family therapy and specialized parenting may also be incorporated into a client's treatment as clinically indicated.

Research on RE-CBT and DBT for Suicide and Self-Harm

Research on RE-CBT for NSSI

Despite the magnitude of suicide and NSSI as worldwide phenomena, there is still a gap in the research between what is known about suicide and RE-CBT as an effective preventive measure in reducing these behaviors. The RE-CBT tradition focuses on cognitive assessment and cognitive intervention. Some application of RE-CBT with NSSI has been described in terms of manualized CBT interventions. Taylor and colleagues (Taylor, Oldershaw, Richards, & Davidson, 2011) developed one of these manualized CBT interventions to treat adolescents called "cutting down" which includes cognitive behavioral assessment, motivational strategies, and coping skills. The results showed following completion of the 8–12-week program a reduction of the NSSI not only at the end of the treatment but also at a 3-month follow-up.

Lately, particular attention in the treatment of RE-CBT for NSSI has been devoted to the crucial importance of the family component. An example of this approach is the integrated CBT (I-CBT) composed of individual CBT sessions, family CBT, and parent training sessions. Esposito-Smythers, Spirito, Kahler, Hurt, and Monti (2011) showed that a CBT treatment program delivered to 40 adolescents with a history of a suicide attempt or severe suicidal ideation and a substance use disorder reduced the number of rehospitalizations and emergency department (ED) visits over the 18-month study period in comparison to those who had treatment as usual (TAU). While NSSI behaviors were not the main target of this study, nearly three-quarters of the adolescents experienced reductions in other challenging behaviors directly related to NSSI.

Research on the Effectiveness of DBT Among Youth Presenting with Suicidality

Much of the early research on DBT was conducted for the comprehensive model used with adults, with the first randomized controlled trial (RCT) of DBT published in 1991. In this trial, Dr. Linehan and her colleagues found that DBT resulted in significant improvements for chronically suicidal and self-injuring women with BPD (Linehan et al., 1991). Since this first RCT, several additional research studies have also demonstrated the effectiveness of DBT for BPD, suicide, and self-harm in adults (e.g., Carter, Willcox, Lewin, Conrad, & Bendit, 2010; Linehan et al., 2015).

In 1995, Miller and Rathus began adopting and adapting Linehan's adult treatment protocol for adolescents. Over the past 20 years, DBT with suicidal and multiproblem adolescents has been found to be more effective than treatment as usual, CBT, and supportive and psychodynamic psychotherapies (McCauley et al., 2018; Mehlum et al., 2014; Miller, Rathus, Linehan, et al., 1997; Miller et al., 2007; Rathus & Miller, 2002). In a randomized controlled trial comparing DBT for adolescents to an enhanced usual care (EUC) condition, Mehlum et al. (2014) found that adolescents receiving DBT had a significant reduction in the number of NSSI episodes as well as a decline in suicidal ideation. At a 3-year follow-up, Mehlum et al. (2019) found that adolescents who engaged in DBT had maintained a reduction in the frequency of NSSI as compared to adolescents who received EUC. Researchers found that a substantial proportion of the effect of DBT on NSSI frequency over the long term was mediated through a reduction in adolescents' experience of hopelessness (Mehlum et al., 2019).

In addition to being adapted for adolescents, DBT has also been applied to preadolescent children with disruptive mood dysregulation disorder (DMDD), a disorder characterized by persistent irritability and behavior outbursts (Perepletchikova et al., 2017). Preliminary outcomes have demonstrated initial acceptability, feasibility, and efficacy of the adapted DBT skills for this population with DMDD (Perepletchikova et al., 2011).

In sum, research has demonstrated the effectiveness of DBT for ages across the life span, and the treatment has also evolved into a more trans-diagnostic treatment by applying the same underlying treatment principles across many different mental health disorders including depression, bipolar disorder, substance use, disordered eating, ADHD, and those with inattention and/or impulse control problems, school refusal problems, and interpersonal difficulties (Miller et al., 2007; Ritschel, Miller, & Taylor, 2013).

Developmental Considerations in Applying RE-CBT and DBT

RE-CBT Considerations

Within its model, RE-CBT posits that rigidity is at the core of psychological disturbance, while flexibility is at the core of psychological health (Dryden, 2009). Therefore, when working with children and adolescents, it is essential to address their innate rigid and irrational thinking. As reported by Bernard (2008, p. 8):

> What moderates the influence of irrationality is the development of rationality and logical reasoning abilities which emerge around the age of six (Piaget's concrete operational stage of development) with abstract reasoning abilities developing more fully around the age of 12 (formal operational stage of development).

As such, irrational beliefs are developmentally expected, and children's irrational beliefs (IBs) are seen with themes related to demandingness, awfulizing, frustration intolerance, self-condemnation, and other condemnation. The identification of IBs among children can be achieved during verbal discussions with the clinician or through utilizing games and vignettes developed to explain to children the variety of IBs, emotions, and behaviors. In addition to some identifying IBs, the RE-CBT clinician may encounter additional challenges when working with children, including (1) finding effective forms of cognitive disputing and (2) generating flexible alternative thoughts. These two challenges are addressed below.

RE-CBT clinicians may find benefit from creative disputing strategies, which will ultimately aid in generating flexible and adaptive thoughts. One such strategy is to help children use the best friend scenario, which minimizes most of the logical complications of the technique of disputation. That is, the RE-CBT clinician would discuss a friend figure who endorses a flexible alternative belief to the child's irrational thought. The goal is to help the child understand that the friend has different emotional experiences as a result of a more healthy and adaptive thought. For example, a child may have a negative thought in response to being left out of a social activity such as "No one wants to be my friend." In response, the clinician may discuss a friend figure who interprets being left out with the thought "They did not want to play with me today." The RE-CBT clinician would use such an example to help the child dispute their rigid or irrational thoughts.

Second, RE-CBT clinicians may face challenges in helping children generate a flexible alternative to their unhealthy thoughts. Developing more flexible alternative beliefs is traditionally done through self-discovery and Socratic questioning, though may not be the most effective strategy with some children. The clinician may use a more didactic style and explicitly offer up examples of healthier ways to consider a situation. RE-CBT clinicians may also utilize the "elegant solution" when working with children; this technique involves accepting irrational beliefs as true rather than disputing or reevaluating the problem. That is, rather than challenging or reevaluating the presenting belief (e.g., by asking questions such as "Did she really reject you? How do you know?"), RE-CBT clinicians work with clients to accept this inference as true/accurate and then look at their evaluation (e.g., "You're right, she rejected you and may not want to be your friend"). This technique helps children to understand the benefits of giving up their unhealthy beliefs, though again, the RE-CBT clinician may need to be more directive in highlighting the problems associated with sticking with the irrational belief.

DBT Considerations

Developmental considerations in applying DBT with children and adolescents largely focus on involving the child's environment directly with children, including their parents. Within the DBT framework, Linehan (1993) identified four characteristic problem areas that were often found among these multiproblem clients: confusion about self, impulsivity, emotional dysregulation, and interpersonal problems. In their work with adolescents and families, Miller et al. (2007) identified a fifth problem area, adolescent-family challenges, characterized by non-dialectical thinking (e.g., black-and-white, all-or-nothing, and inflexible thinking), invalidation (e.g., dismissing, trivializing, and/or minimizing one's emotional experiences, thoughts, and behaviors), and the ineffective application of behavioral principles (e.g., positive reinforcement, extinction, punishment) with one another. This fifth module equally applies to youth interacting with others outside of their families as well, such as school personnel, peers, coaches, and therapists. Rathus and Miller (2002) incorporate parents into a skills training group, such that they receive direct didactic instruction as well, learning the language of DBT. Treatment targets also focus on developmental themes, such as the balance between adolescent strivings for self-determination and parental need for monitoring and discipline, and issues regarding individuation versus dependence on the family (Rathus & Miller, 2002).

Adaptations of RE-CBT and DBT in Schools

Re-CBT

The theory of RE-CBT asserts that unhealthy patterns of thinking (either Beckian automatic thoughts or the IBs of REBT) precede the emotions associated with life-threatening behaviors such as NSSI. Therefore, the professionals working with students would benefit from incorporating cognitive conceptualizations by attempting to challenge and change the students' cognitions directly. As with adults, RE-CBT hypothesizes that children's disturbed emotions are largely generated by their beliefs (Ellis, 1995). The main aim of working with students in schools is to be able to help them identify the cognitive errors that students make and to link them to their emotions. Schools may be the most natural context in which this can occur as any school-specific thoughts are readily accessible and may be more likely to be recalled rather than in a clinician's office a number of days later.

As discussed earlier, RE-CBT clinicians must keep in mind developmental considerations related to identifying and disputing irrational beliefs. Therefore, school-based clinician should consider what approach of disputation to choose to promote cognitive change. DiGiuseppe (1981) pioneered the idea that empirical disputation (e.g., "Where is the evidence that…?") may be an easier and more developmentally appropriate form of disputing irrational beliefs than logical disputing (e.g., "Just because you think…does it follow that…?). School-based clinicians should therefore consider helping students use empirical questions that help students identify evidence for or against irrational thoughts and beliefs. Within a RE-CBT framework, it is also important to implement adaptations that promote behavioral and family system conceptualization (DiGiuseppe & Bernard, 2006). When possible in the school setting, it would be helpful to see the students with their parent(s) together in therapy for the parent(s) to learn how to support the maintenance of the child's rational beliefs.

Another essential adaptation in working in the school is to pay attention to students' developing capacity for emotional regulation, which is in line with some additional CBT-based theories such as DBT. Rational emotive education (REE), the educational derivative of REBT (Knaus, 1974; Vernon, 1989), has been developed to teach young people emotional problem-solving and emotional regulation and is discussed at length in Chap. 20. Finally, another important consideration is the implementation of group therapy when working with children and adolescents. Terjesen and Esposito (2006) described several advantages of using group therapy in the school, and one of the most important is the ability for the students to focus on their thoughts, feelings, and behaviors to help each other change their cognitions, emotions, and actions.

DBT in Schools

Comprehensive school-based DBT (CSB-DBT) was originally designed to target middle to high school-aged students with difficulties with emotion dysregulation (Miller et al., 2007; Rathus & Miller, 2014) and has since been modified for elementary school-aged children. CSB-DBT is defined as having all four modes of DBT in schools: weekly skills group, weekly individual counseling, in-school coaching as needed, and DBT service provider consultation team. These four modes are designed to fulfill the five functions of DBT: (1) acquiring new behavioral skills; (2) increasing student's motivation; (3) generalizing skills to all facets of the student's environment (classroom, lunchroom, home, peers); (4) increasing, motivating, and improving the skills of DBT providers; and (5) structuring the student's environment so that the student can receive comprehensive DBT within the school, which includes protecting time for the student to attend the various modes of DBT as well as possibly engaging caregivers in the DBT experience.

Within the school setting, staff may modify modes of DBT to meet both the needs of students as well as unique barriers (e.g., time, resources) present within a school setting. For example, skills groups may be reduced in terms of duration. While the standard outpatient model holds multifamily skills groups for 2 hours (Rathus & Miller, 2014), groups held within schools may modify content to accommodate 30-, 45-, or 60-minute sessions. Similarly, the length of individual counseling sessions may be modified. DBT clinicians in outpatient therapy directly target life-threatening behaviors (e.g., suicide, self-harm); school-based DBT providers are encouraged to work with their administration and school guidelines in terms of assessment and intervention with suicidal behaviors. That is, school-based DBT providers may be required to follow certain protocols (e.g., notifying parents of risk, using emergency interventions such as calling 911) in a more scripted, protocol-based manner as compared to outpatient providers. School-based providers are encouraged to refer to best practices in suicide risk assessment, as outlined by the National Association of School Psychologists (NASP; see section above). Coaching is also modified to fit the school setting, with teachers, paraprofessionals, and administrators often jumping in to help support students generalize skills during moments of distress throughout the school day. Another difference is the fact that school-based DBT providers are not on call for 24/7 coaching. School-based DBT teams and providers are encouraged to adhere closely to the DBT model, while also making needed changes to translate this evidence-based practice into practice-based evidence.

Case Study

Sarah (name has been changed to protect confidentiality) is a 15-year-old, single female in the tenth grade who was referred for outpatient REBT following her discharge from an inpatient hospitalization. She was hospitalized for 12 days following a suicide attempt in which she overdosed on her mother's prescribed medication. While hospitalized, Sarah was diagnosed with borderline personality disorder. The diagnosis was also informed by Sarah's difficulties with emotion regulation, all-or-nothing thinking with regard to relationships, and sense of emptiness.

Upon her discharge, Sarah was scheduled to see the outpatient REBT therapist for an initial visit and consultation. While her chief complaint was depression at this first visit, she was not able to identify factors contributing to her low mood. Historically, it was reported that Sarah has seen several psychiatrists for pharmacotherapy, though at times, she was not compliant with her medications and ultimately stopped attending the appointments. Additionally, she had been in several psychotherapy treatments before initiating REBT clinical work. Sarah reported experiencing a sense of rejection and abandonment while working with these previous mental health professionals. Sarah stated that when she was taking her medication (Lexapro) regularly, she engaged in fewer NSSI behaviors and experienced more control over her suicidal thoughts. At the beginning of the intake, Sarah reported that she felt anxious about sharing the patterns of her NSSI, though after initial resistance she was able to describe her NSSI as superficial cuts on her forearms or on her legs and that she only does this when she is in the shower using a shaving razor. She reported being able to stop the bleeding from self-harm easily, denying ever needing medical attention for these wounds. Sarah reported that she also has a history of using sharp pins to engage in NSSI, stating that she could "easily hide them." She stated that NSSI helped her to "feel that she was alive" and that NSSI was the only way she could exert control over the intensity of her emotions. At present, Sarah reported more urges to engage in NSSI when alone.

In looking at the context of her behavior, the REBT clinician identified several vulnerability factors and prompting events that led to engaging in NSSI. That is, Sarah engaged in NSSI only in the evening hours when thinking about her depression and how "miserable" her day was. In these moments, she was very self-critical, and her negative thoughts led her to contemplate engaging in NSSI. She also reported that she found cutting in the evening hours more rewarding because she was able to enjoy anticipatory fantasies about that moment earlier in the day. Sarah reported that engaging in NSSI led to both a feeling of excitement and a sense of relief. Given this information obtained in the assessment, it was clear that NSSI primarily served an emotion regulation function.

In working with Sarah, the REBT conceptual framework was based on three key elements: assessment with "understanding the person in the context of her NSSI" (UPCN)," intervention, and, finally, family sessions. Below, the stages of REBT assessment and intervention utilized during Sarah's course of treatment are described.

Assessment Prior to formal assessment, the therapist focused on building a strong therapeutic alliance. This was addressed by defining and agreeing upon the target behaviors/goals and the tasks to achieve these goals and by fostering a purposeful collaborative relationship for clinical care to ensure that she has a degree of confidence in her ability to carry out the treatment strategies.

One of the most crucial aspects of the assessment phase is to identify the primary function(s) of the NSSI, as knowing the function ultimately informs the maintaining mechanisms. Based on assessment with Sarah, NSSI appeared to serve an emotion regulation function and was maintained by removal of negative emotions (negative reinforcement) and increase in positive emotions (positive reinforcement). In order to assess and understand the function(s) of NSSI, clinical work focused on having Sarah recall the latest episode of her NSSI and examine the context (antecedent and consequence) of the NSSI urge and behavior. During this assessment, Sarah reported: "I feel I am alive, and this is the only time I am in control. When I start feeling overwhelmed, I then feel the urge to use the push pin to cut."

The information gathered during the assessment phase was finally integrated into a more in-depth analysis of the NSSI through the use of the UPCN model. The overall conceptualization is of a 15-year-old female client, with limited social relationships, who reports a depressed mood much of the day on most days. She engages in NSSI when alone, during evening hours, and in the context of some emotional dysregulation. She reported that she is looking for a way to be "in control," as she views her NSSI behavior as a coping mechanism for dealing with stress. From an REBT framework, her primary irrational beliefs appeared to be "I don't feel good about myself. I cannot stand living my life like this."

Intervention During the course of clinical work, based on the information gained during the UPCN phase, an REBT treatment sequence consisting of the previously reviewed nine steps (see Table 12.3) was used and is briefly outlined below.

Step 1: Problem Identification This step focuses on gathering additional information about SI, behaviors, and attempts as well as the context for when she experiences the urge to engage in NSSI behaviors. Sarah reported that she knows that something is "building up inside her" and then suddenly feels so overwhelmed with emotions that she has the urge to cut. Problems that were collaboratively agreed upon to be targets of treatment were to provide her with skills to address her depression, reduce isolation, and increase healthy coping strategies aligned with mood regulation.

Step 2: Orientation to REBT Model as It Relates to NSSI This step begins with an introduction to the ABC model of NSSI and assessing Sarah's four major components of her A: past A ("Arguing with my mother"), recent A ("Fighting with a classmate"), present A ("Being by myself in the room"), and immediate A ("I am looking at the push pin on my desk").

Step 3: Assessment of Functional Impairment This step involves clarifying emotional C (depression) and behavioral C (isolation). Sarah reported that these functionally impacted her by reducing meaningful relationships with others, physical inactivity, and lack of personal care. Within the REBT framework, clinicians often look for a secondary emotional disturbance, referred to as a meta-emotional problem, where they may get upset about being upset (DiGiuseppe et al., 2014). It is suggested that the clinician does not investigate at this step any of Sarah's meta-emotional problems because Sarah's overwhelming emotional dysregulation may not allow her to effectively manage the presence of two emotions at the same time. It may be important to ask later in the session, "How do you feel about feeling depressed?"

Step 4: Clarifying Beliefs Related to NSSI Behavior In this step, clinical work is now focused on identifying and assessing Sarah's irrational beliefs. In response to the question: "What were you telling yourself about being by yourself in the room to make yourself feeling depressed and wanting to engage in cutting yourself?"

Sarah reported: "I do not feel good about myself. I cannot stand living my life like this."

Step 5: Making the Belief-Consequence Connection In an effort for Sarah's IBs to be connected with her emotional C and behavioral C, Sarah was asked: "Can you understand that as long as you tell yourself, 'I do not feel good about myself. I cannot stand living my life like this,' you are destined to make yourself feeling depressed and engage in cutting yourself?" While Sarah reported that she understood that idea "in theory," she reported that she thought this would be difficult to truly believe. As such, the clinician continued to reinforce these connections through a number of examples related and unrelated to her B-C connection. The clinician also stressed that a degree of flexibility in her beliefs was at the core of her psychological health. After listening to the examples and at the clinician's invitation to be more aware of her beliefs, Sarah stated: "I guess I need to pay more attention to what I tell myself when I make myself feeling depressed."

Step 6: Challenging and Disputing the Clients IBs Treatment now focused on disputing Sarah's irrational beliefs. While a number of the more traditional disputes reviewed in Table 12.2 were applied, the ones that resonated best with Sarah were the empirical ("Where is the evidence that you *cannot handle* the stress and *must* do the NSSI?") and the functional ("How is it helping you reach your goals of not doing the NSSI behaviors by thinking that way?").

Step 7: Strengthening the Rational Beliefs (RBs) The clinician now helps Sarah to generate a rational alternative RB to her IB. Examples of rational beliefs were "I know it is difficult but I *can handle this*. While I may have the desire to cut myself, I *do not have to*!" These beliefs were collaboratively developed and also were challenged to see how well Sarah could hold onto these beliefs.

Step 8: Putting It All Together This step ensures Sarah can differentiate her unhealthy irrational beliefs from the healthy, realistic rational beliefs. Sarah was asked: "What do you think you'll have to do in order to understand the difference between your thoughts?" She replied: "I do not feel good about myself. I cannot stand living my life like this," and "I would prefer to feel good about myself, but life does not have to be the way I want all the time. I can tolerate it, and it is worth it to me to do so because I do not want to be overly affected about cutting myself." Efforts were made to have her affectively, behaviorally, and cognitively apply her new beliefs and manage her impulses to engage in NSSI behaviors. We developed a crisis intervention plan to help her work toward regulating her affective states and also seeking out support when needed.

Step 9: Long-Term Planning The clinician reinforces the value of implementing everything that was discussed in the sessions. The clinician and Sarah collaboratively worked on setting short-term (complete an ABC self-help form anytime she feels depressed) and long-term goals (reinforce the B-C connection, reduce self-cutting by focusing on alternative activities, and tolerate the urge of wanting to cut herself by asking her parents for emotional support). The most crucial aspect of REBT at this point is to have Sarah PRACTICE the rational belief through as many modalities as possible.

Family Sessions At the beginning of the treatment, Sarah was resistant to the idea of having her family involved. She was afraid that the clinician was going to ally with her parents against her. After several months of individual therapy, the clinician and Sarah had a strong rapport, and she developed trust with the clinician. Sarah then agreed to the involvement of her parents in treatment, acknowledging their role in helping to support treatment gains.

The first component of parent involvement involved providing them with an understanding of some of the core REBT principles to assist with. It was important for the clinician to make sure that Sarah's parents were able to understand her difficulties in terms of the B-C connection. The second part of the family work focused on the understanding of the potential roles they may have in activating and maintaining Sarah's negative beliefs and problem behaviors. Sarah's parents were educated about the natural tendency to inadvertently reinforce and strengthen some of their daughter's challenging behaviors, for example, overly attending to higher levels of distress, while ignoring Sarah's lower-level communication of being upset. Her parents were therefore taught how to thoughtfully give Sarah more emotional space, while also attending to and acknowledging her more skillful communication of her distress.

Summary and Conclusion

Behaviors along the suicide and self-harm spectrums are growing in prevalence among youth, and it can be argued that it is inevitable that school-based mental health staff will work with youth presenting with these behaviors. Comprehensive assessment is needed to best understand students' current and history of SI/NSSI, with a focus being on the function of these behaviors. There are several structured assessment tools that aid in comprehensive assessment, many of which are free to access and utilize. Both REBT and DBT have an evidence base for treating youth exhibiting SI/NSSI. This chapter provided examples of how these interventions can be modified for the school setting; while the research on modifying these treatments for school settings is limited and ongoing, clinical practice and insight suggest that they are promising for school staff in their interventions for youth with complex life-threatening problems. Future research should focus on understanding the most effective ways to adapt these interventions in school-based settings.

Test Yourself Questions

1. There are many factors that are important to assess for and consider when doing a suicide risk assessment. What are some of the key components of a comprehensive risk assessment?
2. You are working with a 15-year-old student who presents with a long history of anxiety and depression. You think RE-CBT would be a good treatment to help this student. What types of interventions will you employ using this model?
3. There are many treatment modes within comprehensive DBT. Define these four modes, including consideration for what these would look like within a school setting.

References

Bernard, M. E. (2008). Paper presented as part of the symposium *"Albert Ellis: A tribute to the grandfather of cognitive behaviour therapy"* (pp. 2), presented at the 43rd Annual Conference of the Australian Psychological Society, Hobart, Tasmania, September, 2008. (39).

Carter, G. L., Willcox, C. H., Lewin, T. J., Conrad, A. M., & Bendit, N. (2010). Hunter DBT Project: Randomized controlled trial of dialectical behaviour therapy in women with borderline personality disorder. *Australian and New Zealand Journal of Psychiatry, 44*, 162–173.

Center for Disease Control and Prevention (CDC). (2017). Death rates due to suicide and homicide among persons aged 10–24: United States, 2000–2017. Retrieved March 1, 2020 from https://www.cdc.gov/nchs/data/databriefs/db352-h.pdf

Chesin, M. S., Galfavy, H., Sonmez, C. C., Wong, A., Oquendo, M. A., Mann, J. J., et al. (2017). Nonsuicidal self-injury is predictive of suicide attempts among individuals with mood disorders. *Suicide and Life-threatening Behavior, 47*(5), 567–579.

Columbia Lighthouse Project (2016). *C-SSRS: About the Protocol.*. Retrieved from https://cssrs.columbia.edu/the-columbia-scale-c-ssrs/about-the-scale/

Cooper, J., Kapur, N., Webb, R., Lawlor, M., Guthrie, E., Mackway-Jones, K., et al. (2005). Suicide after deliberate self-harm: A 4-year cohort study. *American Journal of Psychiatry, 162*, 297–303. (9).

DiGiuseppe, R. (1981). *Using rational-emotive therapy effectively*. Boston: Springer.

DiGiuseppe, R., & Bernard, M. E. (2006). REBT assessment and treatment with children. In *Rational emotive behavioral approaches to childhood disorders* (pp. 85–114). Boston: Springer.

DiGiuseppe, R., Doyle, K., Dryden, W., & Backx, W. (2014). *The practitioners guide to rational emotive behavior therapy* (p. 179). New York: Oxford University Press. (18).

DiGiuseppe, R., Leaf, R., Exner, T., & Robin, M. (1988). *The development of a measure of irrational/rational thinking*. Poster session presented at the World Congress of Behavior Therapy, Edinburgh, Scotland, September 6. (23).

Dryden, W. (1996). *Learning from demonstration sessions*. London, England: Whurr Publisher.

Dryden, W. (1998). Understanding persons in the context of their problems: A rational emotive behavior therapy perspective. In M. Bruch & F. W. Bond (Eds.), *Beyond diagnosis: Case formulation approaches in CBT*. Chichester, UK: John Wiley. (20).

Dryden, W. (2009). *How to think and intervene like an REBT therapist*. London: Routledge.

Ellis, A. (1994). *Reason and emotion in psychotherapy*. New York: Birch Lane Press.

Ellis, A. (1995). Rational emotive behavior therapy. *Current Psychotherapies, 5*, 162–196.

Esposito-Smythers, C., Spirito, A., Kahler, C. W., Hurt, J., & Monti, P. (2011). Treatment of co-occurring substance abuse and suicidality among adolescents: A randomized trial. *Journal of Consulting and Clinical Psychology, 79*, 728–739. (35).

Faye, P. (1995). Addictive characteristics of the behavior of self-mutilation. *Journal of Psychosocial Nursing and Mental Health Services, 33*, 36–39. (12).

Grandclerc, S., De Labrouhe, D., Spodenkiewicz, M., Lachal, J., & Moro, M. R. (2016). Relations between nonsuicidal self-injury and suicidal behavior in adolescence: A systematic review. *PLoS One, 11*(4), 1–15.

Heard, H. L., & Linehan, M. M. (1994). Dialectical behavior therapy: An integrative approach to the treatment of borderline personality disorder. *Journal of Psychotherapy Integration, 4*(1), 55.

Hollander, M. (2017). *Helping teens who cut*. New York: Guilford Publication.

Houston, M. N. (2017). *Treating suicidal clients and self-harm behaviors*. Eau Claire, WI: PESI Publishing & Media. (10).

International Society for the Study of Self-injury. (2018, May). What is self-injury? Retrieved from: https://itriples.org/about-self-injury/what-is-self-injury

Klonsky, E. D. (2009). The functions of self-injury in young adults who cut themselves: Clarifying the evidence for affect-regulation. *Psychiatry Research, 166*(2–3), 260–268.

Knaus, W. J. (1974). *Children's survey of rational beliefs. A manual for elementary school teachers*. New York: Institute for Rational-Emotive Psychotherapy.

Lieberman, R., Poland, S., & Kornfeld, C. (2014). Best practices in suicide prevention and intervention. In P. Harris & A. Thomas (Eds.), *Best practices in school psychology: Systems-level services* (273–288). National Association of School Psychologists.

Linehan, M. M. (1993). Dialectical behavior therapy for borderline personality disorder. Theory and method. *Bulletin of the Menninger Clinic, 51*(3), 261–276. (11).

Linehan, M. M. (2009). University of Washington Risk Assessment Action Protocol: UWRAMP, University of WA, Unpublished Work.

Linehan, M. M. (2014). Linehan risk assessment and management protocol (LRAMP).

Linehan, M. M., Armstrong, H. E., Suarez, A., Allmon, D., & Heard, H. L. (1991). Cognitive-behavioral treatment of chronically parasuicidal borderline patients. *Archives of General Psychiatry, 48*, 1060–1064.

Linehan, M. M., Comtois, K. A., & Ward-Ciesielski, E. F. (2012). Assessing and managing risk with suicidal individuals. *Cognitive and Behavioral Practice, 19*(2), 218–232.

Linehan, M. M., Korslund, K. E., Harned, M. S., Gallop, R. J., Lungu, A., Neacsiu, A. D., et al. (2015). Dialectical behavior therapy for high suicide risk in individuals with borderline personality disorder: A randomized clinical trial and component analysis. *JAMA Psychiatry, 72*, 475–482.

Maris, W. M. (2019). *Suicidology a comprehensive biopsychosocial perspective*. New York: Guilford.

McCauley, E., Berk, M. S., Asarnow, J. R., Adrian, M., Cohen, J., Korslund, K., et al. (2018). Efficacy of dialectical behavior therapy for adolescents at high risk for suicide: A randomized clinical trial. *JAMA Psychiatry, 75*(8), 777–785.

Mehlum, L., Ramleth, R. K., Tørmoen, A. J., Haga, E., Diep, L. M., Stanley, B. H., et al. (2019). Long term effectiveness of dialectical behavior therapy versus enhanced usual care for adolescents with self-harming and suicidal behavior. *Journal of Child Psychology and Psychiatry, 60*(10), 1112–1122.

Mehlum, L., Tørmoen, A. J., Ramberg, M., Haga, E., Diep, L. M., Laberg, S., et al. (2014). Dialectical behavior therapy for adolescents with repeated suicidal and self-harming behavior: A randomized trial. *Journal of the American Academy of Child & Adolescent Psychiatry, 53*(10), 1082–1091.

Miller, A. L., Rathus, J. H., Leigh, E., Landsman, M., & Linehan, M. M. (1997). Dialectical behavior therapy adapted for suicidal adolescents. *Journal of Practical Psychiatry and Behavioral Health, 3*, 78–86.

Miller, A. L., Rathus, J. H., & Linehan, M. M. (2007). *Dialectical behavior therapy with suicidal adolescents*. New York: Guilford. (8).

Miller, A. L., Rathus, J. H., Linehan, M. M., Wetzler, S., & Leigh, E. (1997). Dialectical behavior therapy adapted for suicidal adolescents. *Journal of Psychiatric Practice®, 3*(2), 78.

National Association for School Psychologists (NASP). (2015). *Preventing Suicide: Guidelines for Administrators and Crisit Teams*. Retrieved from: https://www.nasponline.org/resources-and-publications/resources-and-podcasts/school-climate-safety-and-crisis/mental-health-resources/preventing-youth-suicide/preventing-suicide-guidelines-for-administrators-and-crisis-teams

Perepletchikova, F., Axelrod, S. R., Kaufman, J., Rounsaville, B. J., Douglas-Palumberi, H., & Miller, A. L. (2011). Adapting dialectical behaviour therapy for children: Towards a new research agenda for paediatric suicidal and non-suicidal self-injurious behaviours. *Child and Adolescent Mental Health, 16*(2), 116–121.

Perepletchikova, F., Nathanson, D., Axelrod, S. R., Merrill, C., Walker, A., Grossman, M., et al. (2017). Randomized clinical trial of dialectical behavior therapy for preadolescent children with disruptive mood dysregulation disorder: Feasibility and outcomes. *Journal of the American Academy of Child & Adolescent Psychiatry, 56*(10), 832–840.

Posner, K., Brent, D., Lucas, C., Gould, M., Stanley, B., Brown, G., et al. (2008). *Columbia-suicide severity rating scale (C-SSRS)*. New York: Columbia University Medical Center.

Rathus, J. H., & Miller, A. L. (2002). Dialectical behavior therapy adapted for suicidal adolescents. *Suicide and Life-threatening Behavior, 32*(2), 146–157.

Rathus, J. H., & Miller, A. L. (2014). *DBT skills manual for adolescents*. New York: Guilford Publications.

Ritschel, L. A., Miller, A. L., & Taylor, V. (2013). Dialectical behavior therapy for emotion dysregulation. In *Transdiagnostic mechanisms and treatment for youth psychopathology* (pp. 203–232). Guilford Press. https://doi.org/10.1093/oxfordhb/9780199935291.013.10.

Selby, E., Bender, T., Gordon, K., Nock, M., & Joiner, T. (2012). Nonsuicidal self-injury disorder: A preliminary study. *Personality Disorders: Theory, Research, and Treatment, 3*, 167–175. (15).

Shea, S. C. (2002). *The practical art of suicide assessment*. Hoboken, NJ: John Wiley & Sons. (21).

Swann, W. B. (1981). Self-verification processes: How we sustain our self-conceptions. *Journal of Experimental Social Psychology, 17*(4), 351–372.

Swannell, S. V., Martin, G. E., Page, A., Hasking, P., & St. John, N. J. (2014). Prevalence of non-suicidal self-injury in nonclinical samples: Systematic review, meta-analysis and meta-regression. *Suicide and Life-threatening Behavior, 2*, 1–31. (7).

Tatnell, R., Kelada, L., Hasking, P., & Martin, G. (2014). Longitudinal analysis of adolescent NSSI: The role of intrapersonal and interpersonal factors. *Journal of Abnormal Child Psychology, 42*(6), 885–896. (26).

Taylor, L. M. W., Oldershaw, A., Richards, C., & Davidson, K. (2011). Development and pilot evaluation of a manualized cognitive-behavioral treatment package for adolescent self-harm. *Behavioural and Cognitive Psychotherapy, 39*(5), 619–625. (34).

Terjesen, M. D., & Esposito, M. A. (2006). Rational-emotive behavior group therapy with children and adolescents. In *Rational emotive behavioral approaches to childhood disorders* (pp. 385–414). Boston: Springer.

Vaughn, M., Salas-Wright, C., Underwood, S., & Gochez-Kerr, T. (2015). Subtypes on non-suicidal self-injury based on childhood adversity. *Psychiatric Quarterly, 86*, 137–151. (14) and (16).

Vernon, A. (1989). Rational-emotive consultation: A model for implementing rational-emotive education. In R. DiGiuseppe & M. E. Bernard (Eds.), *Rational-emotive consultation in applied settings* (pp. 129–148). Mahwah, NJ: Lawrence Earlbaum Associates.

Whitlock, J. L., Exner-Cortens, D., & Purington, A. (2013). Validity and reliability of the non-suicidal self-injury assessment test (NSSI-AT). Manuscript in preparation.

Williams, F., & Hasking, P. (2010). Emotion regulation, coping and alcohol use as moderators in the relationship between self-injury and psychological distress. *Prevention Science, 11*, 33–41. (13).
World Health Organization (WHO). (2016). *Global Health Observatory. Suicide rates (per 100,000 population)*. Retrieved September 7, 2019 from https://www.who.int/gho/mental_health/suicide_rates/en/

Chapter 13
Cognitive-Behavioral, Rational-Emotive Treatment of Childhood Anger and Conduct Problems

John E. Lochman, Caroline L. Boxmeyer, Shannon Jones, Francesca Kassing, Nicole P. Powell, and Sara Stromeyer

Overview of Anger and Conduct Disorders

Anger and associated conduct problems are some of the most common child mental health referrals, and children with aggressive and disruptive behavior problems are at risk for a variety of negative outcomes. Conduct problems frequently interfere with family functioning, classroom activities, and peer relationships. For example, children with disruptive behavior contribute significantly to their parent's level of stress (Graziano, McNamara, Geffken, & Reid, 2011) and are more likely to experience peer rejection, which in turn predicts lower academic achievement and more aggressive behavior (Ryan & Ladd, 2012). Additionally, aggressive and disruptive behaviors displayed in childhood may develop into more chronic patterns of problem behavior, such as deviant behavior in adolescence and more antisocial behavior later, including substance use, delinquency, and violence (Hinshaw & Lee, 2003).

J. E. Lochman (✉)
Center for Prevention of Youth Behavior Problems at The University of Alabama, Tuscaloosa, AL, USA
e-mail: jlochman@as.ua.edu

C. L. Boxmeyer
College of Community Health Sciences at The University of Alabama, Department of Psychiatry and Behavioral Medicine, Tuscaloosa, AL, USA

S. Jones · N. P. Powell
Center for Youth Development and Intervention, University of Alabama, Tuscaloosa, AL, USA

F. Kassing
Trauma and Grief Center at Baylor College of Medicine/Texas Children's Hospital, Houston, TX, USA

S. Stromeyer
Department of Psychology, University of Alabama, Tuscaloosa, AL, USA

M. Bernard, M. D. Terjesen (eds.), *Rational-Emotive and Cognitive-Behavioral Approaches to Child and Adolescent Mental Health: Theory, Practice, Research, Applications*, https://doi.org/10.1007/978-3-030-53901-6_13

A contextual social-cognitive model provides an ecological framework for identifying risk factors and understanding the etiology of conduct problems among youth. This theory proposes that environmental factors and deficits in social information processing reciprocally interact, leading to disruptive behavior (Lochman & Wells, 2002). With regard to the contextual component, factors related to the family, peer, school, and neighborhood can influence child behavior. Family factors such as abusive or neglectful parenting (Aguilar, Sroufe, Egeland, & Carlson, 2000), inconsistent discipline and low warmth (Stormshak, Bierman, McMahon,, & Lengua, 2000), and high levels of family stress (Leve & Chamberlain, 2004) predict disruptive behavior. Additionally, children who are rejected by prosocial peers due to higher levels of anger and conduct problems are more likely to develop deviant peer relationships, escalating disruptive behavior (Fite, Colder, Lochman, & Wells, 2007). School factors include teacher classroom management (Roland & Galloway, 2002), student-teacher relationship (Rimm-Kaufman et al., 2002), and administrative support for student discipline issues (Mayer, 1995), and a significant neighborhood factor is neighborhood violence (McCabe, Lucchini, Hough, Yeh, & Hazen, 2005).

These contextual factors interact reciprocally with child-level factors, specifically social-cognitive deficits. Children with conduct problems are more likely to perceive peers' ambiguous interactions as intentionally hostile, recall more hostile cues, and expect that aggression will have a positive outcome (Crick & Dodge, 1996; Dodge, Lochman, Harnish, Bates, & Pettit, 1997). These children also tend to generate fewer solutions to social problems and view aggression as an acceptable and effective solution (Lochman & Dodge, 1994).

Assessment and Diagnosis

The two DSM-V diagnostic categories most relevant to anger and conduct problems are oppositional defiant disorder (ODD) and conduct disorder (CD) (American Psychiatric Association, 2013). Oppositional defiant disorder is a persistent pattern of negative, hostile, and defiant behavior that lasts 6 months or more. Children with ODD often lose their temper, argue with adults, actively defy adults' requests, deliberately annoy other people, blame others for their own mistakes, are often touchy or easily annoyed, are often angry and resentful, and are often spiteful or vindictive (APA, 2013). Conduct disorder is characterized by aggressive behaviors (e.g., physical cruelty to animals or people), destruction of property, deceitfulness or theft, and/or major rule violations (e.g., school truancy, running away from home). The most common comorbidities with conduct problems are attention-deficit/hyperactivity disorder, anxiety, depression, and academic underachievement (Matthys & Lochman, 2017), any of which can lead to greater functional impairment and can complicate treatment.

In terms of assessment, it is important to consider both the environmental and developmental contexts of the anger or conduct problems, as well as functional impairment. For instance, some level of anger or aggression may be appropriate and protective in threatening environmental contexts. Furthermore, younger children are more likely to exhibit anger when a goal is blocked, and older children are more likely to exhibit anger when they perceive threats to their self-esteem (Lochman, Powell, Clanton, & McElroy, 2006). Although some level of oppositionality and defiance is developmentally appropriate and observed in all children, both ODD and CD are diagnosed when the frequency and intensity of the symptoms exceed that expected of the developmental level and when the disruptive behaviors impair the child's functioning. In addition to gathering detailed symptomatology and course, detailed clinical interviews should comprise a family history, social history, academic history, and information about neighborhood environment, given the importance of ecological factors.

Rating scales can assess specific symptoms related to the disruptive behavior disorders, such as the Children's Inventory of Anger (Nelson, & Finch, 2000), and can include a range of clinical and adaptive behaviors that are useful in gaining a broad understanding of the child's clinical picture, screening for comorbid conditions, and providing specific information about the type and severity of conduct problems. Use of rating scales with at least three informants (e.g., parent, teacher, child) is also beneficial, in order to gain information about the child's behavior in different contexts (or the child's perception of their own behavior) and to assess for inter-rater reliability or discrepancy. An example of a broad symptom checklist is the Behavior Assessment System for Children (BASC)-3 (Reynolds & Kamphaus, 2015), which has forms for different raters. Rating scales are also useful in tracking progress in treatment over time. To supplement these measures, behavioral observation can assist in identifying antecedents and consequences (O'Neill, Homer, Albin, Storey, & Sprague, 1990). Clinican manuals for Parent Management Training, such as Parent-Child Interaction Therapy (Brinkmeyer & Eyberg, 2003), have examples of observations for clinician use in-session. For school observations, scales such as the BASC-3 Student Observation System (Reynolds & Kamphaus, 2015) can be implemented.

Finally, a key focus of diagnosis should be assessing functional impairment across domains, given that longitudinal studies have indicated that persistent difficulty in adulthood is better predicted by functional impairment than by diagnostic symptoms. A brief measure that assesses functional impairment in peer relations, academic functioning, and classroom behavior is the Children's Impairment Rating Scale (Fabiano et al., 2006).

Research on CBT and RE-CBT with Youth with Anger and Conduct Problems

For preadolescent to mid-adolescent youth, behavioral parent training and child-based treatment using principles evident in cognitive-behavioral therapy and rational-emotive behavior therapy have been shown to effect positive reductions in externalizing behavior problems (Lochman et al., 2012). In a meta-analytic study which focused on the delivery of cognitive-behavioral therapy (CBT) to typically developing children and adolescents with externalizing behavior problems, Sukhodolsky, Kassinove, and Gorman (2004) examined the effectiveness of 40 treatment outcome studies of CBT programs for youth aged 7 to 17 years. Treatment was mainly delivered in a group format, and treatment length was short term, ranging from 8 to 18 hours. The authors reported a moderate effect size (0.67) across all studies. Youth whose problems were categorized in the moderate range appeared to benefit most (effect size of 0.80), compared to children with severe (0.59) or mild (0.57) problems with anger and aggression. Sukhodolsky and colleagues also analyzed different components of CBT, finding the largest effect sizes for social skills development (0.79) and multimodal treatment (0.74), followed by problem-solving (0.67) and affective education (0.36). In another meta-analysis, McCart, Priester, Davies, and Azen (2006) found stronger effects for adolescents than for younger children in their examination of 71 CBT outcome studies and suggested that the effectiveness of CBT interventions may increase with advances in cognitive development.

One example of a CBT program targeting these processes with preadolescent children with anger and aggression problems is the Coping Power Program. It has been empirically supported as an efficacious and effective preventive intervention for children with aggressive and conduct problem behaviors (e.g., Lochman & Wells, 2004), and its effects have been evident through 3-year follow-ups (Lochman et al., 2014; Lochman, Wells, Qu, & Chen, 2013). The program has been designated as a promising program in lists of reviewed empirically proven programs such as Blueprints for Healthy Youth Development, What Works Clearinghouse, and CrimeSolutions.gov. Coping Power is an indicated intervention for preadolescent to early adolescent youth (ages 8–14) delivered in community settings (e.g., schools) to children and parents in a group format. This program has some components that are consistent with rational-emotive behavioral therapy (such as a focus on beliefs and goals) and has been shown to be effective in both school (as preventive interventions) and clinic settings (as treatment interventions) and in diverse national (i.e., North Carolina, Alabama, New York) and international settings (i.e., Canada, Italy, the Netherlands, Pakistan, Puerto Rico; Lochman, Boxmeyer, Andrade, & Kassing, 2019).

Examples of CBT-based programs for adolescents are included in McCart and Sheidow's (2016) review of treatment programs as "well-established" and "probably efficacious." Multisystemic Therapy (Henggeler, Schoenwald, Borduin, Rowland, & Cunningham, 2009) and Treatment Foster Care Oregon (TFCO;

Chamberlain, 2003) are community- and family-based interventions for youth with serious behavior problems that integrate behavior therapy and CBT into their multisystem treatment approaches. "Probably efficacious" treatments for adolescents include Equipping Youth to Help One Another (EQUIP; Gibbs, Potter, & Goldstein, 1995), a multicomponent program taking a cognitive-behavioral approach to group sessions in correctional facilities, and Solution-Focused Group Program (Shin, 2009).

Meta-analytic studies have also investigated the impact of rational-emotive therapies on children's behavioral problems. Gonzalez et al. (2004) included 19 studies in a meta-analysis examining emotional, behavioral, cognitive, and academic effects of rational-emotive treatments for children and adolescents. Findings revealed the strongest effects on disruptive behavior problems (e.g., disruptive classroom behaviors, detentions, referrals to principal's office) with a weighted mean effect size of 1.15. Trip, Vernon, and McMahon (2007) completed a meta-analysis of Rational-Emotive Education studies implemented with school children, examining a range of cognitive, emotional, and behavioral outcomes. The authors found an effect size of 0.85 on behavior modification and "very large" effect sizes on behavioral problems and relationships with others. In its application to anger and conduct disorders, rational-emotive cognitive-behavioral therapy (RE-CBT) has been used with both individuals and groups and in outpatient and school settings (Doyle & Terjesen, 2006; Flanagan, Allen, & Henry, 2010). Programs have been developed for school-aged children (DiGiuseppe & Kelter, 2006) and adolescents (Neamţu & David, 2016). RE-CBT interventions addressing anger and disruptive behavior vary in the degree of parental involvement, with some programs delivered just to youth and others taking a parent-based approach (Gavita & Calin, 2013).

Developmental Considerations

While most programs and interventions are developed for and tested on a specific age range, it is important to consider how they may be effectively adapted to address presenting concerns in other developmental levels. The Coping Power Program, for example, has been adapted and tested with both younger and older children than the intervention's original target population and with children with intellectual disabilities (Stromeyer, Lochman, Kassing, & Romero, 2020). Furthermore, Coping Power has been adapted into different formats, such as those that integrate technological components, in order to increase access and engagement for different diverse developmental age groups. It is important to note that, like other adaptations, these developmental adjustments should be rigorously evaluated.

To make CBT and rational emotive behavior therapy (REBT) programs relevant for younger or developmentally delayed children, activities may have to be more concrete, highly engaging, briefly presented, and make frequent use of stimulating books, puppets, and arts-and-crafts activities. Furthermore, from a prevention standpoint, teaching children social and emotional skills as early as possible is important. Therefore, large-scale randomized controlled trials are currently examining developmental adaptations of Coping Power for preschool-age children (Boxmeyer et al., 2015). In this study, Head Start teachers are being trained to implement the Preschool Promoting Alternative THinking Strategies (PATHS) social emotional curriculum in the classroom, while students' parents are invited to take part in a corollary parent program, which integrates content from both the Coping Power parent program and the preschool PATHS curriculum. Preliminary data indicate that this combined program has benefits for child executive function and classroom behavior, as well as parent and family functioning (Boxmeyer et al., 2015).

Research on prevention programs targeting the early- to mid-adolescence period is lacking, highlighting this as a particularly important gap to fill. As a result, a version of Coping Power has been developed and piloted that extends the program through the middle school years (Coping Power–Early Adolescent version, CP-EA). This version includes increased focus on adolescent issues such as assertive communication, cyberbullying, social media use, and how to repair damaged relationships. It also uses delivery methods more appropriate for adolescents, such as journaling and greater use of video and media content (Lochman et al., 2016).

In addition to creating adaptations for different age groups, it is important to consider how interventions may be adapted for developmentally delayed or intellectually disabled children. Coping Power, for example, has been adapted for and tested in a Dutch sample of children 9 to 16 years old with mild to borderline intellectual disabilities and been shown to lead to reduced children's externalizing behavior and improved parenting behavior and parent–child relationships (Schuiringa, van Nieuwenhuijzen, Orobio de Castro, Lochman, & Matthys, 2017).

The growing interest in adaptations involving technological integration may lead to increased child engagement, particularly for certain age groups. Children and adolescents report that their preferred method of learning involves Internet-based interactive multimedia (Lochman et al., 2017); therefore, inclusion of multimodal methods of delivering session content, with an emphasis on multimedia, may assist program developers in creating engaging adaptations for youth of diverse developmental levels.

Best Practice Guidelines

The National Institute for Health and Care Excellence (NICE) (2013) has a highly regarded and rigorous set of practice guidelines (Andrade et al., 2019). The NICE clinical guideline for antisocial behavior and conduct disorders in children and young people emphasizes integrated and person-centered service delivery with key priority areas. These include recommendations for (1) comprehensive assessment; (2) parent training programs using social-learning frameworks; (3) foster care/guardian training programs; (4) child-focused programs addressing social and cognitive problem-solving; (5) multimodal interventions with interventions for children, the family, and the school and community environment; (6) pharmacological interventions when warranted; and (7) improving access to services. Research recommendations are also provided. The guideline includes general principles of care to consider, such as safety, informed consent, and ways to take into account culture, ethnicity, and social inclusion. Evidence-based interventions, including cognitive-behavioral therapy and rational-emotive behavior therapy, are critically important parts of these practice guidelines.

RE-CBT and CBT in the Treatment of Anger and Conduct Problems

RE-CBT interventions for anger and conduct problems in children follow the established ABCDE model also used with adults. Specifically, activating events (A) lead to beliefs (B), which, in turn, result in emotional and behavioral consequences (C). Individuals learn to dispute (D) nonfunctional erroneous or irrational beliefs, thereby developing an effective (E) rational outlook (Gonzalez et al., 2004). Central to RE-CBT is the principle that an event alone does not lead to an individual's distress; rather, problems with the person's cognitive reaction to the event are responsible for maladaptive emotional and behavioral responses. Children vary in their reactions to the same event, with some making healthy, adaptive interpretations and coping in a functional manner, while other children engage in self-defeating thoughts that result in emotional upset and behavioral disturbances. For example, one child may respond calmly when a peer bumps into her, assuming that the contact was accidental. In contrast, another child may view this as an aggressive act, triggering a belief that she needs to defend herself and a resulting hostile reaction. In the RE-CBT framework, children's variable reactions are thought to be influenced by innate temperamental features and parenting practices (Bernard, 1990).

During RE-CBT treatment for anger and conduct disorders, therapists focus on identifying the faulty beliefs that lead to a child's maladaptive anger and disruptive behaviors. Children are taught to examine whether a particular belief is (a) true, (b) logical, or (c) helpful (Bernard, 1990). Beliefs that do not meet these criteria are recognized as faulty, in that they may provoke strong, maladaptive emotional responses that can interfere with age-appropriate problem-solving and healthy coping. DiGiuseppe and Kelter (2006) identify two types of irrational thinking common in children with anger and disruptive behavior problems. These include demandingness and frustration intolerance. In demandingness, children conceptualize the world in terms of what "should," "ought to," or "must" be. When applied to the behavior of others, demandingness can lead to feelings of anger and rage. For example, a child who believes his older brother "should" always play with him may become enraged when he is not included in his sibling's playdate. An RE-CBT therapist will help the child to recognize that wanting something to be a certain way does not make it a reality. The goal is for the child to view his or her desires as *preferences* (which may or may not be fulfilled) rather than absolute imperatives that *have to* be met. Beliefs consistent with frustration intolerance imply that challenging circumstances are beyond an individual's ability to cope. As a result, a child may become irate and aggressive over a situation that others would experience as merely annoying or uncomfortable. For example, during a quiet classroom test at school, two children may be seated near a classmate who is humming and kicking the table leg. One child may feel somewhat irritated but can accept the situation as less than ideal and focus on her work. In contrast, the other child may think, "There's no way I can do my work with all of this noise! I can't stand it!" An angry outburst may follow. In RE-CBT, such beliefs will be disputed and replaced with helpful, empowering ways of thinking (e.g., "I wish he wouldn't do that but I can handle it").

In a related way, CBT with children with anger and aggression problems attends to broad acquired schema that children have acquired, but the focus is more specifically on emotion regulation and social information processing processes (e.g., Lochman & Dodge, 1994). In a structured CBT program like the Coping Power Program, children use discussion, activities, and role-play to address certain central mechanisms related to their self-control of behavior (Lochman et al., 2019). Children first work on *goal setting* by setting short-term behavior goals and identifying personally meaningful long-term goals to work on (e.g., to improve their relationship with their parents, teacher, or friends). Short-term goals are typically "prosocial opposites" of identified child-specific problem behaviors and are monitored weekly. Goal attainment leads to rewards. As a precursor to learning strategies for managing anger, children enhance their *emotion awareness* by learning to describe various emotions in terms of associated physiological sensations, behaviors, and cognitions. They also learn to identify common trigger situations for specific feelings, and a thermometer task is used to help children recognize the range of intensity of feelings. Children then learn several *emotion regulation* strategies for managing anger arousal, including the use of distraction, relaxation practices, and coping self-statements. Children participate in a number of graded exposure activities, starting with puppets, to practice managing anger arousal. Children with disruptive behavior problems often have an attributional bias that accompanies their anger arousal, leading them to overinterpret others' intentions as hostile. The primary focus in *perspective-taking activities* with aggressive children is on helping them to more accurately encode social cues, addressing these biased attributions. This work sets the stage for children to use *social problem-solving skills*. Children learn to use a stepwise approach to identify interpersonal problems with their peers and family members (from each person's perspective), brainstorm a variety of options for how to solve the problem, anticipate the likely consequences of each solution, and use this information to decide which solution to try first. Children demonstrate their mastery by creating a video illustrating effective social problem-solving in action.

The Coping Power parent group sessions are structured and are conducted in a collaborative manner between group leaders and parents. The parent sessions are largely based on behavioral parent training, although there is also a focus on parents' own stress management and on family problem-solving. The sessions heavily focus on encouraging the use of *positive parenting behaviors*, with an emphasis on parent-child special time activities and the use of parental reinforcement for appropriate behavior. Parents discuss and practice antecedent control of problem situations with children by providing *clear and specific directions* and discuss and use a variety of potential *consequences* for problem behaviors ranging from planned ignoring to use of consistent consequences such as privilege removal, work chores, and time-out.

Case Study

James is a 10-year-old boy whose parents brought him for mental health treatment after they received numerous complaints from James' school about his behavior. The school reported that James frequently lashed out at his peers, talked back to the teacher, and started fights. James' parents had been dealing with his angry outbursts at home for many years. They had become very discouraged and were finding it difficult to maintain their positive affection for James. They finally sought help after James was suspended for a fight that injured one of his classmates.

It took several weeks for James' parents to find a therapist who was covered by their health insurance. While they were waiting, they worried about whether they would be able to get James to open up to a therapist, whether therapy would make a difference, and whether it would be worth the time and financial investment. They were relieved when they found a therapist named Rebecca who had a lot of experience working with children with anger and aggression difficulties. Rebecca said that she used a program called Coping Power to work with children like James and their parents. She shared that she had seen this approach have a lasting positive impact for many children and families.

After taking a thorough history from his parents, Rebecca invested time to develop rapport with James. He was not happy about being made to go to therapy. He opened up a little when he found out that Rebecca was a fan of the same professional baseball team. Rebecca told him that they could spend time chatting about the team's stats at the beginning of each visit. She also told James that he could think of her more like a coach (than a therapist). She explained that she would be teaching him strategies to help him meet his goals, manage his anger, and get in trouble less. Then, they would help James practice using these strategies in his day-to-day life. James especially liked it when Rebecca said that his parents would have to do work in therapy too, not just him. They would have some of their therapy sessions together and some separate.

Rebecca taught James about short-term and long-term goals. She learned that James was hoping to play on his middle school baseball team next year. However, he would not be eligible to play if he got any more detentions or suspensions at school. James and Rebecca agreed that they would work on the strategies from the Coping Power Program to help James learn to manage his anger better and stay out of fights so that he could be eligible to play baseball in middle school.

For the next several sessions, James and Rebecca went over situations in which James had felt angry recently. They used an "anger thermometer" to measure how angry James felt and to record where he felt his anger in his body. They differentiated between situations in which James felt just a little bit irritated or angry (such as when his classmate bumped into his desk), medium angry (such as when his parents gave him an extra chore), and very angry (such as when his teacher got on his case for something that wasn't his fault).

James began to pay attention to the signs of anger in his body. When he was starting to feel a little angry or annoyed, he tended to roll his eyes or make a groaning sound. As he became more angry, he started to feel hot and clench his jaw. When his anger got really high on his anger thermometer, he would raise his voice and yell or hit. Between therapy sessions, Rebecca had James track his anger in real-life situations using anger thermometer worksheets (see Fig. 13.1, as an example). This practice helped James become more adept at catching his anger as it was on the rise, instead of remaining unaware of his escalating anger until it was so strong that it was nearly impossible to avoid lashing out or doing something that would cause problems for himself and others.

Next, Rebecca taught James about the connection between his thoughts and his feelings, including his anger. She explained to James that we all talk to ourselves inside our own head throughout the day. She said that the way we talk to our self makes a big difference in how we feel and how we act, so it is worth paying attention to. James had never heard anyone describe "self-talk" like this before. With Rebecca's prompting, he practiced turning his attention inward and noticing his self-talk more clearly. Rebecca shared examples of her own self-talk as well. James liked drawing comic strips, so he and Rebecca created characters and wrote their internal commentary in thought bubbles, to illustrate different types of self-talk in a range of situations.

At his next visit, Rebecca had James recall a time that he felt angry recently. She drew upon this experience to raise James' awareness of how his thoughts affect his feelings and actions. James shared that the day before, he had been super excited to talk with his friends at lunch about their fantasy baseball teams. On the way to the cafeteria, some of his classmates were talking loudly and getting out of the line. When the teacher saw this, she demanded that they shape up immediately or she would give the entire class silent lunch. James complained to his friend that the teacher wasn't being fair. His teacher overheard this, pulled James aside, and gave him silent lunch. He got so mad he punched the wall. The teacher didn't see James do this, or it surely would have jeopardized his goal of playing on the middle school baseball team.

James and Rebecca used the white board in Rebecca's office to identify James' self-talk in this situation. When the teacher gave James silent lunch, he thought to himself: "She is the meanest teacher ever! It is SO unfair that only I got silent lunch! I wasn't even the one breaking the rules to begin with! I hate school! The teacher has it out for me! She doesn't like me as much as she likes everyone else!" Then they identified some of James' beliefs underlying these thoughts, consistent with a rational-emotive cognitive-behavioral therapy approach. James believed that: "Teachers should treat everyone exactly the same. They should understand exactly

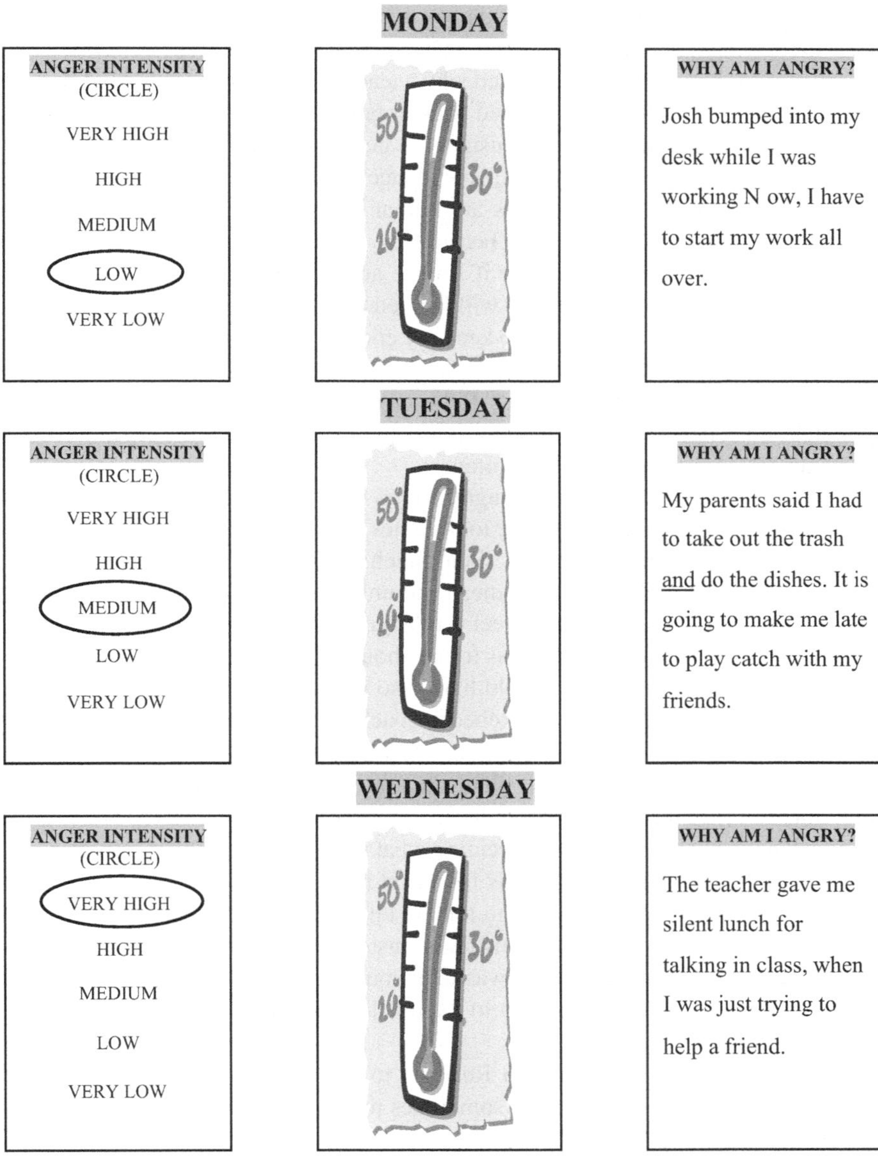

Fig. 13.1 Anger thermometer record form

what is going on at all times, treat everyone fairly, and never make a mistake." They also identified that James believed that his teacher didn't like or care about him at all.

Rebecca led James in an imaginal activity in which he was in charge of guiding an entire class of students from one place to another, to experience the situation from the teacher's perspective. This helped James appreciate how difficult it is for teachers to manage many children at once and to keep track of everything that is going on with each individual child. James realized how easily it could happen for a teacher to single out one child, when many were at fault, when she only had some pieces of information. He also realized why a teacher might be more likely to single out the children who frequently talked back or got in trouble.

James and Rebecca used these insights to generate more rational beliefs about the situation at school. With Rebecca's guidance, James came to expand his beliefs to include the following: "Teachers are human beings with a difficult job. They don't get it right every time. Just because my teacher gives me a consequence doesn't mean she hates me. Maybe if I make an effort to follow the rules and be more respectful, situations like this will happen to me less often. In the future, if a teacher gets on my case, I will try to keep my cool. This will make the teacher's job easier and keep me out of trouble. It is okay to speak up for myself, but I need to do so in the right way, at the right time." Rebecca said that if James can work with his thoughts and beliefs in other situations like he did in this one, it will help him handle his anger better and feel angry less often.

A final strategy that Rebecca taught James was how to stop and think ahead when trying to solve a problem. She took James back to the moment when he realized that his whole class might get silent lunch. This activating event tapped into James' irrational beliefs about how mean and unfair his teacher was and how much she disliked him. This led James to feel very angry and to do the first thing that came to mind, which was to complain to his friend about the teacher. This led to a negative consequence (silent lunch) and could have also jeopardized his goal of playing on the middle school baseball team. Rebecca coached James on brainstorming other choices that might have helped solve this problem better and they acted out each choice. James realized that the problem situation tended to work out best when he took time to 1) see the situation from the teacher's perspective and 2) be really clear about what his goals were, before deciding what to do. In this problem situation, his goals were to be able to talk with his friends at lunch, to feel like his teacher liked him as much as everyone else, and to remain eligible to play on the middle school baseball team. Of all of the solutions he brainstormed, the one that seemed like it would meet all of these goals best was to encourage his classmates to stay in line and remain quiet the rest of the way to the lunch room and to actively model these behaviors himself.

While James was working with Rebecca to learn all of the strategies above, Rebecca also met with his parents (sometimes together with James and sometimes without him present). She explained the skills that James was learning and how his parents could coach and reinforce the same skills at home. Rebecca also consulted with James' teacher for the same purpose. In individual sessions, Rebecca worked with James' parents on positive parenting skills, to help re-establish their positive regard for, and connection with, James and to provide household structures and communication tools to reduce James' angry and aggressive outbursts at home.

Adaptation of CBT and RE-CBT in the Schools for Behavior Problem Children

Tier 1 Interventions Tier 1 interventions in school settings are regarded as universal prevention and are provided to all children in the classroom in an effort to improve overall school behavior (Lochman, Boxmeyer, Andrade, & Kassing, 2019). Examples of classroom-based interventions are the evidence-based PATHS program that focuses on social-emotional learning (Greenberg & Kusche, 2006) and Rational Emotive Behavior Therapy developed as a curriculum for use in school settings (Banks & Zionts, 2009). Targeted interventions such as Coping Power have also been adapted to be delivered to full elementary school classrooms. In early elementary school years, findings showed a significant reduction in overall problematic behaviors and in inattention–hyperactivity problems for the intervention classes compared to the control classes. Students who received Coping Power Program intervention also showed more prosocial behaviors at post-intervention (Muratori, Bertacchi, Giuli, Nocentini, & Lochman, 2017). These universal prevention effects for adaptations of Coping Power have also been extended to preschool classrooms (Muratori et al., 2019) and to adolescents in middle school (Muratori et al., 2019). In the latter study, Coping Power Universal produced significant reductions in adolescents' conduct problems that generalized into the home setting as well as school.

Tier 2 Targeted School Interventions At a secondary, targeted level of intervention support in school settings (i.e., Tier 2), a systematic behavioral screening process is required to identify students requiring additional supports and match evidence-based interventions to student need. Approximately 10–15% of the school population will require some level of targeted support. Children with significant aggressive behavioral problems are one such group. The Coping Power Program can be effectively used as a Tier 2 intervention (Lochman, Boxmeyer, Andrade, & Kassing, 2019; McDaniel et al., 2018). The program is typically delivered to small groups within the school setting. Coping Power can be used with individual students as well (Lochman et al., 2015). When necessary, an abbreviated version of the program can be completed within one school year (Lochman et al., 2014).

To be effectively used as an intervention with behavior problem children in schools, it is essential that the program can be delivered by school psychologists and counselors. As an example, the intensity of training has been found to be critically important in the use of Coping Power in school settings. In a dissemination trial, counselors from 57 elementary schools in Alabama were randomly assigned to one of three conditions: Coping Power-Intensive Training, Coping Power-Basic Training, and Care-as-Usual (Lochman et al., 2009). Counselors in both training conditions received 3 days of training prior to the intervention as well as monthly consultations. The Intensive Training group also received performance feedback based on audio recordings of individual sessions. Training intensity was found to have a significant impact on outcomes, with the Coping Power-Intensive Training group showing significantly greater reductions in teacher-, parent-, and self-reported externalizing behaviors and greater improvements in social and academic behaviors than the other groups (Lochman et al., 2009). A follow-up study of this dissemination trial found that children with counselors who received the Coping Power-Intensive Training experienced smaller declines in language arts grades than children with counselors in the other groups after 2 years (Lochman et al., 2012).

Use with Disadvantaged Students Rational-emotive and cognitive-behavioral programs can also be adapted for use with disadvantaged students. For example, Coping Power has been adapted to address the needs of physically or cognitively disadvantaged groups of students. In a randomized controlled trial of Coping Power Program in a sample of 49 aggressive, deaf children (ages 9–16; 64% African-American, 32% Caucasian, 2% Hispanic) living in a residential school (Lochman et al., 2001), children were screened for aggressive behavior by their teachers and were assigned by classroom to either a Coping Power Program condition or wait-list control condition. The child component of the program was adapted to meet the needs of deaf children, and the parent component, although not used in the study, helped informed training of teachers and residential staff. Based on teacher ratings, children receiving Coping Power demonstrated significant improvements in behavior, social-problem-solving skills, and communication skills compared to children in the control condition (Lochman et al., 2001).

It is often difficult to attain intervention effects with children with low intellectual functioning. Schuiringa et al. (2017) evaluated the effectiveness of Standing Strong Together (SST), a combined group-based parent and child intervention, adapted from Coping Power, for externalizing behavior in 9–16-year-old children with mild to borderline intellectual disabilities (MBID). Children with externalizing behavior and MBID (IQ from 55 to 85) were cluster randomly assigned to SST combined with care as usual or to care as usual only. SST led to a significant benefit on teacher reported but not on parent reported externalizing behavior. SST had significant effects on parent rated positive parenting and the parent-child relationship. The present study shows that a multicomponent group-based intervention for children with MBID is feasible and has the potential to reduce children's externalizing behavior and improve both parenting behavior and the parent-child relationship.

Test Yourself

1. What are some of the contextual factors that clinicians may wish to consider in the assessment, case conceptualization, and treatment of anger among youth?
2. What are some of the core irrational beliefs or cognitions that clinicians may wish to target in the treatment of anger?
3. In consideration of the different tiers of services provided, what programs lend themselves to addressing concerns as it relates to anger among youth?

References

Aguilar, B., Sroufe, L. A., Egeland, B., & Carlson, E. (2000). Distinguishing the early-onset/persistent and adolescence-onset antisocial behavior types: From birth to 16 years. *Development and Psychopathology, 12*, 109–132.

American Psychiatric Association. (2013). *Diagnostic and statistical manual of mental health disorders: DSM-5* (5th ed.). Washington, DC: American Psychiatric Publishing.

Andrade, B. F., Courtney, D., Duda, S., Aitken, M., Craig, S. G., Szatmari, P., et al. (2019). A systematic review and evaluation of clinical practice guidelines for children and youth with disruptive behavior: Rigor of development and recommendations for use. *Clinical Child and Family Psychology Review, 22*, 527–548.

Banks, T., & Zionts, P. (2009). Teaching a cognitive behavioral strategy to manage emotions: Rational emotive behavior therapy in an educational setting. *Interventions in Schools and Clinics, 44*, 307–313.

Bernard, M. (1990). Rational-emotive therapy with children and adolescents: Treatment strategies. *School Psychology Review, 19*(3), 294–303.

Boxmeyer, C., Gilpin, A., DeCaro, J., Lochman, J., Qu, L., Mitchell, Q., & Snead, S. (2015). Power PATH: Integrated two-generation social emotional intervention for Head Start preschoolers and their parents. Online paper collection of the *Association for Public Policy Analysis and Management's 37th Annual Fall Research Conference: The Golden Age of Evidence-Based Policy*. Retrieved from https://appam.confex.com/appam/2015/webprogram/Paper12784.html

Brinkmeyer, M. Y., & Eyberg, S. M. (2003). Parent-child interaction therapy for oppositional children. In A. E. Kazdin & J. R. Weisz (Eds.), *Evidenced-based psychotherapies for children and adolescents* (pp. 204–223). New York: Guilford.

Chamberlain, P. (2003). *Treating chronic juvenile offenders: Advances made through the Oregon multidimensional treatment foster care model*. Washington, DC: American Psychological Association.

Crick, N. R., & Dodge, K. A. (1996). Social information-processing mechanisms on reactive and proactive aggression. *Child Development, 67*, 993–1002.

DiGiuseppe, R., & Kelter, J. (2006). Treating aggressive children: A rational-emotive behavior systems approach. In A. Ellis & M. E. Bernard (Eds.), *Rational emotive behavioral approaches to childhood disorders* (pp. 257–280). Boston: Springer.

Dodge, K. A., Lochman, J. E., Harnish, J. D., Bates, J. E., & Pettit, G. S. (1997). Reactive and proactive aggression in school children and psychiatrically impaired chronically assaultive youth. *Journal of Abnormal Psychology, 106*, 37–51.

Doyle, K. A., & Terjesen, M. D. (2006). Rational-emotive behavior therapy and attention deficit hyperactivity disorder. In A. Ellis & M. E. Bernard (Eds.), *Rational emotive behavioral approaches to childhood disorders* (pp. 281–309). Boston: Springer.

Fabiano, G. A., Pelham Jr., W. E., Waschbusch, D. A., Gnagy, E. M., Lahey, B. B., Chronis, A. M., et al. (2006). A practical measure of impairment: Psychometric properties of the impairment rating scale in samples of children with attention deficit/ hyperactivity disorder and two school-based samples. *Journal of Clinical Child and Adolescent Psychology, 35*, 369–385.

Fite, P. J., Colder, C. R., Lochman, J. E., & Wells, K. C. (2007). Pathways from proactive and reactive aggression to substance use. *Psychology of Addictive Behaviors, 21*(3), 355–364.

Flanagan, R., Allen, K., & Henry, D. J. (2010). The impact of anger management treatment and rational emotive behavior therapy in a public school setting on social skills, anger management, and depression. *Journal of Rational-Emotive & Cognitive-Behavior Therapy, 28*(2), 87–99.

Gavita, O. A., & Calin, A. (2013). RETMAN rational stories versus rational parenting program for the treatment of child psychopathology: Efficacy of two formats of rational-emotive behavior therapy. *Journal of Evidence-Based Psychotherapies, 13*(1), 33–56.

Gibbs, J. C., Potter, G. B., & Goldstein, A. P. (1995). *The EQUIP program: Teaching youth to think and act responsibly through a peer-helping approach*. Champaign, IL: Research Press.

Gonzalez, J. E., Nelson, J. R., Gutkin, T. B., Saunders, A., Galloway, A., & Shwery, C. S. (2004). Rational emotive therapy with children and adolescents: A meta-analysis. *Journal of Emotional and Behavioral Disorders, 12*(4), 222–235.

Graziano, P. A., McNamara, J. P., Geffken, G. R., & Reid, A. (2011). Severity of children's ADHD symptoms and parenting stress: A multiple mediation model of self-regulation. *Journal of Abnormal Child Psychology, 39*, 1073–1083.

Greenberg, M. T., & Kusche, C. A. (2006). Building social and emotional competence: The PATHS curriculum. In S. R. Jimmerson & M. Furlong (Eds.), *Handbook of school violence and school safety: From research to practice* (pp. 395–412). Mahwah, NJ: Lawrence Erlbaum Associates.

Henggeler, S. W., Schoenwald, S. K., Borduin, C. M., Rowland, M. D., & Cunningham, P. B. (2009). *Multisystemic therapy for antisocial behavior in children and adolescents* (2nd ed.). New York: Guilford Press.

Hinshaw, S. P., & Lee, S. S. (2003). Conduct and oppositional defiant disorders. In E. J. Mash & R. A. Barkley (Eds.), *Child psychopathology* (2nd ed., pp. 144–198). New York: Guilford Press.

Leve, L. D., & Chamberlain, P. (2004). Female juvenile offenders: Defining an early-onset pathway for delinquency. *Journal of Child and Family Studies, 13*, 439–452.

Lochman, J.E., FitzGerald, D.P., Gage, S.M., Kannaly, M.K., Whidby, J.M., Barry, T.D., Pardini, D.A., McElroy, H. (2001). Effects of social-cognitive intervention for aggressive deaf children: The Coping Power Program. *Journal of the American Deafness and Rehabilitation Association, 35*, 39–61.

Lochman, J. E., Baden, R. E., Boxmeyer, C. L., Powell, N. P., Qu, L., Salekin, K. L., et al. (2014). Does a booster intervention augment the preventive effects of an abbreviated version of the Coping Power Program for aggressive children? *Journal of Abnormal Child Psychology, 42*, 367–381.

Lochman, J. E., Boxmeyer, C., Andrade, B., & Kassing, F. (2019). Coping power. In B. Fiese, M. Celano, K. Deater-Deckard, E. Jouriles, & M. Whisman (Eds.), *APA handbook of contemporary family psychology, volume 3: Family therapy and training* (pp. 361–376). Washington, DC: American Psychological Association.

Lochman, J. E., Boxmeyer, C. L., Ialongo, N. S., McDaniel, S. C., Pas, E. T., & Powell, N. P. (2019). Tier II family-school partnership programs. In A. Garbacz (Ed.), *Implementing family-school partnerships: Student success in school psychology research and practice* (pp. 88–110). New York: Routledge.

Lochman, J. E., Boxmeyer, C. L., Jones, S., Qu, L., Ewoldsen, D., & Nelson III, W. M. (2017). Testing the feasibility of a briefer school-based preventive intervention with aggressive children: A hybrid intervention with face-to-face and internet components. *Journal of School Psychology, 62*, 33–50. https://doi.org/10.1016/j.jsp.2017.03.010

Lochman, J. E., Boxmeyer, C. L., Powell, N., Qu, L., Wells, K., & Windle, M. (2009). Dissemination of the coping power program: Importance of intensity of counselor training. *Journal of Consulting and Clinical Psychology, 77*, 397–409.

Lochman, J. E., Boxmeyer, C. L., Powell, N. P., Qu, L., Wells, K., & Windle, M. (2012). Coping power dissemination study: Intervention and special education effects on academic outcomes. *Behavioral Disorders, 37*, 192–205.

Lochman, J. E., Boxmeyer, C. L., Powell, N. P., Siddiqui, S., Stromeyer, S. L., & Kelly, M. (2012). Anger and aggression: School-based cognitive-behavioral interventions. In R. B. Mennuti, R. W. Christner, & A. Freeman (Eds.), *Cognitive-behavioral interventions in educational settings: A handbook for practice* (2nd ed., pp. 305–338). New York: Routledge.

Lochman, J.E., Bradshaw, C.P., Powell, N., Debnam, K., Pas, E., & Ialongo, N. (2016, June). Preventing conduct problems in middle schoolers: Preliminary effects of the Early Adolescent Coping Power Program. Paper presented in a symposium (C. Bradshaw, chair) at the 24th Annual Meeting of the Society for Prevention Research, San Francisco.

Lochman, J. E., Dishion, T. J., Powell, N. P., Boxmeyer, C. L., Qu, L., & Sallee, M. (2015). Evidence-based preventive intervention for preadolescent aggressive children: One-year outcomes following randomization to group versus individual delivery. *Journal of Consulting and Clinical Psychology, 83*, 728–735.

Lochman, J. E., & Dodge, K. A. (1994). Social-cognitive processes of severely violent, moderately aggressive and nonaggressive boys. *Journal of Consulting and Clinical Psychology, 62*, 366–374.

Lochman, J. E., Powell, N., Clanton, N., & McElroy, H. (2006). Anger and aggression. In G. Bear & K. Minke (Eds.), *Children's needs III: Development, prevention, and intervention*. Washington, DC: National Association of School Psychologists.

Lochman, J. E., & Wells, K. C. (2002). Contextual social-cognitive mediators and child outcome: A test of the theoretical model in the Coping Power Program. *Development and Psychopathology, 14*(4), 945–967.

Lochman, J. E., & Wells, K. C. (2004). The Coping Power Program for preadolescent aggressive boys and their parents: Outcome effects at the one-year follow-up. *Journal of Consulting and Clinical Psychology, 72*, 571–578.

Lochman, J. E., Wells, K. C., Qu, L., & Chen, L. (2013). Three year follow-up of coping power intervention effects: Evidence of neighborhood moderation? *Prevention Science, 14*, 364–376.

Matthys, W., & Lochman, J. E. (2017). *Oppositional defiant disorder and conduct disorder in childhood* (2nd ed.). Chichester, West Sussex, England: Wiley-Blackwell.

Mayer, G. R. (1995). Preventing antisocial behavior in the schools. *Journal of Applied Behavior Analysis, 28*, 467–478.

McCabe, K. M., Lucchini, S. E., Hough, R. L., Yeh, M., & Hazen, A. (2005). The relation between violence exposure and conduct problems among adolescents: A prospective study. *American Journal of Orthopsychiatry, 75*, 575–584.

McCart, M. R., Priester, P. E., Davies, W. H., & Azen, R. (2006). Differential effectiveness of behavioral parent-training and cognitive-behavioral therapy for antisocial youth: A meta-analysis. *Journal of Abnormal Child Psychology, 34*(4), 527–543.

McCart, M. R., & Sheidow, A. J. (2016). Evidence-based psychosocial treatments for adolescents with disruptive behavior. *Journal of Clinical Child & Adolescent Psychology, 45*, 529–563.

McDaniel, S. C., Lochman, J. E., Tomek, S., Powell, N., Irwin, A., & Kerr, S. (2018). Reducing levels of behavioral risk in late elementary school: A comparison of two targeted interventions. *Behavioral Disorders, 43*, 370–382.

Muratori, P., Bertacchi, I., Giuli, C., Nocentini, A., & Lochman, J. E. (2017). Implementing Coping Power adapted as a universal prevention program in Italian primary schools: A randomized control trial. *Prevention Science, 18*, 754–761.

Muratori, P., Bertacchi, I., Masi, G., , Milone, A., Nocentini, A., Powell, N. P., Lochman, J. E., Jones, S., Kassing, F., & Romero, D. (2019). Effects of a universal prevention program on externalizing behaviors: Exploring the generalizability of findings across school and home settings. *Journal of School Psychology, 77*, 13–23.

Muratori, P., Lochman, J. E., Bertacchi, I., Giuli, C., Guarguagli, E., Pisano, S., et al. (2019). Universal Coping Power for pre-schoolers: Effects on children's behavioral difficulties and pre-academic skills. *School Psychology International, 40*(2), 128–144.

National Institute for Health and Care Excellence (NICE). (2013). *Antisocial behaviour and conduct disorders in children and young people: Recognition and management—Tools and resources*. Retrieved from https://www.nice.org.uk/guidance/cg158/resources.

Neamţu, G. M., & David, O. A. (2016). Coaching emotional abilities in fostered adolescents through rational emotive and cognitive-behavioral education: Efficacy and mechanisms of change of using therapeutic stories. *Journal of Evidence-Based Psychotherapies, 16*(1), 33–56.

Nelson, W. M., III, & Finch, A. J. (2000). *Children's inventory of anger*. Los Angeles, CA: Western Psychological Services.

O'Neill, R. E., Homer, R. H., Albin, R., Storey, K., & Sprague, J. R. (1990). *Functional analysis of problem behaviors: A practical assessment and intervention strategies*. Baltimore: Paul H. Brookes Publishers.

Reynolds, C. R., & Kamphaus, R. W. (2015). *Behavior assessment system for children* (3rd ed.). Bloomington, IL: NCS Pearson, (BASC–3).

Rimm-Kaufman, S. E., Early, D. M., Cox, M. J., Saluja, G., Pianta, R. C., Bradley, R. H., et al. (2002). Early behavioral attributes and teachers' sensitivity as predictors of competent behavior in the kindergarten classroom. *Journal of Applied Developmental Psychology, 23*(4), 451–470.

Roland, E., & Galloway, D. (2002). Classroom influences on bullying. *Educational Research, 44*, 299–312.

Ryan, A., & Ladd, G. (2012). *Peer relationships and adjustment at school*. Charlotte, NC: Information Age Publishing.

Schuiringa, H., van Nieuwenhuijzen, M., Orobio de Castro, B., Lochman, J. E., & Matthys, W. (2017). Effectiveness of an intervention for children with externalizing behavior and mild to borderline intellectual disabilities: A randomized trial. *Cognitive Therapy and Research, 41*, 237–251.

Shin, S.-K. (2009). Effects of a solution-focused program on the reduction of aggressiveness and the improvement of social readjustment for Korean youth probationers. *Journal of Social Service Research, 35*, 274–284. https://doi.org/10.1080/01488370902901079

Stormshak, E. A., Bierman, K. L., McMahon, R. J., Lengua, L. J., & the Conduct Problems Prevention Research Group. (2000). Parenting practices and child disruptive behavior problems in early elementary school. *Journal of Clinical Child Psychology, 29*, 17–29.

Stromeyer, S. L., Lochman, J. E., Kassing, F., & Romero, D. (2020). Cognitive-behavioral therapy with angry and aggressive youth: The Coping Power Program. In R.D. Friedberg & B.Nakamura (Eds.), *Cognitive Behavioral Therapy in Youth: Tradition and Innovation* (pp. 109–124). New York: Springer

Sukhodolsky, D. G., Kassinove, H., & Gorman, B. S. (2004). Cognitive-behavioral therapy for anger in children and adolescents: A meta-analysis. *Aggression and Violent Behavior, 9*(3), 247–269.

Trip, S., Vernon, A., & McMahon, J. (2007). Effectiveness of rational-emotive education: A quantitative meta-analytical study. *Journal of Cognitive & Behavioral Psychotherapies, 7*(1), 81–93.

Chapter 14
Rational-Emotive and Cognitive-Behavioral Treatment for Attention-Deficit/Hyperactivity Disorder Among Youth

Kristene A. Doyle and Mark D. Terjesen

Attention-deficit/hyperactivity disorder (ADHD) is one of the most common disorders of childhood and adolescence, with current estimates conservatively placed at 5% to 7% globally (Polanczyk, de Lima, Horta, Biederman, & Rohde, 2007; Thomas, Sanders, Doust, Beller, & Glasziou, 2015). Researchers have reported that boys are more than twice as likely to be affected by ADHD than girls (American Psychiatric Association [APA], 2013; Hartung & Lefler, 2019; Willcutt, 2012), with there being about a 57% chance of a child having ADHD if their parent does and a 32% chance if their sibling does (Barkley, 2015b).

Diagnostic and Statistical Manual of Mental Disorders (DSM), fifth edition, states that children with this disorder predominantly have difficulty in two major areas: inattention and hyperactivity/impulsivity (American Psychiatric Association, 2013). As indicated in the DSM-5, these symptoms need to be seen in two or more settings, and several of these symptoms must be present before the age of 12. Examples offered of these types of behavior may include difficulty sustaining attention, difficulty following directions, trouble organizing tasks, makes careless mistakes, loses things, is often "on the go," has difficulty waiting their turn, struggles to remain in their seat and adhere to rules in the classroom, and refraining from interrupting (American Psychiatric Association, 2013).

The DSM-5 identifies and describes three types of ADHD (attention-deficit/hyperactivity disorder): predominantly inattentive type, predominantly hyperactive-impulsive type, and combined presentation (American Psychiatric Association, 2013). Children who are diagnosed with the inattentive type of ADHD generally

K. A. Doyle
Albert Ellis Institute, New York, NY, USA
e-mail: krisdoyle@albertellis.org

M. D. Terjesen (✉)
Department of Psychology, St. John's University, Jamaica, NY, USA
e-mail: terjesem@stjohns.edu

M. Bernard, M. D. Terjesen (eds.), *Rational-Emotive and Cognitive-Behavioral Approaches to Child and Adolescent Mental Health: Theory, Practice, Research, Applications*, https://doi.org/10.1007/978-3-030-53901-6_14

exhibit difficulty in organization, following directions, and in sustaining attention while ignoring extraneous/distracting stimuli (Roberts, Milich, & Barkley, 2014). The hyperactive-impulsive type of ADHD lacks the attention difficulties but presents with more hyperactive and impulsive problems (e.g., impatience, acting without thought, excessive fidgetiness, impulsive responding, and difficulty speaking in turn) (Roberts et al., 2014). The combined type of ADHD contains a mixture of the other two categories, with the child exhibiting at least six symptoms that characterize inattention, hyperactivity, and impulsivity (American Psychiatric Association, 2013). In addition, the DSM-5 also states that there must be clear evidence of impairment in social, academic, or occupational functioning (American Psychiatric Association, 2013).

Biological Origin of the Disorder: Primary Symptoms

Unlike many of the other childhood disorders, ADHD is conceptualized as primarily a biological or neurodevelopmental disorder. While precise causes or specific genes linked to ADHD have not been identified as of yet, there is some promising work in identifying specific genomes for ADHD (Biederman & McGough, 2016; Faraone & Larsson, 2019; Nigg, Nikolas, & Burt, 2010). To further support a biological model, the effectiveness of stimulant medication and structural imaging research supports a biological explanation of the disorder. Some research has shown that among students with ADHD, they have significantly smaller volumes in the dorsolateral prefrontal cortex (Seidman, Valera, & Makris, 2005). Further, Rapport et al. (2008) propose that the behaviors demonstrated by students with ADHD are impacted by neural maturation in the cortical regions that are incomplete which is key to the planning and organizational aspects of behavior. Some recent findings may further support the argument to have interventions that target the affective state of students with ADHD beyond medication. Tseng and colleagues (Tseng et al., 2019) used an fMRI to look at the brain activity of 195 youth while they played a computerized attention game that was developed to mimic the type of daily frustration that students experience (e.g., stop playing a game and get ready for bedtime). They found that those who got irritated the most following frustration had more neural activation in the frontal-striatal region of the brain, an area associated with impulse control/inhibition, and regulating attention. Interestingly, there was no difference in brain activation during the frustration experience for those on medication, which the authors suggest that the current medication used to treat ADHD may not be targeting the neural circuits linked to irritability. As such, these findings may lead to the fact that additional interventions are needed to address the irritability component and rational-emotive cognitive-behavioral therapy (RE-CBT) with its focus on targeting frustration intolerance may in fact be that approach.

The secondary features of ADHD (academic underachievement, frustration intolerance (FI), interpersonal difficulties, etc.) are seen as byproducts of the core features (Rapport, Chung, Shore, & Isaacs, 2001). For a more extensive review of ADHD's etiology, please see Barkley (2015b).

RE-CBT Conceptualization of the Secondary Symptoms Associated with ADHD

Along with the core symptoms of ADHD, the majority of students with the diagnosis of ADHD are also diagnosed with at least one other coexisting condition (Elia, Ambrosini, & Berrettini, 2008; Larson, Russ, Kahn, & Halfon, 2011), and many of them manifest subclinical levels that warrant attention. The challenge clinically may be that the symptoms and behaviors of ADHD may obscure the other affective and behavioral concerns. While ADHD may be considered to be more of a biological disorder than many of the other clinical disorders discussed in this edited book, the secondary symptoms, including academic underachievement (DuPaul, Gormley, & Laracy, 2013; National Center for Learning Disabilities [NCLD], 2014), interpersonal difficulties (Hoza et al., 2000), depression and anxiety (Elia et al., 2008), and frustration intolerance (Melegrii et al., 2015), can be explained from a nonbiological perspective.

Academic Underachievement

Children with ADHD tend to experience difficulties with their academic work including academic achievement due to their deficits in attention and their disorganization as well as when they present with comorbid learning disabilities/difficulties. DuPaul (2013) estimates that between 31% and 45% of children with ADHD also have a learning disability (LD). The relationship of ADHD to subsequent academic underachievement is quite strong (Frazier, Youngstrom, Glutting, & Watkins, 2007) and is complicated by lower seatwork completion and more off-task behavior and poorer homework performance than their peers (Mautone, Marshall, Costigan, Clarke, & Power, 2012; Merrill et al., 2017). Academic underachievement is predictable in children with ADHD with or without LD as inattention and/or disorganization and/or impulsivity throws the learner off task.

There are two central aspects as it relates to the academic achievement challenges that students with ADHD experience that we propose the RE-CBT clinician address: namely, ratings of worth (i.e., self-downing) and the resultant affective and cognitive experiences of depression and frustration intolerance which may lead to patterns of work avoidance. In our experience, we have seen that students with ADHD who have experienced a pattern of repeated failure have a greater tendency to rate themselves as "stupid" or view themselves as a "loser." That is, they view their performance, which often may be lower than that of their peers, and develop this type of self-schema. This may then in turn lead students with ADHD to in fact believe this schema and behaviorally engage in a self-fulfilling prophecy (e.g., "Why bother trying? I am stupid and will just fail") and may in fact result in them performing more poorly in school than their normal ability would predict.

Furthermore, these same children have a general approach to learning characterized by frustration intolerance, which manifests itself in many arenas including academic achievement. Students with ADHD may have notable challenges in persistence as a result of both their impulsivity and distractibility as well as based on what they tell themselves. When young people approach their academic work believing, "I can't stand this! It's too hard for me. It should be easier," they are less likely to persevere, and as a result, learning and grades suffer. This frustration intolerance may lead to the avoidance of learning tasks which increases their risk for poor academic performance which in itself may lead to self-downing and depression. The mindset that consists of self-downing and frustration intolerance equips the learner with a mindset that is not conducive to academic achievement.

Difficulties in Interpersonal Relationships

Children with ADHD often experience comorbid social problems and aggressive behavior including, in extreme cases, conduct disorder (e.g., Lewsinson, Shankman, Gau, & Klein, 2004). As students with ADHD may interrupt conversations or engage in a number of negative interpersonal behaviors, they may also experience social rejection (Marshall, Evans, Eiraldi, Becker, & Power, 2014). From an RE-CBT perspective, while some of the social challenges experienced may be a function of the symptoms of ADHD, an understanding of the emotional challenges that they may experience in interpersonal relationships can be further understood by examining the irrational beliefs of those children with ADHD, who also experience interpersonal difficulties. Aduen et al. (2018) reported that the social difficulties students with ADHD often experience are not skill acquisition deficits but rather skill performance deficits. Further, Wells and colleagues (Wells, Day, Harmon, Groves, & Kofler, 2019) showed that while emotion recognition abilities are intact among youth with ADHD, they may have difficulty with misreading ambiguous social cues, making irrational demands, and drawing hostile conclusions. Cognitions such as "I should be included in the game," "They should treat me nicely," "This is terrible" (catastrophizing and awfulizing), "I can't stand to be excluded" (interpersonal FI), and "Peers who treat me unfairly are very bad and deserve to be punished" (e.g., global rating of others) warrant identification, and clinical work with these students may help them develop more healthy beliefs and as a result engage in more adaptive behaviors that may in fact promote greater peer engagement

Depression

As indicated previously, clinical work and case conceptualization of RE-CBT with young people with ADHD may wish to consider the potential secondary experience of depression as a result of repeated failures and rejections. This depression may result from specific beliefs that students may hold about themselves (e.g., "I must be liked/accepted//competent…"), and if they do not, as a result they may conclude in self-depreciating beliefs (e.g., "…and if I'm not, then I'm unlovable/I'm nobody/ I'm incompetent") (Dryden, 2001), which may result in the student experiencing depression. Given many of the attentional and behavioral difficulties inherent in ADHD, some children with this diagnosis may be inclined to have unhealthy beliefs such as demandingness and self-downing which may then lead to feelings of depression.

Assessment and Diagnosis of ADHD

Parents and teachers most often may be the primary referral source for children who present with symptoms that may be seen to be consistent with a diagnosis of ADHD (DuPaul & Kern, 2011). An accurate diagnosis to develop treatment planning is integral to outcome, with diagnosis being derived from an empirically sound, multidimensional approach (Barkley, 2015a).

To guide in the diagnosis and treatment of children with attention-deficit/hyperactivity disorder (ADHD), the American Academy of Pediatrics (AAP, 2019) published a clinical practice guideline that we encourage the reader to consider in conducting a diagnostic assessment. This may assist in the specific choice of modality (interview, observation, rating scales) as well as which ones to consider. A full review of diagnostic and broad and narrow-band measures is beyond the scope of this chapter, but we do wish to highlight a number of considerations for clinicians before they commence with an evaluation.

Prior to beginning any evaluation, we think it important for clinicians to be mindful of a number of factors to consider in a diagnosis of ADHD. First, it is important to consider the purpose of the assessment. We agree that the goal of assessment would be to guide educational and treatment considerations (Pelham, Fabiano, & Massetti, 2005). In so doing, the DSM criteria can also describe behaviors of "normal" children, and as such, it is important for clinicians to consider age-appropriate criteria especially in diagnosing young children (APA, 2013; Terjesen, Sciutto, & O'Brien, 2019). That is, are the behaviors being demonstrated common in many children at this age, and if so, at what point does it become an area of clinical concern?

Another area for clinicians to be mindful of is the fact that the problematic behaviors of ADHD are only considered a disorder when they impair daily functioning in two or more settings (APA, 2013). As such, it is important for the clinician to look at the context in which the child is exhibiting the behaviors and how the environment could be impacting the child's behavior and possibly be maintaining it. Therefore, clinicians would benefit from collecting "data" regarding the potential diagnosis from multiple sources in multiple settings.

The comorbidity of an ADHD diagnosis with other disorder discussed earlier may also interfere with an accurate diagnosis. That is, are some of the symptoms being seen reflective of ADHD or another primary diagnosis? Gathering a thorough history from parents/guardians and teachers may assist in gathering rating scales and determining next step(s) in an assessment and diagnosis. Checklists for rating ADHD symptoms and ruling out other diagnoses and behaviors of concern are often used by clinicians (Pelham et al., 2005) and assist in understanding the age appropriateness of the behaviors as well as how they may lead to functional impairment.

Given the degree of overlap among disorders, the clinician would be well-served to choose assessment measures that specifically address the symptoms that are specific to ADHD as well as assess those symptoms/disorders (i.e., depression, anxiety) that tend to be observed with, or perhaps be a consequence of, the diagnosis of ADHD.

While structured diagnostic interviews are often part of a confirmatory approach for a research diagnosis of ADHD, the research does not support that they add incrementally to an ADHD diagnosis over rating scales (Pelham et al., 2005). Given this along with the time-consuming factor of these interviews, we do not recommend them for diagnostic purposes, but they may assist in gathering additional information about the behavior. A behavioral observation of the target behaviors may include an examination of the antecedents of the behavior as well as the consequences. Conducting a functional analysis of the behavior has been linked to more positive treatment outcomes (Miller & Lee, 2013). Given the behavioral manifestations of ADHD, it stands to reason that these are often the targets for assessment. However, an area that is often overlooked is the cognitions that are frequently associated with it. Having a greater understanding of these beliefs can be important clinically because if they are not successfully addressed, the development of secondary emotional disturbances and possibly further exacerbation of symptoms that are part of the disorder may occur. As such, we will briefly outline the irrational and erroneous beliefs that clinicians may wish to assess and treat in the student with ADHD and their family.

The rational emotive behavior therapy (REBT) and CBT literature is replete with a number of scales (Terjesen, Salhany, & Sciutto, 2009), but many of them have been developed with adults and extended downward for clinical work with youth. Two specific measures that we recommend that are consistent with the REBT and CBT model are the Child and Adolescent Scale of Irrationality (CASI; Terjesen, Kassay, & Anderson, 2017) and the Children's Automatic Thoughts Scale (CATS; Schniering & Rapee, 2002). The CASI was built off of the model of REBT and has 36 items that students are asked to indicate a degree of agreement with the statement that reflects either an irrational or rational belief. The authors reported good reliability and some support for the factor structure of the measure. The CATS assesses negative beliefs in a manner that is consistent with the CBT model and is used for both internalizing and externalizing problems. Given the secondary symptoms that students diagnosed with ADHD may present with, we argue that evaluation of and direct clinical work for these thoughts may help reduce any negative impact on young people's achievement, well-being, and social relationships.

Research on RE-CBT with ADHD

The research on REBT and CBT with ADHD is limited and is not clinically indicated for the core symptoms of ADHD. Pelham (2002) concluded that despite there being a number of studies that examined the effectiveness of cognitive-behavioral approaches for treating ADHD, they do not meet the criteria for empirical support. However, Pelham posits that perhaps cognitive based interventions could have adjunctive treatment benefit for maintenance of behavioral and pharmacologic treatment as well as for treatment of other clinical issues associated with the disorder. In considering the role of cognitive interventions, Hinshaw (2000) emphasized that in work with children diagnosed with ADHD they be linked with behavioral reinforcement strategies.

As we discussed above and outline later in this chapter, we believe that REBT and CBT can play a unique role in the treatment of ADHD that perhaps the pharmacologic, behavioral parent training, and behavior classroom approaches may fail to do: treatment of the secondary symptoms (anger, anxiety, and depression) associated with ADHD. From a research perspective, the exact role of REBT in the treatment of ADHD is an area that still needs to be further examined empirically. Given that we have research which describes the efficacy of behavior management and psychopharmacologic interventions, REBT can be utilized to treat these secondary emotional disturbances often seen in children with ADHD and their accompanying cognitions. Additional research on REBT as a clinical approach toward increasing treatment compliance, managing many of the emotive and social difficulties that may accompany the disorder, preventing further difficulties, and assisting the student and family in reducing difficulties and enhancing the quality of their lives and their relationship is clearly warranted.

Developmental Considerations in Clinical Work with Students with ADHD

With the changes in the DSM (APA, 2013) for symptom presentation (before the age of 12) and number of symptoms as a function of age (one fewer for adolescents), it is important for clinicians to consider a student's age relative to the diagnostic criteria. Age relative to peers is important to consider as well as the fact that students who are the youngest in their classroom tend to be diagnosed much more frequently compared to their classmates. Hyman, DuPaul, and Gormley (2017) argue the importance of using age-based norms when assessing for ADHD to reduce any bias regarding younger students.

A challenge clinically for diagnostic purposes is that in early childhood, many students may exhibit high levels of inattention and hyperactivity, and as such, it may be difficult to differentiate problematic ADHD-related behavior (DuPaul & Kern, 2011). As we move up the developmental continuum, the degree of impairment may increase with age (Barkley, Murphy, & Fischer, 2008).

From an RE-CBT-based model, the age and developmental level of the child are important factors to consider before proceeding with cognitive restructuring (discussed below). Children may lack the cognitive ability to understand certain concepts presented during treatment and may also lack the verbal ability to express their thoughts and feelings. Cognitive restructuring involves disputation of irrational beliefs that may lead to these secondary disturbances which are difficult for children under the age of 11 to comprehend because they have not yet moved into the formal operational thinking stage (Bernard & Joyce, 1984). While not specific to the disorder of ADHD, we have found that students who frequently endorse FI beliefs tend to be less mature and are also not as effective in disputation ("It's too difficult"). We believe that it is important for the clinician to consider both a child's chronological and developmental age when developing disputation strategies. In consideration of application of RE-CBT as a function of developmental level, the reader is referred to Grave and Blisset (2004) and Garber, Frankel, and Herrington (2016).

Best Practice Guidelines in the Treatment of ADHD

As we aim to review the application of RE-CBT in clinical work with ADHD, a complete review of all interventions for ADHD is beyond the scope of this chapter. However, we thought it important to briefly review the evidence-based approaches for ADHD below. The reader is referred to the clinical practice guidelines of the American Academy of Pediatrics (AAP, 2019) for a more comprehensive review.

Pharmacological Treatments

Stimulant medications are considered to be among the more effective approaches for treating children with ADHD and are often considered the first treatment option with over 80% of youth with ADHD having a prescription for stimulants (Visser et al., 2015). Estimates are that up to 90% of children taking stimulant medication will show improvement in ADHD symptoms (Connor, 2015).

There are both short-acting stimulants (e.g., dextroamphetamine and methylphenidate) that show benefits for 3–4 hours and long-acting stimulants (e.g., Concerta and Vyvanse) having a clinical impact for 10–12 hours (Daughton & Kratochvil, 2009). There are a number of non-stimulant medications (Strattera) which the research indicates has smaller effects than those seen through stimulants (Faraone, Biederman, & Mick, 2006) but the change is more gradual (Daughton & Kratochvil, 2009).

While medication does have empirical support, given the high percentage of students who experience side effects (Connor, 2015), there may be some resistance on the part of students and families to use them. Further, not all students respond to medication (Chronis, Jones, & Raggi, 2006), and when not taking the medication, some of the academic, behavioral, and social issues persist.

Behavioral Interventions

Parenting Behavioral Training

Behavioral parent training (BPT) has strong empirical support (Evans, Owens, & Bunford, 2014) and involves clinicians working directly with parents to teach strategies to manage their children's behavior (Altszuler, Macphee, & Merrill, 2017; Raghibi, Fouladi, & Bakhshani, 2014). Altszuler et al. (2017) describe a set of core parent training topics that have been found to be effective across behavioral parent training programs, and these include but are not limited to establishing house rules, effective commands and rewarding compliance, contingent attention, time-out and loss of privileges, home reward systems, and generalizing and maintaining games.

Classroom Behavioral Interventions

Similar to the work done with parents, behavioral interventions in schools are also highly effective and involve teachers implementing behavioral interventions such as token reinforcement or response cost (DuPaul, Eckert, & Vilardo, 2012; Evans, et al., 2014). DuPaul and Stoner (2014) discuss a number of the key steps to be considered in implementing a behavioral intervention in the classroom that integrate many of the same principles of reinforcement in BPT. Self-regulation strategies such as self-monitoring and self-evaluation can be used to facilitate maintenance and generalization of behavioral improvements obtained through a token reinforcement program (DuPaul & Stoner, 2014). For example, students can be prompted at specific intervals to monitor and record their on-task behavior and/or their productivity on academic tasks (Reid, Trout, & Schartz, 2005). The process of self-monitoring involves observing and recording one's behaviors and includes two basic steps. First, the student must determine if the target behavior has occurred, and following that determination, the student must record that occurrence or non-occurrence (Mace, Belfiore, & Hutchinson, 2001). Some variations of this strategy include an initial stage of matching with teacher evaluations followed by gradual transition to self-evaluation alone (DuPaul & Stoner, 2014).

As ADHD behavior needs to be demonstrated across more than one environment, a daily report card (DRC) system is an evidence-based approach to foster home-school communication (Evans et al., 2014; Fabiano et al., 2010).

Organizational Skills Training

Students with ADHD often have difficulty with executive functioning tasks like planning, organization, and time management (Hyman et al., 2017), and these areas of deficit are not addressed via medication (Abikoff et al., 2009). The research is new and promising in executive training for students with ADHD (Langberg, Epstein, & Graham, 2008; Tamm, Nakonezny, & Hughes, 2014) and involves teaching them note-taking strategies, how to complete homework efficiently and accurately, and strategies to organize school materials.

Peer-Based Interventions

Although medication may assist in decreasing impulsive social behaviors of children with ADHD, it does not teach the appropriate social behaviors that may not have been learned at this point. Although Social Skills Training (SST) is often part of a school-based ADHD treatment plan, the evidence behind them is inconsistent (Altsczuler et al., 2017; Evans et al., 2014). However, Altsczuler and colleagues point out that more intensive programs like a Summer Treatment Program (STP) that target social interactions have been shown to impact social behavior.

With a number of evidence-based approaches for treatment of ADHD, the RE-CBT practitioner would also benefit from examining treatment history, child and parental compliance, and perceived treatment acceptability. This may help guide treatment selection as perhaps families who had a low level of adherence to a previous intervention may have done so out of a philosophical disagreement ("I don't believe in medicating children") or because of their own faulty beliefs ("It's too difficult to stick to the token economy plan!").

RE-CBT in the Treatment of ADHD

As mentioned earlier, RE-CBT does not directly treat the core symptoms of ADHD but rather the secondary symptoms or problem behaviors that may be related to their diagnosis and may impact their affective and behavioral states. From an REBT model, we will examine each irrational belief individually and look at the impact of each in clinical work with youth with ADHD.

Frustration Intolerance (FI)

Children and adolescents often demonstrate FI, often referred to as "I can't stand it" (Ellis & MacLaren, 1998) for events when they believe that it is *too* difficult for them to handle/persevere/deal with. Often defined in the REBT literature as having a low tolerance for frustrating situations and a need for immediate gratification, FI is present in various degrees in all children, regardless of diagnosis. In consideration of FI with children with ADHD, it may present itself in extreme forms in both academic and social/interpersonal situations. Academically, when a student with ADHD may have difficulty in the classroom attending to instruction or they are asked to complete a task that may be more challenging for them than most, many children will tell themselves, "This is too hard! I can't stand this. It shouldn't be this difficult." Now for other students without ADHD in the class, it may be true that the work may in fact *be* easier for them, and this difference may be quite obvious to those with the diagnosis. FI may then subsequently lead to work avoidance, and as such, they may fail to meaningfully engage with the learning experience and they may in fact do worse, which often contributes to subsequent self-downing and self-rating (discussed below). FI may also present itself in the challenges that a student with ADHD experiences in social/interpersonal relationships. Their difficulty interpreting and reacting to social cues may lead the student with ADHD to further compound these social deficits as a result of their FI.

As an example of the impact of FI, it is not uncommon when working with children with ADHD to hear that they may have experienced a fight/disagreement with a peer in the school yard. When you probe further, the following Activating Event (A)-Belief (B)-Consequence (C) framework becomes clear:

A: The other students were playing dodgeball during recess, and they said I had to wait for the next game.

B: I can't stand waiting! This is ridiculous. I need to play right now!!!

C: Anger, pushing one's way into the game and then having the subsequent fight.

As children with ADHD demonstrate behaviors that reflect their FI beliefs at the moment, they are less inclined to attend to other important stimuli, such as the verbal and nonverbal behaviors of their classmates. So while they may get what they want in the short term (I got to play the game), as a result, they may experience subsequent peer rejection given their behavior which may trigger further emotional and behavioral difficulties.

Self and Other Rating

As mentioned above, children and adolescents with ADHD, because of the social skills deficits and academic difficulties, upon reflection may view themselves (and not their behavior) poorly and put themselves down. Students may comment that "I'm a loser. Nobody likes me. I'm stupid." These rating of worth beliefs may lead them to experience chronic thoughts of inferiority which can be challenging as they learn to adjust to and cope with ADHD. Estimates are that 15% of children with ADHD may also be diagnosed with depression (Larson et al., 2011) and these students may experience depression and/or thoughts of hopelessness, further withdraw academically and socially, and not experience any further opportunity to develop appropriate skills.

In addition to depression, 41% of students with ADHD experience oppositional defiant disorder (Elia et al., 2008), and 27% with ADHD are diagnosed with a conduct disorder (Larson, 2011). Not taking away any biological factors for this comorbidity, additional contributions may come from how students think about the behavior of others. In the face of rejection or school failure experiences, students may globally rate others (e.g., "They're stupid") which in turn may give rise to extreme feelings of anger, and they may then engage in maladaptive behaviors (e.g., arguing, fighting). This further hinders their efforts to be successful in their schoolwork and relationships.

We recommend that when considering depression, anger, and conduct behaviors, the clinician look at the student's beliefs and work to help them understand the difference between rating oneself or another and rating one's behavior. This is particularly important with ADHD because, at least during the academic years, such individuals may in fact struggle academically and socially. If they rate themselves as *totally stupid*, any academic and social difficulties may be exasperated by such a cognitive style. Further, globally rating a peer, parent, or teacher may further hinder their social development. Unconditional self- and other-acceptance, although difficult concepts to teach adults, should be a focal point of treatment for children and adolescents with ADHD.

Demandingness Beliefs

The REBT model proposes that when students rigidly hold onto beliefs that would be considered to be demands, they may experience negative affective and behavioral outcomes. To be clear, much like the other beliefs, demands are not specific to children with ADHD. Different forms of demandingness are seen in children with and without diagnoses. Students may report demands of self ("I *should be* a better student"; "I *have to* do well in the game") which may lead to feelings of depression. Further, students may endorse demands of others ("I *shouldn't* be told what to do"; "They *should* listen to me"; "I *should* be able to do whatever I want"), and these often will result in unhealthy negative emotions and behavior such as anger and aggression often seen in students with conduct disorder or oppositional defiant disorder. Finally, demands of the world ("Things *shouldn't* be this difficult"; "This *shouldn't* be happening to me?") may lead to both anger and depression. In clinical work with youth, we often look for what the students' hard and fast "rules" are for how they, others, and things should be and then work toward challenging those beliefs.

Awfulizing

The REBT model posits that students experience significant negative affective (anxiety) and behavioral (avoidance) consequences when they engage in patterns of thinking that would be considered to be catastrophizing or awfulizing. That is, they consider past, present, or future events and the consequences of such to be terrible, horrible, and awful. Many children and adolescents with ADHD experience performance and evaluative anxiety. We believe that it is important for the clinician to look at what precedes the anxious behavior in terms of what activating event are they making themselves anxious about; specifically, is it of a social nature or of an evaluative nature? While both involve the child believing the potential consequences to be "awful," the beliefs attached to them may be very distinct. For example, "What if I try and join in on the game and the others reject me? *That would be awful, horrible, the end of the world*" may lead to social anxiety and avoidance, while "What if I tried really hard and did poorly on my test? *That would be horrible and terrible*" may lead to performance anxiety and as such a negative performance on an exam.

The following section provides a review of REBT and allied cognitive-behavioral interventions that are available to practitioners in working with young people with ADHD who experience a range of secondary symptoms and comorbid conditions.

REBT-Based Interventions

Developing a therapeutic alliance with youth is not something specific to ADHD nor RE-CBT, but we think it is important to acknowledge that this can be particularly challenging for the clinician working with the child with ADHD and their family. Oftentimes, children with ADHD are in therapy not because of their own choice but rather because their behavior has now become problematic to others (e.g., parent, teacher) in varied settings. We have found that recognizing this with the students can be helpful as well as providing structure to the therapy session by integrating therapeutic goals and tasks to achieve those goals with something that the child may enjoy. Establishing clear session expectations and developing mechanisms to monitor therapy assignment completion also help develop this relationship and allow the child to experience some success, something that may be missing from other aspects of his/her life.

We have found that incorporating an in-session reward/token economy system to increase attention to clinical work may prove advantageous to make the most out of the session. The use of a game to teach the concept of frustration tolerance has also been helpful for such children. For example, playing a board game allows for both an informal assessment of their problem-solving and affective management strategies and also provides an opportunity for modeling of high frustration tolerance self-statements such as "This is tough but I can get through it!" This assists the student with ADHD in seeing that there is another way that they may think about a problem. Further, the opportunity to provide direct feedback for the child as to how the clinician feels when he/she is interrupted or when the child does not allow turn-taking can be an invaluable step in assisting the child to develop better social skills.

Cognitive Restructuring of Unhealthy Beliefs

Part of an RE-CBT treatment for the secondary difficulties that students with ADHD may experience involves educating them about the role that their thinking plays in their emotional and behavioral problems. Too often clinicians will hear students remark: "He *made* me so angry I had to hit him" or "The situation *makes* me anxious." Before progressing to any disputation of these beliefs, it is important to teach children with ADHD the cognitive model of emotions and behaviors. Teaching the concept that one's beliefs/thoughts/cognitions contribute to feelings/emotions/behaviors is essential. The ABC framework (activating events, beliefs about those events, and subsequent healthy and unhealthy emotions and behaviors) preferably should be the cornerstone of clinical interventions.

We have found that this ABC framework is best taught by incorporating a specific problem the child or adolescent brings into the counseling environment. This makes what can be an abstract concept more concrete and relative to the child. Hence, emotional and behavioral responsibility on the part of the child becomes a primary therapy goal.

Challenging these automatic thoughts and irrational beliefs is key to therapeutic change among youth. Within the REBT framework, these challenges are referred to as disputations, but now may be referred to as discussing, debating, or restructuring. The different types of disputations described in the REBT literature (empirical, logical, heuristic/functional, philosophical, semantic, friend) (see Bernard, 2004) can be used to identify, challenge, and change irrational beliefs to rational beliefs. We offer examples as to how clinicians may wish to challenge frustration intolerance, awfulizing, demandingness of self/others and the world, and self and other global ratings with consideration of working with students with ADHD.

Disputing frustration intolerance is interesting when working with children with ADHD, as there may be some validity to the fact that things may in fact be more difficult for them in comparison to their peers and may be a function of their diagnosis. We recommend that the clinician acknowledge that certain tasks may be more difficult but remind the student that thinking it is *too* difficult will only further serve to have a negative impact upon their performance. We ask children to consider other times when they have thought things are "too difficult and unbearable" and have them discuss whether things were as difficult as they projected. This is more of an evidence-based approach toward challenging their beliefs. We also will use the functional challenge of: "Is thinking this is TOO hard helping you complete this task? Does thinking this way cause you more grief and make the task take even longer?" Having students recognize that it is difficult and they don't like it but can stand it may assist in increasing persistence and perhaps an experience of success.

We have found that when working with children with ADHD, it is often important to dispute "catastrophic" thinking of children and adolescents. Vernon (2002) has a number of techniques and interventions to use to dispute what is referred to as "awfulizing." Here, the clinical work is to have children with ADHD recognize that they make themselves feel anxious about social or academic situations by telling themselves a number of unhealthy thoughts: "It would be the WORST thing ever" if something happened or didn't happen. Working with children to correctly evaluate just how bad the situation would be (empirical) as well as looking at these thoughts from a functional ("Does thinking this way help you deal with this?") and semantic ("How do we define awful? Is it beyond bad? Does this lead to that criterion level?") questions will reduce their level of anxiety.

With disputing of demands, we have found that functional disputes ("How does thinking this way help me reach my goal?") can be especially helpful for a child/adolescent with ADHD. Oftentimes, the empirical ("Where is the evidence for my belief?") and logical ("Does my demand make sense?") disputes pose a challenge to children in terms of comprehension. As an example, a student may think his parent *should* buy him the latest gaming platform because it was reduced in price by 75%. When asked if that belief makes sense/is logical, they may argue back that "Of course it does! Mom always is concerned about money and this is a huge discount. She should get it for me!" Here is where the functional dispute may be among the better choices. By assisting children to help them see that their current way of thinking, especially demandingness, is not working for them and at the same time is *not* changing the reality, this may result in a more flexible style of thinking as well as more adaptive (but possibly negative) affective state.

Disputing global self-ratings (i.e., I'm a loser) is a critical intervention for most young people with ADHD. We have found that with youth, the fruit bowl analogy (DiGiuseppe, Doyle, Dryden, & Backx, 2013) is very effective to teach the concept of unconditional self- and other-acceptance. In this analogy, the clinician presents to the student the idea of a fruit dish, with all different types of fruits, including oranges, apples, pears, and bananas, with one of the bananas having a brown spot on it. The clinician then poses to the student the following question: "What do you do with the fruit dish? Throw it away?" Typically, the student will respond with something to the effect of: "Of course not. Eat around the brown spot, or pick off the brown spot." The clinician then connects the concept of acceptance of self and others with our own brown spots. That is, we have good traits/behaviors and bad traits/behaviors. We do not lose all the positive things about ourselves if we experience something negative. Disputes that use analogies and are more abstract in nature may be more applicable to adolescents. With younger children, perhaps concrete disputations (empirical) with accompanying behavioral/experiential exercises are more appropriate.

Use of Rational Self-Statements

In addition to challenging faulty beliefs when working with children and adolescents with ADHD, the RE-CBT model stresses the importance of developing healthier rational self-statements that will promote greater frustration tolerance and fewer unhealthy affective and behavioral responses. We think it important that the clinician work to have these new beliefs be theoretically and empirically opposite of the unhealthy beliefs while also validating some of the healthy negative affect that they would still experience if they did believe this new way of thinking. As an example, if a student believes that "They *can't stand* having to do dumb homework," after the clinician works with the student to challenge/dispute that belief (e.g., "Is it true that you cannot stand it? How is it helping you to think that way? Do you finish the homework any more quickly?"), we would work with the student on a healthy, rational alternative. We prefer to use the student's own words, but if this does not occur initially, we may provide them with a model: "While I may not like having to do dumb homework, and really would rather not have to do it, *I can stand it.*" We think it is important to model a strong tone and conviction of this new belief at a level above and beyond the level of the irrational belief.

Cognitive-Behavioral Rehearsal/Role Play and Homework

An important consideration is to have clinical gains generalized beyond the counseling office. We have found that while students may agree with the newer healthier beliefs in the therapy session, their ability to adopt and apply this new philosophy in the real world may be challenging. As the irrational beliefs may be their "default" when students are put in similar situations that they struggled with in the past, children and adolescents may tend to go back to faulty patterns of thinking and not recall the new belief system. We have found that through role-playing in the session, an opportunity is provided to test the student's ability to demonstrate their new way of thinking. The clinician may challenge their "new philosophy" by using some of their own words (prior faulty ideas) against them. By having them practice disputation aloud and rehearsing healthier ways of thinking, this may further reinforce the internalizing of their new philosophy. Role-playing also allows the clinician to provide feedback on more effective disputation strategies and observe student behavior in session and provide feedback.

REBT and CBT are very active approaches and often involve having students engage in various activities in between sessions to gather further evidence against their irrational beliefs and reinforce their new philosophy. Rather than calling it homework, we refer to these as "activities" that we will have the students work on between sessions. We think it important that these activities are generated *with* the students as we have found that they are more likely to commit to working on one of these activities if they are also responsible for choosing it. Activities may be assessment driven (e.g., "Write down your thoughts and feelings when you get upset this week"), behavioral/experiential in nature (e.g., "Start conversations with three peers this week"), risk-taking (e.g., "Raise your hand in class when you are not sure of the answer"), or cognitive (e.g., "Practice disputing in front of a mirror five times this week"). We have found that by changing activities weekly, this will often lead to increased compliance and engagement in assignment completion. When generating assignments, we encourage clinicians to look for any barriers (i.e., practical or emotional) that the child or family may think would interfere with completion of this activity this week. Depending on these potential barriers, we may seek to modify the assignment or spend time in session challenging the beliefs that interfere with completion (e.g., "You say that texting others to ask them to do something is TOO hard to do. I know it may be uncomfortable, but maybe we can look at if it really is TOO hard or just difficult"). Typically, we begin the next session by assessing their completion of the between-session assignment and reinforce completion, and if it was not completed, we examine what may have led to non-completion.

Case Study

The case below was treated by the first author (KD).

Robert is a 16-year-old 11th grader who lives with his mother in New York City. Robert's parents divorced when he was 10 years old. Robert came to therapy upon a recommendation made in a comprehensive neuropsychological evaluation he had to assist in educational planning. A review of the neuropsychological report indicated that Robert has an educational classification of Other Health Impaired and receives resource room, integrated co-teaching services in English and intermittent counseling. He also receives accommodations in the form of a copy of class notes for major academic classes and special seating arrangements. Robert was previously diagnosed with attention-deficit/hyperactivity disorder and an anxiety disorder. Robert is also prescribed Sertraline and Concerta by a psychiatrist. Robert's grades were reported to be variable, and it was noted that he was having particular difficulty in the area of writing.

It was reported that Robert's cognitive/intellectual abilities revealed scores consistently within normal limits. Robert's academic abilities fell within the average range. His scores in the areas of *reading* and *mathematics* fell within normal limits. Although *writing* was noted to be an area of weakness for Robert, he performed within normal limits on tasks of written language. An assessment of Robert's memory and learning revealed that Robert has significant difficulty attending to and recalling non-meaningful, rote, sequential information. This score profile is often associated with difficulties with sustained attention.

Difficulties in the areas of sustained attention were revealed, which is consistent with Robert's previous diagnosis of attention-deficit/hyperactivity disorder. Robert had significant deficits in his auditory attention. Not only did Robert have difficulty attending to visual and auditory stimuli, but also on tasks of auditory attention, he made an elevated number of anticipatory errors and had an atypically fast response speed. This indicates that Robert attempted to respond too quickly, and these responses were often inaccurate.

Robert's performance on tasks of executive functioning generally fell within or above normal limits. On a task that required Robert to *inhibit impulsive responding*, his performance indicated that he does have the ability to stop himself from automatically providing a response, but he appears to have to put forth significant cognitive energy when utilizing self-regulation and cognitive self-monitoring in order to inhibit impulsive responding. This increases the amount of time it takes him to complete a task with such demands.

On tasks of *planning, reasoning, and problem-solving*, Robert's performance was consistently at or above the expected levels. Robert's social, emotional, and behavioral functioning was assessed via parent and self-report on the Multidimensional Anxiety Scale for Children – Second Edition (MASC-2), parent report on the Conners 3 Behavior Rating Scale, and a brief clinical interview. Significant symptoms of anxiety were reported based on both parent and self-report measures. According to both Robert and his mother, very elevated scores were obtained in the areas of total anxiety, generalized anxiety, social anxiety, and physical symptoms. This is consistent with Robert's previous diagnosis of anxiety disorder. Robert's mother also completed a general behavior checklist, which revealed concerns regarding Robert's attention, hyperactivity/impulsivity, learning problems, executive functioning, and defiance/aggression. The teacher version of the Conners 3 (short form) was administered to several of Robert's teachers in November 2017. Results revealed elevations on the inattention scale (mathematics, social studies, and English). The hyperactivity/impulsivity scale was elevated according to Robert's math teacher. The learning problems scale was elevated based on the responses of Robert's social studies, science, and English teachers. The defiance/aggression scale was within normal limits according to all teacher reports. The peer relations scale was elevated based on the responses of Robert's mathematics teacher.

Of note, on the self-report scale, Robert's responses yielded very elevated scores in the areas of humiliation/rejection, panic, and generalized anxiety. Robert reported that he often worries about doing something stupid or embarrassing, often worries other people are laughing at him, is often afraid that other kids will make fun of him, is often afraid other people will think he is stupid, and often worries what other people think of him. On the panic scale, Robert reported that he often has sweaty or cold hands, often feels his heart race, sometimes has pains in his chest, and sometimes feels dizzy or faint. The obsessions and compulsions scale was in the elevated range, as Robert endorsed symptoms such as often getting really upset about dirt, germs, chemicals, radiation, or sticky things, often fearing he will be responsible for something bad happening, often checking that nothing terrible has happened, often having to check things several times or more, and sometimes repeating things until it feels just right. These results yielded very elevated scores for both total anxiety and generalized anxiety.

During conversational dialogue during the evaluation process, Robert reported that he often gets what he referred to as "jitters." He reported that his knee will shake when he has the jitters. Robert went on to describe that when he first began to notice that this was happening, he became concerned that he would stand out, but after his mother suggested that he look around at his peers, he realized that many of them also shake their knees. He then described this as "an ADHD thing."

The Conners 3 Behavior Rating Scale - Parent Report was administered to Robert's mother. Responses revealed numerous scales within the very elevated range, which resulted in a very elevated score in the Conners 3 Global Index ($t = 84$), which is an overall measure of behavioral difficulty. The inattention scale ($t = 85$) and the hyperactivity/impulsivity scale were also in a very elevated range ($t = 75$). The executive functioning scale was also very elevated ($t = 77$). Robert's mother reported that he often fails to finish things he starts, often has trouble getting started on tasks or projects, often completes projects at the last minute, is rarely good at planning ahead, and often has trouble organizing tasks or activities. The defiance/aggression scale also fell within the very elevated range ($t = 83$). Robert's mother noted that he is often angry and resentful, often tries to get even with people, very often threatens to hurt others, and very often swears and uses bad language. Some of these behaviors also contributed to a very elevated score on the DSM oppositional defiant disorder scale ($t = 81$). Robert's mother reports that he has a "short fuse and overreacts if he feels slighted." He also is overly sensitive and will avoid activities and shut down if he feels rejected. For example, he stopped attending a theater group he enjoyed because a girl he liked did not share similar feelings.

Based on the results of his most recent evaluation, Robert currently meets DSM-5 diagnostic criteria for attention-deficit/hyperactivity disorder – predominantly inattentive presentation (ICD 10: F90.0/DSM-5: 314.00) and anxiety disorder (ICD-10: F41.9/DSM-5: 300.00). In addition, despite the fact that Robert is currently prescribed medication for both his attention and anxiety, he continues to experience symptoms of both disorders, and they appear to be impacting his academic functioning at this time.

Treatment Plan Based on a review of the neuropsychological evaluation, as well as parent and adolescent interviews, the following treatment goals were established for Robert:

1. Teach Robert the underpinnings of REBT/CBT, including the ABC framework of emotional and behavioral disturbance. This is to help Robert understand the interconnection of his beliefs, feelings, and behaviors to help facilitate more effective emotive and behavioral responses.
2. Ensure Robert assumes emotional and behavioral responsibility.
3. Teach Robert to identify helpful ways of thinking about himself, others, and situations to replace the unhelpful ways he often thinks. Specifically, work on his beliefs about:
    (a) Rating himself globally as a failure or loser due to his attentional problems.

(b) Tasks being *too* difficult or *too uncomfortable* for him (frustration intolerance beliefs) which will serve to negatively impact upon his academic achievement and future occupational endeavors.
(c) Awfulizing about social rejection which may heighten his anxiety and impair his social performance.
(d) Demands of others' behavior, which may lead to social altercations.

4. Explain to Robert's parents the ABC framework to be able to serve as "coaches" at home.
5. Challenge Robert' demandingness of himself and others while emphasizing the rational alternative. Challenging an irrational belief while working on a rational alternative will help Robert internalize a new set of rational beliefs and connect these beliefs with more positive emotions and behaviors.
6. In order to reduce anxiety, dispute Robert's awfulizing about peer rejection, while at the same time providing social skills training and feedback.

Description of Therapy Case

In the initial therapy session, both Robert and his parents were asked to attend. With Robert's parents in the office, the underlying philosophy of REBT/CBT was described to them, using a specific problem highlighting his attentional issues brought up by Robert. The goal of this initial session was to have Robert and his parents leave with the ideas that (1) they are all individually responsible for their beliefs, feelings, and behaviors/actions and (2) it would be most helpful if they accept (albeit not like) Robert's current challenges, rather than make themselves disturbed by it, which only creates additional problems. Through didactic discussion, a coping statement was generated by Robert and his parents that each could employ throughout the week when Robert engaged in the identified problematic behavior of avoiding uncomfortable homework and instead playing video games. For his parents, this was, "While I don't like what is happening, getting overly upset about it by awfulizing will not help get Robert back on track." For Robert, he used the statement, "This homework is going to be annoying but I can tolerate it."

For therapy homework, which was presented as an "activity" to Robert so as to reduce the aversive nature the term "homework" typically carries, I asked him to practice telling himself that statement to increase the chance of success. Because he tended to beat himself up when he encounters academic difficulties, we collaboratively decided that he would also tell himself "Although I may struggle more than other kids in my class, that does not make me a total loser." Robert typed this statement in the Notes app of his iPhone to review throughout the week. In addition, I asked Robert to complete an REBT Self-Help Form (downloadable for free from albertellis.org in multiple languages) if he noticed he was avoiding schoolwork, feeling anxious, or putting himself down which we would review in the next session.

Both Robert and his parents were seen together for the first part of the second session. I followed-up on the activity given. Robert remembered to tell himself the statements "most of the time, when I didn't forget to look at my Notes on my phone." When I asked him how he felt after telling himself the statement, he stated, "Much better than when I call myself a loser!" I reinforced the idea of this helpful thinking (this also served to reinforce the B->C/iB->C connections). We then reviewed the Self-Help form, and it was clear that Robert had a tendency to be impulsive during school and experienced a great deal of frustration intolerance and then subsequent self-downing. Upon reviewing the form, Robert was surprised to see how often he beats himself up during the week. We agreed we would continue to make self-acceptance a priority for our initial sessions.

With respect to the experiment assigned to Robert's parents, they each reported doing better at their emotional responses when things got a bit rough at home, particularly when it was time for Robert to do his schoolwork. They reported that learning the concept of the B->C connection was most helpful for them. The remainder of the session was spent with Robert alone. During this time, as we reviewed a situation at school where Robert concluded he was being left out of a group discussion with his friends and started feeling anxious, I asked him directly, "What was flashing through your mind right before you got anxious"? Robert responded, "They think I have nothing to add to the conversation." When I tried an inference chain with Robert, he kept providing me with inferences and automatic thoughts, rather than an irrational belief. Given the hypothesis-driven nature of the REBT theory, and to avoid Robert from becoming frustrated with my questions, I offered to him that he *might have also been thinking* "They think I have nothing to add to the conversation and that sucks and is horrible." This was a hypothesis based on REBT's theory of anxiety that proposes that awfulizing is at the core of this emotion (Dryden, 2012). As a result, I was able to hypothesize what Robert was telling himself. He looked at me like I was psychic. I basically scored big time with a skeptical teenager! For homework (his activity), we negotiated that Robert Chris self-monitor the times that he catches himself getting anxious, and to see if he is awfulizing.

Subsequent sessions continued to address other irrational beliefs, particularly frustration intolerance about difficult schoolwork as well as self-rating. Robert's ability and willingness to identify his irrational beliefs, challenge them, and replace them with more helpful beliefs all contributed to less avoidance of his schoolwork and reduced fighting with his parents. He reported feeling better emotionally, and his peer relationships also improved. Robert's parents confirmed this report and noted that he appeared more confident. While not perfect, Robert benefited from REBT and understands that he will probably have to continually work on his thinking and behaviors throughout his life. Robert's parents also reported less emotional disturbance in themselves and although divorced often used each other as reminders of what they learned in therapy and assist one another when they "slipped." Robert and his parents reported that although they have a better grip of the problem, they understand that they may need to return to therapy in the future, particularly around times of transition to college.

Adaptation of RE-CBT in the Schools for ADHD

As schools are where ADHD may often be initially identified and where the students are most likely experiencing difficulty, it would be important for the RE-CBT clinician to work collaboratively with the school and also help foster parent-school communication via a Daily Report Card. Educating school personnel as to what ADHD is and how behavioral interventions may be supported with simple rational-emotive and cognitive-behavioral techniques may further enhance success. Creating a list of coping statements that the student may have access to at her desk may also help reduce the frequency and intensity of any negative affective experiences. Working with school personnel to provide opportunities for students to build success while also reinforcing healthier ways of thinking through individual and group-based tasks may be another effective strategy. Finally, we would promote that as schools integrate social-emotional learning in the classroom, they consider an evidence-based approach that has a cognitive component to it to further prevent secondary emotional disturbances that students with ADHD may have.

Test Yourself

1. While medication and behavioral parent training have been effective in treating the core symptoms of ADHD, what other CB-REBT areas would clinicians want to consider in treating the secondary difficulties that are often seen among students with ADHD?
2. It is very important to consider possible alternative explanations for a child's apparent ADHD symptoms. What cognitions/beliefs might affect attention, impulse control, and activity level?
3. Sam is an 8-year-old boy with ADHD combined presentation. Sam's completion of classwork is very inconsistent, and he struggles to stay on task for more than 10 minutes at a time. He gets frustrated very easily and gives up. As a clinician, what beliefs do you think underlie his work effort and how would you go about targeting them from a CB-REBT perspective?

References

Abikoff, H., Nissley-Tsiopinis, J., Gallagher, R., Zambenedetti, M., Seyffert, M., Boorady, R., et al. (2009). Effects of MPH-OROS on the organizational, time management, and planning behaviors of children with ADHD. *Journal of the American Academy of Child & Adolescent Psychiatry, 48*(2), 166–175. https://doi.org/10.1097/CHI.0b013e3181930626

Aduen, P. A., Day, T. N., Kofler, M. J., Harmon, S. L., Wells, E. L., & Sarver, D. E. (2018). Social problems in ADHD: Is it a skills acquisition or performance problem? *Journal of*

Psychopathology and Behavioral Assessment, 40(3), 440–451. http://dx.doi.org.jerome.stjohns.edu:81/10.1007/s10862-018-9649-7
Altszuler, A., Macphee, F., & Merrill, B. (2017). In A. Morrow, W. E. Pelham Jr., & N. K. Schatz (Eds.), *Clinical handbook of psychological disorders in children and adolescents: A step-by-step treatment manual*. New York.
American Academy of Pediatrics, Subcommittee on Children and Adolescents with Attention-Deficit/Hyperactivity Disorder. ADHD: Clinical practice guideline for the diagnosis, evaluation, and treatment of children and adolescents with attention-deficit/hyperactivity disorder. *Pediatrics*, September 30th, 2019.
American Psychiatric Association. (2013). *Diagnostic and statistical manual of mental disorders* (5th ed.). Washington, DC: Author.
Barkley, R. A. (2015a). Emotional dysregulation is a core component of ADHD. In R. A. Barkley (Ed.), *Attention-deficit hyperactivity disorder: A handbook for diagnosis and treatment* (pp. 81–115). New York: The Guilford Press.
Barkley, R. A. (2015b). Etiologies of ADHD. In R. A. Barkley (Ed.), *Attention-deficit hyperactivity disorder: A handbook for diagnosis and treatment* (4th ed., pp. 356–390). New York: Guilford Press.
Barkley, R. A., Murphy, K. R., & Fischer, M. (2008). *ADHD in adults: What the science says*. New York: Guilford.
Bernard, M. E. (2004). *The REBT therapist's pocket companion for working with children and adolescents*. New York: Albert Ellis Institute.
Bernard, M., & Joyce, M. (1984). *Rational-emotive therapy with children and adolescents: Theory, treatment strategies, preventative methods (Wiley series on personality processes)*. New York: Wiley.
Biederman, J., & McGough, J. J. (2016). Advances in the neurobiology of attention-deficit/hyperactivity disorder and related disorders. *Journal of the American Academy of Child and Adolescent Psychiatry,* 55(10). https://doi.org/10.1016/j.jaac.2016.07.173.
Chronis, A. M., Jones, H. A., & Raggi, V. L. (2006). Evidence-based psychosocial treatments for children and adolescents with attention-deficit/hyperactivity disorder. *Clinical Psychology Review, 26*(4), 486–502. https://doi.org/10.1016/j.cpr.2006.01.002
Connor, D. F. (2015). Stimulant and nonstimulant medications for childhood ADHD. In R. A. Barkley (Ed.), *Attention-deficit hyperactivity disorder: A handbook for diagnosis and treatment* (4th ed., pp. 666–685). New York: The Guilford Press.
Daughton, J. M., & Kratochvil, C. J. (2009). Review of ADHD pharmacotherapies: Advantages, disadvantages, and clinical pearls. *Journal of the American Academy of Child & Adolescent Psychiatry, 48*(3), 240–248. https://doi.org/10.1097/CHI.0b013e318197748f
DiGiuseppe, R. A., Doyle, K. A., Dryden, W., & Backx, W. (2013). *A practitioner's guide to rational-emotive behavior therapy*. New York: Oxford University Press.
Dryden, W. (2001). *Reason to change: A rational emotive behaviour therapy (REBT) workbook*. East Sussex: Psychology Press.
DuPaul, G. J., Eckert, T. L., & Vilardo, B. (2012). The effects of school-based interventions for attention deficit hyperactivity disorder: A meta-analysis 1996–2010. *School Psychology Review, 41*(4), 387–412. https://doi.org/10.1080/02796015.2012.12087496
DuPaul, G. J., Gormley, M. J., & Laracy, S. D. (2013). Comorbidity of LD and ADHD: Implications of DSM-5 for assessment and treatment. *Journal of Learning Disabilities, 46*(1), 43–51.
DuPaul, G. J., & Kern, L. (2011). *Young children with ADHD: Early identification and intervention*. Washington, DC: American Psychological Association.
DuPaul, G. J., & Stoner, G. (2014). *ADHD in the schools: Assessment and intervention strategies*. New York: Guilford Publications.
Elia, J., Ambrosini, P., & Berrettini, W. (2008). ADHD characteristics: I. Concurrent co-morbidity patterns in children & adolescents. *Child and Adolescent Psychiatry and Mental Health, 2*, 15.
Ellis, A., & MacLaren, C. (1998). *Rational emotive behavior therapy: A therapist's guide*. Oakland: Impact Publishers.

Evans, S. W., Owens, J. S., & Bunford, N. (2014). Evidence-based psychosocial treatments for children and adolescents with attention-deficit/hyperactivity disorder. *Journal of Clinical Child & Adolescent Psychology, 43*, 527–551. https://doi.org/10.1080/15374416.2017.1390757

Fabiano, G. A., Vujnovic, R. K., Pelham, W. E., Waschbusch, D. A., Massetti, G. M., Pariseau, M. E., et al. (2010). Enhancing the effectiveness of special education programming for children with attention deficit hyperactivity disorder using a daily report card. *School Psychology Review, 39*(2), 219–239. https://doi.org/10.1080/02796015.2010.12087775

Faraone, S. V., Biederman, J., & Mick, E. (2006). The age-dependent decline of attention deficit hyperactivity disorder: A meta-analysis of follow-up studies. *Psychological Medicine, 36*(2), 159–165. https://doi.org/10.1017/S003329170500471X

Faraone, S. V., & Larsson, H. (2019). Genetics of attention deficit hyperactivity disorder. *Molecular Psychiatry, 24*(4), 562–575. http://dx.doi.org.jerome.stjohns.edu:81/10.1038/s41380-018-0070-0

Frazier, T. W., Youngstrom, E. A., Glutting, J. J., & Watkins, M. W. (2007). ADHD and achievement: Meta-analysis of the child, adolescent, and adult literatures and a concomitant study with college students. *Journal of Learning Disabilities, 40*(1), 49–65. https://doi.org/10.1177/00222194070400010401

Garber, J., Frankel, S. A., & Herrington, C. G. (2016). Developmental demands of cognitive behavioral therapy for depression in children and adolescents: Cognitive, social, and emotional processes. *Annual Review of Clinical Psychology, 12*, 181–216. https://doi.org/10.1146/annurev-clinpsy-032814-112836

Grave, J., & Blissett, J. (2004). Is cognitive behavior therapy developmentally appropriate for young children? A critical review of the evidence. *Clinical Psychology Review, 24*, 399–420. https://doi.org/10.1016/j.cpr.2004.03.002

Hartung, C. M., & Lefler, E. K. (2019). Sex and gender in psychopathology: DSM-5 and beyond. *Psychological Bulletin, 145*(4), 390–409. http://dx.doi.org.jerome.stjohns.edu:81/10.1037/bul0000183

Hinshaw, S. P. (2000). Attention-deficit/hyperactivity disorder: The search for viable treatments. In P. C. Kendall (Ed.), *Child & adolescent therapy: Cognitive–behavioral procedures* (pp. 88–128). New York/London: Guilford Press.

Hoza, B., Owens, J. S., Pelham, W. E., Swanson, J. M., Conners, C. K., Hinshaw, S. P., et al. (2000). Parent cognitions as predictors of child treatment response in attention-deficit/hyperactivity disorder. *Journal of Abnormal Child Psychology, 28*, 569–583.

Hyman, S., DuPaul, G. J., & Gormley, M. J. (2017). Evidence-based assessment and intervention for ADHD in school psychology. In M. Thielking & M. Terjesen (Eds.), *Handbook of Australian school psychology*. Cham: Springer. https://doi.org/10.1007/978-3-319-45166-4_16

Langberg, J. M., Epstein, J. N., & Graham, A. J. (2008). Organizational-skills interventions in the treatment of ADHD. *Expert Review Neurotherapeutics, 8*(10), 1549–1561. https://doi.org/10.1586/14737175.8.10.1549

Larson, K., Russ, S. A., Kahn, R. S., & Halfon, N. (2011). Patterns of comorbidity, functioning, and service use for US children with ADHD, 2007. *Pediatrics, 127*(3), 462–470.

Lewsinson, P. M., Shankman, S. A., Gau, J. M., & Klein, D. (2004). The prevalence and comorbidity of sub threshold psychiatric conditions. *Psychological Medicine, 34*, 613–622.

Mace, F. C., Belfiore, P. J., & Hutchinson, J. M. (2001). Operant theory and research on self-regulation. In B. J. Zimmerman & D. H. Schunk (Eds.), *Self-regulated learning and academic achievement: Theoretical perspectives* (pp. 39–65). Mahwah, NJ: Lawrence Erlbaum Associates Publishers.

Marshall, S. A., Evans, S. W., Eiraldi, R. B., Becker, S. P., & Power, T. J. (2014). Social and academic impairment in youth with ADHD, predominately inattentive type and sluggish cognitive tempo. *Journal of Abnormal Child Psychology, 42*(1), 77–90. https://doi.org/10.1007/s10802-013-9758-4

Mautone, J. A., Marshall, S. A., Costigan, T. E., Clarke, A. T., & Power, T. J. (2012). Multidimensional assessment of homework: An analysis of students with ADHD. *Journal of Attention Disorders, 16*(7), 600–609. https://doi.org/10.1177/1087054711416795

Melegari, M. G., Nanni, V., Lucidi, F., Russo, P. M., Donfrancesco, R., & Cloninger, C. R. (2015). Temperamental and character profiles of preschool children with ODD, ADHD, and anxiety disorders. *Comprehensive Psychiatry, 58*, 94–101. http://dx.doi.org.jerome.stjohns.edu:81/10.1016/j.comppsych.2015.01.001

Merrill, B. M., Morrow, A. S., Altszuler, A. R., Macphee, F. L., Gnagy, E. M., Greiner, A. R., et al. (2017). Improving homework performance among children with ADHD: A randomized clinical trial. *Journal of Consulting and Clinical Psychology, 85*(2), 111–122. http://dx.doi.org.jerome.stjohns.edu:81/10.1037/ccp0000144

Miller, F. G., & Lee, D. L. (2013). Do functional Behavioral assessments improve intervention effectiveness for students diagnosed with ADHD? A single-subject meta-analysis. *Journal of Behavioral Education, 22*, 253–282. https://doi.org/10.1007/s10864-013-9174-4

National Center for Learning Disabilities (NCLD). (2014). *The state of learning disabilities: Facts, trends and indicators*. New York: Author.

Nigg, J., Nikolas, M., & Burt, S. A. (2010). Measured gene-by-environment interaction in relation to attention-deficit/hyperactivity disorder. *Journal of the American Academy of Child and Adolescent Psychiatry, 49*(9), 863–873. https://doi.org/10.1016/j.jaac.2010.01.025

Pelham, W. E. (2002). Psychosocial interventions for ADHD. In P. S. Jensen & J. R. Cooper (Eds.), *Attention deficit hyperactivity disorder state of science- best practices* (pp. 12-4–12-7). Kingston, VIC, Australia: Civic Research Institute.

Pelham Jr., W. E., Fabiano, G. A., & Massetti, G. M. (2005). Evidence-based assessment of attention deficit hyperactivity disorder in children and adolescents. *Journal of Clinical Child and Adolescent Psychology, 34*(3), 449–476.

Polanczyk, G., de Lima, M. S., Horta, B. L., Biederman, J., & Rohde, L. A. (2007). The worldwide prevalence of ADHD: A systematic review and meta-regression analysis. *American Journal of Psychiatry, 164*, 942–948. https://doi.org/10.1176/ajp.2007.164.6.942

Raghibi, M., Fouladi, S., & Bakhshani, N. M. (2014). Parent training and behavior therapy on behaviors of children with attention deficit-hyperactivity disorder. *Health Scope, 3*(2), 1–4. https://doi.org/10.17795/jhealthscope-15418

Rapport, M. D., Alderson, R. M., Kofler, M. J., Sarver, D. E., Bolden, J., & Sims, V. (2008). Working memory deficits in boys with attention-deficit/hyperactivity disorder (ADHD): The contribution of central executive and subsystem processes. *Journal of Abnormal Child Psychology, 36*(6), 825–837. https://doi.org/10.1007/s10802-008-9215-y

Rapport, M. D., Chung, K. M., Shore, G., & Isaacs, P. (2001). A conceptual model of child psychopathology: Implications for understanding attention deficit hyperactivity disorder and treatment efficacy. *Journal of Clinical Child & Adolescent Psychology, 30*(1), 48–58. https://doi.org/10.1207/S15374424JCCP3001_6

Reid, R., Trout, A. L., & Schartz, M. (2005). Self-regulation interventions for children with attention deficit/hyperactivity disorder. *Exceptional Children, 71*(4), 361–377. https://search.proquest.com/docview/201228664?accountid=134752

Roberts, W., Milich, R., & Barkley, R. A. (2014). Primary symptoms, diagnostic criteria, subtyping and prevalence of ADHD. In R. A. Barkley (Ed.), *Attention deficit hyperactivity disorder: A handbook for diagnosis & treatment* (4th ed., pp. 51–80). New York: Guilford Press.

Schniering, C. A., & Rapee, R. M. (2002). Development and validation of a measure of children's automatic thoughts: The children's automatic thoughts scale. *Behaviour Research and Therapy, 40*(9), 1091–1109. https://doi.org/10.1016/S0005-7967(02)00022-0

Seidman, L. J., Valera, E. M., & Makris, N. (2005). Structural brain imaging of attention-deficit/hyperactivity disorder. *Biological Psychiatry, 57*(11), 1263–1272. https://doi.org/10.1016/j.biopsych.2004.11.019

Tamm, L., Nakonezny, P. A., & Hughes, C. W. (2014). An open trial of a metacognitive executive function training for young children with ADHD. *Journal of Attention Disorders, 18*(6), 551–559. https://doi.org/10.1177/1087054712445782

Terjesen, M. D., Kassay, K., & Anderson, D. (2017). Evaluation of the psychometric properties of a measure of child irrationality. *Journal of Rational-Emotive & Cognitive-Behavior Therapy, 35*(4), 413–431. https://doi.org/10.1007/s10942-017-0269-z

Terjesen, M. D., Salhany, J., & Sciutto, M. J. (2009). A psychometric review of measures of irrational beliefs: Implications for psychotherapy. *Journal of Rational-Emotive & Cognitive-Behavior Therapy, 27*, 83–96. https://doi.org/10.1007/s10942-009-0093-1

Terjesen, M. D., Sciutto, M. J., & O'Brien, C. (2019). Behavior rating scales and the assessment of ADHD in early childhood: A review of psychometric properties and scale features. *Perspectives on Early Childhood Psychology and Education, 4*.

Thomas, R., Sanders, S., Doust, J., Beller, E., & Glasziou, P. (2015). Prevalence of attention-deficit/hyperactivity disorder: A systematic review and meta-analysis. *Pediatrics, 135*(4), e994–e1001. https://doi.org/10.1542/peds.2014-3482

Tseng, W. L., Deveney, C. M., Stoddard, J., Kircanski, K., Frackman, A. E., Yi, J. Y., et al. (2019). Brain mechanisms of attention orienting following frustration: Associations with irritability and age in youths. *American Journal of Psychiatry, 176*(1), 67–76. https://doi.org/10.1176/appi.ajp.2018.18040491

Vernon, A. (2002). Group counseling: Loss. In D. Capuzzi & D. R. Gross (Eds.), *Introduction to group counseling* (3rd ed., pp. 321–349). Denver, CO: Love Publishing Company.

Visser, S. N., Bitsko, R. H., Danielson, M. L., Ghandour, R. M., Blumberg, S. J., Schieve, L. A., et al. (2015). Treatment of attention deficit/hyperactivity disorder among children with special health care needs. *The Journal of Pediatrics, 166*(6), 1423–1430. https://doi.org/10.1016/j.jpeds.2015.02.018

Wells, E. L., Day, T. N., Harmon, S. L., Groves, N. B., & Kofler, M. J. (2019). Are emotion recognition abilities intact in pediatric ADHD? *Emotion, 19*(7), 1192–1205. http://dx.doi.org.jerome.stjohns.edu:81/10.1037/emo0000520

Willcutt, E. G. (2012). The prevalence of DSM-IV attention-deficit/hyperactivity disorder: A meta-analytic review. *Neurotherapeutics, 9*(3), 490–499. https://doi.org/10.1007/s13311-012-0135-8

Chapter 15
RE-CBT in the Treatment of Autism Spectrum Disorder

Korrie Allen and Veronica Milito

Overview of Autism Spectrum Disorder

Autism spectrum disorder (ASD) is a neurodevelopmental disability characterized by social deficits, communication impairments, and rigid, repetitive behaviors that limit or impair everyday functioning (DSM-V; American Psychiatric Association [APA], 2013). ASD is the fastest growing neurodevelopmental disability in the United States (Perihan et al. 2020), and it occurs in children of different racial, ethnic, and social backgrounds. The global prevalence of ASD has increased 20-fold to 30-fold since the earliest epidemiologic studies were conducted in the 1960s and 1970s (Centers for Disease Control and Prevention [CDC], 2018). The latest prevalence rates estimate the incidence of ASD to be one in every 59 children (one in 38 males, one in 152 females; Baio et al., 2018). Since 2000 alone, prevalence rates have increased by 154% (CDC, 2018), placing the total intervention cost in the United States between $11.5 billion and $60.9 billion and leading ASD to become an urgent public health concern (Baio et al., 2018; Perihan et al., 2020).

Many children with ASD also experience emotional and behavioral problems. Approximately 70% of individuals with ASD have one comorbid mental disorder and 40% have two or more comorbid mental disorders (DSM-V; APA, 2013). Reported prevalence rates of comorbid disorders are considerably higher than in typically developing children (Kerns & Kendall, 2012). Disruptive behaviors and anxiety (e.g., aggression, avoidance, and self-injury) are commonly reported in children with ASD (Bauminger, Solomon, & Rogers, 2010; Farmer & Aman, 2011a; Guttmann-Steinmetz, Gadow, & DeVincent, 2009; Research Units of Pediatric

K. Allen (✉)
Department of Child, Family and School Psychology, University of Denver, Denver, CO, USA

V. Milito
Department of School Psychology, St. Johns University, Queens, NY, USA

M. Bernard, M. D. Terjesen (eds.), *Rational-Emotive and Cognitive-Behavioral Approaches to Child and Adolescent Mental Health: Theory, Practice, Research, Applications*, https://doi.org/10.1007/978-3-030-53901-6_15

Psychopharmacology, 2005). Children with ASD are more likely to engage in aggressive and disruptive behaviors (e.g., tantrums, self-injury) toward themselves, family members, peers, and teachers (Farmer & Aman, 2011a; Kanne & Mazurek, 2011) which represent one of the most common reasons for referral to mental health clinics and emergency departments (Pikard, Roberts, & Groll, 2018).

The presence of clinically significant behavioral problems among children with ASD is widely acknowledged and cited; however, the exact prevalence varies greatly due to the frequent use of clinical samples in studies (for a review, see Fitzpatrick, Srivorakiat, Wink, Pedapati, & Erickson, 2016; Hill et al., 2014; Solomon, Ono, Timmer, & Goodlin-Jones, 2008) and inconsistent or ambiguous definitions of behavior problems (see Hill et al., 2014; Tremblay, Hartup, & Archer, 2005). Some literature has reported that 50–70% of clinically referred children and adolescents with ASD exhibited aggressive behavior to a caregiver, whereas other studies concluded that approximately 90% of study participants with ASD showed some form of challenging behavior (Jang, Dixon, Tarbox, & Granpeesheh, 2011; Kanne & Mazurek, 2011; Mazurek, Kanne, & Wodka, 2013; McTiernan, Leader, Healy, & Mannion, 2011). Additionally, clinically significant anxiety is present in approximately 50% of children with ASD (Wood et al., 2015). Anxiety and disruptive behavior frequently lead to impairment in adaptive functioning and seem to negatively affect quality of life (Steensel, Bogels, & Dirksen, 2012).

Implementing effective treatments in the community, school, and clinic setting for children with ASD and anxiety and/or disruptive behaviors is imperative to enhance functioning across multiple environments. Emerging research has highlighted the use of cognitive-behavioral therapy (CBT) approaches that adhere to evidence-based practices and methods to provide treatment for children with ASD and co-occurring mental health problems, particularly disruptive behavior and anxiety (e.g., Reaven, Blakeley-Smith, Leuthe, Moody, & Hepburn, 2012; White et al., 2013; Wood et al., 2015). The purpose of this chapter is to provide an overview of diagnostic criteria and assessment tools, developmental considerations when treating, and evidence-based cognitive-behavioral interventions for children with ASD and anxiety. This chapter will conclude with a case study and methods to translate the research to school settings.

Diagnostic Progression and Assessment

As indicated earlier, ASD is a neurodevelopmental disorder, meaning that the child's pattern of growth across areas of development is uneven, with skills growing at different rates than each other. For example, a 3-year-old with ASD may read sight words in books but not speak spontaneously. In 1943, Leo Kanner, an Austrian-American psychiatrist and physician, used the term autism to describe children with symptoms of social isolation and linguistic disorders without schizophrenia

(Kanner, 1943). The second edition of the American Psychiatric Association's Diagnostic and Statistical Manual of Mental Disorders (DSM-II; APA, 1952) defined autism as a form of childhood schizophrenia marked by detachment from reality. Not until the DSM-III (APA, 1980) was autism established as a diagnosis separate from schizophrenia and defined as a pervasive developmental disorder. In the DSM-IV, autism was categorized as a spectrum of conditions and included five pervasive developmental disorders (PDDs): autistic disorder, Asperger's syndrome, pervasive developmental disorder-not otherwise specified, Rett's disorder, and childhood disintegrative disorder (APA, 2000). Finally, in 2013, the DSM-5 introduced the term autism spectrum disorder with severity specifiers ranging from "Level 1: requiring support" to "Level 3: requiring very substantial support" (American Psychiatric Association, 2013).

Screening and Evaluation Process The American Academy of Pediatrics (AAP; 2007) recommends that pediatricians screen all 18- and 24-month-old children for ASD. The screening process typically involves gathering initial information about the behaviors of concern and determining the need for a comprehensive evaluation. There are several different screening measures developed for guardians and professionals to provide information regarding the child and his or her functioning (please see Table 15.1). If the screening results indicate the need for further evaluation, often, a multidisciplinary team conducts the evaluation (Harrington & Allen, 2013). A comprehensive evaluation involves collecting a comprehensive review of family and medical history, physical examination, and the use of multiple assessments to determine if a child meets the diagnostic criteria for autism spectrum disorder. The instruments included in the evaluation should be determined on a case-by-cases basis. The evaluation typically involves obtaining information from multiple assessments, observations, and data collection.

The assessment and diagnostic process is often stressful for the family and the child, and studies have shown that parents of children with ASD report higher levels of stress than parents of typically developing children (Baker-Ericzen et al., 2005; Bromley, Hare, Davison, & Emerson, 2004; McStay, Dissanayake, Scheeren, Koot, & Begeer, 2014). Research demonstrates that parents with high levels of irrational thoughts tend to rate their child's symptoms as more stressful and report higher levels of stress (Witt, 2005). The idea that irrational or negative automatic thoughts led to increased stress agrees with the cognitive-behavioral and rational emotive behavior therapy models. Specifically, the finding of a relationship between irrationality and parental stress among parents of children with ASD indicates needs for therapy that targets parental cognitions and the development of rational or positive automatic thoughts (Witt, 2005). The use of rational emotive behavior therapy (REBT; Ellis, 1962) and cognitive-behavioral therapy (CBT; Beck, 1967) to address parental stress and comorbid disorders associated with ASD such as anxiety has emerging research support as outlined below.

Table 15.1 Screening and diagnostic measures

Measure	Acronym	Age range	Description
Screening measures			
Infant and toddler checklist, also called communication and symbolic behavior scales developmental profile	ITC CSBS-DP	9–24 months	Designed to screen for communication delays but recently has tested well for early autism screening http://www.brookespublishing.com/store/books/wetherby-csbsdp/checklist.htm
Modified checklist for autism in toddlers	M-CHAT	16–30 months	A 23-item yes/no questionnaire based on earlier CHAT www.firstsigns.org and www.m-chat.org
Screening tool for autism in toddlers and young children	STAT	24–36 months	Empirically based, interactive measure developed to screen for autism. The STAT consists of 12 items that take approximately 20 minutes to administer. http://stat.vueinnovations.com
Social communication questionnaire	SCQ	4 years, with a mental age over 2 years	Brief instrument completed by a parent or primary caregiver that helps evaluate communication skills and social functioning in children who may have autism. Composed of 40 yes or no questions
Diagnostic measures			
Autism diagnostic interview-revised	ADI-R	Children and adults with mental ages above 18 months	Clinical diagnostic instrument that focuses on behavior in three main areas: Reciprocal social interaction, communication and language, and restricted and repetitive interests and behaviors
Autism diagnostic observation schedule-second edition	ADOS-2	12 months through adulthood	Semi-structured, standardized assessment of social interaction, communication, play, and imaginative use of materials. Consists of four 30-minute modules administered to different individuals according to their level of expressive language
Gilliam autism rating scale-second edition	GARS-2	3 years to 22 years	Norm-referenced instrument that assists teachers and clinicians in identifying and diagnosing autism and in estimating the severity of the child's disorder
Childhood autism rating scale-second edition	CARS-2	2 years and up	Brief assessment to identify children with autism and determine symptom severity through quantifiable ratings based on direct observation

Research on REBT and CBT for Children with ASD

Currently, the majority of REBT and CBT research among children with ASD focuses on treating comorbid disorders rather than the core symptoms of the ASD. Preliminary findings from randomized controlled trials examining CBT to treat the core symptoms of ASD demonstrate improvement in the areas of social problem-solving, peer engagement, and pro-social behavior (Wood et al., 2009); however, the majority of studies examine the impact of CBT to reduce anxiety and improve social skills. Treating the co-occurring mental health conditions for children with ASD is often critical to improving their functioning at home and school. Individuals with ASD often struggle with emotional regulation, and this may manifest as an externalizing disorder (e.g., disruptive behavior disorder) or an internalizing disorder (e.g., anxiety, depression) (Wood et al., 2017). Children with ASD and behavior problems may have difficulties enrolling and remaining in schools (Chalfant et al., 2007; Kanne & Mazurek, 2011). Aggressive behaviors also cause risk for physical harm, reduce quality of life, and are the greatest predictor of parental stress (Baker, Blacher, Crnic, & Edelbrock, 2002; Kanne & Mazurek, 2011). Failure to address behavioral problems and anxiety in children with ASD during early- to mid-childhood allows these behaviors to become established. Without intervention, problem behaviors are unlikely to ameliorate (Horner, Carr, Strain, Todd, & Reed, 2002; Oliver, Murphy, & Corbett, 1987; Rojahn, 1994). Finally, the presence of behavioral problems among children with ASD impedes developmental progress and the acquisition of key skills emphasized by early intensive behavioral interventions (Jang et al., 2011). When behavioral problems are addressed and decreased, children with ASD are more likely to comply with more intense and focused therapies (Masse, McNeil, Wagner, & Chorney, 2007).

Over the past 20 years, the research on anxiety and ASD has grown considerably. Wood and Gadow (2010) estimate that 7% to 57% of children with ASD experience anxiety compared to 2.2–27% among the general population. Anxiety among children with ASD has the potential to impact functioning across multiple environments as well as the ability to interact socially with others (Reaven et al., 2012). Specifically, excessive worry or rumination about social situations may compound the core deficits of ASD. Failing to treat children with ASD and anxiety may lead to limited social interactions or rejection, difficulties in the school setting, and underemployment as an adult.

The development of effective interventions to treat both disruptive behaviors and anxiety among youth with ASD is an important healthcare and educational priority (Perihan et al., 2020). Over the past decade, the research using CBT among children with ASD and anxiety has demonstrated positive outcomes (e.g., Reaven et al., 2012; White et al., 2013; Wood et al., 2015).

CBT was originally developed by Beck (1967) to address the causes of anxiety and depression. The primary goal of CBT is to teach individuals to identify irrational beliefs, monitor automatic thoughts, and replace negative automatic thoughts with more realistic and adaptive ones (Kendall and Hedtke, 2006). Programs typically involve using structured cognitive and behavioral techniques with specific sessions and instructions (Perihan et al., 2020). CBT is viewed as the gold standard approach for treating typically developing children with anxiety; therefore, researchers have studied the impact of using CBT among children diagnosed with ASD to reduce anxiety.

A primary principle of cognitive-behavioral intervention is that thoughts, feelings, and behaviors interact and significantly impact each other. Parental involvement in the treatment of children with ASD and anxiety seems to yield positive outcomes as well (e.g., Chalfant et al., 2007; Wood et al., 2015).

Predescu, Dobrean, Pop, Miclutia, and Sipos (2013) conducted a study to assess the presence of irrational beliefs among mothers of children with ASD based on the theory of REBT. Similar to CBT, REBT is an action-oriented approach to managing cognitive, emotional, and behavioral disturbances that places an emphasis on the present; individuals are taught how to examine and challenge their unhelpful thinking, which creates unhealthy emotions and self-defeating/self-sabotaging behaviors (Ellis & Bernard, 2006). The study found that parents of children with ASD experience higher levels of emotional distress that are associated with irrational thinking and limited coping skills. In addition, Witt (2005) also found that parents with high irrational beliefs rated their child's symptoms as more stressful. Not only are CBT and REBT beneficial for children, but including the parents in the treatment is likely to improve outcomes (e.g., White et al., 2013; Wood et al., 2009).

Because of the similarities between the behavioral problems exhibited by children with ASD and those displayed by typically developing children, it is appropriate to identify evidence-based treatments for disruptive behavior and anxiety that could be translated to an ASD population for the treatment of behavioral problems. REBT and CBT may reduce anxiety and improve behavior and consequently increase compliance with intense and focused ASD therapies such as Applied Behavior Analysis (ABA) or speech and occupational therapy across a range of modalities. Therefore, REBT and CBT should not supersede other therapies for ASD; rather, they may be used in conjunction as a first-line treatment to prepare ASD children for these other therapies by targeting comorbid disorders.

Developmental Considerations When Using REBT and CBT

Currently, many of the studies evaluating the impact of CBT focus on children with high functioning ASD. Children with ASD are more likely than typically developing children to exhibit intellectual delays, think rigidly, and exhibit difficulty interacting with peers. Thinking abstractly and forming relationships are often two difficult areas for children with ASD. Rotheram-Fuller and Hodas (2015) outline the importance of identifying a child's cognitive and behavioral functioning prior to starting an intervention to determine adaptations needed to make the intervention work best with the child. CBT requires the ability to think abstractly in order to engage in important aspects of the treatment such as cognitive restructuring, developing anxiety management skills, and participating in behavioral exposure to anxiety-provoking situations. In addition, process variables such as positive engagement and child-therapist alliance improve CBT outcomes.

In the area of cognitive functioning, the CDC (2018) reported that 31% of children with ASD were classified as having IQ scores in the range of intellectual disability (IQ ≤70), 23% in the borderline range (IQ = 71–85), and 46% in the average or above average range of intellectual ability (IQ >85). Recent research has been published demonstrating the effectiveness of CBT in Adults with an Intellectual Disability, but the research among children with ASD and intellectual delays is limited. Grave and Blissett (2004) found that typically younger children (preoperational) are less responsive to CBT than older children and adolescents and that age seems to mediate the efficacy of the treatment. Therefore, taking into account age and the cognitive ability of the child helps to determine whether rational-emotive cognitive-behavioral therapy (RE-CBT) is a viable treatment option or if adaptations to the treatment are warranted.

Additionally, positive engagement is important for beneficial outcomes, particularly when treating children with anxiety and ASD who tend to present as inhibited and withdrawn (Chu & Kendall, 2004). The therapist may have to use nontraditional strategies to develop a positive and warm relationship to engage the child in the therapeutic process (McLeod & Weisz, 2005). For example, engaging the child in an area of interest often helps them start to talk and engage in a more back-and-forth discussion. Other potential features of ASD that may impact CBT include difficulties with emotion recognition, causal reasoning, perspective taking, and empathy (Rotheram-Fuller & Hodas, 2015).

Best Practices and Evidence-Based Therapies to Treat Core Features of ASD

There are several established behavioral and educational therapies and treatments available to treat the core symptoms of autism. These include Applied Behavior Analysis (ABA), UCLA Young Autism Project, Pivotal Response Training (PRT), TEACCH Method, and DIR/Floortime. In addition, a body of research supports the use of pharmacological treatment to address irritability, aggression, and disruptive behavior. Below is a brief overview of the primary components of each treatment approach (for a comprehensive review, see Rogers & Vismara, 2008).

Behavioral Treatments The behavioral intervention literature has strong support for the effectiveness of comprehensive services for children with ASD. Established behavioral and educational therapies/treatments are available, including Applied Behavior Analysis (ABA), Early Intensive Behavioral Intervention (the UCLA Young Autism Project), Pivotal Response Training, Early Start Denver Model, Learning Experiences and Alternative Program for Preschoolers and their Parents, Treatment and Education of Autistic and Communication Handicapped Children

(TEACCH Method), Positive Behavior Support (PBS), and DIR/Floortime (Carroll & Kodak, 2019; Masse et al., 2007; Smith & Iadarola, 2015). These focused therapies employ a number of techniques to increase socially appropriate behaviors; decrease challenging behaviors; and improve language, social, and behavioral deficits in children with ASD (Carroll & Kodak, 2019).

Pharmacological Treatments

Several recent studies have established the short-term efficacy of antipsychotic medications (i.e., risperidone and aripiprazole) in the treatment of the acute symptoms of aggressive behaviors among children with ASD (Farmer & Aman, 2011a, 2011b; Volkmar, 2001). In addition, two recent studies examined the effectiveness of a combined medication plus parent training approach in treating children with ASD and challenging behavior (Aman et al., 2009; Frazier et al., 2010). In both studies, the greatest reduction in aggressive behaviors was reported in the combined treatment group when compared to medication alone. However, these studies did not examine the effectiveness of a behavior intervention alone, complicating the interpretation of the relative benefits of each treatment and the delineation of specific benefits, which may be present only when behavior management treatments are provided in the absence of medication. It is impossible to determine if the combination of treatments is synergistic or the same as one of the modalities used alone.

REBT and CBT in the Treatment of ASD and Anxiety and Disruptive Behavior

As stated above, due to the increase in prevalence of ASD and comorbid disorders, research studies evaluating the impact of cognitive-behavioral interventions have increased over the past decade. Three meta-analyses have been conducted over the last 8 years demonstrating the growth in research evaluating the efficacy of manualized interventions for children with ASD and anxiety. Specifically, Sukhodolsky, Bloch, Panza, and Reichow (2013) conducted a meta-analysis of cognitive-behavioral therapy for anxiety in children with high-functioning autism that included eight studies. The studies yielded significant effects of CBT relative to waitlist or treatment-as-usual control conditions in children with ASD, and the results were similar to the effects of CBT for anxiety in typically developing children. Most recently, a meta-analysis was conducted by Perihan et al. (2020) that included 23 studies evaluating the effect of CBT for reducing anxiety in children with high-functioning ASD. Results of each of the meta-analysis demonstrated the positive effects of CBT for children with ASD; however, Perihan et al. (2020) found that compared to CBT treatment for anxiety in typically developing children, the results were less robust among children with ASD, which differs from the findings of the two previous studies. Perihan et al. (2020) speculate that this finding indicates that children with ASD may not respond to CBT as well as their peers. Therefore, adaptation or individualization may be needed for children with ASD to better benefit from CBT (Keefer et al., 2017; Perihan et al., 2020).

Outlined below are specific manualized treatment programs including Behavioral Interventions for Anxiety in Children with Autism, Exploring Feelings, Face Your Fears, and Multimodal Anxiety and Social Skill Intervention for Adolescents with ASD. Each of the programs has been found efficacious in a minimum of one RCT, and overviews are presented in Table 15.2. The research is expanding and supports the continued adaptation of rational-emotive and cognitive-behavioral strategies in higher-functioning children with ASD.

The most widely studied intervention that utilizes CBT in work with children with ASD is a family-based CBT program, Behavioral Interventions for Anxiety in Children with Autism (BIACA; Fujii et al., 2013; Storch et al., 2013; Wood et al., 2009, 2015, 2017). The BIACA program was one of the first comprehensive interventions that included elements of both ASD and anxiety CBT programs for children. BIACA was originally developed based on the Building Confidence CBT program (Wood, McLeod, Hiruma, & Phan, 2008). The Building Confidence program was designed to treat anxiety in typically developing children. The BIACA manual includes psychoeducation, coping skills, and in vivo exposure as well as several parent-training components designed to help parents learn techniques to teach their children to cope with anxiety. In addition, the manual includes "enhancements" to address common deficits associated with ASD such as social and adaptive skills, poor attention and motivation, and rigid behavior. To date, four randomized controlled trials have been conducted demonstrating the efficacy of the program making it a well-established treatment.

The Exploring Feelings program was designed to reduce anxiety and anger among children with ASD (Sofronoff et al., 2005). Two randomized studies have been conducted in the clinical setting and demonstrated promising results with parent reported improvements in their child's anxiety and anger and children showing an increase in strategies to manage anxiety (Sofronoff et al., 2005).

The Facing Your Fears program is a group therapy intervention designed to manage anxiety for children between the ages of 7 and 14 years with high-functioning ASD (Reaven et al., 2012). The children meet in small groups once a week for approximately 12 weeks. The 90-minute sessions focus on psychoeducation, development of coping skill such as deep breathing, emotion regulation strategies, problem-solving, cognitive restructuring, and graded exposures. One randomized controlled trial has been conducted, and the results indicated that participants demonstrated significant reductions in parent-reported anxiety (Reaven et al., 2012). In addition, a recent study was conducted adapting the intervention to the school-based setting, and the results indicated significant reductions in both youth and parent reported anxiety symptoms post intervention (Drmic, Aljunid & Reaven, 2017).

The Multimodal Anxiety and Social Skills Intervention for Adolescents with ASD is a program that addresses both anxiety and social disability deficits. The dual aspect of the treatment is based on the premise that "unaddressed anxiety problems

Table 15.2 Examples of RE-CBT interventions

Treatment	Therapy format	Primary RE-CBT components
Multimodal anxiety and social skill intervention for adolescents with ASD (White et al., 2013)	Age range: 12–17 years Format: Individual and group Number of sessions: Up to 13 Duration: Varies depending on module, 60–75-minute meetings	Psychoeducation, coping skills, problem-solving, exposure, and social skills development
Exploring Feelings (Sofronoff, Attwood, & Hinton, 2005)	Age range: 9–13 years Format: Individual Number of sessions: 6 Duration: 6 weeks, 120-minute meetings	Relaxation techniques, anger recognition, emotional release, and social contact
STAMP (stress and anger management program) (Scarpa & Reyes, 2011)	Age range: 5–7 years (depends on the developmental level-should be between preschool and first grade) Format: Group Number of sessions: 9 Duration: 9 weeks, 60-minute meetings	Affective education, cognitive restructuring, and creating an emotional toolbox
Face your fears (Reaven, Blakelu-Smith, Culhane-Shelburne, & Hepburn, 2012)	Age range: 7–14 years Format: Group Number of sessions: 12 Duration: 90-minute meetings	Psychoeducation, developing coping skills, emotion regulation strategies, problem-solving, cognitive self-control, and graded exposure
Behavioral interventions for anxiety in children with autism (Storch et al., 2013; Wood et al., 2009, 2015)	Age range: 7–15 years Format: Individual Number of sessions: 16 Duration: 60–90-minute meetings	Psychoeducation, developing of coping and positive social behavior skills, and in vivo exposure
Adapted for children with ASD		
Cool kids (Chalfant, Rapee, & Caroll, 2007)	Age range: 7–17 years Format: Group Number of sessions: 12 (9 weekly; 3 booster) Duration: 160-minute meetings	Recognition of anxious feelings and somatic reactions to anxiety, cognitive restructuring, coping self-talk, exposure to feared stimuli, and relapse prevention
Coping cat (Keehn et al., 2013)	Age range: 8–14 years Format: Individual Number of sessions: 16 Duration: 90-minute meetings	Coping techniques, emotion recognition and understanding, cognitive restructuring, self-evaluation, and self-reinforcement

(continued)

Table 15.2 (continued)

Treatment	Therapy format	Primary RE-CBT components
Discussing + doing = daring (Steensel & Bogels, 2015)	Age range: 7–18 years Format: Group Number of sessions: 12 Duration: 90-minute meetings	Psychoeducation, cognitive restructuring, relaxation, exposure, and relapse prevention

can undermine the benefits that might otherwise be realized with a pure social skills intervention" (White et al., 2013, p. 2; White, Koenig, & Scahill, 2010). In addition, the intervention utilizes a unique model that includes a manual-based modular treatment program delivered via three modalities: individual therapy (up to 13 sessions), group social skills training (seven sessions), and parent coaching (after each individual session). The therapist selects the most appropriate treatment modules from the individual sessions based on the child's anxiety and social difficulties. The program allows for efficient delivery of a treatment tailored to the individual needs of the child. The results from the RCT found an improvement in social skills and a reduction in anxiety (White et al., 2013).

Overall, RE-CBT programs for treating anxiety among children with ASD involve a combination of behavioral and cognitive strategies. Most programs start with a psychoeducation component for both the child and parent, followed by cognitive restructuring and the development of positive or rational belief systems. The development of coping and relaxation techniques helps the child respond to graded exposure to stressful situations. Self-monitoring and relapse prevention are also typically used in the treatment of anxiety and may include booster sessions to promote the continued use of skills. Lastly, each of the programs includes various levels of parental involvement to support the child and expand parental coping mechanisms. To further demonstrate the use of the RE-CBT, a case study is included below.

Case Study

Frank is a 12-year-old boy referred to a psychologist by his parents due to generalized anxiety and frequent outbursts in the school and home settings. Frank was diagnosed with high-functioning ASD as a 4-year-old and received Applied Behavior Analysis (ABA) for 2 years until he started first grade. He achieved his motor milestones within normal limits; however, he received weekly speech therapy due to a speech and language delay. The transition to seventh grade has been difficult. Academically, he is in the gifted and talented program and earns primarily A's; however, recently he has started to voice concerns about going to school. He reports to his parents that he feels scared and that the other students hate him. His mother reported that before school in the morning, he cries, pleads, and begs to stay home.

After coaxing Frank out of the house, he often walks into school agitated and volatile.

Frank reported that he feels nervous talking to new people and he thinks they all hate him. He reported that he feels overwhelmed when people speak to him and he wants to scream and run out of the room. Frank's behavior seems to escalate during lunch and electives, and he often runs out of the classroom. His teachers report that Frank seems agitated and when angry, he will yell "shut up" to other students. Frank reports that he often spends a majority of his day hiding in the bathroom to avoid interacting with the students.

Frank's parents contacted a therapist to help him better cope with school and reduce his anxiety and stress. They found a psychologist that specialized in treating children with ASD and anxiety. After an intake session, the psychologist indicated that Frank's anxiety seemed to be impairing his functioning and that he would benefit from cognitive-behavioral therapy. During the intake session based on the Behavior Assessment System for Children Second Edition Self Report Form (BASC-2 SRP; Reynolds & Kamphaus, 2004) on the anxiety scale, Frank scored in the clinically significant range. The psychologist explained that she planned to use REBT to address Frank's maladaptive cognitions and promote healthier emotional and behavioral responses (David & Szentagotai, 2006).

During the first session, the psychologist explained REBT to Frank and his parents. The primary factors of REBT with children are skills acquisition and learning to cope with increasingly complex problems (Vernon, 2007). Children rarely have control over the things that affect their lives. REBT "empowers children by arming them with knowledge and skills, emphasizing that this information can be used in present as well as future problematic situations" (Vernon, 2007, p.109). The foundation of REBT is based on the Ellis (1962) ABC model—the internal or activating event (A), which results in feelings and behaviors (C, consequences) that are created by rational or irrational beliefs (B). Essentially, irrational beliefs result in negative feelings and behaviors. Irrational beliefs take the following forms: (1) awfulizing—the belief that a situation is more than 100 bad (e.g., It would be horrible if the kids do not like me); (2) low frustration tolerance—the belief that they cannot imagine handling a situation (e.g., I cannot stand middle school); (3) demanding of self or others (e.g., I have to be the best in the class); and (4) global evaluation of worth (e.g., If someone is mean to me, I am a loser and will never make friends). It became clear when speaking with Frank that he had developed two primary irrational beliefs related to low frustration tolerance and global evaluation of worth. First, he stated numerous times that he could not stand middle school and second that because a girl was mean to him he must be a loser and nobody would ever like him. The primary goal became to help Frank develop rational or flexible beliefs, such as "It is not my first choice of a school, but I can handle it" and "Even if someone is mean to be, they do not define who I am."

The next session began by teaching Frank about another key component of REBT, disputation and challenging irrational beliefs. There are different types of disputation such as empirical, logical, semantic, and pragmatic disputing (DiGiuseppe, Doyle, Dryden, & Backx, 2013). The therapist used empirical disputing and followed an approach developed by Bernard, Ellis, and Terjesen (2006) that required Frank to provide examples of behaviors that would either support or "debunk" that belief that nobody liked him. Frank enjoyed writing and frequently wrote in a small notebook throughout the day. The therapist asked him to record any behaviors that indicated someone might like him such as a student saying hello, opening a door for him, sitting next to him at lunch, asking him to join a group during class, and/or walking with him in the hallway. Frank demonstrated limited ability to recognize nonverbal communication; therefore, many examples were provided of behavior that would indicate a positive interaction.

During the third session, Frank was excited to share the results of his "data." He seemed genuinely shocked to report 126 incidences where another student or teacher seemed to like him and only 14 incidences of a negative interaction. From here, the therapist used this information to help Frank challenge his irrational beliefs and work toward developing a healthier thought such as "While I would like others to like me, and it would be disappointing if they don't, I can handle it." In addition, the therapist strived to teach Frank that being liked does not define him as a person. Over the course of the school year, Frank had stopped inviting friends over or going to clubs he had attended previously. During this session, Frank was asked to engage in behavioral activities to further enhance the cognitive restructuring. He developed a social fear hierarchy and would challenge himself to climb a step up the ladder each week. He decided to start by attending one Boy Scouts meeting. The therapist and Frank spent the remainder of the session role-playing possible scenarios to help prepare him.

Over the next three sessions, Frank and the therapist continued to work on cognitive restructuring and developing new effective beliefs to cope with difficult situations. Collecting empirical evidence and role-playing were a vital part of the treatment. Frank seemed to demonstrate limited social skills, and practicing the skills prior to engaging in a behavioral challenge helped him feel prepared. In addition, following each session, the therapist met with the parents to provide psychoeducation regarding anxiety and cognitive restructuring and to ensure they could support the weekly homework assignments. Frank's parents also helped him work through the ABC model when he was upset. By the conclusion of the treatment, Frank and his parents reported that he felt more comfortable at school and started to invite new friends to his house. He was also re-administered the BASC-2 SRP and no longer scored in the clinical range on the anxiety scale. All of his initial symptoms were improved.

Adaptation of REBT and CBT in the Schools for Children with ASD

The research on the use of REBT and CBT among children with ASD in the school setting is limited. Two recent studies demonstrate the effectiveness of school-based CBT intervention for anxiety in children with ASD (Drmic et al., 2017; Luxford et al., 2017). Drmic et al. (2017) found preliminary evidence that adapting the Facing Your Fears program to the school setting yielded a reduction in child and parent reported anxiety. Another encouraging aspect of the study was that the program was implemented by non-clinician school staff and achieved positive outcomes.

Children with ASD have high service utilization rates because of the complexity and early onset of the disorder, lifelong prevalence, and associated impairments. As stated above, many children also have co-occurring disruptive behaviors (e.g., aggression, tantrums, and self-injury) which are one of the most common reasons for referral to pediatric and mental health clinics (Masse et al., 2007). Administrators and teachers face enormous pressure to ensure the academic success of all students. Teachers are challenged with the arduous task of maintaining high academic standards for all students while simultaneously managing problem behaviors that are disruptive to the learning environment. Although school systems are not responsible for meeting all the needs of the students, schools must meet the need when the problem impacts learning for individual children or hampers the learning environment for the greater school community. Christner, Forrest, Morley, and Weinstein (2007) point out that "though there is considerable documentation to suggest a need for providing mental services in schools, there are a number of factors that make fitting these services into the culture of the school difficult" (p. 175).

Over four decades ago, Bronfenbrenner (1979) developed the ecological context perspective demonstrating that schools represent a key component of the child's microsystem. Schools are one of the most proximal influences on a child's life and not surprisingly represent the primary setting where children exhibit impairment (Ginsberg, Becker, Kingery, & Nichols, 2008). Therefore, providing evidence-based interventions in the school setting is imperative to effectively prevent and treat mental health problems.

The response-to-intervention framework uses a multi-tiered model of intervention that involves universal, targeted, and intensive levels of intervention in an effort address problems school-wide. This model applies to instructional as well as behavioral, emotional, and social problems. The research indicates that programs using cognitive-behavioral interventions based on the work of Ellis, Beck, and others demonstrate the largest beneficial effects across all levels of intervention (e.g., Mennuti, Freeman, and Christner, 2006). For example, there are over 150 different universal prevention programs currently available (Hallfors & Goddette, 2002). Programs that involve teachers employing cognitive-behavioral and behavioral modification strategies with the guidance of a school psychologist or other mental health professionals demonstrate the largest beneficial effects (Wilson, Lipsey, & Derzon, 2003). Teachers can markedly influence a child's behavior by modeling and reinforcing pro-social attitudes and behaviors within the classroom.

Research further demonstrates that school-based cognitive-behavioral interventions that focus on small groups or individual students yield improvements in emotional, behavioral, social, and academic functioning (Weisz & Kazdin, 2010). Moreover, in a comprehensive review conducted by Chambless and Ollendick (2001), they found that approximately 80% of the treatments for specific disorders described as having research support used cognitive-behavioral therapy. Cognitive-behavioral therapy focuses on how the child interprets his experiences and how these thoughts ultimately influence his or her emotional behavior (Reinecke & Simons, 2005). Mennuti, Freeman, and Christner (2006) indicate that the solution-focused and time-limited model of cognitive-behavioral therapy makes it a good match for the school setting. School-based interventions provide a naturalistic setting to practice new thoughts and evaluate emotional behavior change. Although there is a large body of research on universal prevention programs, the field is only beginning to implement RE-CBT to the school setting for children with ASD.

Overall, the research using RE-CBT to treat children with ASD and comorbid disorders such as anxiety is promising. Current studies demonstrate that when using cognitive-behavioral strategies, both parent and child reported symptoms of anxiety are reduced and the functioning of the child improves (e.g., White et al., 2013; Wood et al., 2015). Recent studies have even expanded interventions to the school setting and maintained the postive outcome of reducing child anxiety (Drmic et al., 2017). Due to the increase in prevalence of ASD, developing and/or adapting treatments to treat comorbid disorder will be vital to the functioning of these children.

Test Yourself Questions

1. What age does the American Academy of Pediatrics recommend children are screened for autism spectrum disorder?
2. While ABA has been effective in treating the core symptoms of ASD, what are common treatments for comorbid disorders such as anxiety?
3. Elisa is a 14-year-old girl with ASD and anxiety. She is refusing to go to school because she thinks the other students do not like her and the work is too hard. As her therapist, what irrational beliefs do you think are leading to her emotional distress? What RE-CBT strategies could you use to reduce her anxiety and improve her functioning?

References

Aman, M. G., McDougle, C. J., Scahill, L., Handen, B., Arnold, L. E., Johnson, C., et al. (2009). Medication and parent training in children with pervasive developmental disorders and serious behavior problems: Results from a randomized clinical trial. *Journal of the American Academy of Child and Adolescent Psychiatry, 48*, 1143–1154.

American Psychiatric Association. (1952). *Diagnostic and statistical manual of mental disorders* (2nd ed.). Washington, DC: Author.

American Psychiatric Association. (1980). *Diagnostic and statistical manual of mental disorders* (3rd ed.). Washington, DC: Author.

American Psychiatric Association. (2000). *Diagnostic and statistical manual of mental disorders* (4th ed. -text rev ed.). Washington, DC: Author.

American Psychiatric Association. (2013). *Diagnostic and statistical manual of mental disorders* (5th ed.). Washington, DC: Author.

Baio, J., Wiggins, L., Christensen, D. L., Maenner, M. J., Daniels, J., Warren, Z., et al. (2018). Prevalence of autism Spectrum disorder among children aged 8 years - autism and developmental disabilities monitoring network, 11 sites, United States, 2014. *MMWR Surveillance Summaries, 67*(6), 1–23.

Baker, B. L., Blacher, J., Crnic, K. A., & Edelbrock, C. (2002). Behavior problems and parenting stress in families of three-year-old children with and without developmental delays. *American Journal of Mental Retardation, 107*, 433–444.

Baker-Ericzén, M. J., Brookman-Frazee, L., & Stahmer, A. (2005). Stress levels and adaptability in parents of toddlers with and without autism spectrum disorders. *Research and Practice for Persons with Severe Disabilities, 30*(4), 194–204.

Bauminger, N., Solomon, M., & Rogers, S. J. (2010). Externalizing and internalizing behaviors in ASD. *Autism Research, 3*, 101–112.

Beck, A. T. (1967). *Depression: Clinical, experimental, and theoretical aspects*. New York: Hoeber.

Bernard, M. E., Ellis, A., & Terjesen, M. (2006). *Rational-emotive behavioral approaches to childhood disorders: History, theory, practice and research*. Springer Science+ Business Media.

Bromley, J., Hare, D. J., Davison, K., & Emerson, E. (2004). Mothers supporting children with autistic spectrum disorders: Social support, mental health status and satisfaction with services. *Autism, 8*, 409–423.

Bronfenbrenner, U. (1979). *The ecology of human development*. Harvard University Press.

Carroll, R. A., & Kodak, T. (2019). Evidence-based treatment models for autism spectrum disorder. In C. B. McNeil, L. B. Quetsch, & C. Anderson (Eds.), *Handbook on parent-child interaction therapy for children on the autism spectrum*. New York: Springer.

Centers for Disease Control and Prevention [CDC]. (2018). Prevalence of autism spectrum disorder among children aged 8 years–autism and developmental disabilities monitoring network, 11 sites, United States, 2014. *Morbidity and Mortality Weekly Report Surveillance Summaries, 67*(6), 1–23.

Chalfant, A. M., Rapee, R., & Caroll, L. (2007). Treating anxiety disorders in children with high functioning autism spectrum disorders: A controlled trial. *Journal of Autism and Developmental Disorders, 37*, 1842–1857.

Chambless, D. L., & Ollendick, T. H. (2001). Empirically supported psychological interventions: Controversies and evidence. *Annual Review of Psychology, 52*, 685–716.

Christner, R. W., Forrest, E., Morley, J., & Weinstein, E. (2007). Taking cognitive behavior therapy to the school: A school-based mental health approach. *Jounal of Contemporary Psychotherapy, 37*, 175–183.

Chu, B. C., & Kendall, P. C. (2004). Positive association of child involvement and treatment outcome within a manual-based cognitive-behavioral treatment for children with anxiety. *Journal of Consulting and Clinical Psychology, 72*(5), 821.

David, D., & Szentagotai, A. (2006). Cognitions in cognitive-behavioral psychotherapies; toward an integrative model. *Clinical Psychology Review, 26*, 284–298.

DiGiuseppe, R., Doyle, K. A., Dryden, W., & Backx, W. (2013). *A practitioner's guide to rational-emotive behavior therapy*. Oxford: Oxford University Press.

Drmic, I., Aljuined, M., & Reaven, J. (2017). Feasibility, acceptability and preliminary treatment outcomes in a school-based CBT intervention program for adolescents with ASD and anxiety in Singapore. *Journal of Autism and Developmental Disorders, 47*, 3909–3929.

Ellis, A. (1962). *Reason and emotion in psychotherapy*. Sacaucus, NJ: Citadel.

Ellis, A., & Bernard, M. E. (Eds.). (2006). *Rational emotive behavioral approaches to childhood disorders: Theory, practice and research*. New York: Springer.

Farmer, C. A., & Aman, M. G. (2011a). Aggressive behavior in a sample of children with autism spectrum disorders. *Research in Autism Spectrum Disorders, 5*, 317–323.

Farmer, C. A., & Aman, M. G. (2011b). Aripiprazole for the treatment of irritability associated with autism. *Expert Opinions in Pharmacotherapy, 12*, 635–640.
Fitzpatrick, S. E., Srivorakiat, L., Wink, L. K., Pedapati, E. V., & Erickson, C. A. (2016). Aggression in autism spectrum disorder: Presentation and treatment options. *Neuropsychiatric Disease and Treatment, 12*, 1525–1538.
Frazier, T. W., Youngstrom, E. A., Haycook, T., Sinoff, A., Dimitrious, F., Knapp, J., et al. (2010). Effectiveness of medication combined with intensive behavioral intervention for reducing aggression in youth with autism spectrum disorder. *Journal of Child and Adolescent Psychopharmacology, 20*, 167–177.
Fujii, C., Renno, P., McLeod, B. D., Lin, C. E., Decker, K., Zielinski, K., & Wood, J. J. (2013). Intensive cognitive behavioral therapy for anxiety disorders in school-aged children with autism: A preliminary comparison with treatment-as-usual. *School Mental Health, 5*(1), 25–37.
Ginsburg, G. S., Becker, K. D., Kingery, J. N., & Nichols, T. (2008). Transporting CBT for childhood anxiety disorders into inner-city school-based mental health clinics. *Cognitive and Behavioral Practice, 15*(2), 148–158.
Grave, J., & Blissett, J. (2004). Is cognitive behavior therapy developmentally appropriate for young children? A critical review of the evidence. *Clinical Psychology Review, 24*(4), 399–6420.
Guttmann-Steinmetz, S., Gadow, K. D., & DeVincent, C. J. (2009). Oppositional defiant and conduct disorder behaviors in boys with autism spectrum disorder with and without attention-deficit hyperactivity disorder versus several comparison samples. *Journal of Autism and Developmental Disorders, 39*, 976–985.
Hallfors, D., & Godette, D. (2002). Will thePrinciples of Effectiveness' improve prevention practice? Early findings from a diffusion study. *Health Education Research, 17*(4), 461–470.
Harrington, J., & Allen, K. (2013). The Clinician's Guide on Autism. *Pediatrics in Review, 35*, 62–78.
Hill, A. P., Zuckerman, K. E., Hagen, A. D., Kriz, D. J., Duvall, S. W., van Santen, J., et al. (2014). Aggressive behavior problems in children with autism spectrum disorders: Prevalence and correlates in a large clinical sample. *Autism Spectrum Disorder, 8*(9), 1121–1133.
Horner, R. H., Carr, E. G., Strain, P. S., Todd, A. W., & Reed, H. K. (2002). Problem behavior interventions for young children with autism: A research synthesis. *Journal of Autism and Developmental Disorders, 32*, 423–446.
Jang, J., Dixon, D. R., Tarbox, J., & Granpeesheh, D. (2011). Symptom severity and challenging behavior in children with ASD. *Research in Autism Spectrum Disorders, 5*, 1028–1032.
Kanne, S. M., & Mazurek, M. O. (2011). Aggression in children and adolescents with ASD: prevalence and risk factors. *Journal of Autism and Developmental Disorders, 41*, 926–937.
Kanner, L. (1943). Autistic disturbances of affective contact. *The Nervous Child, 2*(3), 217–250.
Keefer, A., Kreiser, N. L., Singh, V., Blakeley-Smith, A., Duncan, A., Johnson, C., ... & Vasa, R. A. (2017). Intolerance of uncertainty predicts anxiety outcomes following CBT in youth with ASD. *Journal of Autism and Developmental Disorders, 47*(12), 3949–3958.
Keehn, R. H., Lincoln, A. J., Brown, M. Z., & Chavira, D. A. (2013). The coping cat program for children with anxiety and autism spectrum disorder: A pilot randomized controlled trial. *Journal of Autism and Developmental Disorders, 43*(1), 57–67.
Kendall, P. C., & Hedtke, K. A. (2006). *Cognitive-behavioral therapy for anxious children: Therapist manual*. Ardmore, PA: Workbook Publishing.
Kerns, C. M., & Kendall, P. C. (2012). The presentation and classification of anxiety in autism spectrum disorder. *Clinical Psychology: Science and Practice, 19*(4), 323–347.
Luxford, S., Hadwin, J. A., & Kovshoff, H. (2017). Evaluating the effectiveness of a school-based cognitive behavioural therapy intervention for anxiety in adolescents diagnosed with autism spectrum disorder. *Journal of Autism and Developmental Disorders, 47*(12), 3896–3908.
Masse, J. J., McNeil, C. B., Wagner, S. M., & Chorney, D. B. (2007). Parent-child interaction therapy and high functioning autism: A conceptual overview. *Journal of Early and Intensive Behavior Intervention, 4*, 714–735.

Mazurek, M. O., Kanne, S. M., & Wodka, E. L. (2013). Physical aggression in children and adolescents with autism spectrum disorders. *Research in Autism Spectrum Disorders, 7*(3), 455–465.

McLeod, B. D., & Weisz, J. R. (2005). The therapy process observational coding system-alliance scale: measure characteristics and prediction of outcome in usual clinical practice. *Journal of Consulting and Clinical Psychology, 73*(2), 323.

McStay, R. L., Dissanayake, C., Scheeren, A., Koot, H. M., & Begeer, S. (2014). Parenting stress and autism: The role of age, autism severity, quality of life and problem behavior of children and adolescents with autism. *Autism, 18*(5), 502–510.

McTiernan, A., Leader, G., Healy, O., & Mannion, A. (2011). Analysis of risk factors and early predictors of challenging behavior for children with autism spectrum disorder. *Research in Autism Spectrum Disorders, 5*(3), 1215–1222.

Mennuti, R., Freeman, A., & Christner, R. (2006). *Cognitive-behavioral interventions in educational settings*. New York: Routledge.

Oliver, C., Murphy, G. H., & Corbett, J. A. (1987). Self-injurious behavior in people with mental handicap: A total population study. *Journal of Mental Deficiency Research, 31*, 147–162.

Perihan, C., Burke, M., Bowman-Perrott, L., Biver, A., Gallup, J., Thompson, J., et al. (2020). Effects of cognitive behavioral therapy for reducing anxiety in children with high functioning ASD: A systematic review and meta-analysis. *Journal of Autism and Developmental Disabilities, 50(6), 1958–1972.*

Pikard, J., Roberts, N., & Groll, D. (2018). Pediatric referrals for urgent psychiatric consultation: clinical characteristics, diagnoses and outcome of 4 to 12 year old children. *Journal of the Canadian Academy of Child and Adolescent Psychiatry, 27*(4), 245.

Predescu, E., Dobrean, A., Pop, C., Miclutia, I., & Sipos, R. (2013). Cognitive Coping Strategies and Emotional Distress in Mothers of Children with Autism Spectrum Disorder. *Applied Medical Informatics, 32*, 14–21.

Reaven, J., Blakeley-Smith, A., Culhane-Shelburne, K., & Hepburn, S. (2012). Group cognitive behavior therapy for children with high-functioning autism spectrum disorders and anxiety: A randomized trial. *Journal of Child Psychology and Psychiatry, 53*(4), 410–419.

Reaven, J., Blakeley-Smith, A., Leuthe, E., Moody, E., & Hepburn, S. (2012). Facing your fears in adolescence: Cognitive-behavioral therapy for high-functioning autism spectrum disorders and anxiety. *Autism Research and Treatment*. https://doi.org/10.1155/2012/423905

Reinecke, M. A., & Simons, A. (2005). Vulnerability to depression among adolescents: Implications for cognitive-behavioral treatment. *Cognitive and Behavioral Practice, 12*, 166–176.

Research Units of Pediatric Psychopharmacology (RUPP) Autism Network. (2005). Risperidone treatment of autistic disorder: longer-term benefits and blinded discontinuation after 6 months. *American Journal of Psychiatry, 162*, 1361–1369.

Reynolds, C. R., & Kamphaus, R. W. (2004). *Behavior assessment system for children* (2nd ed.). Bloomington, MN: Pearson Assessments.

Rogers, S. J., & Vismara, L. A. (2008). Evidence-based comprehensive treatments for early autism. *Journal of Clinical Child and Adolescent Psychology, 37*, 8–38.

Rojahn, J. (1994). Epidemiology and topographic taxonomy of self-injurious behavior. In T. Thompson & D. Gray (Eds.), *Destructive behavior in developmental disabilities: Diagnosis and treatment* (2nd ed., pp. 49–67). Thousand Oaks, CA: Sage Publication.

Rotheram-Fuller, E., & Hodas, R. (2015). Using CBT to assist children with autism spectrum disorders/pervasive developmental disorders in the school setting. In *Cognitive and behavioral interventions in the schools* (pp. 181–197). New York: Springer.

Scarpa, A., & Reyes, N. M. (2011). Improving emotion regulation with CBT in young children with high functioning autism spectrum disorders: A pilot study. *Behavioral and Cognitive Psychotherapy, 39*(4), 495–500.

Smith, T., & Iadarola, S. (2015). Evidence base update for autism spectrum disorder. *Journal of Clinical Child & Adolescent Psychology, 44*(6), 897–922.

Sofronoff, K., Attwood, T., & Hinton, S. (2005). A randomized controlled trial of a CBT intervention for anxiety in children with Asperger syndrome. *Journal of Child Psychology and Psychiatry, 46*(11), 1152–1160.

Solomon, M., Ono, M., Timmer, S., & Goodlin-Jones, B. (2008). The effectiveness of Parent-Child Interaction Therapy for families of children on the autism spectrum. *Journal of Autism and Developmental Disorders, 38*, 1767–1776.

Steensel, F. J., & Bögels, S. M. (2015). Cbt for anxiety disorders in children with and without autism spectrum disorders. *Journal of Consulting and Clinical Psychology, 83*(3), 512–523.

van Steensel, F. J., Bögels, S. M., & Dirksen, C. D. (2012). Anxiety and quality of life: Clinically anxious children with and without autism spectrum disorders compared. *Journal of Clinical Child & Adolescent Psychology, 41*(6), 731–738.

Storch, E. A., Arnold, E. B., Lewin, A. B., Nadeau, J. M., Jones, A. M., Nadai, A. S., et al. (2013). The effect of cognitive- behavioral therapy versus treatment as usual for anxiety in children with autism spectrum disorders: A randomized, controlled trial. *Journal of the American Academy of Child & Adolescent Psychiatry, 52*(2), 132–142.e2.

Sukhodolsky, D. G., Bloch, M. H., Panza, K. E., & Reichow, B. (2013). Cognitive-behavioral therapy for anxiety in children with high- functioning autism: A meta-analysis. *Pediatrics, 132*(5), e1341–e1350.

Tremblay, R. E., Hartup, W. W., & Archer, J. (Eds.). (2005). *Developmental origins of aggression*. New York: Guilford Press.

Vernon, A. (2007). Application of rational emotive behavior therapy to groups within classrooms and educational settings. In R. W. Christner, J. Stewart, & A. Freeman (Eds.), *Handbook of cognitive-behavior group therapy with children and adolescents*. New York: Routledge.

Volkmar, F. R. (2001). Pharmacological interventions in autism: theoretical and practical issues. *Journal of Clinical Child Psychology, 30*, 80–87.

Weisz, J. R., & Kazdin, A. E. (Eds.). (2010). *Evidence-based psychotherapies for children and adolescents*. Guilford Press.

White, S. W., Koenig, K., & Scahill, L. (2010). Group social skills instruction for adolescents with high-functioning autism spectrum disorders. *Focus on Autism and Other Developmental Disabilities, 25*(4), 209–219.

White, S. W., Ollendick, T., Albano, A. M., Oswald, D., Johnson, C., Southam-Gerow, M. A., et al. (2013). Randomized controlled trial: multimodal anxiety and social skill intervention for adolescents with autism spectrum disorder. *Journal of Autism and Developmental Disorders, 43*(2), 382–394.

Wilson, S. J., Lipsey, M. W., & Derzon, J. H. (2003). The effects of school-based intervention programs on aggressive behavior: A meta-analysis. *Journal of Consulting and Clinical Psychology, 71*(1), 136.

Witt, K. (2005). *The role of parental irrationality and child autism characteristics on parental stress level*. New York: St. John's University.

Wood, J. J., Drahota, A., Sze, K., Har, K., Chiu, A., & Langer, D. A. (2009). Cognitive behavioral therapy for anxiety in children with autism spectrum disorders: a randomized, controlled trial. *Journal of Child Psychology and Psychiatry, 50*(3), 224–234.

Wood, J. J., Ehrenreich-May, J., Alessandri, M., Fujii, C., Renno, P., Laugeson, E., et al. (2015). Cognitive behavioral therapy for early adolescents with autism spectrum disorders and clinical anxiety: A randomized, controlled trial. *Behavior Therapy, 46*(1), 7–19.

Wood, J. J., Klebanoff, S., Renno, P., Fujii, C., & Danial, J. (2017). Individual CBT for anxiety and related symptoms in children with autism spectrum disorders. In *Anxiety in children and adolescents with autism spectrum disorder* (pp. 123–141). Academic Press.

Wood, J. J., & Gadow, K. D. (2010). Exploring the nature and function of anxiety in youth with autism spectrum disorders. *Clinical Psychology: Science and Practice, 17*(4), 281–292.

Wood, J. J., McLeod, B. D., Hiruma, L. S., & Phan, A. Q. (2008). *Child anxiety disorders: A family-based treatment manual for practitioners*. New York: WW Norton & Co.

Chapter 16
Treatment of Sleep Disorders in Children and Adolescents: A Rational-Emotive, Cognitive-Behavioral Approach

Robin J. Sakakini, Mark D. Terjesen, and Mayra Reyes-Ruiz

Sleep and healthy sleep habits are essential behaviors among youth with insufficient or disruptive sleep resulting in daytime difficulties (Meltzer & McLaughlin-Crabtree, 2015). Perfect and colleagues (Perfect, Frye, & Sakakini, 2019) describe sleep insufficiency as probably among the most challenging sleep-related issues seen among youth. This gets further complicated when you consider the impact of insufficient sleep on child academic (Pagel & Kwiatkowski, 2010; Roberts, Roberts, & Duong, 2009; Silva et al., 2011) and social-emotional (El-Sheikh, Kelly, Buckhalt, & Hinnant, 2010; Perfect, Levine-Donnerstein, Archbold, Goodwin, & Quan, 2014) functioning. The American Academy of Sleep Medicine (AASM, 2014) recommends ranges of sleep by developmental age: 10 to 13 hours (preschool aged), 9 to 12 hours (school-aged: 6–12 years), and 8 to 10 hours (13 years and older) (AASM, 2014). Regrettably, the amount of sleep time among youth has been declining (Perfect et al., 2019). Further, there is also an increase in sleep-related problems seen among youth with diagnoses and/or mental health difficulties (Perfect, et al., 2019). This may exacerbate their preexisting conditions and may further complicate accurate assessment and treatment. This is further complicated by the fact that most clinicians report minimal training in pediatric behavioral sleep medicine (Mindell et al., 2009, 2011, 2013). This chapter aims to provide clinicians with an overview of behavioral sleep problems seen among youth, with a specific focus on assessment and intervention strategies from a rational-emotive and cognitive-behavioral therapy (RE-CBT) approach. A review of the research and best practices for intervention will be linked to developmental considerations as well as work with parents. Finally, a case study will highlight the strategies reviewed.

R. J. Sakakini
Oaks Christian School, Westlake Village, CA, USA

M. D. Terjesen (✉) · M. Reyes-Ruiz
St. John's University, Queens, NY, USA
e-mail: Terjesem@stjohns.edu

M. Bernard, M. D. Terjesen (eds.), *Rational-Emotive and Cognitive-Behavioral Approaches to Child and Adolescent Mental Health: Theory, Practice, Research, Applications*, https://doi.org/10.1007/978-3-030-53901-6_16

Defining Sleep, Sleep Problems, and the Impact on Functioning Among Youth

There are a number of theories that propose explanations for the purpose of sleep (Frank & Benington, 2006), but there is no considerable evidence to support these theories. What we do know is that sleep promotes brain plasticity and the areas most impacted by sleep are attention, cognition, and mood (Frank & Benington, 2006. Raven, Van der Zee, Meerlo, & Havekes, 2018).

Sleep-related problems among youth may be overshadowed by other clinical disorders (Sadeh, Raviv, & Gruber, 2000), and as such, the sleep-related problems or disorders may go unnoticed. This is further complicated by the fact that there is no universally agreed upon definition of sleep problems (Sakakini, 2011). Harvey (2016) proposed a transdiagnostic approach to sleep disorders where they are seen as common processes across a range of psychological disorders. We like this model, especially in that it would promote competence across a greater number of clinical interventions, but are concerned that without sufficient knowledge among clinicians about sleep problems among youth, these areas may be neglected from a diagnostic and then subsequent intervention perspective.

The *International Classification of Sleep Disorders – Third Edition* (*ICSD-III*) provides standardized definitions and criteria for 83 different conditions, including sleep disorders occurring exclusively during childhood (American Academy of Sleep Medicine [AASM], 2014).

For the purpose of this chapter, the definition of a sleep problem put forth by Owens and colleagues will be utilized. They define a sleep problem as a condition that interferes with the initiation and maintenance of normal sleep, and "that is viewed as a problem by the child or caregiver, the significance of [which] may be characterized by its severity, chronicity, and frequency and associated impairment in daytime function in the child or family" (Owens, 2005, p.49).

Medical and Behavioral Sleep Problems

With approximately 25% of children demonstrating a sleep problem (Mindell & Owens, 2015), it stands to reason that this is an important clinical concern. The types of sleep difficulties seen among youth can be broadly characterized into medically and behaviorally based sleep problems. While the focus of this book chapter is on the assessment and treatment of behaviorally based problems, it is important to address those medically based ones so that appropriate referral to a sleep specialist can be made. These include narcolepsy, obstructive sleep apnea (OSA), restless legs syndrome (RLS), and periodic limb movement disorder (PLMD).

Narcolepsy is considered to be a neurological disorder that initially presents as extreme daytime sleepiness despite having a sufficient opportunity to sleep at night (Maski & Owens, 2016; Meltzer & McLaughlin-Crabtree, 2015). While relatively rare, the highest severity is among children when onset is abrupt (American Psychiatric Association, 2013). However, the initial onset of narcolepsy typically occurs in adolescents, but it often is not identified until adulthood (Meltzer & McLaughlin-Crabtree, 2015). Obstructive sleep apnea (OSA) occurs when upper airway obstructions disrupt sleep and may lead to learning and/or behavioral difficulties along with daytime sleepiness. Estimates of OSA are approximately 0–5.7% of youth (Marcus et al., 2012). Restless leg syndrome (RLS) and periodic limb movement disorder (PLMD) often co-occur (AASM, 2014; Meltzer & McLaughlin-Crabtree, 2015) and involve discomfort followed by the repeated urge to move one's leg occurring primarily during bedtime/sleep (AASM, 2014). These disruptions in sleep can impact daytime functioning and lead to the child demonstrating behaviors that are more often linked to ADHD (Meltzer & McLaughlin-Crabtree, 2015). RLS has a prevalence of approximately 2 to 6% overall among youth (Picchietti et al., 2007, 2013), but many consider this an underestimate (Meltzer & McLaughlin-Crabtree, 2015). All the above-mentioned disorders and their symptoms do warrant consideration during a clinical assessment as well as appropriate referral to a physician or sleep medicine specialist. When the medical issue is addressed, consideration of other strategies (RE-CBT, behavioral parent training) may be warranted.

Behaviorally based sleep disorders occur across all age groups and are more common than the medically based sleep disorders (Honaker & Meltzer, 2016; Meltzer & McLaughlin-Crabtree, 2015). Insomnia is experienced when a child has difficulty initiating and/or maintaining sleep. One to 6% of youth experience insomnia, with higher estimates for youth with mental health or developmental difficulties (Mindell, Emslie et al., 2006; Roberts, Roberts, & Duong, 2008). However, the research reflects considerable variability among adolescents with prevalence rates ranging from 3 to 36% (Meltzer & McLaughlin-Crabtree, 2015).

One of the more common sleep-related challenges seen among youth is that of daytime sleepiness, with greater than one-third of youth either struggling to stay awake or reporting that they fall asleep during activities throughout the day (Dewald, Meijer, Oort, Kerkof, & Bogels, 2010). Daytime sleepiness is the result of insufficient sleep that can be caused by a sleep disorder (Perfect et al., 2019). Many adolescents demonstrate a preference for a later sleep onset time and as a result a later wake time (Jenni & Carskadon, 2007; Perfect et al., 2019). This may impact their natural internal circadian rhythm which may lead to delayed sleep-wake phase disorder (DSWPD). This then conflicts with early school start times, and as a result, students may experience insufficient sleep (Lundgren, 2020; Perfect et al., 2019). Parasomnias occur during sleep and may include sleep walking, night terrors, or confusional arousal (Proserpio & Nobili, 2017). While fairly common in childhood (Stallman & Kohler, 2016), most cases resolve without treatment by adolescence (Laberge, Tremblay, Vitaro, & Montplaisir, 2000; Perfect et al., 2019).

Impact of Sleep Problems on Student Functioning

Poor or insufficient sleep can have a deleterious impact on children and adolescents across a range of areas including academic functioning and social-emotional well-being. One of the functions of sleep is to assist in consolidating memories (Kopasz et al., 2010), and as a result of insufficient sleep, children and adolescents may have more difficulties with consolidating material learned in school and executive functioning (Beebe, Ris, Kramer, Long, & Amin, 2010; Drake et al., 2003; Perfect et al., 2014; Wong, Rowland, & Dyson, 2014).

In addition to academics, sleep problems also impact students overall social-emotional functioning (Gruber et al., 2012; Vriend et al., 2012; Winsler, Deutsch, Vorona, Payne, & Szklo-coxe, 2015). A number of health-related outcomes (e.g., sadness, suicidal ideation) have been shown to be related to sleep insufficiency (Alfano, Zakem, Costa, Taylor, & Weems, 2009; Gangwisch et al., 2010; Winsler et al., 2015), although it is important to note that the relationship is most likely bidirectional. In addition to the affective relationship with sleep problems, there are a number of interpersonal (e.g., bullying, aggression) factors that are also related to sleep (Aronen, Paavonen, Fjällberg, Soininen, & Törrönen, 2000; Kubiszewski, Fontaine, Potard, & Gimenes, 2014; McKnight-Eily et al., 2011). Given the strong relationship of sleep to these crucial developmental factors, it is important that clinicians assess for and deliver evidence-based interventions for sleep when appropriate.

Assessment and Diagnosis of Sleep Problems

We think it is important that clinicians provide a comprehensive evaluation of not just the sleep problems but of the larger academic and social-emotional issues that were previously reported to be linked to sleep difficulties. More importantly, we think it is essential for clinicians to consider and ask questions related to sleep for *any* initial referral for clinical services. The rationale for this is based on the premise that sleep difficulties may not be the first thing the person making the referral reports. That is, the parent or teacher may report that the student is having difficulty paying attention or seems lethargic. If we automatically jump to assess for ADHD or depression without considering the role of sleep, we may be engaging in some diagnostic foreclosure and miss an important area that may be related to functioning. While a comprehensive review of sleep assessment measures and their psychometric properties is beyond the focus of this chapter, we thought it is helpful to briefly discuss important assessment procedures and measures to consider. For a thorough review, the reader is referred to Meltzer and McLaughlin (2015) and Sadeh (2015).

To begin, we think it is important to gather information from three main sources: child, parent, and school. While parents can report on sleep initiation and potentially problems experienced during the night, sleep quality is subjective and gathering the perception from the child may be more clinically helpful. Teachers are an essential source of information in terms of the impact on daily functioning. Gathering a comprehensive sleep history can be initially conducted through an interview. We support the recommendations of Sadeh (2015) in looking at sleep quality, quantity, and sleep schedule. Sleep architecture (i.e., REM sleep stages) is not something one has the capacity to assess at initial intake. In addition to gathering information about issues related to sleep (i.e., diet, use of technology), it is critical to also determine how the parent responds to the specific behaviors demonstrated. A sleep diary may be completed by the child and the parent and is fairly common as an outcomes assessment measure in sleep intervention research (Sadeh, 2015). See Table 16.1 for a sample sleep diary.

Depending on the type of sleep problem you are assessing, there exist a number of well-established rating scales/questionnaires that clinicians may wish to consider using. Ji and Liu (2016) and Sadeh (2015) provide comprehensive reviews of these measures. Some of the measures that we recommend are the Sleep Disturbance Scale for Children (SDSC; Bruni et al., 2006; Ferreira et al., 2009), Children's Sleep Habits Questionnaire (CSHQ; Owens, Spirito, & McGuinn, 2000), and Sleep Disorders Inventory for Students (SDIS; Luginbuehl, 2005). All of these measures provide important information about the sleep difficulties that students may experience and do not require specific technology (i.e., actigraph). While the data gathered from an actigraph is objective and provides valuable information about sleep-wake behaviors (Meltzer, Walsh, Traylor, & Westin, 2012), they are cost prohibitive at present.

Research on RE-CBT in the Treatment of Sleep Problems

Rational-emotive and cognitive-behavioral therapies have been broadly applied to a number of psychological disorders and have shown significant positive outcomes among children and adolescents (Esposito, 2009; Gonzalez et al., 2004). More of the research on rational emotive behavior therapy (REBT) and cognitive therapy

Table 16.1 Sleep Diary

Date:	1/1/2020
Naps (how many and length)	1–60 minutes
Time you got in bed at night	10:30 pm
Time you fell asleep at night	12:15 am
Nightwakings (how many and length)	2–20 minutes and 8 minutes
Time you woke up in the morning	6:08 am
How well did you sleep last night (1 is very good/restful and 5 is horrible, I am exhausted)?	4
Notes (medications, feelings, caffeine, exercise, etc.)	Stressed; coffee at 11 am, soccer practice

(CT) as they relate to treatment of sleep has primarily been associated with treatment of nightmares and insomnia, with a limited number of studies focusing on the treatment of sleep problems among youth.

Cognitive behavioral therapy for insomnia (CBT-I) is considered to be an evidence-based clinical intervention for insomnia in adults (Okajima & Inoue, 2018). CBT-I incorporates a number of interventions (i.e., stimulus control and sleep restriction) seen with brief behavioral therapy for insomnia (BBTI; Germain & Buysse, 2011). The added components of CBT-I include cognitive restructuring as some clients may have unhealthy or negative beliefs about their sleep difficulties. In addition to cognitive restructuring, the core components of CBT-I include relaxation training, sleep hygiene psychoeducation, stimulus control (i.e., bed being only associated with sleep), and sleep restriction by limiting the total time in bed (Jacobs, 2007).

A small number of studies have provided support for CBT-I as an intervention for treating insomnia in adolescence (de Bruin, Bögels, Oort, & Meijer, 2015; Schlarb, Liddle, & Hautzinger, 2010). However, a meta-analysis of CBT-I among children and adolescents by Ma and colleagues (Ma, Shi, & Deng, 2018) reported positive effects for CBT-I on sleep onset latency and sleep efficiency but not for wake after sleep onset and total sleep time. They conclude that CBT-I might be effective in the treatment of insomnia in children and adolescents, but that more large-scale randomized clinical trials are needed. In looking at this review as well as through a search in treatment of insomnia among youth, there did not appear to be any research conducted to evaluate the impact of REBT in treatment of insomnia among youth.

Another area that is related to sleep is students who have nighttime anxiety or fears. This may reflect a worsening of anxiety as it gets closer to bedtime with students ruminating about the events (e.g., social, academic) without distractions that may help ameliorate these worries (Meltzer & McLaughlin-Crabtree, 2015). While the worries here are not specific to sleep, they do impact sleep. Clinicians would benefit from integrating and having a healthy bedtime routine reinforced in combination with more traditional RE-CBT-based approaches toward treatment of anxiety.

Developmental Considerations in the Treatment of Sleep Problems Among Youth

Honaker and Meltzer (2016) report that across all age groups, behaviorally based sleep disorders are the most common. However, the type of sleep problems seen among youth does vary as a function of age. Meltzer and McLaughlin-Crabtree (2015) report that in the preschool years, you begin to see an increase in bedtime struggles which may be a result of their greater independence. Further, as their cognitive skills begin to develop, there may also be an increase in fears at night. These nighttime fears may lead to greater bedtime resistance. Among the school-age group, there may be more children who report daytime sleepiness. This may be a function of delayed-sleep onset as well as the fact that many school start times are early (Keller et al., 2015). Insufficient sleep among adolescents may be due to a myriad of factors including school start time (Minges & Redeker, 2016), technology (Bartel, Gradisar, & Williamson, 2015; Fuller, Lehman, Hicks, & Novick, 2017), and delayed circadian rhythm (Donaldson & Owens, 2006). Further, it is important for clinicians to consider the developmental age of the youth when designing clinical interventions to treat sleep problems among children and adolescents. This may also involve considering the source of information as to sleep problems that is from child, parent, or teacher, as well as who will be implementing the intervention. Many of the behaviorally oriented strategies will involve parents serving as the direct interventionist to promote sleep hygiene as well as limiting behaviors that may reinforce the sleep problem. In direct work with youth, Meltzer and McLaughin-Crabtree (2015) propose that in implementing cognitive interventions, younger children appear to benefit from strategies that are more concrete in nature, whereas adolescents may be better able to engage in cognitive restructuring through an approach such as RE-CBT. Having younger children rehearse rational coping statements related to their specific worries ("I've got this. The dark isn't that bad. My room is safe") may be more helpful than the traditional identification, challenging, and changing of irrational beliefs that are used with adolescents and will be described below in the treatment section and in the case study.

Best Practice Guidelines in the Treatment of Behavioral Sleep Problems Among Youth

Behavioral sleep disorders respond fairly well to behavioral sleep interventions (Meltzer & Mindell, 2014; Sakakini, 2011). All sleep interventions start with a consistent, positive bedtime routine with healthy sleep hygiene habits. We have provided guidelines of effective sleep hygiene practices that you may wish to use in your work with families (see Table 16.2).While this can sometimes alone be effective in treating behavioral insomnia of childhood (Mindell, 1999), often, further behavioral intervention is required. Below we provide a brief description of commonly used behavioral sleep interventions that have demonstrated efficacy.

Extinction is an efficacious treatment for behavioral insomnia of childhood and nightwakings (Kuhn & Elliot, 2003; Mindell, Kuhn et al., 2006). Extinction refers to intentionally ignoring a child's attempts to gain interaction during bedtime and the night (e.g., crying, screaming, calling out for parent) until the undesired behavior is extinguished (Donaldson & Owens, 2006). If parents adhere to the treatment, they will typically achieve success quite quickly (Donaldson & Owens, 2006). Graduated extinction is typically more favorable for parents and allows the parent to briefly respond to distress from a child on a progressively less frequent basis (Donaldson & Owens, 2006).

Table 16.2 Sleep hygiene tips

Have a *regular bedtime and wake time*, even on the weekends
Exercise daily for 20–30 minutes, ideally in the morning and afternoon, not too close to bedtime
Limit *caffeine* consumption, particularly after 4 pm (for kids, this can include chocolate)
Create a calming, consistent *bedtime routine*
Do the rituals in the same order
Begin the routine at the same time every night
Give child a 10-minute warning
Let child know this is the last activity of the day
Have a period of winding down
Avoid stimulating activities
Have a *light snack* before bedtime. It is best to go to bed neither starving nor stuffed
Make a *bedroom* a quiet and dark oasis for sleep
Bed is a sleep only zone – no homework or other activities in bed
Comfortable temperature
Lights off
White noise or soft music can be soothing
Turn off *screens* in the hour before bed and dim lights
The light from a screen can interfere with the production of the sleep-promoting hormone melatonin
Remove screens (phone, tablets, computers, TVs, gaming systems) from the bedroom

Limit setting and checking can be utilized with children who display bedtime resistance and involve consistently implementing clearly developed rules for appropriate bedtime behaviors. The "Bedtime Pass Program" (Moore, Friman, Fruzzetti, & MacAleese, 2007) is a limit-setting intervention that includes a set number of "passes" that the child can exchange for appropriate requests (e.g., drink, cuddle). The parent ignores any requests from the child once all of the passes have been used. Any unused passes can be exchanged for a reward.

Graded exposure can help children who require parental presence to fall asleep and involves utilizing an exposure "hierarchy" of gradually withdrawing the parent from the bedroom (if the parent is present in the child's room at bedtime) or gradually moving the child out of the parent's bed/room. Positive reinforcement is given when each step is attained. Graded exposure has been effective with school-age children (e.g., Paine & Gradisar, 2011).

Faded bedtime with response cost is appropriate for children who have difficulty falling asleep or staying asleep and closely resembles a combination of two behavioral interventions with the strongest treatment efficacy for chronic adult insomnia: sleep restriction and stimulus control (Kuhn & Elliot, 2003). Once a consistent bedtime routine is in place, bedtime is delayed aiding with rapid sleep initiation (Mindell, Kuhn, Lewin, Meltzer, & Sadeh, 2006). If the child does not fall asleep in a prescribed amount of time, the parents then take the child out of bed for set periods of time. Once the child is falling asleep quickly, the bedtime is moved earlier by 15- or 30-minute increments over successive nights until a preestablished bedtime goal is achieved (Mindell, Kuhn et al., 2006). During this intervention, a scheduled wake time is enforced and daytime sleep is not permitted, with the exception of age-appropriate naps (Mindell, Kuhn et al., 2006).

Bright light therapy combined with chronotherapy is an evidence-based treatment for delayed sleep phase disorder (DSPD). The adolescent follows a sleep-wake schedule based on their natural waking time and is exposed to natural light or a light box for 30–60 minutes upon waking. Over the course of days or weeks, their bedtime and wake time are advanced until the desired schedule is achieved (Gradisar, Smits, & Bjorvatn, 2014).

From an RE-CBT approach, we do think it is important to educate parents when having them deliver a behavioral sleep intervention that there is the possibility of an "extinction burst" where parents may see an increase in undesired behaviors at the initiation of treatment before clinical improvement is seen (Donaldson & Owens, 2006). As an example, when parents attempt to set limits on bedtime and extinguish bedtime resistance, their child may fight back and the noncompliance may escalate. When parents are inconsistent with their limit setting, the negative behavior may be reinforced, and it is important for parents to be consistent in limits in order for them to be effective (Donaldson & Owens, 2006). Parents may benefit from reassurance and coping thoughts/strategies to maintain these limits despite how stressful the child's behavior may be (Sakakini, 2011).

RE-CBT in the Treatment of Sleep Problems

Treatment of behavioral sleep problems that integrates an RE-CBT component often involves direct work with the student as well as working with the parent. While the work often overlaps, we will discuss RE-CBT for cognitive restructuring among youth first followed by RE-CBT work with parents to handle sleep problems and promote healthy sleep behaviors.

Often, students with sleep difficulties may endorse a number of irrational beliefs or negative/distorted thoughts related to sleep that impact sleep behavior. RE-CBT work with students with sleep problems promotes healthy sleep behaviors by challenging the thoughts that interfere with their follow-through of these behaviors. The constant worry about sleep that younger ("I can't fall asleep alone! I *need* my parents in my room. They *have to* lay with me. Bedtime is *awful*") and older students may have ("I *have* to fall asleep! What's wrong with me? I have a big day tomorrow and it will be *terrible* if I do not fall asleep!) can unfortunately make one night of restlessness transform into more chronic difficulties. While it can be helpful to examine precipitating variables (e.g., exams, peer conflict) that may have an impact on insufficient sleep, we want to look for the maintaining thoughts that continue to impact upon successful sleep.

Cognitive Restructuring: Dispute, Debate, and Discuss

From our experience, there are a number of common unhealthy negative thoughts (UNTs) or irrational beliefs (IBs) that interfere with sleep. Our goal is to work with students to identify, challenge, and change these IBs to then have them develop more healthy, rational beliefs (RBs) which improve sleep functioning. These thoughts may vary as a function of sleep problem type (e.g., insomnia vs. delayed sleep onset), but the approaches to challenging these thoughts remain the same.

One thought that can significantly interfere with insomnia is referred to as awfulizing or catastrophizing (DiGiuseppe, Doyle, Dryden, & Backx, 2013). Here, while trying to fall asleep, the student may be awfulizing about an event that happened earlier ("It's terrible that I made such a social mistake"), or as linked to sleep, they may be looking at their clock and catastrophizing the consequences of not falling sleep ("I cannot believe I am not asleep yet; my day tomorrow will now be *awful*!). The RE-CBT clinician would work with the student to be an emotional detective and try and look for evidence behind that belief ("How BAD do we know your day will be if you get less sleep?), if the belief makes sense ("Is it logical to think that just one bad night sleep, while it may have an impact on your day, would make it the WORST day?") as well as from a functional challenge ("Does saying my day will be awful help me fall asleep any faster?). Having students catch and then challenge these thoughts provides for an opportunity to develop a helpful coping statement ("Even if I have difficulty falling asleep, the worst thing that would happen is I will struggle a little bit tomorrow. I have had bad nights before and survived them").

Students may also have demands about their inability to fall asleep that may cause additional stress and impact on sleep onset and quality. Demands were considered by Ellis to be the primary irrational belief (DiGiuseppe et al., 2013) and consist of thoughts about how one *must* behave. With regard to sleep, younger students may think: "I need one of my parents in my room to fall asleep!" and older students may think: "I *have to* get to sleep! I *should* have fallen asleep 20 min ago! I have a big day tomorrow and I *need* to get to sleep! The RE-CBT clinician would work to challenge these needs from an empirical ("What do we know? We know there have been other times when you have fallen asleep without one of your parents in your room, you may have had difficulty sleeping, but you survived"), a semantic ("Yes, you want to fall asleep, but is getting that desired amount a necessity for survival?), and a functional perspective ("Does stressing about the need for sleep help you reach your goal: falling asleep?"). Coping thoughts that recognize the importance of sleep but may help reduce stress and improve sleep behavior may consist of statements like: "While it probably would be better for me to get more sleep tonight, I don't need to and only telling myself that I have to have this much sleep makes me even more stressed and less likely to fall asleep."

Oftentimes, demandingness overlaps with other related irrational beliefs like frustration intolerance (DiGiuseppe et al., 2013) that may interfere with healthy sleep behaviors. Frustration intolerance beliefs are when students believe that something that they are dealing with is completely unbearable or cannot be tolerated.

Students may have certain rigidly held beliefs about other life variables that get intertwined with frustration intolerance that may lead to delayed sleep onset. Examples may be about sleep time ("I *should* be allowed to stay up later! All my friends do. *I can't stand this*!!") or about use of technology ("I *need to* have my phone. I *have to* be able to connect with my friends! I *can't handle* not knowing what is going on!"). Here too, the RE-CBT clinician would integrate the empirical ("Can you really NOT stand it? I know you do not like it, but can you stand it?), semantic ("I understand wanting a later bedtime or technology access, but are they truly "needs"?), and functional ("How does it help you to get upset? Do you get your phone/later bedtime? Does fighting with your parents help you fall asleep better or have better quality of sleep?"). We think it important to validate what the students *wants*, without reinforcing their beliefs about *needs* which impact on their sleep behaviors. These wants can be used in developing coping thoughts to manage their frustration and promote better sleep ("While I really want my phone and think it's not fair that I cannot have it, getting upset doesn't get me it and it also doesn't help me sleep well"). These healthier coping thoughts may help reduce elevated nighttime affective states and sleep onset and promote heathier sleep.

Work with parents has been shown to be effective in treating behavioral sleep problems (Sakakini, 2011). We do think it important to discuss certain beliefs that the parents may endorse that may interfere with parents sticking to behavioral strategies outlined above. Rather than going through beliefs related to each specific behavioral intervention, we will discuss four core beliefs as they relate to compliance with healthy sleep behaviors. In looking at sleep hygiene, some student sleep behaviors get reinforced. For example, students who get into their parents' bed in the middle of the night may not be redirected by their parents to return to their own bed. While parents may know that it is better for their child to sleep in their own bed, based on their history, they may know that this will be a struggle and may lead to crying/arguing and it is just easier to allow them to stay in their bed. Parents may have beliefs of frustration intolerance ("I can't stand the idea of repeatedly getting up and bringing her back to her room") as well as awfulizing ("If this leads into a 30-minute middle-of-the-night meltdown, that would be terrible for her and for me") that block effective behavioral sleep practices.

Bedtime fading and having positive bedtime routines have shown to be effective for children who have problems falling asleep, but being consistent in these routines can be challenging for parents. Their beliefs ("yes, I know this is important, but I have had a rough day and I need a break") may interfere with how the intervention is implemented and as such may further reinforce the negative sleep habits. Graduated extinction where the parent provides scheduled reassurance may also be complicated by parent beliefs when they try and ignore their child's efforts to gain their attention by crying or calling for them. Ratings of worth may interfere with application of the intervention as parents may think they are a "horrible person for letting their child be upset."

This is where we think RE-CBT can be a significant added component to promoting healthier sleep habits among children: through work with their parents to improve implementation of well-established behavioral strategies. By helping parents identify and change irrational beliefs that may contribute to unhealthy parent affect and poor sleep decisions, it may improve overall sleep hygiene among children and adolescents.

Case Study: Jessica's Insomnia (RE-CBT-Insomnia)

Jessica is a 15-year-old attending a private high school, who was referred for psychotherapy by her high school guidance counselor due to concerns with dropping grades, changes in mood, and her tendency to appear sleepy/fall asleep in class. Jessica has no history of hospitalizations or psychiatric treatment and is not on any medications. Six months prior to this referral for treatment, Jessica saw a therapist to process grief and focused on mindfulness techniques. Jessica is enrolled in several Advanced Placement (AP) courses and has a history of being a high-achieving student at the top of her class. Jessica and her mother reported that she experiences fatigue during the day, difficulty sustaining attention in classes, increasing irritability, and low frustration tolerance leading to increased conflicts with her parents and friends.

In the initial clinical interview with Jessica and her mother, they shared that Jessica's cousin died from a progressive illness a few years prior and that she had a delayed emotional response to the loss. Jessica reported that she has been thinking about her cousin more in the last year especially at night when she is trying to sleep. Jessica's cousin was a year younger than her, and now that she is in high school, Jessica finds herself thinking about her cousin's "unfulfilled life potential and high school experiences" and how it is wrong and not fair that this happened. Jessica reported that she has problems sleeping and frequently worries about her "life purpose" in relation to her cousin's death. Jessica reports sadness and that she is often awake at night thinking about how her problems are insignificant compared to her cousin's death yet desires to make the most of the life that her cousin did not have the opportunity to live.

In addition to a clinical interview with Jessica and her mother, in order to gather data about her sleep onset, duration, quality, and potential sleep disorders, Jessica's mother completed the Sleep Disorders Inventory for Students-Revised-Adolescent (SDIS-R-A). The SDIS-R-S is a screening tool for sleep disturbance disorders including sleep-related breathing disorder (SRBD), periodic limb movement disorder (PLMD), restless legs syndrome (RLS), delayed sleep phase syndrome (DSPS), and narcolepsy (NARC). On this measure, Jessica's mother rated her sleep, and overall her scores did not indicate a sleep disturbance disorder. Her mother did endorse that Jessica is almost always up past one in the morning and she grinds her teeth and snores while she sleeps. A recommendation/referral to a physician was made to rule out any medical factors that may be contributing to her difficulties due to the reporting of Jessica snoring and grinding her teeth. Data from Jessica's self-report interview revealed that in recent months, Jessica has been sleeping an average of 2.5 hours a night with significant difficulty initiating sleep. On at least two nights a week, she does not sleep at all, goes to school, and takes 4-hour naps after school, then she may sleep for 3 hours the following night.

While results of the SDIS-R-A ruled out a sleep disturbance disorder, based on Jessica's self-report, her symptoms are consistent with a presentation of insomnia. Jessica reports dissatisfaction with the quantity of sleep on most nights which has persisted for over 3 months, and it is impacting her behaviorally and emotionally. Jessica recognizes how her lack of sleep is impacting her grades and her general presentation and mood. She is more easily distracted in class, and as a result, she is not meeting her expectations for academic performance in the AP classes as compared to the last academic year. Jessica also compared her sleep and morning routine this year to that of last school year. She used to sleep an average of 7 hours each night and would spend almost an hour getting herself ready for school each day including doing her make-up, curling her hair, and eating breakfast. This year, she reported that she rushes to put her uniform on and get out the door within a half-hour, skipping all the grooming activities she did last year. In the last few months, Jessica has had several incidents in which low frustration tolerance and irritability have affected her relationship with her mother. Her skirt zipper broke at school, she called her mother, but when her mother was not able to help her, she screamed at her saying "you don't care about me, you are never there to help me, you said I could call you and you'd be available!" Jessica is motivated for treatment, recognizing the impact her insomnia is having on her life.

Treatment for Jessica's insomnia began with psychoeducation based on the Jacobs (2007) manual included informing Jessica of research-based recommendations for sleep hygiene, sleep duration, and ramifications of sleep deprivation. Jessica learned that those who experience sleep loss have an impaired daytime functioning in the areas of mood, attention, and memory. Jessica was tasked with completing a sleep diary between sessions in which she tracked the time she got in bed, the time she thinks she fell asleep, and the time she woke up. Jessica also logged caffeine consumption, exercise, and daytime naps.

Cognitive restructuring work with Jessica required her to describe her thoughts prior to going to sleep and any feelings she had in anticipation of sleeping. When Jessica took naps after school, she thought that she had ruined her sleep, would never fall asleep and would have a terrible day the next morning. She also would engage in some retrospective awfulizing ("It's terrible what happened to my cousin; I'm not who I was last year") as well as some prospective awfulizing ("If I cannot fall asleep now, tomorrow will be a terrible day!"). She reported that when she would go to bed, she would often look at her clock throughout the night and think thoughts that reflected frustration intolerance ("*I can't stand* that I have been in bed for 3 hours and still have not fallen asleep!") as well as demandingness ("I *have* to get to sleep!"). She was taught to identify these thoughts and challenge them. More specifically, she worked on using more functional disputes ("How is it helping me to think, I *have* to get to sleep and if I don't, tomorrow would be *terrible*?") as well as empirical disputes and coping statements ("Regrettably, there have been other nights I struggled with sleep, while I may struggle the next day, I will handle it").

In addition to the cognitive restructuring work, behavioral homework included work on improving her sleep hygiene. Jessica would often do homework in her bed as well as play music and watch television while in bed. Her sleep routine included at least 2 hours of being in bed with her phone on mindlessly scrolling through social media, then ruminating about her role in society, whether she had a purpose in life, and pressuring herself to minimize her problems in light of her cousin's death. Behavioral work included asking her to only use her bed for sleep (i.e., stimulus control) and find other spaces to complete her homework. Her behavioral bedtime protocol was to set her 15-minute white noise app, and if she was still awake at the end, she needed to get up, sit at her desk, drink water, read or draw, but not pick up her phone. Then when she felt sleepiness, she could return to her bed and reset the white noise app. Jessica's mother was enlisted to monitor her afterschool routine to limit napping, in order to reserve her sleep for nighttime. If needed, naps were limited to 20–30 minutes but would not exceed 1 hour. These were monitored throughout the course of therapy with a focus on limiting/minimizing naps in terms of frequency and duration.

After 5 weeks of cognitive-behavioral therapy for insomnia, Jessica's average daily sleep duration increased to 7 hours a night, and she was no longer napping after school. The sleep diaries helped Jessica became more aware of her actual sleep duration and reduced her guilt about ruining her sleep. She also reported improvement in her ability to focus on her schoolwork during the day and reduced irritability during interactions with her parents and friends. She indicated that she still experienced some sadness as it related to her cousin and also had some moments of concern when she had difficulty falling asleep, but that she did not get too upset in both circumstances to the point that it impacted her sleep and subsequently her socialization and academics. While some of her other challenges still warranted intervention, integrating an RE-CBT treatment protocol for sleep into clinical work has helped reduce the impact of deficient sleep on these other areas of concern and increased her ability to benefit from therapy.

Adaptation of RE-CBT for Sleep Problems in Schools

There are a few areas that we think are important to consider as they relate to the assessment and treatment of sleep problems in school. First, we would encourage school-based practitioners to consider the role of sleep in student affect and behavior, as insufficient sleep may exacerbate symptoms of another disorder and may lead to unnecessary evaluations or accommodations/interventions. That is, before conducting a psychoeducational evaluation for a student because his grades have decreased and his teacher described him as "lazy," perhaps consider the relationship of sleep with academics (Buckhalt, El-Sheikh, Keller, & Kelley, 2009; Pagel &

Kwiatkowski, 2010) and prioritize sleep as one of the first areas to examine. As sleep problems are common among students with ADHD and autism (Cortese, Faraone, Konofal, & Lecendreux, 2009), we think it is important to also consider sleep with students who have a diagnosis/educational classification, as a sleep problem may exacerbate their symptoms. Similar to academics, given the relationship of sleep difficulties with a number of social-emotional outcomes (Roberts et al., 2008), we encourage that a sleep assessment be a mainstay of all school-based evaluations. If sleep problems are identified early enough and appropriate intervention is delivered, it may ameliorate the long-term impact of some of these difficulties.

We also agree with Owen and colleagues (Owens et al., 2014), who suggest that schools provide students, parents, teachers, and school nurses with information regarding sleep. We think schools may want to incorporate sleep hygiene and education into the curriculum in the school. We also think that given the negative correlation between early school start times and academic performance (Dunster et al., 2018; Lewin et al., 2017), school-based practitioners may also want to advocate for a later school start time where appropriate.

Finally, we think it is important that a collaborative team-based approach (parent, school-based practitioner, educator, medical staff) be developed to help identify the appropriate course of action for treatment. Being mindful of the role and training of school-based practitioners, caution is offered in having the school setting be the first choice of intervention for more significant sleep problems among youth. Psychoeducation and collaboration among the school staff, parents, and students are essential to most effectively address sleep problems among youth. Integrating core concepts of RE-CBT may enhance treatment compliance and teach students and their parents strategies to most effectively manage sleep problems.

Test Yourself Questions

1. While behavioral interventions have been effective in treating behavioral sleep problems, what other CB-REBT areas would clinicians want to consider when working with a student and parents to treat a student's sleep problem?
2. What cognitions/beliefs might affect a parent trying to implement consistent positive bedtime routines?
3. Justin is a 16-year-old who plays on his phone at bedtime then tosses and turns in bed for hours before finally falling asleep, only having to wake up a few hours later for school. As a clinician, what beliefs do you think underlie his bedtime behaviors and insomnia and how would you go about targeting them from a CB-REBT perspective?

References

Alfano, C. A., Zakem, A. H., Costa, N. M., Taylor, L. K., & Weems, C. F. (2009). Sleep problems and their relation to cognitive factors, anxiety, and depressive symptoms in children and adolescents. *Depression and Anxiety, 26*(6), 503–512. https://doi.org/10.1002/da.20443

American Academy of Sleep Medicine. (2014). *International classification of sleep disorders*. Darien, IL: American Academy of Sleep Medicine.

American Psychiatric Association. (2013). *Diagnostic and statistical manual of mental disorders (DSM-5®)*. Washington, D.C.: American Psychiatric Pub.

Aronen, E. T., Paavonen, E. J., Fjällberg, M., Soininen, M., & Törrönen, J. (2000). Sleep and psychiatric symptoms in school-age children. *Journal of the American Academy of Child and Adolescent Psychiatry, 39*(4), 502–508. https://doi.org/10.1097/00004583-200004000-00020

Bartel, K. A., Gradisar, M., & Williamson, P. (2015). Protective and risk factors for adolescent sleep: A meta-analytic review. *Sleep Medicine Reviews, 21*, 72–85. https://doi.org/10.1016/j.smrv.2014.08.002

Beebe, D. W., Ris, M. D., Kramer, M. E., Long, E., & Amin, R. (2010). The association between sleep disordered breathing, academic grades, and cognitive and behavioral functioning among overweight subjects during middle to late childhood. *Sleep, 33*, 1447–1456.

Bruni, O., Ferini-Strambi, L., Russo, P. M., Antignani, M., Innocenzi, M., Ottaviano, P., et al. (2006). Sleep disturbances and teacher ratings of school achievement and temperament in children. *Sleep Medicine, 7*(1), 43–48.

Buckhalt, J. A., El-Sheikh, M., Keller, P., & Kelley, R. (2009). Concurrent and longitudinal relations between children's sleep and cognitive functioning. *Child Development, 80*, 875–892. https://doi.org/10.1111/j.1467-8624.2009.01303.x

Cortese, S., Faraone, S. V., Konofal, E., & Lecendreux, M. (2009). Sleep in children with attention-deficit/hyperactivity disorder: Meta-analysis of subjective and objective studies. *Journal of the American Academy of Child & Adolescent Psychiatry, 48*, 894–908. https://doi.org/10.1097/CHI.0b013e3181ac09c9

de Bruin, E. J., Bögels, S. M., Oort, F. J., & Meijer, A. M. (2015). Efficacy of cognitive behavioral therapy for insomnia in adolescents: A randomized controlled trial with internet therapy, group therapy and a waiting list condition. *Sleep, 38*, 1913–1926. https://doi.org/10.5665/sleep.5240

Dewald, J. F., Meijer, A. M., Oort, F. J., Kerkof, G. A., & Bogels, S. M. (2010). The influence of sleep quality, sleep duration and sleepiness on school performance in children and adolescents: A meta-analytic review. *Sleep Medicine Reviews, 14*, 179–189. https://doi.org/10.1016/j.smrv.2009.10.004

DiGiuseppe, R. A., Doyle, K. A., Dryden, W., & Backx, W. (2013). *A practitioner's guide to rational emotive behavior therapy (3rd addition)*. New York: Oxford University Press.

Donaldson, D. L., & Owens, J. A. (2006). Sleep and sleep problems. In G. G. Bear & K. M. Minke (Eds.), *Children's needs III: Development, prevention, and intervention* (pp. 1025–1039). Bethesda, MD: National Association of School Psychologists.

Drake, C., Nickel, C., Burduvali, E., Roth, T., Jefferson, C., & Badia, P. (2003). The pediatric daytime sleepiness scale (pdss): Sleep habits and school outcomes in middle-school children. *Sleep: Journal of Sleep and Sleep Disorders Research, 26*(4), 455–458.

Dunster, G. P., de la Iglesia, L., Ben-Hamo, M., Nave, C., Fleischer, J. G., Panda, S., et al. (2018). Sleepmore in Seattle: Later school start times are associated with more sleep and better performance in high school students. *Science Advances, 4*(12), 1–7. https://doi.org/10.1126/sciadv.aau6200

El-Sheikh, M., Kelly, R. J., Buckhalt, J. A., & Hinnant, J. B. (2010). Children's sleep and adjustment over time: The role of socioeconomic context. *Child Development, 81*, 870–883. https://doi.org/10.1111/j.1467-8624.2010.01439.x

Esposito, M. A. (2009). *REBT with children and adolescents: A meta-analytic review of efficacy* (Publication No. 3361233) [Doctoral Dissertation, St. John's University]. ProQuest Dissertations Publishing.

Ferreira, V. R., Carvalho, L. B., Ruotolo, F., de Morais, J. F., Prado, L. B., & Prado, G. F. (2009). Sleep disturbance scale for children: Translation, cultural adaptation, and validation. *Sleep Medicine, 10*(4), 457–463. https://doi.org/10.1016/j.sleep.2008.03.018. doi: S1389-9457(08)00104-4[pii].

Frank, M. G., & Benington, J. H. (2006). The role of sleep in memory consolidation and brain plasticity: Dream or reality? *The Neuroscientist, 12*(6), 477–488. https://doi.org/10.1177/1073858406293552

Fuller, C., Lehman, E., Hicks, S., & Novick, M. B. (2017). Bedtime use of technology and associated sleep problems in children. *Global Pediatric Health, 4*, 1–8. https://doi.org/10.1177/2333794X17736972

Gangwisch, J. E., Babiss, L. A., Malaspina, D., Turner, J. B., Zammit, G. K., & Posner, K. (2010). Earlier parental set bedtimes as a protective factor against depression and suicidal ideation. *Sleep, 33*(1), 97–106. https://doi.org/10.1093/sleep/33.1.97

Germain, A., & Buysse, D. J. (2011). Brief behavioral treatment of insomnia. In M. Perlis, M. Aloia, & B. Kuhn (Eds.), *Practical resources for the mental health professional, behavioral treatments for sleep disorders* (pp. 143–150). Academic Press.

Gonzalez, J. E., Nelson, J. R., Gutkin, T. B., Saunders, A., Galloway, A., & Shwery, C. S. (2004). Rational emotive therapy with children and adolescents: A meta-analysis. *Journal of Emotional and Behavioral Disorders, 12*(4), 222–235. https://doi.org/10.1177/10634266040120040301

Gradisar, M., Smits, M. G., & Bjorvatn, B. (2014). Assessment and treatment of delayed sleep phase disorder in adolescents: Recent innovations and cautions. *Sleep Medicine Clinics, 9*, 199–210.

Gruber, R., Michaelsen, S., Bergmame, L., Frenette, S., Bruni, O., Fontil, L., et al. (2012). Short sleep duration is associated with teacher-reported inattention and cognitive problems in healthy school-aged children. *Nature and Science of Sleep, 4*, 33–40. https://doi.org/10.2147/NSS.S24607

Harvey, A. G. (2016). A Transdiagnostic intervention for youth sleep and circadian problems. *Cognitive Behavioral Practice, 23*, 341–355.

Honaker, S. M., & Meltzer, L. J. (2016). Sleep in pediatric primary care: A review of the literature. *Sleep Medicine Reviews, 25*, 31–30. https://doi.org/10.1016/j.smrv.2015.01.004

Jacobs, G. D. (2007). *Clinical training manual for a CBT program for insomnia*. Sudbury, MA: Somnus.

Jenni, O. G., & Carskadon, M. A. (2007). Sleep behavior and sleep regulation from infancy through adolescence: Normative aspects. *Sleep Medicine Clinics, 2*(3), 321–329.

Ji, A., & Liu, J. (2016). Subjective sleep measures for adolescents: A systematic review. *Child Care Health Development, 42*(6), 825–839.

Keller, P. S., Smith, O. A., Gilbert, L. R., Bi, S., Haak, E. A., & Buckhalt, J. A. (2015). Earlier school start times as a risk factor for poor school performance: An examination of public elementary schools in the commonwealth of Kentucky. *Journal of Educational Psychology, 107*(1), 236–245. https://doi.org/10.1037/a0037195

Kopasz, M., Loessl, B., Hornyak, M., Riemann, D., Nissen, C., Piosczyk, H., et al. (2010). Sleep and memory in healthy children and adolescents — A critical review. *Sleep Medicine Reviews, 14*(3), 167–177. https://doi.org/10.1016/j.smrv.2009.10.006

Kubiszewski, V., Fontaine, R., Potard, C., & Gimenes, G. (2014). Bullying, sleep/wake patterns and subjective sleep disorders: Findings from a cross-sectional survey. *Chronobiology International, 31*(4), 542–553. https://doi.org/10.3109/07420528.2013.877475

Kuhn, B. R., & Elliot, A. J. (2003). Treatment efficacy in behavioral pediatric sleep medicine. *Journal of Psychosomatic Research, 54*, 587–597. https://doi.org/10.1016/S0022-3999(03)00061-8

Laberge, L., Tremblay, R. E., Vitaro, F., & Montplaisir, J. (2000). Development of parasomnias from childhood to early adolescence. *Pediatrics, 106*, 67–74. https://doi.org/10.1542/peds.2004-0815F

Lewin, D. S., Wang, G., Chen, Y. I., Skora, E., Hoehn, J., Baylor, A., et al. (2017). Variable school start times and middle school student's sleep health and academic performance. *Journal of Adolescent Health, 61*(2), 205–211. https://doi.org/10.1016/j.jadohealth.2017.02.017

Luginbuehl, M. (2005). *Sleep disorders inventory for students – children's form*. Clearwater, FL: Child Uplift.

Lundgren, D. (2020). *Examining Start Times among Schools in New York State: Patterns, Rationale, and Implications*. [Doctoral Dissertation, St. John's University]. ProQuest Dissertations Publishing.

Ma, Z., Shi, L.-J., & Deng, M.-H. (2018). Efficacy of cognitive behavioral therapy in children and adolescents with insomnia: A systematic review and meta-analysis. *Brazilian Journal of Medical and Biological Research, 51*(6), e7070. Epub May 21, 2018.https://doi.org/10.1590/1414-431x20187070

Marcus, C. L., Brooks, L. J., Davidson Ward, S., Draper, K. A., Gozal, D., Halbower, A. C., et al. (2012). Diagnosis and management of childhood obstructive sleep apnea syndrome. *Pediatrics, 130*(3), 714–755. https://doi.org/10.1542/peds.2012-1672

Maski, K., & Owens, J. A. (2016). Insomnia, parasomnias, and narcolepsy in children: Clinical features, diagnosis, and management. *The Lancet Neurology, 15*(11), 1170–1181. https://doi.org/10.1016/S1474-4422(16)30204-6

McKnight-Eily, L. R., Eaton, D. K., Lowry, R., Croft, J. B., Presley-Cantrell, L., & Perry, G. S. (2011). Relationships between hours of sleep and health-risk behaviors in us adolescent students. *Preventive Medicine, 53*, 271–273. https://doi.org/10.1016/j.ypmed.2011.06.020

Meltzer, L. J., & McLaughlin-Crabtree, V. (2015). *Pediatric sleep problems: A clinician's guide to behavioral interventions*. Washington, DC: American Psychological Association. https://doi.org/10.1037/14645-000

Meltzer, L. J., & Mindell, J. A. (2014). Systematic review and meta-analysis of behavioral interventions for pediatric insomnia. *Journal of Pediatric Psychology, 39*(8), 932–948. https://doi.org/10.1093/jpepsy/jsu041

Meltzer, L. J., Walsh, C. M., Traylor, J., & Westin, A. M. (2012). Direct comparison of two new actigraphs and polysomnography in children and adolescents. *Sleep, 35*, 159–166. https://doi.org/10.5665/sleep.1608

Mindell, J., & Owens, J. (2015). *A clinical guide to pediatric sleep: Diagnosis and management of sleep problems* (3rd ed.). Philadelphia: Lippincott Williams & Wilkins.

Mindell, J. A., Bartle, A., Ahn, Y., Ramamurthy, M. B., Huong, H. T. D., Kohyama, J., et al. (2013). Sleep education in pediatric residency programs: A cross-cultural look. *BMC Research Notes, 6*(1), 130.

Mindell, J. A., Bartle, A., Wahab, N. A., Ahn, Y., Ramamurthy, M. B., Huong, H. T. D., et al. (2011). Sleep education in medical school curriculum: A glimpse across countries. *Sleep Medicine, 12*(9), 928–931.

Mindell, J. A., Emslie, G., Blumer, J., Genel, M., Glaze, D., Ivanenko, A., et al. (2006). Pharmacological management of insomnia in children and adolescents: Consensus statement. *Pediatrics, 117*, e1223–e1232. https://doi.org/10.1542/peds.2005-1693

Mindell, J. A., Kuhn, B., Lewin, D. S., Meltzer, L. J., & Sadeh, A. (2006). Behavioral treatment of bedtime problems and night wakings in infants and young children. *Sleep, 29*, 1263–1276.

Minges, K. E., & Redeker, N. S. (2016). Delayed school start times and adolescent sleep: A systematic review of the experimental evidence. *Sleep Medicine Reviews, 28*, 86–95. https://doi.org/10.1016/j.smrv.2015.06.002

Moore, B. A., Friman, P. C., Fruzzetti, A. E., & MacAleese, K. (2007). Brief report: Evaluating the bedtime pass program for child resistance to bedtime – A randomized, controlled trial. *Journal of Pediatric Psychology, 32*, 283–287.

Okajima, I., & Inoue, Y. (2018). Efficacy of cognitive behavioral therapy for comorbid insomnia: A meta-analysis. *Sleep and Biological Rhythms, 16*, 21–35. https://doi.org/10.1007/s41105-017-0124-8

Owens, J. (2005). Insomnia in children and adolescents. *Journal of Clinical Sleep Medicine, 1*(04), e454–e458.

Owens, J., & Adolescent Sleep Working Group, & Committee on Adolescence. (2014). Insufficient sleep in adolescents and young adults: An update on causes and consequences. *Pediatrics, 134*, 921–932. https://doi.org/10.1542/peds.2014-1696

Owens, J. A., Spirito, A., & McGuinn, M. (2000). The children's sleep habits questionnaire (CSHQ): Psychometric properties of a survey instrument for school-aged children. *Sleep, 23*, 1–9.

Pagel, J. F., & Kwiatkowski, C. F. (2010). Sleep complaints affecting school performance at different educational levels. *Frontiers in Neurology, 1*, 1–6.

Paine, S., & Gradisar, M. (2011). A randomized controlled trial of cognitive-behavior therapy for behavioral insomnia of childhood in school-aged children. *Behavior Research and Therapy, 49*, 379–388.

Perfect, M. M., Frye, S. S., & Sakakini, R. J. (2019). Sleep problems. In A. G. Dempsey (Ed.), *Pediatric health conditions in schools: A clinician's guide for working with children, families, and educators*. New York: Oxford University Press.

Perfect, M. M., Levine-Donnerstein, D., Archbold, K., Goodwin, J. E., & Quan, S. F. (2014). The contribution of multiple sleep disturbances on school and psychosocial functioning. *Psychology in the Schools, 51*, 273–295. https://doi.org/10.1002/pits.21746

Picchietti, D., Allen, R. P., Walters, A. S., Davidson, J. E., Myers, A., & Ferini-Strambi, L. (2007). Restless legs syndrome: Prevalence and impact in children and adolescents- the peds rest study. *Pediatrics, 120*(2), 253–266. https://doi.org/10.1542/peds.2006-2767

Picchietti, D. L., Bruni, O., Weerd, A., Durmer, J. S., Kotagal, S., Owens, J. A., et al. (2013). Pediatric restless legs syndrome diagnostic criteria: An update by the international restless legs syndrome study group. *Sleep Medicine, 14*(12), 1253–1259.

Proserpio, P., & Nobili, L. (2017). Parasomnias in children. In S. Nevšímalová & O. Bruni (Eds.), *Sleep disorders in children*. Switzerland: Springer International Publishing.

Raven, F., Van der Zee, E. A., Meerlo, P., & Havekes, R. (2018). The role of sleep in regulating structural plasticity and synaptic strength: Implications for memory and cognitive function. *Sleep Medicine Reviews, 39*, 3–11. https://doi.org/10.1016/j.smrv.2017.05.002

Roberts, E., Roberts, C., & Duong, H. T. (2009). Sleepless in adolescence: Prospective data on sleep deprivation, health and functioning. *Journal of Adolescence, 32*, 1045–1057. PMID: 1936185.

Roberts, R. E., Roberts, C. R., & Duong, H. T. (2008). Chronic insomnia and its negative consequences for health and functioning of adolescents: A 12-month prospective study. *Journal of Adolescent Health, 42*, 294–302. https://doi.org/10.1016/j.jadohealth.2007.09.016

Sadeh, A. (2015). Sleep assessment methods. *Monographs of the Society for Research in Child Development, 80*(1), 33–48. https://doi.org/10.1111/mono.12143

Sadeh, A., Raviv, A., & Gruber, R. (2000). Sleep patterns and sleep disruptions in school-age children. *Developmental Psychology, 36*, 291–301.

Sakakini, R. (2011). *Behavioral treatments for sleep problems in youth: A meta-analytic review* (Doctoral dissertation). Retrieved from ProQuest. (3452590).

Schlarb, A. A., Liddle, C. C., & Hautzinger, M. (2010). JuSt - a multimodal program for treatment of insomnia in adolescents: A pilot study. *Nature and Science of Sleep, 3*, 13–20. https://doi.org/10.2147/NSS.S14493

Silva, G. E., Goodwin, J. L., Parthasarathy, S., Sherrill, D. L., Vana, K. D., Drescher, A. A., et al. (2011). Longitudinal association between short sleep, body weight, and emotional and learning problems in Hispanic and Caucasian children. *Sleep, 34*, 1197–1205. https://doi.org/10.5665/SLEEP.1238

Stallman, H. M., & Kohler, M. (2016). Prevalence of sleepwalking: A systematic review and meta-analysis. *PLoS One, 11*(11), e0164769. https://doi.org/10.1371/journal.pone.0164769

Vriend, J. L., Davidson, F. D., Corkum, P. V., Rusak, B., McLaughlin, E. N., & Chambers, C. T. (2012). Sleep quantity and quality in relation to daytime functioning in children. *Children's Health Care, 41*(3), 204–222. https://doi.org/10.1080/02739615.2012.685039

Winsler, A., Deutsch, A., Vorona, R. D., Payne, P. A., & Szklo-coxe, M. (2015). Sleepless in fairfax: The difference one more hour of sleep can make for teen hopelessness, suicidal ideation, and substance use. *Journal of Youth and Adolescence, 44*(2), 362–378. https://doi.org/10.1007/s10964-014-0170-3

Wong, M. M., Rowland, S. E., & Dyson, R. B. (2014). Sleep problems, academic performance and substance use among adolescents. *North American Journal of Psychology, 16*(3), 629–648.

Chapter 17
Using RE-CBT with Transgender and Gender-Expansive Children and Youth

Jamie M. Joseph, Samantha Busa, and Breanne Taylor

Overview

Gender identity is a self-defined concept of being male, female, or other gender and can differ from what is assigned to someone at birth based on their chromosomes and external genitalia (American Psychological Association [APA], 2015). "Transgender" is an adjective that is an inclusive umbrella term that describes someone whose gender self-concept is different from their biological sex, whereas "cisgender" people's gender self-concept is consistent with their biological sex (APA, 2015). It is estimated that 1.4 million adults identify as transgender (0.6% of the population; Williams Institute, 2017). The prevalence of transgender youth is challenging to estimate given barriers to research, treatment, and disclosure (APA, 2012). Estimates of transgender youth have varied over time. The first study to provide population estimates for youth who identify as transgender in each of the 50 states and the District of Columbia indicated that 0.7% of youth ages 13–17 years or 150,000 youth identify as transgender in the United States (Herman, Flores, Brown, Wilson, & Conron, 2017). The most recent estimate of transgender high school students from the Centers for Disease Control and Prevention is 2% (Johns et al., 2019).

Transgender children and youth may experience gender dysphoria, which is a diagnostic label in the Diagnostic and Statistical Manual of Mental Disorders (DSM-5; American Psychiatric Association, 2013), describing the distress related to

J. M. Joseph (✉)
Cognitive Behavior Therapy & Evaluation, Coral Springs, FL, USA

S. Busa
Department of Child and Adolescent Psychiatry, Hassenfeld Children's Hospital at NYU Langone, New York, NY, USA

B. Taylor
Nova Southeastern University, Fort Lauderdale, FL, USA

M. Bernard, M. D. Terjesen (eds.), *Rational-Emotive and Cognitive-Behavioral Approaches to Child and Adolescent Mental Health: Theory, Practice, Research, Applications*, https://doi.org/10.1007/978-3-030-53901-6_17

the disconnect between an individual's body and gender self-concept. It is important to stress that being transgender is not by itself a pathological difficulty. What can be the focus of treatment is the psychological dysphoria that results from the incongruency between the physical body and gender identity. Affirmative treatment of children and youth's self-defined understanding of their gender is the focus of current standards of care by major professional associations such as the World Professional Association for Transgender Health (WPATH, 2011), the American Psychological Association (APA, 2015), and the Endocrine Society (Hembree et al., 2017).

Transgender children and youth have higher rates of psychological difficulties and a greater risk of suicide compared to their cisgender peers (Toomey, Syversten, & Shramko, 2018). Cognitive Behavioral Therapy (CBT) and specifically Rational Emotive Behavior Therapy (REBT), the combination of which can be called RE-CBT, are proposed by the authors to be an affirmative therapeutic modality to assist gender diverse and transgender children and youth to live happier, healthier, emotional lives. The current literature is lacking in the application of CBT and REBT when working with transgender and gender-expansive (TGGE) children and youth, and this chapter is the first of its kind. Some specific RE-CBT principles for coping are outlined for individual therapy and system wide when applied in the school system, and a case study that reflects clinical applications of RE-CBT in working with TGGE is provided. Social and medical transitions are briefly discussed.

Overview of Transgender and Gender-Expansive (TGGE) Youth and Introduction to Gender-Related Terms and Concepts

Sex and gender are often conflated by the general public as they are seen as intertwined; however, these concepts are unique and are worth defining. *Sex or sex assigned at birth* is a person's biological status, which is largely categorized as male, female, or intersex (i.e., atypical combinations of features that usually distinguish male from female). Some indicators of biological sex are chromosomes, gonads, internal reproductive organs, and external genitalia (APA, 2012). *Gender*, on the other hand, is culturally defined. It refers to attitudes, feelings, and behaviors a particular culture associates with a person's biological sex. Behavior that is compatible with cultural expectations is referred to as *gender normative*; behaviors that are viewed as incompatible with these expectations constitute *gender nonconformity* (APA, 2012).

A person's *gender identity* is their individual and subjective sense of being a boy or a girl, or male or female, neither or other. It is a self-defined, internal conception of oneself and is not necessarily visible to others (APA, 2015). Importantly, a person's gender identity may or may not align with their sex assigned at birth. *Cisgender* is an adjective which refers to a person whose internal conception of their self as male or female aligns with the sex assigned to them at birth (APA, 2015).

Transgender is an adjective, used as a collective term, to describe the full range of people whose gender identity differs from that which would be typically associated with the sex they were assigned at birth (APA, 2015). The authors posit that that "transgender," "gender diverse," "gender expansive," and "gender nonconforming" are inclusive terms that describe any individual whose gender identity does not align with the sex that was assigned to them at birth. The single term "transgender" is consistent with current nomenclature to designate inclusivity of the multiplicity of transgender identities. These include nonbinary (gender identities that are not exclusively masculine or exclusively feminine), genderqueer (individuals who defy all categories of culturally defined gender and self-identify as gender-free, gender neutral, or outside of gender altogether) (Chen, Edwards-Leeper, Stancin, & Tishelman, 2018), gender fluid (a person who does not identify themselves as having a fixed gender), and agender (a person who does not identify themselves as having a particular gender) identities to name a few. Terms are often changing, and it is important to ask each client how they define their own gender rather than placing a label on them.

Sexual orientation and *gender identity* are not the same. These concepts are often confused for one another, and understanding how they are related, but different, is important. Sexual orientation refers to an individual's physical, sexual, romantic, and/or emotional attraction to someone else (APA, 2015). For example, a person may be sexually, romantically, and physically attracted to others of the same gender, different gender, both genders, neither gender, people who are genderqueer, androgynous, or have other gender identities (APA, 2015). Transgender people may be heterosexual, homosexual, or bisexual, similar to that of cisgender people. Often, sexual orientation is confabulated and confused with the term gender identity, which is a person's internal sense of being male, female, nonbinary, or something else. Gender identity is how one sees their gender in terms of male, female, nonbinary, or anything else. It is not about who they are attracted to; it is about their own identity. As such, this chapter will only consider gender identity and transgender youth as it relates to RE-CBT.

Assessment and Diagnosis of Gender Dysphoria in Children and Youth

Gender dysphoria refers to the distress and discomfort that may exist for some people whose gender identity differs from their sex assigned at birth (Fisk, 1974; Knudson, De Cuypere, & Bockting, 2010). Although not all people whose gender identity differs from the sex they were assigned at birth will experience psychological manifestations of distress, others do experience anywhere from mild to severe levels of gender dysphoria (APA, 2015). In 2013, the Diagnostic and Statistical Manual of Mental Disorders, Fifth Edition, classified gender dysphoria as its own diagnosis category (American Psychiatric Association, 2013), replacing the diagnosis of gender identity disorder in the previous version (American Psychiatric Association, 2000). This reclassification of the term marked a transition to seeing transgender identities as non-pathological, emphasizing that it is the distress the person feels as a result of the disconnect between their gender identity and their sex assigned at birth as the target of intervention, not the gender identity itself at all. The diagnosis of gender dysphoria is complex, involves interviews with parents, children, and schools, and requires an understanding of gender identity development, though there is no standard of assessment (WPATH, 2011). It is recommended by the World Professional Association for Transgender Health (WPATH) that those who are diagnosing gender dysphoria have expertise in this subject matter and have had specific training in gender dysphoria, such as a minimum of foundational training provided by WPATH with subsequent supervision.

Regardless of age, transgender and gender diverse populations are at higher risk for psychological distress that is co-occurring with potential gender dysphoria. This is evident when looking at the data from a national study, where 40% of transgender adults surveyed reported having made a suicide attempt in their lifetime. Moreover, 92% of these individuals reported having attempted suicide before the age of 25. This is a stark comparison to the general population, in which the suicide attempt rate is estimated around 4.6% (James et al., 2016). A study of adolescents aged 11–19 showed that nearly 14% of all adolescents report a suicide attempt, though there are differences in rates based on gender identity. Cisgender females (17.6%) and cisgender males (9.8%) have statistically significant lower suicide attempt rates than all transgender and questioning youth. In addition, transgender male (50.8%) and nonbinary youth (41.8%) have higher rates of suicide attempt rates than transgender females (29.9%) and questioning youth (27.9%; Toomey et al., 2018).

Further, there are emerging studies indicating that at least a portion of transgender and gender-expansive (TGGE) youth are at increased risk for anxiety, depression, academic and behavioral problems, social isolation, eating disorders, substance abuse, self-harming behaviors, bullying, high risk sexual practices, suicide attempts, and completed suicides when compared with same aged cisgender peers (Grossman & D'Augelli, 2007; Reisner et al., 2015). TGGE youth with gender dysphoria also have high rates of co-occurring mental health diagnoses (American Psychiatric Association, 2013; de Vries et al., 2011). Among a clinical sample of transgender adolescents and emerging adults, 30.3% reported a history of at least one suicide attempt, and 41.8% reported a history of self-injurious behaviors. Spack et al. (2012) reported that almost 44% of transgender youth presenting for gender management at their program in Boston had diagnoses of anxiety-related disorders and severe mood disorders. Becerra-Culqui et al. (2018) found that in an electronic medical records review of the mental health of transgender and gender-expansive children and adolescent compared to cisgender peers, there was a higher frequency of mental health conditions, with most worrisome results being suicidal ideation and self-inflicted injuries with prevalence estimates higher in TGGE children and adolescents than in matched cisgender reference groups.

When we compare transgender and cisgender youth, we see higher rates of mental health concerns for transgender youth. This includes depression, anxiety, suicidal ideation and attempts, non-suicidal self-injurious behaviors, as well as higher rates of inpatient and outpatient psychological treatment (Reisner et al., 2015). It is important to note that the majority of transgender youth do not have a co-occurring mental health condition; however, in one sample of gender dysphoric adolescents, while 67.6% had no DSM-IV Axis I diagnosis, 32.4% had at least one DSM-IV Axis I diagnosis and 15.2% had at least two diagnoses (de Vries et al., 2011). This indicates that transgender youth have a higher rate of co-occurring diagnoses that exceeds the cisgender population.

The research suggests that estimates for transgender youth with depressive symptoms range from 6% to 42% (Holt et al., 2016; Skagerberg et al., 2013; Wallien et al., 2007). In addition, approximately 25–30% of transgender adolescents report attempting suicide in their lifetimes (Grossman, Park, & Russell, 2016; Olson, Schrager, Belzer, Simons, & Clark, 2015), compared to 8.6% of all adolescents (Centers for Disease Control and Prevention [CDC], 2018). Finally, high rates of anxiety disorders and disruptive behavior disorders are also observed in transgender individuals than the cisgender population (de Vries et al., 2011; Mustanski, Garofalo, & Emerson, 2010; Wallien et al., 2007). In addition to co-occurring mood and anxiety disorder, some developmental disorders have also been linked to gender dysphoria. Specifically, autism spectrum disorder has been observed to co-occur frequently with gender dysphoria (Janssen, Huang, & Duncan, 2016; May, Pang, & Williams, 2016; Strang et al., 2016).

One hypothesis related to the high rates of symptomatology for transgender youth is that minority stress and subsequent internalized transphobia make transgender youth more at risk for anxiety and depression (Chodzen, Hidalgo, Chen, & Garofalo, 2019). Minority stress is the concept that being a member of a marginalized or oppressed group puts one at risk for experiencing discrimination, violence, and other negative social outcomes that lead to increased rates of psychopathology (Cohen, Feinstein, Rodriguez-Seijas, Taylor, & Newman, 2016; Mustanski et al., 2010; Puckett, Maroney, Levitt, & Horne, 2016). TGGE youth report social exclusion, parental rejection, and high levels of discrimination, bullying, and violence (Bauer, Scheim, Pyne, Travers, & Hammond, 2015; Kahn, Johnson, Lee, & Miranda, 2018). With the high rates of mental health concerns mentioned previously for TGGE youth, in addition to the unique stressors that transgender youth experience, it is important to consider the treatment options for youth who are experiencing anxiety and depression.

Research on General CBT in Treating Gender Dysphoria in TGGE Youth

Empirical research exploring the impact of specific affirmative psychological and mental health treatment modalities and their impact on the adjustment and functioning of transgender children and adolescents is lacking. For cisgender children and adolescents, the gold standard treatment is cognitive behavioral therapy (CBT; e.g., Hoffman, Asnaani, Vonk, Sawyer, & Fang, 2012). When working with minority populations, it is important to consider adaptations and the efficacy of treatment for these individuals. Research investigating the impact of evidence-based therapies for TGGE youth is sparse. Currently, there are few published studies assessing how treatments like CBT can and should be adapted for transgender youth (Busa, Janssen, & Lakshman, 2018). Austin and colleagues (Austin, Craig, & D'Souza, 2018) published work on a CBT coping skills group intervention for gender and sexual minority youth. The intervention was meant to provide affirming spaces for gender and sexual minority youth using CBT interventions. The adaptations included provided support related to minority stress and explicitly discussed the fact that it was an affirmative space. This group was meant to address depressive symptoms in a diverse sample of youth, which included diverse gender identity and sexual identities. The study looked at a subsample of transgender youth who participated in the program and found that the aforementioned adaptations to the treatment were significantly effective in decreasing depressive scores and can improve coping among transgender youth (Austin et al., 2018).

At present, there are no studies that specifically address the use of REBT with transgender youth. In later sections, this chapter aims to highlight and outline how REBT can be used in the treatment of gender dysphoric youth.

Developmental Considerations

Gender diverse people may become aware of their expansive gender identity at any age. Some people will identify as different from the sex they were assigned at birth from a very early age such as childhood; others will become aware and explore at later times in life, be it adolescence or adulthood (APA, 2015). Although the discussion of the evolution of a transgender identity in adulthood is beyond the scope of this chapter, it is important to realize that not all gender diverse individuals will have established their affirmed gender identity before childhood and adolescent ages are surpassed. There is no wrong time or time that is too late for a person to fully understand their gender identity, and this understanding and evolution can be a longer process for some than others.

In line with the age range considered in this chapter, developmental considerations for children and youth in terms of gender fall into three distinct cohorts: (1) prepubescent TGGE children, (2) early pubertal TGGE youth, and (3) late pubertal TGGE adolescents. Understanding the different social, medical, and/or surgical treatment options for each of these groups is important for mental health professionals working in this area of expertise (Chen et al., 2018). The Endocrine Society and WPATH have put forth clinical guidelines outlining the medical interventions that are considered the standard of care for treating TGGE children and youth. Importantly, the Endocrine Society Guidelines emphasize the role of specialized, qualified mental health professionals working alongside the endocrinologist, youth, and caregivers when making these treatment recommendations and decisions on a highly individualized, case-by-case basis (Hembree et al., 2017; WPATH, 2011).

In consideration of both the developmental trajectory of a TGGE youth's journey and working with gender-expansive people of all ages, it cannot be stressed enough how essential an interdisciplinary collaborative care model is to best meet the needs of individuals. We recommend that treating teams should include experts in working with gender diverse populations within the fields of mental health and all areas of medicine, the youth, and their family/guardians in addition to community resources in the schools, faith systems, and legal systems as well.

Prepubescent TGGE Children: For children that have not achieved the start of puberty, there is no need for medical intervention. The role of the mental health professional in this developmental range includes providing psychoeducation about gender development, working on family, cultural, educational environments in how to best support the child's overall well-being. There is rightfully a growing consensus that conversion therapy, which attempts to force a child's gender identity toward their sex assigned at birth, is harmful and unethical and it is being deemed illegal for minors in many areas of the United States (SAMHSA, 2015). Changes here usually revolve around a "social transition," which is a nonmedical intervention for gender dysphoria in which an individual adopts an affirmed name, hair length/style, clothing, and pronouns that are aligned with their gender identity rather than the sex they were assigned at birth (Olson, Durwood, Demeules, & McLaughlin, 2016).

Early Pubertal TGGE Youth: Those who have been determined by a mental health professional specializing in gender diverse care to have a pervasive and intense pattern of gender nonconformity which may worsen with the onset of puberty are afforded the option to undergo treatment with gonadotropin-releasing hormone analogues (GnRHa – also known as puberty blockers) to temporarily suppress the development of their secondary sex characteristics. Administration of GnRHa is a medical intervention that is typically prescribed in the early stages of puberty to prevent the development of unwanted physical sex characteristics. This in essence is a pause on their puberty development and allows the youth the chance to continue to have ongoing gender exploration without the distress of their bodies going through unwanted puberty. This medical treatment is considered to be fully reversible. For youth who do not choose to continue a transgender identity, ending the GnRHa will allow the puberty of their assigned sex at birth to proceed. Those who continue to identify as a gender differing from their sex assigned at birth face other choices after their extended exploration of gender and halted puberty comes to a closure.

Pubertal TGGE Adolescents: The Endocrine Society Clinical Practice Guidelines (Hembree et al., 2017) indicate that gender-affirming hormones (GAH – medical intervention that involves exogenous testosterone or estrogen administration to cause the wanted secondary sex characteristics of the youth's affirmed gender) can be an appropriate treatment for certain TGGE youth. Those meeting criteria for treatment with GAH must have been diagnosed by a qualified mental health professional specializing in the management and treatment of gender diversity that there is a confirmed and consistent diagnosis of gender dysphoria and that any co-occurring psychological or social problems that could interfere with treatment have been addressed and are under control. Additionally, the youth must exhibit the mental capacity to consider the consequences of GAH (some of which are irreversible) and side effects of treatment (potential fertility loss and consideration of options to preserve fertility if possible) and have given their assent to treatment, and for those under the legal age of giving medical consent, parents or legal guardians must consent to the GAH treatment. Finally, to qualify for GAH treatment, there must be no other medical contraindications (i.e., cardiovascular concerns, bone health, family history, health habits, and other comorbidities).

As outlined by Chen et al. (2018), criteria for gender-affirming surgeries affecting fertility include:

> (a) Persistent, well-documented GD [Gender Dysphoria], (b) legal age of majority in the given country, (c) continuously and responsibility using GAH for 12 months (assuming there is no medical contraindication for GAH), (d) successful continuous full-time living in the affirmed gender role for 12 months, (e) significant medical or mental health concerns (if present) are well controlled, and (f) demonstrable knowledge of all practice aspects of surgery including cost, required lengths of hospitalization and postsurgical rehabilitation. (p. 79)

These same authors point out that the Endocrine Society Guidelines (Hembree et al., 2017) and WPATH Standards of Care (Coleman et al., 2012) allow an age exception for gender affirming chest surgeries such as breast augmentation or chest masculinization, both of which do not affect fertility. Affirming top surgeries are allowable for minors who have been living in their affirmed gender for 12 continuous months, with parental or legal guardian consent, as per WPATH Guidelines, SOC 7.

Best Practice Guidelines for Treatment of Gender Dysphoria in TGGE Youth

Affirmative social and medical transition to one's affirmed gender identity is considered by many professional organizations as the modern-day standard of care to treat and reduce gender dysphoria. Policy statements have been released by organizations such as the APA (American Psychological Association, 2015) and the WPATH (WPATH, 2011). Recommendations for psychologists generally include: (1) have knowledge and understanding of gender identity and how this relates and differs from sexual orientation; (2) understand the barriers, stigma, and discrimination that transgender individuals experience on a day-to-day basis and how this impacts them long term; (3) understand that gender identity development occurs across the life span and that children specifically can have a transgender identity; (4) know that affirmative medical interventions can vastly decrease gender dysphoria for transgender individuals; and (5) gender affirmative psychotherapy is essential for transgender people if they are seeking out services.

In the gender affirmative model, positive gender development and psychological health are defined by "a child's opportunity to live in the gender that feels most real or comfortable to that child and to express that gender with freedom from restriction, aspersion, or rejection" (Hidalgo et al., 2013 p. 286). When children and youth are prevented from living their self-defined identity by outside controls, such as family, peers, school, religion, and culture, they are at increased risk to develop a multitude of psychological adversities including low self-esteem, depression, self-harm, suicidal ideation and attempts, PTSD, isolation, homelessness, and incarceration (D'Augelli, et al., Garofalo, Deleon, Osmer, Doll, & Harper, 2006; Hidalgo et al., 2013; Roberts, Rosario, Corliss, Koenen, & Bryn Austin, 2012; Skidmore, Linsenmeier, & Bailey, 2006; Toomey, Ryan, Díaz, Card, & Russell, 2010; Travers et al., 2012).

The gender affirmative model is a method of therapeutic care that recognizes children of any age can be aware of and know their gender identity as authentic. With the child or adolescent being the expert on their own gender identity, the gender affirmative model acknowledges that a social transition in gender can be beneficial at any stage of development (Ehrensaft, 2017). In this model, the child or adolescent is seen as the one who is the expert on their gender, and it is not up to parents, clinicians, or other adults in the child's life to tell them what their gender is based on external genitalia, chromosomes, and cultural, religious, social, or family norms and expectations.

Basic premises of the gender affirmative model are eloquently highlighted by several different authors to include the premises that (1) variation and diversity in gender is not a pathological disorder; (2) gender presentation varies across cultures; gender involves an interplay between biology, time, development, socialization, and context; (3) gender is fluid and not binary being female and male only; (4) if psychological/psychiatric disorders are present, they are often a result of negative interpersonal and cultural reactions to the child; (5) gender pathology lies more in the external culture than in the person; and (6) the job of the professional is to assist the child or adolescent to live in the gender that feels most authentic and comfortable to them (Edwards-Leeper, 2017; Edwards-Leeper, Leibowitz, & Sangganjanavanich, 2016; Ehrensaft, 2017; Hidalgo et al., 2013). Among the main therapeutic goals of the gender affirmative model is to assist the child or adolescent in facilitating an authentic gender self, alleviate gender distress and stress, build gender resilience, and enlist social supports (Ehrensaft, 2017). Emerging research reports that many transgender children who have been affirmed in their gender identity by their families and those with affirmative support mature into well-adjusted adults and can be as psychologically healthy as their cisgender peers indicating a need for affirmative approaches (De Vries et al., 2014; Olson et al., 2016).

In terms of affirmative psychological approaches, cognitive behavioral therapy can be used to potentiate an individual with gender dysphoria's ability to manage the distress associated with the chasm between their assigned sex and their affirmed gender identity. Another crucial role of the psychologist or mental health professional is to be part of a larger multidisciplinary team. This team should be comprised of medical providers including endocrinologists, adolescent medicine doctors, psychiatrists, surgeons, fertility specialists, as well as a network of primary care doctors who are well versed in gender-affirming care. It is also helpful for psychologists to be aware of laws in their state related to name changes and to have referrals available for lawyers, schools, and support groups.

REBT for the Treatment of Gender Dysphoria in TGGE Youth

In consideration of the current state of affirmative psychological interventions with transgender children and adolescents, Spivey and Edwards (2019) underscore the fact that:

> Affirmative psychological interventions have the potential to strengthen existing resiliency and lessen transgender individual's psychological distress over the course of development, which could save transgender individuals' time and financial resources and reduce health disparities associated with chronic stress and psychological distress. (p. 11).

In line with this assertion, the present authors propose that REBT is an ideal philosophy and practical clinical approach to assist transgender children and adolescents to cope with the unique challenges and adversities they may face in addition to assisting them in achieving their own personal goals for the trajectory of their lives into adulthood.

REBT, developed in 1955 by Dr. Albert Ellis (Ellis, 1955, 1958,1962), is a specific action-oriented form of cognitive behavioral therapy that teaches individuals to identify, challenge, and replace their self-defeating beliefs about themselves, others, and the world with healthier ones that promote emotional well-being and achievement of one's goals. "From its inception, Albert Ellis pioneered the application of REBT with children and adolescents, stressing, in particular the importance of teaching young client's positive mental health concepts that would promote their social, emotional, behavioral and cognitive development" (Vernon, 2019, p. 243). Additionally, REBT has been taught to children in school settings, where it has accompanied the standard academic curriculum along with a specialized rational emotive behavior curriculum designed to teach healthy emotional literacy (Knaus, 1974; Trip, Vernon, & McMahon, 2007). When used in this manner, REBT concepts can be not only considered an "intervention" to dealing with the difficulties encountered by gender dysphoric individuals, it can also be considered "preventative" and "inoculating" to emotional maladjustment for all youth.

Research and theoretical literature on specifically REBT-based techniques and practice in working with transgender youth is nonexistent. This mirrors a similar dearth of literature on REBT-based practices when working with LGBTQ (lesbian, gay, bisexual, transgender, queer) clients in general, regardless of age and sexual orientation (Moody, 2019). To date, the only other REBT-related publication even mentioning work with transgender individual is Moody (2019), which addresses adults, not children or adolescents, and also combines LGBTQI (lesbian, gay, bisexual, transgender, queer, and intersex) all together, not specifically addressing unique concerns to the transgender population. Given the REBT literature's dearth of attention thus far to the transgender population in general and here, specifically children and adolescents, the present authors propose for the first time that affirmative REBT for gender diverse and transgender children and adolescents and their caregivers is an interventional therapy and philosophy that can be used to potentiate transgender youths' ability to manage possible distress associated with the discrepancy between their assigned sex and their affirmed gender identity, in addition to navigating and thriving in all areas of their life, society, and adjustment.

Clinical Applications of REBT in Working with Transgender Children and Adolescents

Unconditional Self-Acceptance (USA)

REBT is affirmative in and of its own right. Tenants of REBT are inherent to the gender affirmative model of care. Teaching gender diverse youth unconditional self-acceptance (USA) is perhaps the most important key REBT concept for reducing anxiety, depression, and other emotional distress. Transgender youth are often told by themselves and others that they have an inherent flaw due to the difference in their gender concept and their sex identified at birth. This cis-normative message can create tremendous distress emotionally. In contrast, REBT stresses the concept of unconditional self-acceptance as a character trait leading to emotional good health (DiGiuseppe, Doyle, Dryden, & Backx, 2013; Ellis, Wolfe, & Moseley, 1968; Knaus, 1974). Ellis et al. (1968) directed to teach children that they are all capable human beings and are likable in their own ways. Moreover, that not one trait, behavior, or situation can define their entire existence as a human being. USA teaches children to accept themselves in an emotionally healthy way, without rating themselves and degrading themselves based on any trait, behavior, or characteristic of themselves. Rational emotive counseling methods are valuable in teaching youth to challenge their self-depreciation and to establish their own unconditional self-acceptance, ultimately leading to less internalization of distress. For example, gender identity is one aspect of the whole self, which is a complex constellation of many different traits, behaviors, and self-identification.

The A-B-C Model and Rational Versus Irrational Beliefs

In teaching gender diverse youth the ABCs of REBT, they are empowered to become aware of the impact of their thoughts and beliefs on their own emotions and behaviors. In teaching that activating events (A's) are only partially responsible for emotional and behavioral consequences (C's), we make the way for teaching youth the influential power of their own belief system (B's). In highlighting the difference between rational thinking (helpful) leading to functional, healthy, and adaptive emotions and irrational (unhelpful) thinking leading to disturbed, dysfunctional, maladaptive emotions (reference), we can teach gender-expansive youth that they have options within their control that can assist them in determining how they feel. Teaching the difference between rational and irrational beliefs equips gender diverse youth with a coping tool to empower them to choose their emotional reactions to adverse events, situations, and circumstances. For example, a gender-expansive youth who tells themselves that "it is awful" that they were assigned a specific gender at birth that is different from their self-defined gender is likely to feel depressed and anxious about their situation. A more helpful belief is that "it is unfortunate that my body has different features than the way I see my gender, but it is far from awful and although I don't like it, it is the body that I have and I can modify it if I chose to medically and express my gender in many ways that are not defined by my physical body."

Teaching the Difference Between Healthy and Unhealthy Negative Emotions

In working with gender diverse populations, it is of great importance to show acceptance of the youth's realistic situation. That is, their biological sex and body are not aligned with their gender identify and self-concept. This disconnect is accepted as a fact in affirmative treatment. However, the REBT principle of healthy negative emotions vs. unhealthy negative emotions can empower individuals with either adaptive coping or distress and overwhelming psychological ramifications. In working with youth who factually acknowledge that their bodies are not alighted with their gender identity, it is important to validate that as a reality for that person. Yes, it is unfortunate and not a desirable situation. However, the REBT principle of teaching youth that they have a choice in how they think about this disconnect and approach it from a logistical, rational, and problem-solving stance vs. one of despair, distress, and destruction can be dictated by healthy negative emotions vs. unhealthy negative emotions. By teaching rational, flexible thinking, it is possible to empower youth with the acceptance of their bodies as they were at birth, while working at educational empowerment of modern-day scientific and medical advances that can help individuals to take steps and measures to medically transform their hormones, bodies, and lives to their affirmed gender, rather than overly disturbing themselves with being imprisoned by their birth sex.

Teaching TGGE Youth to Dispute Irrational Beliefs

In focusing on the specific concerns about which a transgender individual with gender dysphoria is distressed, REBT addresses unhelpful attitudes and unhelpful negative emotions (e.g., unhealthy anger, depression, anxiety, guilt, etc.) and maladaptive behaviors (e.g., procrastination, addictive behaviors, aggression, unhealthy eating, sleep disturbance, etc.) that can negatively impact a transgender person's perception of their self-worth, life satisfaction, and view of others and the world in general. To modify this, REBT practitioners work closely with people with gender dysphoria to identify their individual set of beliefs (attitudes, expectations, and personal rules) that lead to their unhelpful emotional distress.

REBT utilizes a variety of methods to help an individual with gender dysphoria to reformulate their unhelpful, sabotaging beliefs into sensible, realistic, and helpful ones. One specific and critical REBT technique is called "disputing." In disputing dysphoric transgender individuals' unhealthy negative beliefs and replacing them with more rational and helpful views of themselves and the world, REBT ultimately assists gender diverse individuals in developing a philosophy and approach to living that can help to decrease their own personal distress and increase their skills and effectiveness in communicating and in coping with a world that is still wrought with transphobic attitudes, micro-aggressions, and real dangers. For example, "it will be impossible for me to have a happy life in any way because I was born in the wrong body." Disputation of this type of black and white thinking could involve the therapist asking the client to discuss a time that they did feel pleasure, satisfaction, or happiness in the past on any level, showing them that it is possible to be gender diverse and satisfied at the same time.

Case Study with Gender Dysphoria in TGGE Youth

Brief Background and Diagnosis

To protect the anonymity of the client and family, all names have been changed and details have been modified. Alexandra is a 14-year-old youth living with her parents and 10-year-old sister in a suburban, middle class town in the United States. At birth, Alexandra was biologically identified female and she was raised as a girl. As a young child, Alexandra enjoyed playing with dolls, cars, and glittery art supplies, and her favorite color was yellow. She played equally well with males and females and was well liked by her teachers, always performing well in school. She tended to prefer dressing in more gender-neutral colors and clothing growing up.

As her natal female puberty approached and she began development of secondary sex characteristics of breast growth, she became dysphoric and unhappy with her body. Her mood began to change with increases in dysthymia, agitation, anxiety, and irritability. Alexandra confided in her parents that she did not feel like "she was a girl in her heart and mind" and that she was becoming consumed with fear and dread of her body's growing breast buds and widening hips. She was frustrated and angry with her body for changing in this way and feeling worse about herself and each day was becoming more challenging. Alexandra's parents sought treatment to determine how to understand and best support their child. After performing a comprehensive affirming and gender-informed assessment of gender (Liebowitz & Janssen, 2018), Alexandra was diagnosed with gender dysphoria.

Treatment Plan

In addition to the fundamentals of CBT and REBT, treatment was designed and tailored in line with best practices as recommended by the WPATH (2012), APA (2012) and the Endocrine Society (Hembree et al., 2017). Psychoeducation and consultation about gender identity were provided to Alexandra and her family. Alexandra requested that going forward, the affirmed name "Alex" be used and that the male pronouns he, him, his be used in lieu of female pronouns. Sessions were conducted as a combination of individual and parent/sibling included as needed to assist Alex, his parents, and sister in exploring their thoughts and concerns about the gender exploration and social transition.

Goals and Objectives of Treatment

Diagnosis and Alliance with Client and Family

1. Assemble a multidisciplinary treatment team consisting of an REBT trained psychologist, pediatrician, pediatric endocrinologist specializing in gender care, parents, school support personnel, and community support agencies specializing in gender diversity.

Teach REBT Framework

2. Teach Alex and his parents to understand the REBT/CBT framework, including the interconnection of thoughts, feelings, and behaviors to help facilitate more effective emotional and behavioral responses.
3. Teach Alex that he is largely responsible for his thoughts, feelings, and behaviors.
4. Show Alex that he can unconditionally accept himself (teach USA) as a complex human being despite the physical genitalia with which he was born.

5. Teach Alex that when he is less emotionally distressed about the effects of his natal development, practical and logical decisions can be made in line with modern affirmative social and medical interventions.
6. Assist Alex and his parents in accessing and being assertive, sharing information about the gender social transition with peers, teachers, and community and not awfulizing about possible rejection, but teaching skills to deal with possible negative feedback or reactions.

Progress Monitoring and Outcome Assessment

7. Continue to explore gender identity and exploration over time, while natal puberty is suppressed with blockers.
8. Ongoing assessment and monitoring of mood, behavior, gender identity, and social transition to provide continued consultation to Alex and family for possible cessation of blockers and return to natal puberty vs. transition to affirmed gender with cross gender hormone treatment.

Unconditional Other Acceptance: An Adaptation of RE-CBT in Schools System-Wide for TGGE Youth to Find Affirmation of Gender Diversity

The individual needs of transgender students in schools and learning environments will vary greatly depending on many different factors inherent to the student, community, staff, parents, and legal system to name a few. However, despite this myriad of factors, every student, regardless of their gender, has a basic right to learn in a safe and accepting school environment. "Just as a transgender youth's transition is a journey, so too is the process of supporting that transition and creating an affirming school environment for them" (Gender Spectrum, 42). Students who are bullied and harassed by peers or school staff are less likely to succeed academically (Kosciw, Greytak, Palmer, & Boesen, 2014), and gender-based bullying impacts all youth, not just those who identify as transgender. A system-wide intervention in creating a school environment that respects and affirms not only gender diversity but also all types of diversity and empowers all students will perhaps make the most impact for TGGE youth within the context of their academic institution. "Gender-inclusive messages encourage greater acceptance of diversity and discourage children from expressing judgments about people based on factors like race, class, sexuality, gender, family structure, ethnicity and religion" (Gender Spectrum, 11).

The REBT concept of "Unconditional Other Acceptance" (UOA) is at its very core, a vehicle to instill acceptance of diversity of all students in the school community, whether it is about gender identity or any other variable by which humans exhibit differences and diversity. A major goal for the teaching of REBT concepts within the school community is to teach students, faculty, staff, and parents the value of UOA. In teaching UOA, we teach the acceptance of diversity of all humans on all variable traits that everyone has good and not so good traits and qualities and that giving someone a total rating based on anyone variable is an overgeneralization and does not define the individual. Rather, accepting others as different than oneself but not rating them bad or good opens the door for them to be accepted just because they exist and not globally rating them based on a "difference" they may have over oneself. Different is not good or bad; it just is. It is what we tell ourselves about those differences that create labeling, other ratings, overgeneralizations, and faulty conclusions about others based on a diverse trait or difference.

Conclusion

Gender diverse children and youth can find empowerment in managing distress experience by an incongruence between their gender identity and physical body manifestation. Teaching RE-CBT skills such as unconditional self-acceptance, unconditional other acceptance, the A-B-C model, and differentiating between rational and irrational beliefs are the first steps in empowering children and youth to develop emotional self-regulation and therefore happier, more productive and successful lives. Additionally, RE-CBT coping skill development enables youth to be able to better deal with interpersonal interactions and navigate their social and emotional environments. It is the hope of the present authors that this is the first of many works that elaborate on RE-CBT in working with transgender children and youth.

Test Yourself Questions

1. What is the difference between assigned sex at birth and gender identity?
2. In consideration of the experiences unique to gender-expansive youth and children, how would you use an REBT framework to address their emotional concerns?
3. What is the significance of a multidisciplinary treatment team in working with gender diverse children and youth?
4. How are gender identity and sexual orientation different concepts?

References

American Psychiatric Association. (2000). *Diagnostic and statistical manual of mental disorders* (4th ed., Text Revision ed.). Washington, DC: Author.

American Psychiatric Association. (2013). *Diagnostic and statistical manual of mental disorders* (5th ed.). Arlington, VA: Author.

American Psychological Association. (2012). Guidelines for psychological practice with lesbian, gay, and bisexual clients. *American Psychologist, 67*(1), 10–42. https://doi.org/10.1037/a0024659

American Psychological Association. (2015). Guidelines for psychological practice with transgender and gender nonconforming people. *American Psychologist, 70*(9), 832–864. https://doi.org/10.1037/a0039906

Austin, A., Craig, S. L., & D'Souza, S. A. (2018). An AFFIRMative cognitive behavioral intervention for transgender youth: Preliminary effectiveness. *Professional Psychology: Research and Practice, 49*(1), 1.

Bauer, G. R., Scheim, A. I., Pyne, J., Travers, R., & Hammond, R. (2015). Intervenable factors associated with suicide risk in transgender persons: A respondent driven sampling study in Ontario, Canada. *BMC Public Health, 15*, 525. https://doi.org/10.1186/s12889-015-1867-2

Becerra-Culqui, T. A., Liu, Y., Nash, R., Cromwell, L., Flanders, W. D., Getahun, D., et al. (2018). Mental health of transgender and gender nonconforming youth compared with their peers. *Pediatrics, 141*(5), e20173845.

Busa, S., Janssen, A., & Lakshman, M. (2018). A review of evidence based treatments for transgender youth diagnosed with social anxiety disorder. *Transgender Health, 3*(1), 27–33.

Centers for Disease Control and Prevention (CDC). (2018). 1991–2015 high school youth risk behavior survey data.

Chen, D., Edwards-Leeper, L., Stancin, T., & Tishelman, A. (2018). Advancing the practice of Pediatric psychology with transgender youth: State of science, ongoing controversies, and future directions. *Clinical Practice in Pediatric Psychology, 6*(1), 73–83.

Chodzen, G., Hidalgo, M. A., Chen, D., & Garofalo, R. (2019). Minority stress factors associated with depression and anxiety among transgender and gender-nonconforming youth. *Journal of Adolescent Health, 64*(4), 467–471.

Cohen, J. M., Feinstein, B. A., Rodriguez-Seijas, C., Taylor, C. B., & Newman, M. G. (2016). Rejection sensitivity as a transdiagnostic risk factor for internalizing psychopathology among gay and bisexual men. *Psychology of Sexual Orientation and Gender Diversity, 3*(3), 259.

Coleman, E., Bocking, W., Botzer, M., Cohen-Kettenis, P., DeCuypere, G., Feldman, J., et al. (2012). Standards of Care for the health of transsexual, transgender, and gender nonconforming people. Version 7. *International Journal of Transgenderism, 13*(4), 165–232. https://doi.org/10.11080/15532739.2011.700873

de Vries, A. L., Doreleijers, T. A., Steensma, T. D., & Cohen-Kettenis, P. T. (2011). Psychiatric comorbidity in gender dysphoric adolescents. *Journal of Child Psychol Psychiatry, 52*(11), 1195–1202. https://doi.org/10.1111/j.1469-7610.2011.02426.x.

De Vries, A. L. C., McGuire, J. K., Steensma, T. D., Wagenaar, E. C. F., Doreleijers, T. A. H., & Cohen-Kettenis, P. T. (2014). Young adult psychological outcome after puberty suppression and gender reassignment. *Pediatrics, 134*, 4.

DiGiuseppe, R. A., Doyle, K. A., Dryden, W., & Backx, W. (2013). *A practitioner's guide to rational-emotive behavior therapy*. Oxford University Press.

Edwards-Leeper, L. (2017). Affirmative care of TGNC children and adolescents. In A. A. Singh & L. M. Dickey (Eds.), *Affirmative counseling and psychological practice with transgender and gender nonconforming clients*. Washington, DC: APA.

Edwards-Leeper, L., Leibowitz, S., & Sangganjanavanich, V. F. (2016). Affirmative practice with transgender and gender nonconforming youth: Expanding the model. *Psychology of Sexual Orientation and Gender Diversity, 3*(2), 165–172. https://doi.org/10.1037/sgd0000167

Ehrensaft, D. (2017). Gender nonconforming youth: Current perspectives. *Adolescent Health, Medicine and Therapeutics, 8*, 57–67.
Ellis, A. (1955). New approaches to psychotherapy techniques. *Journal of Clinical Psychology Monograph Supplement, 11*, 1–53.
Ellis, A. (1958). Rational psychotherapy. *Journal of General Psychology, 59*, 35–49.
Ellis, A. (1962). *Reason and emotion in psychotherapy*. Secaucus, NJ: Lyle Stuart.
Ellis, A., Wolfe, J., & Moseley, S. (1968). *How to raise an emotionally happy, healthy child.* New York: Albert Ellis Institute.
Fisk, N. M. (1974). Editorial: Gender dysphoria syndrome--the conceptualization that liberalizes indications for total gender reorientation and implies a broadly based multi-dimensional rehabilitative regimen. *The Western Journal of Medicine, 120*(5), 386–391.
Garofalo, R., Deleon, J., Osmer, E., Doll, M., & Harper, G. W. (2006). Overlooked, misunderstood and at-risk: Exploring the lives and HIV risk of ethnic minority male-to-female transgender youth. *Journal of Adolescent Health, 38*, 230–236.
Gender Spectrum. Schools in transition a guide for supporting transgender students in K-12 schools. Available at genderspectrum.org.
Grossman, A. H., & D'Augelli, A. R. (2007). Transgender youth and life-threatening behaviors. *Suicide and Life-threatening Behavior, 37*, 527–553.
Grossman, A. H., Park, J. Y., & Russell, S. T. (2016). Transgender youth and suicidal behaviors: Applying the interpersonal psychological theory of suicide. *Journal of Gay & Lesbian Mental Health, 20*(4), 329–349.
Hembree, W. C., Cohen-Kettenis, P. T., Gooren, L., Hannema, S. E., Meyer, W. J., Murad, M. H., et al. (2017). Endocrine treatment of gender-dysphoric/gender-incongruent persons: An Endocrine Society Clinical Practice Guideline. *The Journal of Clinical Endocrinology & Metabolism, 102*(11), 3869–3903. https://doi.org/10.1210/jc.2017-01658
Herman, J. L., Flores, A. R., Brown, T. N. T., Wilson, B. D. M., & Conron, K. J. (2017). *Age of individuals who identify as transgender in the United States*. Los Angeles, CA: The Williams Institute.
Hidalgo, M. A., Ehrensaft, D., Tishelman, A. C., Clark, L. F., Garofalo, R., Rosenthal, S. M., et al. (2013). The gender affirmative model: What we know and what we aim to learn. *Human Development, 56*(5), 285–290. https://doi.org/10.1159/000355235
Hofmann, S. G., Asnaani, A., Vonk, I. J. J., Sawyer, A. T., & Fang, A. (2012). The efficacy of cognitive behavioral therapy: A review of meta-analyses. *Cognitive Therapy and Research, 36*(5), 427–440.
Holt, V., Skagerberg, E., & Dunsford, M. (2016). Young people with features of gender dysphoria: Demographics and associated difficulties. *Clinical Child Psychology and Psychiatry, 21*(1), 108–118.
James, S. E., Herman, J. L., Rankin, S., Keisling, M., Mottet, L., & Anafi, M. (2016). *The Report of the 2015 U.S. Transgender Survey*. Washington, DC: National Center for Transgender Equality.
Janssen, A., Huang, H., & Duncan, C. (2016). Gender variance among youth with autism spectrum disorders: A retrospective chart review. *Transgender Health, 1*(1), 63–68. https://doi.org/10.1089/trgh.2015.0007
Johns, M. M., Lowry, R., Andrzejewski, J., Barrios, L. C., Demissie, Z., McManus, T., et al. (2019). Transgender identity and experiences of violence victimization, substance use, suicide risk, and sexual risk behaviors among high school students — 19 States and Large Urban School Districts, 2017. *MMWR Morbidity and Mortality Weekly Report, 68*, 67–71. https://doi.org/10.15585/mmwr.mm6803a3
Kahn, E., Johnson, A., Lee, M., & Miranda, L. (2018). LGBTQ Youth Report 2018.
Knaus, W. J. (1974). *Rational emotive education: A manual for elementary school teachers*. New York: Albert Ellis Institute.
Knudson, G., De Cuypere, G., & Bockting, W. (2010). Recommendations for revision of the DSM diagnoses of gender identity disorders: Consensus statement of the World Professional Association for Transgender Health. *International Journal of Transgenderism, 12*(2), 115–118.

Kosciw, J. G., Greytak, E. A., Palmer, N. A., & Boesen, M. J. (2014). *The 2013 National School Climate Survey: The experiences of lesbian, gay, and transgender youth in our Nation's schools*. New York: GLSEN.

Liebowitz, S., & Janssen, A. (2018). Affirming and gender-informed assessment of gender diverse and/or transgender youth across development. In A. Janssen & S. Liebowitz (Eds.), *Affirmative Mental Health Care for Transgender and Gender Diverse Youth* (pp. 1–29). Cham, Switzerland: Springer International Publishing AG, Part of Springer Nature 2018.

May, T., Pang, K., & Williams, K. J. (2016). Gender variance in children and adolescents with autism spectrum disorder from the National Database for autism research. *International Journal of Transgenderism, 18*(1), 7–15. https://doi.org/10.1080/15532739.2016.1241976

Moody, R. L. (2019). REBT with LGBTQ clients. In W. Dryden & M. E. Bernard (Eds.), *REBT with Diverse Client Problems and Populations* (pp. 359–381) Springer Nature Switzerland AG.

Mustanski, B. S., Garofalo, R., & Emerson, E. M. (2010). Mental health disorders, psychological distress, and suicidality in a diverse sample of lesbian, gay, bisexual, and transgender youths. *American Journal of Public Health, 100*(12), 2426–2432. https://doi.org/10.2105/AJPH.2009.178319)

Olson, K. R., Durwood, L., Demeules, M., & McLaughlin, K. A. (2016). Mental health of transgender children who are supported in their identities. *Pediatrics, 137*(3), e20153223.

Olson, J., Schrager, S. M., Belzer, M., Simons, L. K., & Clark, L. F. (2015). Baseline physiologic and psychosocial characteristics of transgender youth seeking care for gender dysphoria. *Journal of Adolescent Health, 57*(4), 374–380.

Puckett, J. A., Maroney, M. R., Levitt, H. M., & Horne, S. G. (2016). Relation between gender expression, minority stress, and mental health in cisgender sexual minority women and men. *Psychology of Sexual Orientation and Gender Diversity, 3*(4), 489.

Reisner, S. L., Vetters, R., Leclerc, M., Zaslow, S., Wolfrum, S., Shumer, D., & Mimiaga, M. J. (2015). Mental health of transgender youth in care at an adolescent urban community health center: a matched retrospective cohort study. *Journal of Adolescent Health, 56*(3), 274–279.

Roberts, A. L., Rosario, M., Corliss, H. L., Koenen, K. C., & Bryn Austin, S. (2012). Childhood gender nonconformity: A risk indicator for childhood abuse and posttraumatic stress in youth. *Pediatrics, 129*, 410–417.

SAMHSA. (2015). *Ending conversion therapy: supporting and affirming LGBTQ youth*. Rockville, MD: Author.

Skagerberg, E., Parkinson, R., & Carmichael, P. (2013). Self-harming thoughts and behaviors in a group of children and adolescents with gender dysphoria. *International Journal of Transgenderism, 14*(2), 86–92.

Skidmore, W. C., Linsenmeier, J. A. W., & Bailey, J. M. (2006). Gender nonconformity and psychological distress in lesbians and gay men. *Archives of Sexual Behavior, 35*, 685–697.

Spack, N. P., Edwards-Leeper, L., Feldman, H. A., Leibowitz, S., Mandel, F., Diamond, D. A., et al. (2012). Children and adolescents with gender identity disorder referred to a pediatric medical center. *Pediatrics, 129*, 418–425. https://doi.org/10.1542/peds.2011-907

Spivey, L. A., & Edwards-Leeper, L. (2019). Future directions in affirmative psychological interventions with transgender children and adolescents. *Journal of Clinical & Adolescent Psychology, 48*(2), 343–356. https://doi.org/10.1080/15374416.2018.1534207

Strang, J. F., Meagher, H., Kenworthy, L., de Vries, A. L., Menvielle, E., Leibowitz, S., et al. (2016). Initial clinical guidelines for co-occurring autism spectrum disorder and gender dysphoria or incongruence in adolescents. *Journal of Clinical Child and Adolescent Psychology*, 1–11. https://doi.org/10.1080/15374416.2016.1228462

Toomey, R. B., Ryan, C., Díaz, R. M., Card, N. A., & Russell, S. T. (2010). Gender-nonconforming lesbian, gay, bisexual, and transgender youth: School victimization and young adult psychosocial adjustment. *Developmental Psychology, 46*, 1580–1589.

Toomey, R. B., Syvertsen, A. K., & Shramko, M. (2018). Transgender adolescent suicide behavior. *Pediatrics, 142*(4), e20174218.

Travers, R., Bauer, G., Pyne, J., Bradley, K., Gale, L., & Papadimitriou, M. (2012). *Impacts of strong parental support for trans youth: A report prepared for Children's Aid Society of Toronto and Delisle Youth Services*. http://transpulseproject.ca/wp-content/uploads/2012/10/Impacts-of-Strong-Parental-Support-for-Trans-Youth-vFINAL.pdf.

Trip, S., Vernon, A., & McMahon, K. (2007). Effectiveness of rational-emotive education: A quantitative meta-analytical study. *Journal of Cognitive and Behavioral Psychotherapies, 7*(1), 81–93.

Vernon, A. (2019). REBT with children and adolescents. In W. Dryden & M. E. Bernard (Eds.), *REBT with diverse client problems and populations* (pp. 243–263). Cham, Switzerland: Springer Nature Switzerland AG.

Wallien, M. S., Swaab, H., & Cohen-Kettenis, P. T. (2007). Psychiatric comorbidity among children with gender identity disorder. *Journal of the American Academy of Child & Adolescent Psychiatry, 46*(10), 1307–1314.

WPATH. (2011). *Standards of care for the health of transsexual, transgender, and gender nonconforming people, seventh version* (Vol. 2017). Minneapolis, MN: World Professional Association for Transgender Health.

Chapter 18
Rational Emotive, Cognitive Behavioral Therapy with Sexual Minority Youth

Angelica Terepka and Leonell Torres-Pagán

Chapter Overview

Adolescents who identify as sexual minorities, or lesbian, gay, bisexual, or queer/questioning, may experience unique difficulties related to this identity, which can affect their mental health and well-being (Russell & Fish, 2016). As such, it is crucial that all clinicians have an understanding of factors impacting sexual identity development in childhood and adolescence, non-heteronormative sexual identities, and how to engage in effective therapeutic work with sexual minority populations. The following chapter will provide a general understanding of how clinicians address sexual orientation in clinical practice through the use of rational emotive behavior therapy (REBT) developed by Albert Ellis and other cognitive behavioral therapies (CBTs).

Historical Debates and Current Progress

Following review of literature written by Albert Ellis regarding homosexuality, the authors conclude that Dr. Ellis was a proponent of gay rights but his writing and commentary were constricted by the social zeitgeist of that time. Ellis (1965) clearly stated, "there is nothing intrinsically immoral or wicked about homosexuality" (p. 96), and further suggested a more fluid approach to sexuality labeling humans as "plurisexual creatures" (p. 96). As a result of his early work in a text

A. Terepka (✉)
Columbia University Irving Medical Center, New York, NY, USA

L. Torres-Pagán
New York Presbyterian Hospital, Columbia University Medical Center, Queens, NY, USA

M. Bernard, M. D. Terjesen (eds.), *Rational-Emotive and Cognitive-Behavioral Approaches to Child and Adolescent Mental Health: Theory, Practice, Research, Applications*, https://doi.org/10.1007/978-3-030-53901-6_18

titled "Homosexuality: Its causes and cure" (Ellis, 1965) and provocative commentary suggesting that homosexuality involved behavior that was deviant from the heterosexual norms hence creating anxiety and tension in homosexual individuals, Ellis was previously regarded as an antagonist of lesbian, gay bisexual (LGB) rights. However, a closer examination of his work elucidates that the late psychologist argued that the heteronormative reality of society (at the time of his life) accurately creates displeasure and annoyance in LGB individuals and suggested that LGB individuals can utilize these sentiments to "calmly work to change [social] regulations" (Ellis, 1964, p. 11). While the authors of this chapter acknowledge that Ellis' previous work contains harsh language regarding sexuality, which is not surprising given the provocative style for which he is best known, the authors commend Ellis for his ability to hold a dichotomous view acknowledging that sexuality is a domain that individuals struggle with because of the inflexible heteronormative views of society. In our chapter, we hope to expand on the application of REBT concepts including the connection between beliefs and emotional/behavioral consequences, as well as unconditional self-acceptance, as psychotherapeutic domains that can promote the well-being of LGB individuals.

Diverse Sexual Orientations: Definitions, Prevalence, and Development

Sexual orientation is broadly defined as romantic or sexual attraction to others. A deeper understanding of sexual orientation considers three main components: *behavior*, or the actual sexual behaviors an individual engages in; *attraction* which indicates physical or romantic attraction to another individual; and *identity*, which encompasses an individual's understanding of their sexuality and any affiliated labels of that understanding (Human Rights Campaign, 2012). Contemporary understandings of sexual orientation propose that these components fluctuate over time and may or may not be congruent with each other. In other words, not all youth who engage in same-sex sexual behavior or experience same-sex attraction adopt a label to describe their sexual orientation outside of the heteronormative (i.e., "straight" or only attracted to members of the opposite sex) classification (Morgan, 2013). In the same light, it is important to remember that adopting a certain identity does not preclude the individual from engaging in other types of same-sex or opposite sex behavior (Morgan, 2013). For example, a female youth may identify as a lesbian indicating same-sex attraction to other females but may have engaged in sexual behavior with males in the past. Therefore, a general guideline is to accurately assess sexual behavior in youth by asking about *partners* rather than *boyfriend* or *girlfriends*, self-identified attraction to others, and allowing youth to describe their own sexual orientation (depending on their knowledge of terminology), rather than assuming or assigning a sexual orientation based on behavior and same-sex attraction (Gold & Terepka, 2019).

Generally speaking, minority sexual orientation identities include those of lesbian, gay, bisexual, transgender, queer/questioning, intersex, and asexual (LGBTQIA) identity. Transgender and intersex identity is often included when discussing sexual minority populations, but there is an important distinction related to gender identity, rather than sexual orientation that makes these subpopulations unique; as such, clinical practice with individuals identifying as transgender is outside the scope of this chapter and is discussed in another chapter in this edited volume. For the purposes of this chapter, sexual minority populations will be referred to as SMY (sexual minority youth) or lesbian, gay, and bisexual (LGB) individuals.

It benefits clinicians to understand that comprehension of sexual orientation involves an evolving knowledge of the consistently changing spectrum of terminology used to describe sexual orientation. Descriptions range from traditional labels (e.g., heterosexual, lesbian, gay, and bisexual) to more contemporary labels (e.g., pansexual, queer, demisexual, asexual, etc.) (McInroy & Craig, 2012). The Human Rights Campaign (HRC) provides a comprehensive list of terms and can be easily referenced by clinicians (Human Rights Campaign, 2012). Contemporary labels such as pansexual (30%), bisexual (26%), and queer (21%) are more utilized as descriptors of sexual orientation than traditional descriptions such as gay (16%), lesbian (16%), or others (Craig et al., 2017).

Youth have been shown to develop awareness of non-heterosexual identity as early as 12 years of age (Pew Research Center, 2013) with average age of awareness being 15 to 16 years of age (Floyd & Bakerman, 2006). More recent research suggests that sexual minority youth are becoming aware of their sexual orientation at earlier ages than past generations (Morgan, 2013) and are more likely to adopt non-heterosexual identities prior to experimentation with same-gender sexual behaviors. Furthermore, identification as a sexual minority, regardless of when that identification occurs, is relatively stable over time, with only about 5% of sexual minorities shifting to a heterosexual identity later in development (Rosario, Schrimshaw, Hunter, & Braun, 2006). As such, sexual identity development plays an important role in early adolescence and even young adulthood as youth engage in relationships.

Some early models of sexual development (Cass, 1979) indicate a linear process (i.e., recognition of same-sex attraction, moving into disclosure of attraction and adoption of LGB identity, and entering an LGB community); however, these proposed models lack generalizable clinical and empirical support and do not account for cultural and socioeconomic variability. Therefore, clinicians are advised to normalize all sexual orientation identities and work to gain an understanding of the client's idiosyncratic development of their sexual identity rather than apply a specific theory of development to the client (Chun & Singh, 2010). This is particularly relevant when considering additional identities clients encompass including cultural, religious, socioeconomic, and gender identity which may impact clients' awareness and acceptance of sexual orientation. Client-centered demographics which can result in differences regarding sexuality and sexual identity development (Fukuyama & Ferguson, 2000) are important to consider and make clinicians' efforts to rely on a specific model of sexual orientation development futile.

Mental Health Disparities Among SMY

Overall, LGB individuals are at greater risk for poorer mental health compared to their heterosexual counterparts. Studies of adult LGB persons indicate higher rates of depression and mood disorders (Bostwick, Boyd, Hughes, & McCabe, 2010; Cochran, Sullivan, & Mays, 2003) and anxiety disorders (Cochran et al., 2003). LGB individuals also experience higher rates of post-traumatic stress disorder (Hatzenbuehler, 2009) and suicidal ideation and attempts (Cochran et al., 2003). Substance abuse disorders are also more prevalent in LGB populations compared to heterosexual populations (Burgard, Cochran, & Mays, 2005). These disproportionate rates of symptomology, psychological distress, and mental health disorders are also seen among LGB youth populations (Fish & Pasley, 2015; Needham, 2012). Of great concern is research indicating that SMY are almost three times as likely to report suicidality (including ideation and attempts) compared to their heterosexual counterparts (Marshal et al., 2011; Mustanski, Garofalo, & Emerson, 2010).

Furthermore, research has highlighted some population specific differences in mental health concerns and sexual orientation. Specifically, sexual minority males are more likely to attempt suicide than sexual minority females (Marshal et al., 2011), sexual minority females are more likely to report substance use concerns compared to heterosexual females and sexual minority males (Fish & Pasley, 2015; Needham, 2012), and youth questioning their sexuality report poorer mental health than lesbian or gay identified counterparts (Birkett, Koenig, & Espelage, 2009). Research is lacking in examining mental health among individuals with multiple minority statuses (Russell & Fish, 2016). However, it is hypothesized that additional minority status further contributes to minority stress experiences, which has been linked to poorer mental health outcomes (Fukuyama & Ferguson, 2000).

Minority Stress Theory

Minority stress theory (Meyer, 2003) suggests that LGB individuals experience stress as a result of their stigmatized social status which may explain the increased risk of psychological distress in LGB populations. Minority stress includes experiences of victimization, harassment, and discrimination based on sexual orientation or other individual characteristics (i.e., distal/external stressors). This may also include expectations of rejection, concealment of sexual orientation, and internalized heterosexism or homonegativity (i.e., proximal/internal stressors). D'Augelli and colleagues (1998, 2002) identified four types of victimization experienced by LGB youth which are directly linked to external environments including limited opportunities to explore identity (e.g. marginalization), negative reactions about their sexuality from family or peers, increased risk of sexually transmitted infections, and direct attacks of violence and harassment (D'Augelli, Pilkington, & Hershberger, 2002). External minority-based stressors are heavily influenced by the individual's environment; although adult LGB individuals have more agency in changing their environment to relieve some minority stress experiences, SMY have less capability to alter their environments (e.g. school, living situation, etc.). Moreover, these stressors are also difficult to change in the course of therapy unless one is working with family members and other individuals within the client's environment.

Hatzenbuehler (2009) further contributed to the understanding of the impact of minority stress by proposing potential mechanisms that influence its relationship with negative mental health outcomes. Minority stress impacts proximal or internal factors such as coping and emotional regulation strategies, interpersonal functioning (i.e., expectation of rejection and discrimination), and cognitive processes including the development of belief systems and perception and interpretation of experiences (Hatzenbuehler, 2009). Internalized homonegativity, as well as rejection sensitivity and expectations of rejection in social settings, to plays a roll in the relationship between discrimination experiences and mental health difficulties (Feinstein, Goldfried, & Davila, 2012).

Given the research on minority stress and its relationship to mental health in SMY, it is believed that RE/CBT approaches can facilitate improvement for SMY experiencing distress. In contrast with external stressors, internal stressors such as expectations of rejection and internalized homonegativity are better controlled by the individual and therefore can be more amenable to change via psychotherapy. It is believed that interventions focused on improving these mechanisms (e.g. coping, emotional regulation, and cognitive process) can help ameliorate the negative impact of minority stress and help improve the mental health of SMY.

Application of RE/CBT: Current Research and Needs of SMY

Cognitive behavioral therapy (CBT) and rational emotive behavior therapy (REBT) have consistently demonstrated effectiveness in the treatment of numerous mental health diagnoses for children and adolescents from diverse populations, including LGB youth (Moody, 2019; Pachankis, Hatzenbuehler, Rendina, Safren, & Parsons, 2015; Russell & Fish, 2016). In the past, REBT faced some scrutiny due to the lack of efficacy studies on diverse population and overall perceptions of this modality ignoring culture-specific issues and practical interventions (Weinrach, 2006). Some of these limitations remain today, as at the moment of this review, most of the work published from earlier 2010 to present day on the subject is limited to case illustrations, brief overviews of literature, and guidelines from other therapeutic modalities (Bernard, 2011; Moody, 2019). Such findings are consistent with a recent publication on REBT with diverse populations (Moody, 2019) indicating the lack of randomized clinical trials (RCTs) testing the effectiveness of REBT with minority groups. In spite of the limitations, Moody (2019) listed a few tenets inherent to the ABC model that may be beneficial for treatment with LGB populations, including increasing attention on irrational beliefs, highlighting differences between unhealthy and healthy emotional/behavioral consequences, unconditional acceptance, and incorporating brief behavioral exercises.

Moreover, the REBT concept of unconditional acceptance has played an important role in the development of frameworks like acceptance and commitment therapy (ACT) and other affirmative therapies often used for LGBTQ+ communities to address internalized homophobia (Dryden & David, 2008; Moody, 2019; O'Shaughnessy & Speir, 2018). Research has found that in addition to the dispute of global attributions, practicing unconditional acceptance can also lead to increases in self-efficacy among the LGB population (Russell & Fish, 2016). To an extent, minority stress theory allows for comprehensive conceptualization that encompasses intersectionality of identities, and an REBT approach to therapy emphasizes acknowledgment and acceptance of these unique experiences as they pertain to SMY.

REBT holds promising directions as a treatment modality in the treatment of SMY. Future research can advance the understanding of several limitations in REBT treatment such as working with activating events, developing rational and healthy attributions, and assessing mechanisms of change from a transdiagnostic approach (David, Cotet, Matu, Mogoase, & Stefan, 2018; Moody, 2019; Weinrach, 2006). Research directions could include the application of qualitative research designs such as case studies (Yin, 2014), which underscore a systematic approach to inquiry of the contextual factors in relation to the individual. There is also a need to develop gold standard research designs like RCTs to test the effectiveness and efficacy of the REBT interventions specific to the population (Hariton & Locascio, 2018; Pachankis et al., 2015). Data obtained from RCTs can help clinicians deliver evidence-based treatment and promote better practices, policies, and training. Subsequent research on REBTs could potentially also provide more insight on treatment disparities in different settings (e.g., schools, outpatient, and inpatient) and diverse community strata.

Best Practices in RE/CBT with SMY

REBT and CBT protocols adapted for treatment with SMY populations benefit from encompassing a multicultural approach. Multicultural competence entails three components: awareness (insight into personal assumptions, values, and biases), knowledge (understanding of clients' cultural world views and factors impacting clients of a particular population), and skill (development and effective use of techniques necessary for working with clients of various diverse populations) (Sue & Torino, 2005). As such, it is important that assessment and treatment of sexual minority youth in clinical practice take into account these domains.

At the outset, appropriate multicultural counseling entails an understanding of both client and therapist factors that influence treatment. Therefore, clinicians engaging LGB youth in treatment are encouraged to assess their own assumptions, values, and biases regarding sexual orientation. Even the best-intentioned therapists functioning from assumptions about LGB populations may engage in microaggressions which can be harmful within the context of therapy (Nadal et al.,

2011). Therefore, assessment of personal biases around sexual orientation and gender expression is encouraged as such practice can allow the practitioner to minimize potential issues that may limit the effectiveness of therapy (Moody, 2019). Measures such as the Lesbian, Gay, Bisexual, and Transgender Development of Clinical Skills Scale (LGBT-DOCSS; Bidell, 2017) and the Sexual Orientation Counselor Competency Scale (SOCCS; Bidell, 2015) are particularly suited for clinicians as they measure biases, as well as clinical knowledge and preparedness relevant to working with LGB populations.

General guidelines for providing therapy to clients with minority status, including individuals in the LGB youth population, begin with rapport building and assessment of presenting concerns (Safren & Rogers, 2001). One distinctive consideration when working with LGB youth is that of consent. Although confidentiality in treatment with LGB youth is addressed in a separate section of this chapter regarding developmental concerns, general guidelines for clinicians working with youth emphasize the importance of discussing limits to confidentiality with the client and their caregiver at the start of therapy.

Thoroughly crafted assessment of the clients' identity formation, mental health concerns or presenting problems, safety and risk concerns, and strengths and support is also a vital component of the initial part of therapy. Following assessment, multicultural competent therapy typically emphasizes treatment that is affirming of diverse identities (Hays, 2009) and aims to reduce the effect of experienced minority stressors (Pachankis, 2014). Specifics on how therapists can incorporate multicultural competent practices into their use of REBT interventions will be detailed throughout the remainder of this chapter.

Developmental Considerations Working with SMY

Youth are exposed to LGB-related topics at various points in their development including communication from family members, entering school systems with diverse populations, or exposure via LGB-related media sources. Individuals raising or working with youth are encouraged to address these issues in developmentally appropriate manners. For younger children who do not have an understanding of physical attraction or sex, definitions of LGB identity can be explained through emphasis on the emotional connection between same-gendered individuals. For instance, the following statements may be helpful in explaining LGB relationships to a younger child: "The word 'gay' is used to describe two boys who love each other the way [insert names of romantic couple known to child]" or "many people of all genders can fall in love with someone, anyone, and decide that they want to get married and take care of each other as a family." When questions about procreation in LGB communities arise, statements such as "families can be created in many different ways (e.g. adoptions, remarriage, etc.)" can help a child understand the diversity of family ties. For older youth who have an understanding of sexual attraction, definitions of LGB that incorporate sexual and romantic attraction can be used. One general rule in addressing questions from youth about LGB identity is to respond in a short, clear, and positive answer which will help display acceptance and openness to discussion of the topic (Human Rights Campaign, 2012).

Some youth may not bring LGB issues to their caregivers for various reasons. However, caregivers can approach their youth about LGB-related topics in several ways including identifying sexual minority friends, neighbors, or relatives who are out to their children and discussing their relationship or sharing stories of instances where gender expectations are not adhered to by the caregiver themselves. Furthermore, intentional exposure to diversity through Pride celebrations or media, books, and television with LGB themes or characters can provide sexual minority youth with visible examples and role models. Lastly, caregivers can work to actively address any hateful or discriminatory statements made by anyone in the youth's environment (including the youth themselves) by providing education about LGB identity and the negative effects of using derogatory language to describe others. Therapists working with youth who have questions about LGB themes or are in the initial stages of identity exploration are encouraged to use similar developmentally appropriate language within their work.

Navigating an Ethical Dilemma: Parental Disclosure

An important area of consideration when working with LGB youth is the consideration of disclosure to parents and guardians. To begin, sexual minority clients who fear that their identities may be disclosed to their caregivers may not openly discuss their sexual orientation with therapists. Therefore, sharing limits to confidentiality with the client and their caregiver at the start of therapy is encouraged. It would behoove clinicians to be aware of the regulations within their state of practice as they relate to confidentiality with youth. Some states differ in right to confidentiality based on who provides consent to treatment (i.e., parent/caregiver or youth), as well as age of the client. Thorough understanding of jurisdictional regulations also implies ascertaining when and if treatment information can be withheld even if caregivers are consenting to treatment. For example, in some states, information can be withheld if it is likely to cause harm to the minor client (English, Bass, Boyle, & Eshragh, 2010).

Exercising sharp clinical judgement when working with LGB youth and balancing the risks of disclosure vs. maintaining confidentiality are important for clinicians to consider. For example, disclosure of a youth's sexual orientation to caregivers may result in potential for harm (e.g. rejection by parents, verbal or physical abuse, etc.) if family members are not accepting; however, nondisclosure of risky sexual behavior (e.g. engagement in sexual activity with multiple partners, high risk of sexually transmitted infection, etc.) also carries the potential for harm. Thorough assessments of sexual activity can help clinicians make appropriate decisions.

Assessment with SMY

Given the layered factors of sexual orientation previously discussed, it is recommended that clinicians accurately assess all three of the components relevant to sexual orientation: attraction, identity, and sexual behavior (Saewyc et al., 2004). It is important to note that youth will present with various levels of knowledge of different sexual orientations and sexual health behaviors. For example, younger adolescents coming from conservative families with limited access to social media may not know terms such as "sexual orientation" or "LGBTQIA community"; therefore, therapists are encouraged to ask broad questions to determine their client's understanding of nuances within this population. A question such as "tell me about the kinds of people that you find yourself attracted to or interested in romantically" allows clinicians to obtain information regarding sexual attraction without utilizing categorical labels that the client may not be aware of. Furthermore, such a question can be followed by a more specific inquiry about identity such as "how do you identify your sexual orientation?" For clients who are less aware of the nuances and definitions related to sexual orientation, such a question could provide a space for psychoeducation about what sexual orientation is and normalization of common labels such as gay, bi, and questioning.

To assess sexual behavior, clinicians are encouraged to ask questions about engagement of sexual activity, descriptions of past sexual partners, frequency of sexual encounters, number of partners, use of safe-sex practices such as condom usage or regular testing for sexually transmitted diseases, and identification of other risky sexual behavior (e.g. engagement of sexual activity while under the influence of substances, sexual activity with strangers, etc.) (Solomon, Heck, Reed, & Smith, 2017). Clinicians should use gender neutral language and labels in assessment of potential romantic partners. Assessment of sexual behavior can include inquiries such as "have you engaged in sexual activity in the past?" and if so, "can you tell me a little bit about your past/current partner(s)?" Knowledge about "safe-sex" practices, as acquired from peers, parents, media, and formal education, should also be assessed. Additionally, clinicians are encouraged to assess how LGB youth meet sexual partners. Recent research highlights SMY's usage of social media and internet dating websites as a primary medium for romantic and sexual relationships (Macapagal et al., 2018). The role of technology in access to relationships within the LGB youth community for various reasons (e.g. romantic/sexual relations, high-risk sexual behavior, platonic support systems, connection to role models, etc.) may be considered as well.

Additionally, it is recommended that clinicians assess additional domains relevant to sexual orientation such as cultural contexts, levels of disclosure or "coming out" to others (i.e., peers, family, etc.), experiences of stigma or victimization, and self-appraisals of sexual orientation and potential internalized homonegativity (Solomon et al., 2017). Given the increased risk of mental health concerns and specifically suicidality, clinicians are advised to thoroughly assess for suicidal ideation and attempts. Standardized formal assessments of suicidality, such as the

Table 18.1 Sample questions and prompts for intake interviews with LGBTQ youth

Topic	Sample questions/prompts
Sexual identity	Tell me about the kinds of people that you've found yourself attracted to or interested in romantically. Do you identify as straight, gay, bi, or something else?
Gender identity	What name do you go by? What are your pronouns?
Coming out	Who have you told that you are (insert identity)? Tell me about how that went. Are there other people you have thought about telling?
Cultural contexts	How do you feel your cultural group views (insert identities)? How do your spiritual views influence your identity as (insert identity)?
Experiences of stigma	What do you hear people around you saying about people who are (insert identity)? How do (or would) your parents feel about you being (insert identity)?
Internalized homo/transnegativity	How do *you* feel about your identity? What was it like for you as you came to realize you were (insert identity)?
Safe-sex practices	What have you learned about "safe sex" from school or from your parents? Your peers? Do you have access to condoms? How often do you use them?
Suicidal ideation	Many people have thoughts like "I wish I was dead" or "I don't want to be around anymore." Have you ever had thoughts like that? If the client endorses suicidal thoughts: What do you do when you have those thoughts? How do you deal with them? Have they ever been more than just thoughts? Have you ever acted on them?
Strengths and protective factors	Who do you feel comfortable talking about your identity with? Do you know about any LGBTQ resources at your school or in your town? What do you feel are the positive things about being (insert identity)?

Note: Reprinted from Solomon et al. (2017). Reprinted with permission

Columbia Suicide Severity Rating Scale (Mundt et al., 2013), can be integrated into the overall initial assessment process to capture past suicidal ideation as well as potential risk for suicide. Furthermore, assessment of strengths, social supports, and protective factors is highly encouraged because these can be utilized to support the individual throughout therapy. Solomon et al. (2017) offer several prompts clinicians can utilize to obtain information during assessment with LGB youth (see Table 18.1).

RE/CBT for SMY

Several authors have proposed key components for gay affirmative approaches, including cognitive based therapy, for sexual minority youth (Craig, Austin, & Alessi, 2013; Pachankis, 2014; Safren & Rogers, 2001). At the start of therapy, practitioners are encouraged to affirm the identities of SMY during the assessment process by being knowledgeable about LGB populations and promote a collaborative treatment process by providing clear description of rationale for therapy. Such practices contribute to fostering a strong therapeutic rapport with SMY, creating a good foundation for more specific CBT/REBT treatment. The aforementioned information in this chapter can assist clinicians in developing the necessary knowledge base for working with LGBT youth populations.

Subsequent sessions focus on addressing the impact of stigma, oppression, and homonegativity on lived experiences. The REBT therapist can assist clients in recognizing how experiences of oppression have influenced their worldviews and how these belief systems apply to activating events. In doing so, REBT therapists can provide psychoeducation on the ABC model of therapy by using examples of stigma influenced beliefs and thinking patterns, its influence on neutral activating events, and the resulting consequences of that interaction. An example demonstrating the ABC model utilized in REBT approaches can be seen in Fig. 18.1; the diagram also includes an example of disputation and a new, more adaptive, cognitive and emotional effect resulting from the therapeutic technique.

The REBT therapist can help clients distinguish between environmentally driven concerns and those that stem from dysfunctional cognitive processes. Maladaptive

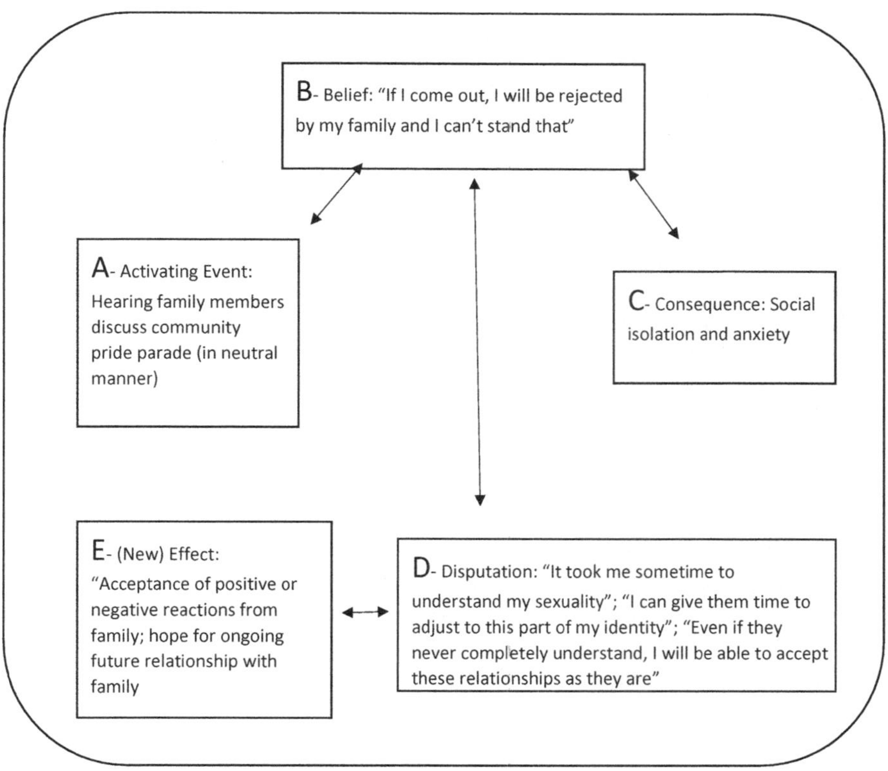

Fig. 18.1 Even if they never completely understand, I will be able to accept these relationships as they are

or dysfunctional cognitive process can be addressed through validation of self-reported experiences of discrimination and cognitive restructuring or disputation. REBT focuses on irrational or dysfunctional beliefs associated with activating events (e.g. rejection, oppression, etc.) rather than changing the activating event itself. This is especially useful in therapy with SMY who experience less agency in altering environmental influences than do adult patients. Specific cognitive patterns can be labeled and explored in session, including faulty inferences, absolutes, evaluations (awfulizing, global ratings of self or others), and causal attributions. Moody (2019) recommends that the REBT therapist focus on irrational beliefs pathologizing sexual minority identities and gender variant expression (e.g. internalized gender biases related to cultural backgrounds) to create a broader base for personal exploration in therapy. Particularly when working with individuals of minority identity status, clinicians are encouraged to question the helpfulness or functionality of thoughts and beliefs rather than questioning the validity of thoughts (Craig et al., 2013) when engaging in cognitive based techniques. Additionally, clinicians can aim toward developing elegant solutions with clients at any age by incorporating a more dichotomous view of life events (e.g., "my parents may be surprised by my coming out, but it does not necessarily mean they will not accept me as I am") and developing an understanding that such a perspective increases tolerance of emotions linked to difficult events (Young, 2006).

Furthermore, therapists can help clients examine emotions of shame and guilt surrounding LGB identity, same-sex attractions, and behavior. Albert Ellis (1968, 1964) in particular targeted emotions of shame and guilt through the course of REBT via acceptance techniques and shame attacking techniques. With regard to the latter, shame attacking exercises (e.g. assignments where clients test social norms by defying social expectations) need to be carefully considered by both therapist and client before assignment of such therapeutic tasks due to the increased risk of assault in LGB populations (D'Augelli et al., 2002). Furthermore, affirmative therapy for diverse clientele recognizes that anger can be an emotional response to oppression (Ross, Doctor, Dimito, Kuehl, & Armstrong, 2007); therefore, validation of anger and other emotions stemming from minority stress experiences is vital, and therapists are encouraged to help clients to find functional uses for such emotions (e.g. activism) (Moody, 2019).

In addition to a focus on identifying and adapting irrational beliefs and tolerating difficult emotions, REBT is particularly well suited for treatment for the sexual minority youth population because of its focus on unconditional self-acceptance. The REBT therapist themselves can be used as an agent of unconditional self-acceptance by serving as a therapeutically relational model of acceptance of the client; the lived example of the accepting therapeutic relationship can then be applied to a development of accepting relationships outside of therapy. Further, semantic techniques common to REBT can also help increase self-acceptance and decrease self-deprecating thoughts. Young (2006) suggests one semantic exercise where the clinician explains the difference between "a person with less" and being "less of a person." For example, youth who are struggling to meet friends because of fear of being rejected may benefit from incorporating self-talk that suggests they are "a person with less confidence in social situations" rather than being "less of a person" because of their past history of rejection. Moreover, such play on semantics can combat maladaptive cognitive patterns and help clients identify specific goals for treatment (e.g., improve confidence in social situations). Self-compassion exercises may also be useful in promoting self-acceptance in LGB youth experiencing shame (Petrocchi, Matos, Carvalho, & Baiocco, 2016). A crucial element of acceptance when working with the SMY population involves helping the client to "develop an understanding that acknowledging and accepting the world for what it is (e.g., the client's parents will not come to their wedding because of who they are marrying) does not mean that the client is approving of the world" (Moody, 2019, p. 361).

REBT's focus on distress tolerance serves as another major contributor to affirmative therapy with SMY. General identity establishment in adolescence involves uncertainty and navigation of peer rejection/acceptance; increasing youth's ability to tolerate uncertainty and rejection and acceptance of such situations is a key component to REBT practice with SMY. Therapists can remind LGB youth of the ABC model and identifying differences between thoughts and emotions, highlighting that the youth does not need to act on or internalize certain emotions. Additionally, identification of strategies (e.g., distraction methods, relaxation techniques, journaling, etc.) to help cope with difficult emotions can also be beneficial. Behavioral exercises exposing SMY to experiences of uncertainty (i.e., social situations where the possibility of acceptance or rejection by peers is present) can be assigned and processed in session to help patients develop their capability to cope with uncertainty and other emotional outcomes resulting from the behavioral exercises.

Clients and practitioners can collaboratively work on increasing behaviors to reduce stress, increase personal strengths and supports, and build social skills to ameliorate environmentally based concerns. Identifying personal strengths and support networks is vital in assessment and throughout treatment with SMY (Craig et al., 2013). REBT/CBT therapists can help youth identify venues where social networks and peer support may be available to clients. Modification of this component of treatment to the client's level of disclosure of sexual identity to family and peers, as well as their comfort level with association with LGB support systems, is encouraged. For example, an SMY who is not out to parents or peers may fear being inadvertently outed by attending a specific LGB support center/gathering. To accommodate the lack of disclosure to others, the therapist may recommend that the patient explore their identity by private exposure to publicly out individuals via social media, television, YouTube, or autobiographies (Craig et al., 2017). To further bolster the therapeutic aim of social support, clinicians can focus on improving communication skills in LGB youth clientele. Techniques such as role play can help patients learn to express themselves accurately, prepare for social experiences (e.g., coming out to parents, meeting new friends, etc.), and learn how to advocate for themselves and others within the LGB community.

As with most cognitive therapies, clients are encouraged to complete homework assignments that will link cognitive insights gained in therapy to active practice and application of new ways of thinking, feeling, and behaving. LGB youth can be assigned generalized tasks such as cognitive monitoring of negative thought patterns, as well as tasks more specific to identity exploration and integration such as observation of role models within the LGB community, engagement in LGB supportive groups, and identification of values across their multiple identities.

Case Illustration

The following condensed case example illustrates use of REBT/CBT techniques when working with LGB youth. For the purpose of this case illustration, names or potential identifiers were changed to protect client identity.

Gabrielle, a 16-year-old female, was referred by her parents and teachers for anxiety. Symptoms of anxiety include social withdrawal and worries about being rejected in social situations; difficulty falling asleep at night and experiences of increased heart rate related to worrying were also reported. At the start of therapy, Gabrielle identifies as a female, Guatemalan, raised in the Catholic religious tradition. She reports having "crushes on girls" but identifying as "heterosexual" because she could "never actually marry a girl." Gabrielle is heavily involved in her religious community and is an active member of a local Latinx cultural center. She has not disclosed her same-gender attraction to her family members, or peers within her religious community. Gabrielle is a high achieving student and participates in school clubs and extracurricular activities; recently, she has started attending her school's new Gender and Sexuality Alliance (GSA) because she is interested in a future career in public policy. While participating in the GSA, she develops friendships with several peers who openly identify as sexual minority youth; however, she keeps her participation in the GSA a secret from her parents. Gabrielle agrees to attend therapy because she is experiencing increasing anxiety and has recently started to feel as though she is "leading a double life."

Case Conceptualization

Despite never disclosing her attraction to female peers, Gabrielle's parents and community inadvertently informed her of expected roles and expectations for relationships (i.e., beliefs) through the following cultural messages she was exposed to within several cultural contexts: a woman *needs* a man to take care of her; a woman *must* learn to cook well to take care of her husband and family; being "gay" results in people "going to hell" (ratings of worth); and LGB individuals are confused. Her recent exposure to the LGB identity, and self-acknowledgment of attraction to same-gendered peers, has created tension in her worldview defined by strong adherence to gender roles, religious identity, and desire to maintain familial harmony. Examples of irrational beliefs as described in REBT are provided in Table 18.2, highlighting maladaptive thinking patterns as well as their more adaptive alternatives.

Table 18.2 Case example of irrational/maladaptive beliefs and their rational alternatives

Inflexible demands	Alternative outlook
My family must accept my sexuality	*Preferred:* I want my family to accept me completely, but I do not control their level of acceptance
Awfulizing: If my family rejects me, I will be homeless My family must accept me, and if they don't, they are total jerks If I am gay, I am going to hell	*Anti-awfulizing belief:* My family may reject me, but they will continue to allow me to live with them I want my family to accept me, but I know it may be difficult for them I believe that God made me in his "likeness and image"; that includes my attraction to others
Low frustration tolerance belief: I cannot bear it if my family rejects my sexuality	*High frustration tolerance belief:* It would be hard for me to deal with my family's rejection of me, but I will be able to find sources of love and acceptance
Depreciation belief: If my family rejects me, it would prove that I am an unlovable person	*Acceptance belief:* I am worthy of love despite my family's reaction to what type of relationship I have

Treatment Process

Initial sessions following the intake focus on general psychoeducation of sexual orientation and LGB identity, most of which Gabrielle is familiar with due to her participation in the GSA. The therapist also explores how this information sits with her. Gabrielle acknowledges her sense of being "split" between two worlds. She identifies specific thoughts such as "this identity is okay for my friends but not for my family." The clinician discusses the connection between emotional reactions and cognitive processes (ABC model) either through verbal description or visual explanation using the cognitive triangle common to RE-CBT. The clinician and Gabrielle collaboratively discuss how the model is relevant to Gabrielle's life and she identifies how her thoughts often result in increased anxiety.

Sessions following initial assessment, collaboration on treatment goals, and psychoeducation about sexuality in general include a focus on REBT/CBT specific techniques. The following is an example of a therapeutic session where Gabrielle explores the connection between cognitive process and emotional consequences. Additionally, the client and clinician engage in disputation or challenging of maladaptive thoughts. In doing so, the clinician also fosters a sense of self-acceptance.

Excerpt from Mid-session of Treatment

Therapist: Okay, so last week we talked about how your thoughts are closely linked with your feelings of anxiety and the tension and panic you've been experiencing. You discussed some of the specific thoughts you have that really raise your anxiety. Do you mind sharing the ones that seem most relevant to you this week?

Gabrielle: Sure. Well, this week, I hung out with my church friends. We didn't talk about anything too deep and definitely not about gay people, but I found myself wondering what they think about gay people.

Therapist: What do you imagine they think about gay people?

Gabrielle: Well, I think they think like me; gay people are going to hell.

Therapist: Tell me, when you have that thought, how does it make you feel?

Gabrielle: Well, panicked. Uncomfortable. Scared. What if I am going to hell because I keep having crushes on girls more and more.

Therapist: Well, I can definitely understand how you may be scared and uncomfortable thinking about your crushes on girls, especially if you believe that anyone who is gay is going to hell. Do you think we can talk a little more about your beliefs?

Gabrielle: Sure.

Therapist: Gabrielle, what does your religion teach about God's love for humanity in general?

Gabrielle: You mean like, all people?

Therapist: Yes, like all people.

Gabrielle: Well, most importantly it teaches that we are all created by God in his "likeness and image" and that we are always loved, and we will always be forgiven.

Therapist: Wow. That's pretty powerful. Do you feel that love?

Gabrielle: Well, I used to be sure of it. But now, I'm worried God won't love me anymore.

Therapist: Help me understand: you believe that God has created you and all human beings, but you are worried that God won't love someone he himself created – you are worried he won't love you?

Gabrielle: Well, when you put it that way, I guess it doesn't make sense, does it? He does love me … but … he doesn't want me to be gay.

Therapist: That's a possibility. Gabrielle, if we had to break down that thought into two different statements: (a) God loves me and (b) God doesn't want me to be gay, what emotions are tied to each one for you?

Gabrielle: Well, if I think about the second one, God not wanting me to be gay, I feel anxious and worried and alone because well, I think I may be gay. But, when I focus on that first thought, that God loves me, I feel so happy and loved.

Therapist: With that in mind, which thought do you think is more helpful to you?

Gabrielle: That God loves me.

Therapist: I would agree.

Gabrielle: To be honest, I believe that one more – that God loves me. Mostly because of what we just discussed a few minutes before, this idea that if God created me, gay and all, how could he hate me?

Therapist: It sounds like you are challenging the thought that "if you are gay, God does not love you, and so you may go to hell," more and more.

Gabrielle: Well, yeah. It's kinda like you said. It doesn't seem like that thought is helping me figure all this out. But these other thoughts that I've also always

> known, that "God loves me" and has "created me exactly how I should be," well those help me feel loved and connected to my faith. It feels better to focus on that way of thinking. And what's more is that when I think about God's love for me, I am reminded that my family and friends too love me, and I am hopeful that that won't change even if I am gay. It may not be true, maybe they won't love me, but at least that thought helps me keep the hope of acceptance alive.

It is important to note that within this excerpt, the therapist empowered Gabrielle to explore and dispute her own beliefs without directly challenging her beliefs. Additionally, the therapist utilized language consistent with the client's description of herself and her beliefs. Most importantly, Gabrielle was not made to "rethink" her belief system, or to assert validity for her religious beliefs; rather, she was encouraged to acknowledge the dichotomy present in most belief systems and choose to engage in a thinking pattern that is more helpful and adaptive.

In addressing any of these multicultural identities, the therapist demonstrates respect for Gabrielle's views while initiating a collaborative approach to understand how these beliefs factor (or not) into her distress, rather than direct disputation of these beliefs. Practitioners are encouraged to help the client determine the workability and helpfulness of beliefs rather than their accuracy (i.e., "How does this style of thinking about [insert multicultural belief] impact your distress?").

RE-CBT Adaptation in School for SMY: Looking Ahead

Over the past decades, there has been a growing interest to address mental health in school settings. A number of mental disorders and chronic stress reported among the student population have been linked to academic concerns such as drop-out, lower grades, poorer health outcomes, and the risk of substance abuse and/or severe mental illness in adulthood (Perou et al., 2013). These outcomes are expected to be far worse for sexual minority youth. Recent studies have found that LGBTQ+ are at greater risk of being isolated and bullied and experience depression and suicidal behaviors in contrast to other students in schools (Birkett, Newcomb, & Mustanski, 2015; Kann et al., 2016). As such, there is an ongoing opportunity to consider potential mental health programs within schools as one of the most important environments for the children and adolescents' cognitive, emotional, and social development (Atkins, Hoagwood, Kutash, & Seidman, 2010).

Although there are few programs that address the mental health disparities reported for the LGB youth population, there are promising applications for modalities based on rational emotional therapy in schools. Albert Ellis proposed one of the earliest forms of educational program based on mental health for schools. Since the early 1970s, literature and curriculums developed for children/adolescents have incorporated the ABC's paradigm to foster critical thinking skills and ways to tackle irrational beliefs (Vernon, 2006). Ellis's work in schools emphasized a focus on social-emotional learning based on rational emotive behavior therapy's tenets which led to the Rational Emotive Education (REE) programs (Vernon, 2006). The REE served as a prevention curriculum with lessons on effective coping skills, which included dispute of faulty thinking, developing healthy behaviors, and better interpersonal relationships (Vernon, 2006). This is particularly important for the LGB students who face internalized homophobia which has been linked to difficulties in emotional, behavioral expression and suicidal ideation (Berg, Munthe-Kass, & Ross, 2015; McLauren, 2016). In addition, many inflexible schemas can emerge from experiencing internalized homophobia during the early years of development which can impact the coming out process and social connections (Frost & Meyer, 2009). Application of REE can lead to identification and management of core irrational beliefs about self, guilt, shame, and low-distress tolerance in youth as a result of internalized homophobia.

The practice of acceptance is critical in order to amend the emotional experience and the learning of healthier responses when working with students who experienced internalized stigmatization of their sexuality. According to the work conducted in schools from REE and similar frameworks, acceptance involves helping students to become aware of their strengths and the full spectrum of their emotional experience, including those considered negative (Vernon, 2006). It is recommended that interventions focused on increasing acceptance aim at helping LGB youth understand their experience of microaggressions and minority stressors, as well as the connection between these activating events and how they contribute to their worldviews. However, youth should not be encouraged to simply accept discrimination and negative treatment by others but rather understand its presence in the world and learn to adaptively cope with this reality by utilizing cognitive and emotional coping strategies.

As part of these efforts, REE principles can be taught to school stakeholders (e.g., teachers, school counselors and other school personnel) to promote the well-being of LGB children and adolescents (Vernon, 2006). Effective implementation of the model within schools relies on stakeholders' commitment toward the learning and practice of these concepts through implementation such as informal or structured emotional regulation educational lessons, integrated into school-wide curriculums (Vernon, 2006). Integration of REE tenets allows school personnel to ensure a safe and diverse school environment. In doing so, school personnel can help identify their own biases and generalizations that impact their view of their students. In contrast to the early years of the REE in schools, emerging institutional policies can potentially support school personnel with program implementation by focusing on inclusive curriculums, establishment of Gay-Straight Alliances, staff training, the use of pronouns, dress codes, and public restrooms, among others (APA, 2015; Kosciw, Greytak, Bartkierwicz, Boesen, & Palmer, 2012). As mental health disparities and oppression among SMY populations remain an ongoing issue, the commitment to improving mental health and education from different fronts in school settings is of paramount responsibility.

Conclusion

Emerging proposals for the applicability of RE/CBT for therapy with LGB youth such as this chapter highlight ethical, clinical, developmental, cultural, and contextual considerations when working with SMY populations. The increasing recognition of conceptual frameworks such as the minority stress model and the relationship with the experiences of historically marginalized populations (Moody, 2019) result in ongoing improvement of clinical work and applicability among RE/CBT practitioners. As we illustrated early in this chapter, many of the early debates on sexuality and diversity were brought by Albert Ellis (1990) inciting the beginning of a revolution of acceptance of sexual minority identity as a healthy variant of sexuality. It is imperative to acknowledge that there is a long road ahead and much of the progress requires commitment from practitioners and researchers alike. The use of RE/CBT is expected to grow exponentially among practitioners, requiring RE/CBT specific training, which should include examining the intersection of culture, systemic barriers, families, school, social strata, and gender in treatment with SMY. These efforts are considered to be part of best practices in the field and promote a better understanding of the needs of youth, particularly those with marginalized identities.

Test Yourself

1. What are some important aspects of initial assessment unique to working with SMY?
2. Which components of RE/CBT are particularly suited for therapeutic work with SMY?
3. Carlos is a seventh grader who identifies as Latino and gay and attends an all-male school. Male peers physically and verbally harass Carlos because of their suspicions that he is attracted to males. As a result, he denies his sexual orientation from friends and family. What are important factors to consider when working with Carlos? As an RE/CBT clinician, how would you approach Carlos's fears of "coming out" to friends and family?

References

American Psychological Association. (2015, September 1). Supporting transgender and gender diverse students in schools. *Key Recommendations for School Administrators.* https://www.apa.org/pi/lgbt/programs/safe-supportive/lgbt/school-administrators.pdf.

Atkins, M. S., Hoagwood, K. E., Kutash, K., & Seidman, E. (2010). Toward the integration of education and mental health in schools. *Administration and Policy in Mental Health, 37*(1–2), 40–47. https://doi.org/10.1007/s10488-010-0299-7

Berg, R., Munthe-Kass, H., & Ross, M. (2015). Internalized homonegativity: A systematic mapping review of empirical research. *Journal of Homosexuality, 63*(4), 541–558. https://doi.org/10.1080/00918369.2015.1083788
Bernard, M. (2011). Homosexuality. In B. Michael (Ed.), *Rationality and the pursuit of happiness: The legacy of Albert Ellis* (pp. 173–185). West Sussex, UK: Wiley-Blackwell.
Bidell, M. (2015). Using the sexual orientation counselor competency scale (SOCCS) in mental health and healthcare settings: An instructor's guide. *MedEdPORTAL, 11*, 10040. https://doi.org/10.15766/mep_2374-8265.10040
Bidell, M. P. (2017). The lesbian, gay, bisexual, and transgender development of clinical skills scale (LGBT-DOCSS): Establishing a new interdisciplinary self-assessment for health providers. *Journal of Homosexuality, 64*(10), 1432–1460. https://doi.org/10.1080/00918369.2017.1321389
Birkett, M., Koenig, B., & Espelage, D. L. (2009). LGB and questioning students in schools: The moderating effects of homophobic bullying and school climate on negative outcomes. *Journal of Youth and Adolescence, 38*(7), 989–1000. https://doi.org/10.1007/s10964-008-9389-1
Birkett, M., Newcomb, M. E., & Mustanski, B. (2015). Does it get better? A longitudinal analysis of psychological distress and victimization in lesbian, gay, bisexual, transgender and questioning youth. *The Journal of Adolescent Health, 56*(3), 280–285.
Bostwick, W. B., Boyd, C. J., Hughes, T. L., & McCabe, S. E. (2010). Dimensions of sexual orientation and the prevalence of mood and anxiety disorders in the United States. *American Journal of Public Health, 100*(3), 468–475. https://doi.org/10.2105/AJPH.2008.152942
Burgard, S. A., Cochran, S. D., & Mays, V. M. (2005). Alcohol and tobacco use patterns among heterosexually and homosexually experienced California women. *Drug and Alcohol Dependence, 77*(1), 61–70. https://doi.org/10.1016/j.drugalcdep.2004.07.007
Cass, V. C. (1979). Homosexual identity formation: A theoretical model. *Journal of Homosexuality, 4*(3), 219–235. https://doi.org/10.1300/J082v04n03_01
Chun, K., & Singh, A. A. (2010). The bisexual youth of color intersecting identities development model: A contextual approach to understanding multiple marginalization experiences. *Journal of Bisexuality, 10*(4), 429–451. https://doi.org/10.1080/15299716.2010.521059
Cochran, S. D., Sullivan, J. G., & Mays, V. M. (2003). Prevalence of mental disorders, psychological distress, and mental health services use among lesbian, gay, and bisexual adults in the United States. *Journal of Consulting and Clinical Psychology, 71*(1), 53–61. https://doi.org/10.1037//0022-006x.71.1.53
Craig, S. L., Austin, A., & Alessi, E. (2013). Gay affirmative cognitive behavioral therapy for sexual minority youth: A clinical adaptation. *Clinical Social Work Journal, 41*(3), 258–266. https://doi.org/10.1007/s10615-012-0427-9
Craig, S. L., McInroy, L. B., D'Souza, S. A., Austin, A., McCready, L. T., Eaton, A. D., et al. (2017). Influence of information and communication technologies on the resilience and coping of sexual and gender minority youth in the United States and Canada (project #queery): Mixed methods survey. *JMIR Research Protocols, 6*(9), e189. https://doi.org/10.2196/resprot.8397
D'Augelli, A. R., Hershberger, S. L., & Pilkington, N. W. (1998). Lesbian, gay, and bisexual youth and their families: Disclosure of sexual orientation and its consequences. *The American Journal of Orthopsychiatry, 68*(3), 61–71. https://doi.org/10.1037/h0080345
D'Augelli, A. R., Pilkington, N. W., & Hershberger, S. L. (2002). Incidence and mental health impact of sexual orientation victimization of lesbian, gay, and bisexual youths in high school. *School Psychology Quarterly, 17*(2), 148–167. https://doi.org/10.1521/scpq.17.2.148.20854
David, D., Cotet, C., Matu, S., Mogoase, C., & Stefan, S. (2018). 50 years of rational-emotive and cognitive-behavioral therapy: A systematic review and meta-analysis. *Journal of Clinical Psychology, 74*(3), 304–318. https://doi.org/10.1002/jclp.22514
Dryden, W., & David, D. (2008). Rational emotive behavior therapy: Current status. *Journal of Cognitive Psychotherapy, 22*(3), 195–209. https://doi.org/10.1891/0889-8391.22.3.195
Ellis, A. (1964). A guide to rational homosexuality. *Archives of Sexuality & Gender, 4*(8), 1–6.
Ellis, A. (1965). *Homosexuality: Its causes and cure*. New York: L. Stuart.

Ellis, A. (1968). Homosexuality: The right to be wrong. *The Journal of Sex Research, 4*(2), 96–107.

Ellis, A. (1990). Rumors about my anti-homosexual views: A reply to Kristin Gay Esterberg. *The Journal of Sex Research, 27*(4), 645–646.

English, A., Bass, L., Boyle, A. D., & Eshragh, F. (2010). *State Minor Consent Laws: A Summary* (3rd ed.). Chapel Hill, NC: Center for Adolescent Health and the Law.

Feinstein, B. A., Goldfried, M. R., & Davila, J. (2012). The relationship between experiences of discrimination and mental health among lesbians and gay men: An examination of internalized homonegativity and rejection sensitivity as potential mechanisms. *Journal of Consulting and Clinical Psychology, 80*(5), 917–927. https://doi.org/10.1037/a0029425

Fish, J. N., & Pasley, K. (2015). Sexual (minority) trajectories, mental health, and alcohol use: A longitudinal study of youth as they transition to adulthood. *Journal of Youth and Adolescence, 44*(8), 1508–1527. https://doi.org/10.1007/s10964-015-0280-6

Floyd, F. J., & Bakerman, R. (2006). Coming-out across the life course: Implications of age and historical context. *Archives of Sexual Behavior, 35*, 287–297. https://doi.org/10.1007/s10508-006-9022-x

Frost, D. M., & Meyer, I. H. (2009). Internalized homophobia and relationship quality among lesbians, gay men, and bisexuals. *Journal of Counseling Psychology, 56*(1), 97–109. https://doi.org/10.1037/a0012844

Fukuyama, M. A., & Ferguson, A. D. (2000). Lesbian, gay, and bisexual people of color: Understanding cultural complexity and managing multiple oppressions. In R. M. Perez, K. A. DeBord, & K. J. Bieschke (Eds.), *Handbook of counseling and psychotherapy with lesbian, gay, and bisexual clients* (pp. 81–105). Washington, DC: American Psychological Association.

Gold, M., & Terepka, A. (2019). Interviewing adolescents. In J. Meschan (Ed.), *Promoting mental health in children & adolescents: Primary care and advocacy* (pp. 71–95). Itasca, IL: American Academy of Pediatrics.

Hariton, E., & Locascio, J. J. (2018). Randomised controlled trials - the gold standard for effectiveness research: Study design: Randomised controlled trials. *BJOG : An International Journal of Obstetrics and Gynaecology, 125*(13), 1716. https://doi.org/10.1111/1471-0528.15199

Hatzenbuehler, M. L. (2009). How does sexual minority stigma "get under the skin"? A psychological mediation framework. *Psychology Bulletin, 135*(5), 707–730. https://doi.org/10.1037/a0016441

Hays, P. A. (2009). Integrating evidence-based practice, cognitive behavior therapy, and multicultural therapy: Ten steps for culturally competent practice. *Professional Psychology: Research and Practice, 40*(4), 354–360. https://doi.org/10.1037/a0016250

Human Rights Campaign. (2012). *Welcoming schools: Professional development tools.* Washington, DC: Human Rights Campaign (HRC) Foundation. www.welcomingschools.org/2012/03/professional-development/

Kann, L., Olsen, E. O., McManus, T., et al. (2016). Sexual identity, sex of sexual contacts, and health-related behaviors among students in grades 9–12 – United States and selected sites, 2015. *MMWR Surveillance Summary, 65*(9), 1–202. https://doi.org/10.15585/mmwr.ss6509a1

Kosciw, J. G., Greytak, E. A., Bartkiewicz, M. J., Boesen, M. J., & Palmer, N. A. (2012). *The 2011 National School Climate Survey: The experiences of lesbian, gay, bisexual and transgender youth in our nation's schools.* New York: GLSEN.

Macapagal, K., Moskowitz, D. A., Li, D. H., Carrion, A., Bettin, E., Fisher, C. B., et al. (2018). Hookup app use, sexual behavior, and sexual health among adolescent men who have sex with men in the United States. *Journal of Adolescent Health, 62*(6), 708–715. https://doi.org/10.1016/j.jadohealth.2018.01.001

Marshal, M. P., Dietz, L. J., Friedman, M. S., et al. (2011). Suicidality and depression disparities between sexual minority and heterosexual youth: A meta-analytic review. *The Journal of Adolescent Health, 49*(2), 115–123. https://doi.org/10.1016/j.jadohealth.2011.02.005

McInroy, L., & Craig, S. L. (2012). Articulating identities: Language and practice with multiethnic sexual minority youth. *Counseling Psychology Quarterly, 25*(2), 137–149. https://doi.org/10.1080/09515070.2012.674685

McLauren, S. (2016). The interrelations between internalized homophobia, depressive symptoms, and suicidal ideation among Australian gay men, lesbians, and bisexual women. *Journal of Homosexuality, 63*(2), 156–168. https://doi.org/10.1080/00918369.2015.1083779

Meyer, I. H. (2003). Prejudice, social stress, and mental health in lesbian, gay, and bisexual populations: Conceptual issues and research evidence. *Psychological Bulletin, 129*(5), 674–697. https://doi.org/10.1037/0033-2909.129.5.674

Moody, R. (2019). REBT with LGBTQ clients. In W. Dryden & M. Bernard (Eds.), *REBT with diverse clients problems and populations* (pp. 350–381). New York: Springer.

Morgan, E. M. (2013). Contemporary issues in sexual orientation and identity development in emerging adulthood. *Emerging Adulthood, 1*(1), 52–66. https://doi.org/10.1177/2167696812469187

Mundt, J. C., Greist, J. H., Jefferson, J. W., et al. (2013). Prediction of suicidal behavior in clinical research by lifetime suicidal ideation and behavior ascertained by the electronic Columbia-suicide severity rating scale. *Journal of Clinical Psychiatry, 74*(9), 887–893. https://doi.org/10.4088/JCP.13m08398

Mustanski, B. S., Garofalo, R., & Emerson, E. M. (2010). Mental health disorders, psychological distress, and suicidality in a diverse sample of lesbian, gay, bisexual, and transgender youths. *American Journal of Public Health, 100*(12), 2426–2432. https://doi.org/10.2105/AJPH.2009.178319

Nadal, K. L., Issa, M., Leon, J., Meterko, V., Wideman, M., & Wong, Y. (2011). Sexual orientation microaggressions: "Death by a thousand cuts" for lesbian, gay, and bisexual youth. *Journal of LGBT Youth, 8*(3), 234–259. https://doi.org/10.1080/19361653.2011.584204

Needham, B. L. (2012). Sexual attraction and trajectories of mental health and substance use during the transition from adolescence to adulthood. *Journal of Youth and Adolescence, 41*(2), 179–190. https://doi.org/10.1007/s10964-011-9729-4

O'Shaughnessy, T., & Speir, Z. (2018). The state of LGBQ affirmative therapy clinical research: A mixed-methods systematic synthesis. *Psychology of Sexual Orientation and Gender Diversity, 5*(1), 82–98. https://doi.org/10.1037/sgd0000259

Pachankis, J. E. (2014). Uncovering clinical principles and techniques to address minority stress, mental health, and related health risks among gay and bisexual men. *Clinical Psychology: A Publication of the Division of Clinical Psychology of the American Psychological Association, 21*(4), 313–330. https://doi.org/10.1111/cpsp.12078

Pachankis, J. E., Hatzenbuehler, M. L., Rendina, H. J., Safren, S. A., & Parsons, J. T. (2015). LGB-affirmative cognitive-behavioral therapy for young adult gay and bisexual men: A randomized controlled trial of a transdiagnostic minority stress approach. *Journal of Consulting and Clinical Psychology, 83*(5), 875–889. https://doi.org/10.1037/ccp0000037

Perou, R., Bitsko, R., Blumberg, S., et al. (2013). Mental health surveillance among children—United States, 2005–2011. *MMWR. Morbidity and Mortality Weekly Report, 62*(2), 1–35.

Petrocchi, N., Matos, M., Carvalho, S., & Baiocco, R. (2016). Compassion-focused therapy in the treatment of shame-based difficulties in gender and sexual minorities. In M. D. Skinta & A. Curtin (Eds.), *Mindfulness and acceptance for gender and sexual minorities* (pp. 69–86). Oakland, CA: Context Press.

Pew Research Center. (2013, September 16). *A survey of LGBT Americans: Attitudes, experiences, and values in changing times*. https://www.pewsocialtrends.org/wp-content/uploads/sites/3/2013/06/SDT_LGBT-Americans_06-2013.pdf.

Rosario, M., Schrimshaw, E. W., Hunter, J., & Braun, L. (2006). Sexual identity development among gay, lesbian, and bisexual youths: Consistency and change over time. *Journal of Sex Research, 43*(1), 46–58. https://doi.org/10.1080/00224490609552298

Ross, L. E., Doctor, F., Dimito, A., Kuehl, D., & Armstrong, M. S. (2007). Can talking about oppression reduce depression? *Journal of Gay and Lesbian Social Services, 19*(1), 1–15. https://doi.org/10.1300/J041v19n01_01

Russell, S. T., & Fish, J. N. (2016). Mental health in lesbian, gay, bisexual, and transgender (LGBT) youth. *Annual Review of Clinical Psychology, 12*, 465–487. https://doi.org/10.1146/annurev-clinpsy-021815-093153

Saewyc, E. M., Bauer, G. R., Skay, C. L., Bearinger, L. H., Resnick, M. D., Reis, E., et al. (2004). Measuring sexual orientation in adolescent health surveys: Evaluation of eight school-based surveys. *Journal of Adolescent Health, 35*(4), 345e1–345e.15. https://doi.org/10.1016/j.jadohealth.2004.06.002

Safren, S. A., & Rogers, T. (2001). Cognitive-behavioral therapy with gay, lesbian, and bisexual clients. *In Session: Psychotherapy in Practice, 57*(5), 629–643. https://doi.org/10.1002/jclp.1033

Solomon, D. T., Heck, N., Reed, O. M., & Smith, D. W. (2017). Conducting culturally competent intake interviews with LGBTQ youth. *Psychology of Sexual Orientation and Gender Diversity, 4*(4), 403–411. https://doi.org/10.1037/sgd0000255

Sue, D. W., & Torino, G. C. (2005). Racial-cultural competence: Awareness, knowledge, and skills. In R. T. Carter (Ed.), *Handbook of racial-cultural psychology and counseling: Training and practice* (2nd ed., pp. 3–18). Hoboken, NJ: Wiley.

Vernon, A. (2006). REBT with children and adolescents. In W. Dryden & M. Bernard (Eds.), *REBT with diverse clients problems and populations* (pp. 241–263). New York: Springer.

Weinrach, S. (2006). Reducing REBT's wince factor: An insider perspective. *Journal of Rational-Emotive and Cognitive-Behavioral Therapy, 24*(3), 183–198. https://doi.org/10.1007/s10942-006-0044-z

Yin, R. (2014). *Case study research. Design and methods*. Thousand Oaks, CA: Sage Publications.

Young, H. (2006). REBT assessment and treatment with adolescents. In A. Ellis & M. E. Bernard (Eds.), *Rational emotive behavioral approaches to childhood disorders: Theory, practice, and research* (pp. 115–132). New York: Springer.

Chapter 19
Academic Procrastination and Educational Underachievement: How REBT Works

Michael Bernard

Research reveals external assets (home, school, community) including positive environment (e.g., Banerjee, 2016), parental attachment (e.g., Chen, 2017), participation in organized, extracurricular activities (e.g., Darling, 2005), support, empowerment, boundaries-expectations, and constructive use of time (e.g., Benson, 2007) to be associated with academic procrastination and educational underachievement.

Internal assets mitigating academic procrastination include the personality traits of conscientiousness (e.g., White, Graham, & Blass, 2018), achievement motivation (e.g., Meese & Agger, 2018), character strengths such as hope (Alexander & Onwuegbuzie, 2007), attitudes including frustration intolerance beliefs (Harrington, 2005), commitment to learning, academic self-efficacy (e.g., Bandura, 1997; Klassen & Kuzucu, 2009), growth mindset (e.g., Dweck, 2006, 2016), as well as coping skills such as self-regulation (e.g., Zimmerman & Schunk, 2001). Additionally, internal affective states such as self-worth/self-esteem (e.g., Topcu & Leana-Tascılar, 2018) and academic anxiety have been found associated with procrastination. It has been argued that the internal assets of young people moderate the influence of their external environment (e.g., Chen & Chang, 2016; Christens & Peterson, 2011).

When I worked in schools as a consultant educational/school psychologist and applied REBT as my primary modality for understanding, assessing, and intervening with childhood problems when working with referred students and consulting with their parents and teachers, many students referred for lack of motivation and poor achievement at all levels of schooling manifested signs and symptoms of work procrastination. And some but not all referred students who displayed primary emotional issues (anxiety, depression) and behavioral problems concomitantly displayed work procrastination.

M. Bernard (✉)
University of Melbourne, Melbourne Graduate School of Education, Melbourne, Australia
e-mail: m.bernard@unimelb.edu.au

M. Bernard, M. D. Terjesen (eds.), *Rational-Emotive and Cognitive-Behavioral Approaches to Child and Adolescent Mental Health: Theory, Practice, Research, Applications*, https://doi.org/10.1007/978-3-030-53901-6_19

At that time, I investigated what research revealed about the cognitive, emotional, and behavioral characteristics of students who demonstrated academic procrastination. The work of Solomon, Rothblum, and colleagues (e.g., Rothblum, Solomon, & Murakami, 1986; Solomon & Rothblum, 1984) was particularly illuminating in helping me identify different cause of academic procrastination that guided my assessment of a referred student. While early research in the area of academic procrastination had focused on the absence of study skills in procrastinators, these researchers examined the cognitive and emotional characteristics of high and low academic procrastinators. Solomon and Rothblum (1984) found two main psychological factors associated with procrastination:

1. *Fear of failure*, which includes anxiety about meeting others' expectations (evaluation anxiety), concerns about meeting one's own standards (perfectionism), lack of self-confidence, lack of assertion, and low self-esteem
2. *Task aversiveness*, which relates to the unpleasantness of the task and laziness

Solomon and Rothblum found that there were two distinct groups of procrastinators. The first is a small homogeneous group who experience various symptoms surrounding fear of failure. The second group is larger and more heterogeneous; it includes those students who procrastinate due to the aversiveness of the task. Rothblum et al. (1986) found that in comparison with low academic procrastinators, high academic procrastinators experience more anxiety, are more likely to attribute success on exams to external and fleeting circumstances (rather than their own ability and effort), have lower self-efficacy, and have less control over their emotional reactions.

Defining Educational Underachievement

There are a variety of meanings of the term "underachievement." Schaefer and Millman (1981) describe underachievers as children who see little personal meaning in school or who have not developed achievement motivation and related goal setting and success behaviors. Brophy (1996) discusses underachievement as reflected in children who do a minimum to just "get by" and who (a) are indifferent to school, (b) do minimum amounts of work, and (c) are not challenged by schoolwork and are poorly motivated.

I defined the construct of educational underachievement as follows (Bernard, 2006):

> Educational underachievement means that a student's school performance as seen in grades or test results is lower than we would predict from a student's age, ability and potential....Some signs of educational underachievement are when a student: a) performs much better on a test of ability than in schoolwork, b) performs well at one time and then does poorly at another, c) performs well in some subjects, but doesn't do well in other subjects, d) occasionally reveals in what they say or do good academic or creative ability relative to their usual performance, and e) demonstrates one or more of the following

characteristics: low self-esteem, fear of failure, discouragement, lack of confidence, lack of motivation and effort, goals which are too low or too high, poor time management, rebelliousness, and poor study techniques.

Underachievement is sometimes mistakenly operationalized as students not achieving minimum academic standards in one or more subjects at any grade level. Schools and school districts sometimes calculate the percentage of underachievers as the ratio of students not achieving standards in comparison with those that do. However, I believe there is considerable consensus in the field toward defining underachievement as a discrepancy between academic aptitude and achievement (classroom grades, standardized achievement test scores). So, for example, a student of high ability may underachieve even though s/he has achieved grade level expectations. Alternatively, a student with very low academic ability who works very hard but does not achieve grade level expectations would be considered an "achiever." Hard-working students with low ability would be considered "low achievers" but not "underachievers" because they are performing to potential.

Different Types of Underachievers

Underachievers are a heterogeneous group with individual underachievers displaying unique patterns of symptoms and causal factors. The literature identifies several distinct "types" of underachievers. It is useful when conducting a rational emotive behavior therapy (REBT) assessment of students who underachieve to consider the extent to which s/he resembles one of the following types.

Rebellious/Aggressive Type Typified by the "You can't make me do this," these young people believe they should be able to do what they want to do. This attitude may result from the way their parents raised them, their unique temperament (e.g., feisty), or a combination of both. They have lots of power struggles with their families and in particular big battles over homework. These young people may use nonschool performance as a way of punishing their parents for real or imagined injustices ("I'll fix their wagon!").

Immature/Dependent/Anxious Type These emotionally immature young people are very reluctant to do things on their own when they are young and tend to hover around their parents and teachers asking lots of questions. They are very concerned about what adults think of them if they make mistakes. In school, they rely too much on their teachers asking lots of questions and frequently showing their teacher their work. They have a high need for approval, and they fail to develop the independence to try new or hard things.

Helpless-Discouraged-Depressed Type These students may have been a bit "immature" when starting school and have limited academic aptitude or a learning disability. They fall behind quickly and experience many fewer positive reinforcements for their schoolwork. They begin to see a disconnect between their efforts and positive achievement outcomes and, as a consequence, develop a negative view of themselves and cannot see themselves accomplishing much at school in the future. Low academic self-concept and poor self-efficacy for most school subjects accompany this type of underachiever throughout the years of schooling.

The Perfectionistic Type These students demand unrealistically high standards of themselves. They have the idea that to be successful and worthwhile, they must do things perfectly at school. When they anticipate not performing perfectly in an area, they can underperform by not putting in the effort. Lack of effort provides them with a convenient rationalization for lack of perfection ("I simply didn't try very hard. If I did, I would have been perfect"). They can waste a lot of time getting started because they are afraid of not getting it right. They selectively achieve in areas where they have excellent talent and often underperform in areas of perceived weakness. Perfectionists also tend to restrict their activities to only those where they have a better than average chance of achieving very high results.

Peer-Conforming Type The underachieving lifestyle is becoming institutionalized as a subculture with many young people. Young people witness powerful and respected peer models with great prestige not valuing their schoolwork and who put pressure on students who appear to value their work. Bart Simpson, a very recognizable TV personality who is the prototypical underachieving student, is still revered almost 20 years after being born on "The Simpsons." In many schools, there can be great peer pressures beginning in middle primary grades on students not to do their work. While some who endorse this lifestyle do so for reasons more associated with the culture of hedonism so prevalent in western society today, others conform to an anti-achieving lifestyle for fear if they did not, they would be rejected by their peers.

Low Frustration Tolerance Type While a vast majority of underachievers have very little ability to tolerate normal levels of frustration, some have particularly abysmally low levels of frustration tolerance. Some of these young people whom we used to call "lazy" appear to have an allergy to hard or boring schoolwork while carrying on successfully in other areas of their lives. Frequently, these students are born with an easily frustratable temperament which they battle with for much of their lives. Combined with a smothering, overprotective, or permissive style of parenting, these young people fail to develop the frustration tolerance and delay of gratification needed to meet the responsibilities of school and, in some cases, life. They frequently tell themselves: "Life should be fun and exciting all the time. I can't be bothered doing this. It's unfair that I have to do this. This is too hard. I cannot stand it." Additionally, they tend to be chronically disorganized failing to keep track of assignments, deadlines, and time and have no patience for filing things away including learning material and resources.

Non-achievement/Peter Pan Syndrome These frequently good-natured students are motivated to do anything possible to avoid doing schoolwork; that is, these students are strongly motivated to avoid success. They believe that doing schoolwork successfully will reveal to others their true capabilities and will result in having to assume unwanted responsibilities and the sacrifice of fun.

A variety of techniques and strategies have been employed to combat underachievement. Some are comprehensive and involve teacher-parent collaboration in using behavior modification (e.g., behavioral contracting, daily/weekly school-home report card). Other approaches work directly with the student employing a variety of techniques (including study skills, goal setting, time management, self-monitoring, disputing irrational beliefs, use of positive self-statements, emotional self-management, coping skills). It appears that while many diverse treatments have met with success in ameliorating targeted symptoms (e.g., anxiety, self-esteem, poor study skills, social relationships), only comprehensive programs involving parents, teachers, and the student and which address the full array of symptoms observed in the student are effective in influencing student engagement in work and subsequent achievement. Different treatment protocols are typically employed in the treatment of the different types of underachievement outlined above.

REBT Analysis of Academic Procrastination and Underachievement

Guiding my understanding from an REBT perspective of academic procrastination and underachievement in the early days was Bill Knaus who wrote an incredibly insightful chapter "Children and Low Frustration Tolerance" (LFT) in my edited book with Ellis, *Rational Emotive Approaches to the Problems of Childhood* (1983), and in the same book, Jim Bard and Harold Fisher who wrote a chapter "A Rational-Emotive Approach to Underachievement."

Knaus (1983, 2006) sounded the alarm alerting educators and mental health practitioners to be more aware of the pernicious effects of LFT on young people. LFT is frequently neglected in books of childhood psychopathology.

> Children exhibiting low frustration tolerance and weak frustration management skills may go through life inconsistently responding to challenge, having problems in organizing, demonstrating impatience, inhibiting competencies, giving up easily, procrastinating and agitating themselves about their frustration.

Here is Knaus' articulation of a child development and mental health principle that still rings true today: "The greater the deviation from age-expectant behaviour towards low frustration tolerance, the greater the child's vulnerability" (p. 139).

Knaus' explanation of frustration paints the picture of LFT:

> Frustrations erupt when we face an impediment. They exist when our wants, wishes, and desires get thwarted or interrupted. Frustration begins with a feeling of discomfort and ranges from imperceptible to powerful. If sufficiently intense, frustration can disrupt memory functions and result in disorganized thinking and behaving.... Most children are adaptable and improve their frustration management skills as they grow older. Others display a marked aversion for frustrating circumstances and either try to shelter themselves or try to

> expediently remove the source of tension. Chronically frustrated youngsters are often labelled troubled, behaviour problem, inhibited or *burnt-out*.

He discussed *frustration disturbances* indicating they are largely self-created. According to Knaus, some young children are afraid of almost any negative sensation. When frustrated, these sensation-sensitive youngsters try to squelch the feeling rather than confront the problem. LFT, a strong urge to throw off discomfort, occurs with little forethought and involves: (a) a young person viewing situations as frustrating when he or she cannot do what he or she wants to do; (b) a young person exaggerating the importance of avoiding discomfort and who predicts the situation will be *too* uncomfortable; (c) the prediction happens very quickly and the young person's response is inhibited or impulsive; (d) the young person generating an LFT language system including expletives, avoidance phrases ("I don't want to"), intolerance phrases ("I can't stand it"), distress phrases ("I am overwhelmed), self-downing phrases ("I'm a loser"), and extrapunitive phrases ("It's his/her fault"); (e) the LFT language system intensifies visceral sensations and cognitive disorganization leading to unpleasant feelings that can stimulate further LFT self-talk; and (f) the visceral language reciprocal process distracts from the child's ability to cope and consequently, and as a result of poor coping and poor school performance, feeds into the development and maintenance of self-concept disturbance.

In conclusion, one of Knaus' many contributions to REBT theory and applications with young people (e.g., the foremost being Rational Emotive Education, Knaus, 1974) is his linking of LFT disturbances with self-concept disturbances and how the interactivity of each results in self-defeating behaviors such as procrastination and underachievement.

Perhaps, the most erudite discussion of the causes of underachievement in children and adolescents in the REBT literature was provided by Bard and Fisher (1983). Bard and Fisher define underachievement as poor academic performance resulting mainly from students' beliefs that are false and incompatible with the educational system. These authors identified five different irrational and/or erroneous beliefs that give rise to the problem and associated family characteristics that contribute to the dysfunctional belief systems of children.

"Everything Will Turn Out OK Whether I Work or Not." This unrealistic belief leads students to "dodge the bullet" when it comes to completing work on time, and extended deadlines, negotiated homework assignments, and makeup exams are the rule rather than the exception. The delay and avoidance tactics of these non-hostile happy-go-lucky students are justified by their naive belief that they will be looked after.

According to Bard and Fisher (1983), this belief may result in some children from the experience of being overindulged and may originate in a parenting style where children are rewarded first rather than being rewarded after they have expended effort. "Instead of promising a reward after work has been completed, they deliver the reward first and then expect the task to be done thereafter" (p. 198). A key aspect of parents whose children cling onto these dysfunctional beliefs is that for different reasons, they do as much as they can to bail their children out of difficult situations so that things do not turn out badly for their children even if they have not done their work.

Three phases of therapy are advocated to change this dysfunctional belief. First, the establishment of a reliable school-home communication system where children's poor work performance and ensuing negative consequences are clear to all so that the child cannot pretend that things are improving. Second, serious work needs to occur so that the child can see through hard (and painful) evidence that the belief is very dubious and probably false. Here, parents and teachers alike refrain from bailing out the child with extending deadlines, and the full brunt of failing grades is experienced by the child in the form of logical consequences (repeating a class/grade level, being grounded, and not receiving the latest video game). It is important for the therapist or counselor to have concrete evidence on hand to dispute the erroneous belief. Third, once the child sees that his/her philosophy will not work, a process of reconstruction of belief is initiated where the child is supported in coming up with what they really want in life (e.g., success, better self-concept, fewer hassles), and which new beliefs will enable them to achieve their goals.

"Everything Should Be Entertaining and/or Enjoyable and There Should Be No Unpleasantness Whatsoever." According to Bard and Fisher, this belief may exist in combination with the first belief or can stand by itself. This belief which Ellis refers to as *low frustration tolerance* is one of the most difficult to modify. The performance of students who endorse this belief tends to be very uneven with strong achievement in evidence when the student is studying high interest material suited to his/her cognitive strengths and underachievement occurring when the student encounters someone or something that is not entertaining or enjoyable.

Features of parents associated with this belief include permissive and powerless parenting ("Children should not be frustrated," "It's too hard to be a strong parent"), inconsistent parenting (one parent setting very strict standards, the other who subverts the standards and subscribes to more permissive style), overindulgence and overprotectiveness (making excuses and covering up for the child), and lack of assertion in carrying through on standards.

"Talk" therapy for students with an *LFT* philosophy often proves problematic. The regime is to meet with parents and have them clarify and communicate expectations (home rules) and to develop their emotional resilience in order to enforce consequences firmly but kindly. The therapeutic alliance is crucial in working with these difficult customers. If children with *LFT* believe that their therapist is on their side and seek your approval, then it becomes possible to shift their *hedonic calculus* away from overfocusing on short-term pleasures and avoidance of short-term discomforts to one where they consider the long-term costs to their eventual success of avoiding short-term pain.

"To Do Well in School Would Betray Relationships I Have with My Friends." Bard and Fisher (1983) propose that students who endorse this belief have been turned off and alienated by the policies and practices of their parents and turned on by a set of principles that diverge from their family tradition. There are notable instances of students who due to lack of effort fail academically in order to meet a peer group standard that does not exist (other students in peer group do not mind if the students get good grades). An alternative or complimentary explanation is that some students who find themselves attracted to peers with nonconforming lifestyles as a way of rebelling against their parents and who believe they need the approval of their peers make conscious decisions not to do schoolwork despite an underlying desire to be successful in order to avoid rejection.

Oftentimes, parents of this group of underachievers tend to have conservative values with an emphasis on "proper" customs including hard work and self-discipline. These parents communicate to their children a rigid set of "shoulds" concerning behavior with little discussion or rationale provided. Children who endorse the values of what they perceive to be an anti-achieving peer group do so as a way of rejecting arbitrary, traditional values.

In therapy, it is important for the practitioner to establish him/herself as independent from representing the party line of the parents and as someone who is impartial and reasonable. This can be accomplished by questioning some of the more rigid standards for behavior held by the parents. Once credibility has been established, the therapist can discuss with the child the influence of the peer group. In particular, the therapist can employ *empirical disputation* to establish whether the peer group would, indeed, reject the young person who begins to demonstrate pro-academic work behavior. If the young person can see that the peer group will not reject him/her for doing schoolwork and if doing schoolwork does not represent in the young person's mind a victory for parents, then the young person may be motivated to start to engage in schoolwork. If the young person encounters evidence that s/he will be rejected by peers, then fruitful discussions can be held concerning whether peers in the group are really friends and whether an alternative peer group might be more suitable.

"It Is Demeaning, Dishonorable, and Destructive of My Personal Integrity to Cooperate with Authority in Any Way." Young people who endorse this anti-achieving philosophy tend to be very self-centered and reject in very hostile ways attempts of society to regulate their behavior. This type of anti-achiever may demonstrate their ability to resist authority and for others to do little about it through a variety of destructive and nonconforming behaviors.

According to Bard and Fisher, the common feature of parenting style associated with this belief system is powerless parenting that refers to parents' inability to enforce home rules or policies. The fact of parental helplessness serves to support the idea that "No one can make me do what I do not want to do." At a certain point in the power struggle between children and parents, the anti-achieving child makes up his/her mind that no matter how much his/her parents yell, scream, and abuse, they cannot control his/her behavior. Frequently, such abuse is combined with unloving parental behavior.

It is difficult to get these difficult customers to agree to therapy as it is perceived as authority. Sometimes, if the young person is in trouble with the law, the student can be induced by an agent of the juvenile court to see a practitioner. Therapy involves the therapist using the full range of his/her persuasive powers to convince the young person that there is personal benefit in cooperating with others and doing schoolwork in particular.

"Nothing I Do at School Will Ever Benefit Me." Oftentimes, students who hold this philosophy enter school expecting little and are surprised that academic achievement is expected of them. These students are often hard to identify because they may do poorly from the very beginning of school. These students often are not noticed as teachers tend to hold low expectations for their school performance.

Bard and Fisher observe that families from lower socioeconomic circumstances are more likely than other families to encourage this attitude toward school. High expectations for student achievement and the importance of student effort or not in evidence in parent-child communication.

In order for this belief to be challenged, it is vital that young people are provided with tangible benefits that the school offers to him/her and his/her family. That is, conventional psychotherapy will not be sufficient to change the mindset of young people coming out of home backgrounds where the value of education as cultural capital is not recognized.

In my 2004 book, *The REBT Therapist's Pocket Companion for Working with Children and Adolescents,* I spelled out the typical ABCs of work procrastination associated with educational underachievement in younger populations (Table 19.1).

One final important aspect in understanding, assessing, and treating procrastination-driven underachievement is the ways people who procrastinate use self-deception to justify their self-defeating, procrastinating behavior. Ellis and Knaus (1979) and Bernard (1991) discussed the following common rationalizations of procrastinators in general that are often in evidence in clinical work with young people who underachieve:

- "I'll do it later."
- "I'll do it later when I'm more in the mood."
- "I need to relax."
- "Make hay while the sun shines."
- "No one cares whether I do this or not."

Table 19.1 ABCs of procrastination

*A*ctivating events: tedious, time-consuming, frustrating classwork and homework
*B*eliefs: Inferences (conclusions, predictions): Difficult tasks are impossible. Everything will turn out okay whether I work or not. To do this work would be a violation of my personal integrity. Nothing I do at school will benefit me Absolutes (shoulds, oughts, musts, needs): I shouldn't have to do things I do not feel like doing. School should be comfortable and fun and never boring Evaluations: This work I have to do is the worst thing in the world. I can't stand having to do it. School is the worst place in the world for forcing me to do this work
*C*onsequences (emotions, behaviors): forgetfulness, daydreaming, delays in getting started and finishing schoolwork, anger when forced to do things s/he doesn't feel like doing, impatience, impulsiveness, avoidance tactics, laziness, diffuse anxiety

- "I only work best under pressure, so I'll wait until the last minute before beginning."
- "I achieved a good result before when I did my work at the last minute."

REBT for Combatting Educational Underachievement

Factors contributing to individual young person's underachievement are varied and idiosyncratic. As such, a toolbox approach is often best to employ as one needs to very flexible and creative in addressing the idiosyncratic needs of individual underachievers. What follows now are suggestions for working with different types of young people who underachieve.

Before initiating an intervention of any sort, an initial assessment needs to substantiate the concerns of the referring parent or teacher that the young person is underachieving. That is, be sure to gather your own data before determining the existence of underachievement. During this process, you will want to note whether the young person underachieves in all subjects or in select classes. If not available, you may want to administer an individual intelligence test to get an objective gauge of academic aptitude. An examination of previous and current report cards as well as standardized achievement tests is the surest way to determine the existence and extent of underachievement. You will also be on the lookout for discrepancies in achievement in classes that call for similar abilities. For example, if a young person is achieving well in history but not in English, the underachievement alarm bell rings. Similarly, the bell can ring if you notice a dramatic drop in achievement in one or more classes from one year to the next.

It is not easy to detect underachievement in some young people. The ones that coast along achieving acceptable standards as well as the creative students sometimes show their teachers little to indicate that they are more capable. This is especially the case of the non-achievement syndrome young person described above who covers up underachievement with multiple excuses.

Here are illustrations of the applications of REBT to the modification of procrastination in order to reduce the discrepancy between a young person's academic aptitude of achievement as measured by class grades and standardized tests of achievement.

Low Frustration Tolerance (Task Aversiveness) As discussed in this chapter, some underachieving students not only have not developed high frustration tolerance associated with work persistence and effort, they have extremely low levels of frustration tolerance and have limited abilities to delay gratification. As a consequence, they avoid many developmentally appropriate responsibilities in all areas of their lives including school. They put off doing tasks and chores because they are frustrating, boring, or hard and give up easily after starting to do something because they find it hard or boring. They spend a lot of time having fun and enjoying themselves especially when there is work to be done.

When seeking to challenge the beliefs of underachievers who avoid responsibility and display symptoms of distractibility and low frustration tolerance as well as who appear to lose interest in even the briefest of discussions, I recommend against pushing their limits of attention. I employ more interactive, engaging, and practical cognitive, emotive, and behavioral methods for challenging their irrational beliefs.

Here is an example of how a practitioner-in-training who followed this advice is designing an activity to dispute the irrational beliefs of a sixth-grade underachieving student, Winston. Winston appeared to have undiagnosed ADHD. In this excerpt, the practitioner describes her approach to tackling Winston's beliefs that science is boring and it should not be so.

In order to dispute Winston's belief (inference) that science is boring, I performed two simple science experiments with him. Both illustrated static electricity through the use of a balloon. In the first experiment, we used a balloon and water from a faucet. In the second one, we used a balloon and a piece of Fruit Loops cereal on a string. The static electricity on the balloon made the water from the faucet and the cereal move toward the balloon. I then asked Winston if he thought the experiments were cool or boring. In both instances, he replied he thought both experiments were cool. I then told him that we had just conducted a science experiment and, therefore, we had just disproved his previously stated belief that science was boring. I also stated that his favorite hobby, skateboarding, was just applied scientific concepts so he could not possibly really think science was all that boring.

Winston also was found to hold the belief that all class work *should* be fun and if it wasn't, he *shouldn't* have to do it. Once again, a disputing strategy was devised that did not involve simple didactic or Socratic "talk" therapy.

Winston stated that he found his class work boring and that he shouldn't have to do it so I thought it might be good to try something different with him. I told the school counselor, Mr. K., that I wanted to bring Winston into his office during the session and just ask him if his job was fun and exciting all the time. Of course, when we did this, Mr. K. stated that it wasn't and that even as a counsellor he had to do things at times that he did not want to do. He also reiterated to Winston that he gets a report card just like Winston does and his goal was to do well on his report card. I asked Mr. K. if the principal asked him to do something that he felt was boring and not fun, could he tell the principal he wasn't going to do it since it was boring and he shouldn't have to do it? Of course, he stated he could not. When we got back to the counseling room, I asked Winston why we went to see Mr. K., and he said to show that school is not fun all the time, but you have to do your work. I told him that no matter how old you are, you will always have to do things that are not considered fun, but in order to achieve your goals, you have to do them. I told him that I'm sure his mom has to do things every day at work that she thinks are not fun, but because she has to take care of him, she does them. I then focused attention on disputing Winston's irrational statement that he could not stand doing boring schoolwork. I asked him if he had completed boring work before to which he replied affirmatively. I asked him did his eyeballs fall out. Did he pass out or faint when he did boring work? He laughed and said "Yes". I reiterated to him that he was able to complete boring work just like he had done before. I also stated that if he had different, rational thoughts about boring schoolwork, he may have a different attitude about schoolwork. I reminded him about what Mr. K. stated about having to complete boring work even when he did not desire to do so. I reiterated that boring work is part of life, but we can do things to make boring work more tolerable. I asked Winston what are some of things we talked about in the past that can help us complete boring work? He stated we can do it right away. I then asked him, "What if the principal asked Mr. K. to do a report on all the kids in the school and he did not want to do it, what are some things he could do to make it easier to do? Winston's homework for this week was to talk to one adult and one classmate and ask them if they thought school/work is fun and exciting all the time and what they do when it is not.

I asked Winston if breaking the assignment into smaller parts might make a boring assignment easier to do? He responded that it would. In my example, I stated maybe if Mr. K. broke up the reports he was doing by doing the sixth-grade girls first, then the sixth-grade boys, then the seventh-grade girls, etc., then it may make doing a boring assignment easier to complete. I asked Winston if breaking an assignment into smaller pieces may make a boring assignment more manageable to him? He stated that it would. Prior to our meeting, I asked Winston's science teacher for a science textbook and the page they were working on. I then had Winston turn to the page in the science textbook that they were on and told him when his science teacher told him to read five pages, he could break it up into smaller parts and that may make it easier to do. I then had him read the first two paragraphs on the first page and told him to stop for 1 minute and then read the next two paragraphs. He was able to do this easily. He said doing work this way might help him to complete his work instead of thinking about having to do the whole assignment at once.

I then asked Winston that during our science experience, if we did not put the balloon near the water or near the piece of cereal, would we have seen the effects of static electricity? He stated no. I then told him that sometimes after we start an assignment, it becomes more interesting than we thought. I stressed that in order to find this out though, we have to be willing to participate in our class work. I did this because Winston's science teacher stated that he sometimes does not even try in class, even when they are doing group projects. I told Winston that even when we think things are boring, if we try to participate in them anyway, we may discover they are not so boring after all.

We then compiled the following list of strategies Winston can employ when undertaking boring class work: Do it right away, break the assignment into smaller parts, do the easiest parts first, and participate more often, even if the work is boring.

I asked Winston if the following rational thought would help him complete boring schoolwork: While I would prefer this schoolwork not be boring, I have to do

Table 19.2 Cognitive, emotive, and behavioral methods for working with underachieving students who display low frustration tolerance

1. Help to organize the students' home and school study environment by making a checklist of materials that need to be taken to school and home each day
2. Check the student's notebooks on a regular basis to ensure that papers and work are correctly organized
3. Incorporate the student's interests in the content of assignments
4. Design short-term and long-term assignments with success built in for the student
5. Help the student break down long-term assignments and projects into easier, short-term steps
6. Help the student schedule assignment steps on weekly and semester/term calendars
7. Be sure the student understands the directions before beginning his/her work
8. Communicate high, realistic expectations for work to the student
9. Do not accept poor work from the student
10. Help the student set daily and short-term goals
11. Discover the type of tangible reinforcements that the student prefers
12. Provide strong, immediate reinforcement for effort the student puts toward work that he/she finds hard or boring
13. Provide prompt and immediate feedback on the student's progress toward daily and short-term goals
14. Give the student a free day on Friday if he/she has worked hard during the week
15. Negotiate with the student and establish a behavioral contract
16. Provide positive reinforcements when the student edits or proofs his/her work
17. Structure appropriate competition in the classroom
18. Encourage the student to join an existing, work-oriented, peer study group
19. Encourage the student to join a study skills group

it to pass this class. He said he liked the statement we had come up in a previous session that stated: When it's done, I can have some fun. I asked him if repeating this statement helped him complete his work in the past, to which he replied that it had. We then role-played Winston first repeating this statement to himself then reading two paragraphs of his science textbook.

Tips for working with students who demonstrate LFT are presented in Table 19.2.

Anxiety (Fear of Failure) There are different forms of anxiety that result in procrastination and underachievement. There are the *perfectionists* who subconsciously sabotage their success by avoiding schoolwork. Their rationalization for lack of perfection can be found in their decision to procrastinate ("I wasn't perfect because I didn't try hard enough"). Suggestions for working with perfectionists are found in Table 19.3. Then there are the *approval seekers* who create so much anxiety for themselves worrying (catastrophizing) about what others (peers, parents, teachers) will think of them; they dodge the discomfort by putting their work out of their minds altogether until the last minute. Oftentimes, feelings of helplessness and depression accompany their anxiety.

What follows are two case studies that reveal how anxiety can work to stimulate procrastination and underachievement and the importance of identifying and challenging irrational beliefs that give rise to anxiety-related underachievement.

Table 19.3 Methods for working with underachieving students who are perfectionists

1. Help the student become more aware of his or her perfectionism and the negative costs of this habit of the mind on his/her emotions (e.g., anxiety) and behavior (e.g., avoidance of activities that he/she anticipates not doing perfectly)
2. Teach the student about famous people or role models who stumbled and fumbled their way to success. Point out that these individuals needed to make mistakes and take risks in order to succeed (e.g., Edison)
3. Have the student list the things he/she has always wanted to do but has been afraid of not doing perfectly. Have the student agree to try one of these activities
4. Encourage the student to identify his/her areas of weakness. Have them agree to try activities in these areas. When the student has attempted such an activity, point out that the student now has evidence that he/she can tolerate doing things imperfectly
5. Encourage the student to stop ruminating about his/her grades. Encourage him/her to get involved in activities unrelated to school
6. Teach the student that there is a continuum of achievement; achievement is not an all (perfection) or nothing (complete failure). Help the student set goals at a place on the achievement continuum where he/she does not have to be the best in order to learn something and have fun
7. Constantly challenge the student's perfectionist habit of the mind (i.e., "I must do everything perfectly all the time"). Encourage the student to give him/herself permission to make mistakes
8. Help the student to accept and become comfortable with doing things that are ambiguous and about which there is uncertainty about how to proceed
9. For long-term projects and assignments, require the student to hand in the beginning portion (e.g., introductory paragraph, outline) well in advance. Explain that what is important is that he/she does some work, not that the work be done perfectly
10. Help the student to see tasks as a series of parts that have to be completed one after another rather than as a whole chunk that must be completed perfectly
11. Teach the student the importance of having all materials necessary for completing that portion of the assignment done on hand
12. Encourage the student to get organized by laying out or outlining the different parts of the work that have to be done
13. Provide rewards for the student as he/she completes each portion of an assignment
14. Reward the student for attempting things and not doing them perfectly
15. Help the student enjoy the pleasure of doing new activities. Encourage him/her to reward him/herself for trying new things
16. Reduce competition in class
17. Establish classroom expectations that are not too rigid

Case Study. Consider the case of Michael, a bright but highly anxious and moderately depressed 12-year-old who was underachieving in most of his classes in grade 6.

In exploring issues surrounding his anxiety and depression, assessment data revealed that Michael was avoiding completing any schoolwork because when he did, his teacher would write red comments on his work which his mother would view at home. At those times, his mother would become extremely angry with Michael who interpreted such behavior in terms of his mother not loving him. You can see that Michael's irrational cognitions ("My mother doesn't love me. She'll never love me again. I need my mother's approval and recognition for everything that I do. I'm a loser") that were challenged using REBT did not exist in a psychological vacuum but rather occurred simultaneously with unhealthy emotions (high anxiety, depression) and self-defeating behavior (avoiding schoolwork).

The intervention involved sharing with Michael's mother how Michael interpreted her angry behavior and the impact of her behavior on Michael's underachievement. In a combined meeting, his mother disputed Michael's irrational belief assuring him that even when she gets angry with him, she still loves him very much. This turning point in the case leads to Michael restructuring his irrational beliefs with concurrent changes occurring in his emotions and behaviors. In addition, direct 1:1 interventions lead to an increase in his tolerance for the discomfort he felt when being criticized by his mother. A discussion with his teacher concerning the need to change the color of his ink when making comments on Michael's assignments and to provide more positive written feedback also helped allay his mother's anxieties about Michael and her own success or failure as a parent.

Case Study. I was also referred Darren, a 17-year-old, in the second to the last year of secondary school, who was underachieving in physics, a subject needed as a prerequisite for his proposed university program that he very much wanted to attend. Data gathering revealed, in fact, that Darren had turned in only two of 12 practicum assignments since the beginning of the year where he received an average grade.

It was clear to everyone that Darren had enough ability to perform at a reasonable level on these assignments, but to everyone's consternation and amazement given the physics assignment's importance to his future, he simply did not produce the goods. During the third session, Darren was asked about his physics teacher's perceptions concerning his lack of work completion. "Well," said Darren, "he probably thinks I'm lazy, but at least he doesn't think I'm stupid." It turned out that Darren had a high need for approval of his teacher and awfulized about his teacher thinking that he was unintelligent. Laziness was the excuse for lack of intelligence, and this Darren could live with. Once again, irrational beliefs, unhealthy emotions (anxiety), and self-defeating behavior (lack of work completion), a social and emotional disability, were conspiring together to produce underachievement.

The REBT intervention involved disputing his need for approval from his teacher and helping him reformulate his need into a preference or desire along with a series of anti-awfulizing exercises including the use of the catastrophe scale to help Darren not blow disapproval out of proportion. Darren was also given behavioral homework assignments to risk the displeasure of his teacher by asking his teacher for a plan to make up the missing assignments as well as emotive change skills of relaxation and rational emotive imagery to help lessen his physiological arousal. These cognitive behavioral elements together helped to dramatically lessen and for all intents and purposes eliminate anxiety as a social and emotional disability. Darren handed in enough of his missing assignments to achieve a credible grade at the end of the year.

Non-achievement Syndrome (Fear of Growing Up) This type of underachiever is generally an adolescent who is afraid to grow up. I have found that this type of young person frequently holds irrational beliefs involving the need for comfort which had better be disputed as being counterproductive to most young people's expressed desire to be successful established early on in the therapeutic sequence. Cognitive, emotive, and behavioral methods for working with this type of underachiever can be found in Table 19.4.

Anger/Chronic Misbehavior This social and emotional blocker leading to underachievement involves young people breaking important home and school rules including destroying property and hurting others. They act defiantly toward

Table 19.4 Methods for working with underachieving students who display the non-achievement syndrome

1. Do not become discouraged when the student does not follow through with what he/she promised to do
2. Do not provide the student with solutions for solving problems. Give the problem-solving responsibility to the student
3. Hold a private conference with the student
4. Make an agreement with the student concerning the goal of getting better grades
5. Offer the student assistance in achieving the goal of doing better in school
6. Obtain from the student's other teachers information about the specific work requirements, which assignments the student has completed and which the student has not completed. Record this information without evaluative comments and discuss it with the student privately. Record the specific problems and excuses that the student offers as his/her reasons for each incomplete assignment
7. Select a class in which the student has an incomplete assignment and the excuse that he/she uses to explain his/her failure to finish it. Record the exact details of the problem that hinders the student's achievement of better grades, including how often the problem has occurred in the past
8. Inform the student of the consequences that will ensue if the problem continues. Confirm whether the student still has the goal of getting better grades
9. Ask the student to generate different solutions to the problem that is blocking his/her path to better grades. Discuss things that could interfere with each solution, and have the student come up with countermeasures for these interferences. Give the student the responsibility for thinking through the steps necessary to solve the problem
10. Ask the student what he/she proposes to do now in light of the discussion about specific solutions. Once the student selects a solution, discuss the specifics of when, how, and how long the student will implement it
11. Do not expect the student to have done everything in the proposed solution. Continue the above process of confrontation and have the student identify solutions and make plans to implement them until progress is evident
12. As the student takes on more responsibility, use less confrontation and more supportive gestures. Help the student answer questions about him/herself and the future

Adapted from Mandel, Marcus, and Mandel (1992)

people in authority and may get very angry when faced with people blocking them from getting what they want. Irrational beliefs typically held by these sorts of underachieving students include *other-downing* ("People should always treat me fairly and considerately in the way I treat them, and when they behave poorly or look or act differently from me, I can't stand it and I believe they are losers and totally bad") combined with *cognitive impulsivity* defined by the absence of reflection about different ways to handle interpersonal conflict, the consequences of different courses of action, and how someone else will feel after you have chosen to act in a certain way.

The preferred treatment approach for young people of any age who display extreme anger and chronic misbehavior is to work with their parents and teachers to set up contingency arrangements whereby the young person becomes explicitly aware of extreme penalties associated with rule breaking, especially harmful behavior to others or the environment as well as the beneficial effects of compliant behavior. When working with young people whose underachievement is due to anger management issues, direct 1:1 intervention that addresses their irrational beliefs and employs cognitive, emotive, and behavioral strategies is recommended.

Case Study. What follows is a running commentary provided by a practitioner-in-training who successfully disputed the irrational beliefs of a 14-year-old boy, Aaron, who was refusing to work in science due to problems he was having with his teacher. Aaron would become furious with his teacher when he perceived he was being unfairly picked in and refused to do his work. Here, the practitioner focuses on the disputing of key irrational beliefs of Aaron, but rather than confronting the adolescent with a forceful argument, humor was used to make the point and to avoid putting the adolescent on the defensive.

In order to dispute Aaron's irrational thoughts regarding Ms. H., I stressed the concept of human fallibility by disputing Aaron's global rating of others (Ms. H.). I used both logical and semantic disputation to dispute irrational thoughts regarding Ms. H. I presented a Happening → Thinking → Feeling → Behaving → Consequences chart, on which I had summarized some of Aaron's irrational thoughts he had communicated to me regarding Ms. H. His thoughts were as follows: "Ms. H. is unfair so I should not have to follow class rules or do class work." He also clearly stated that he cannot stand it when Ms. H. acts unfairly and that Ms. H. was a total bitch. Aaron confirmed that these statements accurately captured his thoughts about Ms. H. I then discussed with Aaron the difference between irrational and rational thoughts. I then restated the following irrational thought with Aaron to see if he agreed with it: "My teacher acts unfairly towards me all the time. He should act fairly all the time in order for me to do my work and follow rules." Aaron stated he agreed with this statement as well. I then discussed with him whether this statement was true, logical, or helpful and if not maybe we needed to change it. Aaron stated that Ms. H. treats him unfairly all the time. I then used semantic disputation to correct his incorrect inference. I stated if that were true then the minute he hit the door, she would begin to accuse him of doing things he did not do. I began to imitate how

Ms. H. would have to behave if she acted that way all the time. Aaron thought this was funny. I then asked Aaron if this was how Ms. H. acted all the time, to which he laughed and said "yes." I then disputed this empirically by saying if she treated him this way all the time, she would not have time to teach. He then acknowledged that she did not act like that all the time but sometimes. I then asked Aaron when he first learned a new skateboarding trick, did he do it perfectly the first time? He responded negatively to this. I then drew the pie chart so we could list both Ms. H.'s positive and negative characteristics (I only put four spaces in case Aaron could not come up with any positive comments about Ms. H.). I told Aaron that Ms. H. always spoke very highly of him when I spoke to her and that was a positive characteristic. I then stated that the one negative characteristic I could state about Ms. H. was that as a new teacher who is still learning, she makes mistakes along the way like we all do when we are learning something new. I then asked him if he got a brand new skateboard and noticed that it had a small scratch on the wheel, would he throw it in the trash? He responded negatively to this. I then stated that is how we are as human beings. We all have our little scratches, but we still have value as human beings. I then asked him to give me a positive characteristic about Ms. H., and to my surprise, he was able to produce one fairly easily. We then came up with the following rational statement: Ms. H. is a new teacher, and while I would prefer she not act unfairly, that's sometimes how teachers act. I then still need to pass this class so I can deal with it. I asked Aaron if he repeated this to himself when he felt Ms. H. was being unfair, would it at least allow him to decrease his anger so he would be able to do his work? He stated that he would still be angry but thinking this thought might help him reduce his anger.

Developing Social-Emotional Strengths to Overcome Procrastination and Underachievement

In addressing the needs of young people who have academic problems including those who underachieve, cognizance needs to be placed not only on eradicating psychosocial barriers to learning (e.g., LFT, anxiety, anger), but also a strength-building productive focus is needed in order to develop the social and emotional skills including their rational beliefs of students who underachieve (e.g., Ozer, Demir, & Ferrari, 2013). REBT clearly illuminates the irrational beliefs and concomitant unhealthy emotions and unhelpful behaviors that need to be identified, challenged, and changed in order to help remove the barriers to learning. But as Albert Ellis has said, there is also the need to develop rational beliefs and attendant positive emotion and behaviors that support motivation and school success. Young people can underachieve as a result of having underdeveloped social and emotional capabilities due to a combination of cultural, parenting, and biological-temperament factors. They may not present with any psychosocial or mental health problems. These young people, as well as the young people with social and emotional blockers described in the previous section, will greatly profit from a variety of social and emotional learning experiences designed to accelerate their social and emotional development. These social and emotional skills include academic confidence, work persistence, work organization, and teamwork skills.

As part of my social-emotional learning (SEL) program, You Can Do It! Education, I founded over 20 years ago, my colleagues and I have developed over the years a number of resources (classroom curricula) that REBT/CBT and other school practitioners including teachers, mentors, and student welfare officers are using to teach these social and emotional skills to groups and individual students. Chief among these is the online, digital *NEW Program Achieve (years 1–6; years 7–12). A social-emotional learning curriculum* (https://youcandoiteducation.com.au/).

The psychoeducational principles to teach these social and emotional skills are relatively straight forward.

1. Assess young person's academic confidence, work persistence, work organization, and teamwork skills and identify those that need further development. This can be accomplished through the use of available surveys.
2. Set goal for improvement working on one SEL at a time. Select one that is easiest to improve first.
3. Help young person identify and rip up any rationalizations s/he may hold that block motivation to apply social and emotional skills (keys for success). Examples of these rationalizations include:

    - I'll do it later.
    - I will only get a low mark so what's the point in trying.
    - I'm too tired.
    - No one else is doing it. Why should I?
    - I need to relax.
    - I don't know how to do this.

4. Clearly define the SEL for the young person, provide examples, and review/discuss rational beliefs that help the young person develop the area.
5. Discuss the "ins and outs" of using the targeted SEL in subjects/classes where young person is underachieving.
6. Use cognitive, emotive, and behavioral activities to deepen young person's knowledge and skill of the targeted SEL.
7. Complete a weekly goal setting homework form where the young person agrees to practice two or three examples of behavior that represent examples of the targeted SEL (see Table 19.5).
8. Review progress at the beginning of next session in achieving goals. Provide the young person with feedback for using the targeted key (e.g., "You really showed persistence this week") as well as feedback for use of rational beliefs and self-talk (e.g., "You really seem to be getting the idea that success comes through effort. Giving effort is becoming part of your approach to schoolwork").

Table 19.5 Example of a weekly, goal-setting homework form

Name of Student Linda Suarez Date March 3

Name of Counsellor Laura Thompson

1. Which of the Foundations ~~do you want~~ to learn or practice (circle one)?

   confidence persistence (organization) getting along emotional resilience

2. My goal this week is (be specific):

   - write down complete details of homework assignments
   - remember to bring all books I need for class

3. List obstacles that might stop you from achieving your goal and how you will deal with them.

   - rushing
   - lazy

4. Write down any positive self-talk that will help you achieve your goal.

   "Being organized feels good!"

5. Date by which you want to achieve goal March 10

6. Your Signature Linda Suarez

   Signature of Mentor *Laura Thompson*

Result a week later:

Did you achieve your goal? ☒ yes ☐ no ☐ almost

Talk about what you learned, including the positives that happened when you achieved the goal or the negatives that occurred by not achieving your goal.

Final Comment: Opportunity Knocks

My sense is that while achievement is front and center of schools' radar screens (and missions), underachievement as a construct and problem is not recognized. Over the past decade, research into underachievement and its causes has diminished. The same observation holds for the awareness and study of academic procrastination; educators as well as student service personnel are as literate in understanding and remediating the causes of procrastination and underachievement. There is little question that REBT is a strong platform for advancing literacy of professionals into the causes and cures of the widespread challenge of combatting academic procrastination and its consequence of underachievement.

Test Yourself

1. There are a number of factors that have historically been linked to academic underachievement. How might a clinician consider these factors in development of a case formulation and for treatment planning?
2. What are some of the core beliefs that students may have that interfere with their academic effort and performance?
3. Consider how you would modify your educational and clinical work dependent on the type of cognitive, behavioral, and affective state (LFT, perfectionist, non-achievement syndrome) that the youngster presents with.

References

Alexander, E. S., & Onwuegbuzie, A. J. (2007). Academic procrastination and the role of hope as a coping strategy. *Personality and Individual Differences, 42*, 1301–1310.

Banerjee, P. A. (2016). A systematic review of factors linked to poor academic performance of disadvantaged students in science and maths in schools. *Journal of Cogent Education, 3*(1), 1–17.

Bandura, A. (1997). *Self-efficacy: The exercise of control*. New York: W.H. Freeman.

Bard, J., & Fisher, H. R. (1983). A rational emotive approach to academic underachievement. In A. Ellis & M. E. Bernard (Eds.), *Rational-emotive approaches to the problems of childhood*. New York: Plenum Press.

Benson, P. L. (2007). Developmental assets: An overview of theory, research, and practice. In R. K. Silbereisen & R. M. Lerner (Eds.), *Approaches to positive youth development* (pp. 33–58). Thousand Oaks, CA: Sage.

Bernard, M. E. (1991). *Procrastinate later! How to motivate yourself to do it now*. Melbourne, Australia: Information Australia.

Bernard, M. E. (2006). Working with the educational underachiever: A social and emotional developmental approach. In A. Ellis & M. E. Bernard (Eds.), *Rational Emotive Behavioral Approaches to Childhood Disorders* (pp. 310–366). New York: Springer.

Brophy, J. (1996). *Teaching problem students*. New York: Guilford Press.

Chen, B.-B. (2017). Parent–adolescent attachment and academic adjustment: The mediating role of self-worth. *Journal of Child and Family Studies, 26*, 2070–2076.

Chen, B.-B., & Chang, L. (2016). Procrastination as a fast life history strategy. *Evolutionary Psychology, 14*, 1–5.

Christens, B. D., & Peterson, N. A. (2011). The role of empowerment in youth development: A study of sociopolitical control as mediator of ecological systems' influence on developmental outcomes. *Journal of Youth and Adolescence, 41*, 623–635.

Darling, N. (2005). Participation in extracurricular activities and adolescent adjustment: Cross-sectional and longitudinal findings. *Journal of Youth and Adolescence, 34*, 493–505.

Dweck, C. S. (2006, 2016). *Mindset: The new psychology of success*. New York: Ballantine Books.

Ellis, A., & Knaus, W. J. (1979). *Overcoming procrastination*. New York: New American Library.
Harrington, N. (2005). It's too difficult! Frustration intolerance beliefs and procrastination. *Personality and Individual Differences, 39*, 873–883.
Klassen, R. M., & Kuzucu, E. (2009). Academic procrastination and motivation of adolescents in Turkey. *Educational Psychology, 29*, 69–81.
Knaus, W. J. (1974). *Rational emotive education. A manual for elementary school teachers*. New York: Albert Ellis Institute.
Knaus, W. J. (1983). Children and low frustration tolerance. In A. Ellis & M. E. Bernard (Eds.), *Rational-emotive approaches to the problems of childhood*. New York: Plenum Press.
Knaus, W. J. (2006). Frustration tolerance training for children. In A. Ellis & M. E. Bernard (Eds.), *Rational emotive behavioral approaches to childhood disorders*. New York: Springer Science +Business Media.
Mandel, H., Marcus, S. I., & Mandel, D. (1992). *Helping the non-achievement syndrome student: A clinical training manual*. Toronto, ON: Institute on Achievement and Motivation Publication, York University.
Meese, J., & Agger, C. (2018). *Achievement motivation in education*. Oxford, UK: Oxford Research Encyclopedias.
Ozer, B. U., Demir, A., & Ferrari, J. R. (2013). Reducing academic procrastination through a group treatment program: A pilot study. *Journal of Rational-Emotive and Cognitive-Behavior Therapy, 31*, 127–135.
Rothblum, E. D., Solomon, L. J., & Murakami, J. (1986). Affective, cognitive and behavioural differences between low and high procrastinators. *Journal of Counselling Psychology, 33*, 388–394.
Schaefer, C., & Millman, H.L. (1981). *How to help children with common problems*. New York: Plume.
Solomon, L. J., & Rothblum, E. D. (1984). Academic procrastination: Frequency and cognitive-behavioural correlated. *Journal of Counselling Psychology, 31*, 503–509.
Topcu, S., & Leana-Tascılar. (2018). The role of motivation and self-esteem in the academic achievement of Turkish gifted students. *Gifted Education International, 34*, 3–18.
White, S., Graham, L. J., & Blass, S. (2018). Why do we know so little about the factors associated with gifted underachievement? A systematic literature review. *Educational Research Review, 24*, 55–66.
Zimmerman, B. J., & Schunk, D. H. (2001). *Self-regulated learning and academic achievement: Theoretical perspectives* (2nd ed.). Mahwah, NJ: Erlbaum.

Part III
Applications

Chapter 20
Rational Emotive Education as Social–Emotional Learning

Ann Vernon and Michael Bernard

The recent report by the "From a Nation at Risk to a Nation of Hope" (2019) prepared by the Aspen Institute, National Commission on Social, Emotional, and Academic Development, has, again, confirmed what most now regard not as a fad, but as common sense; namely:

> …Children require a broad array of skills, attitudes, character traits, and values to succeed in school, careers, and life. They require skills such as paying attention, setting goals, collaboration, and planning for the future. They require attitudes such as internal motivation, perseverance, and a sense of purpose. They require values such as responsibility, honesty, and integrity. They require the abilities to think critically, consider diverse views, and problem solve. And these social, emotional, and academic capacities are increasingly demanded in the American workplace, which puts a premium on the ability to work in diverse teams, grapple with difficult problems, and adjust to rapid change.

More than ever before, there is a need in schools today for evidence-based, comprehensive, developmentally based school-wide programs designed to promote social and emotional competence as well as to prevent and/or reduce behavior and emotional problems including educational under-achievement. Fortunately, there now exists an increasing number of "promising" school-based programs being implemented that focus on the social and emotional learning of children and adolescents that are designed to equip young people with an array of social and emotional capabilities seen as intrinsic to academic success, emotional well-being, and positive relationships and which lead to reductions in existing problems.

A. Vernon (✉)
University of Northern Iowa, Tucson, AZ, USA

M. Bernard
Melbourne Graduate School of Education, University of Melbourne, Melbourne, VIC, Australia
e-mail: m.bernard@unimelb.edu.au

M. Bernard, M. D. Terjesen (eds.), *Rational-Emotive and Cognitive-Behavioral Approaches to Child and Adolescent Mental Health: Theory, Practice, Research, Applications*, https://doi.org/10.1007/978-3-030-53901-6_20

Successful school-based social and emotional learning programs share common characteristics. Good practice has teachers with the support of psychologists and counselors teaching social and emotional skills in formal lessons as an integrated component of the curriculum. However, it is recognized that in order for students to generalize these skills, social and emotional learning experiences need to be present throughout the school day including during academic instruction and throughout the school year. Other characteristics of social emotional education programs include (a) are of longer duration, (b) synthesize a number of successful approaches, (c) incorporate a developmental model, (d) provide greater focus on the role of emotions and emotional development, (e) provide increased emphasis on generalization techniques, (f) provide ongoing training and support for implementation, and (g) utilize multiple measures and follow-ups for assessing program effectiveness.

Albert Ellis pioneered the application of rational emotive behavior therapy (REBT) to the treatment of children and adolescents in the mid-1950s, and from its inception, REBT has been psycho-educational in nature. A long-time proponent of the use of REBT in schools, Ellis has always stressed the importance of a prevention curriculum designed to help young people help themselves by learning positive mental health concepts (Ellis, 1971, 1972). From 1971 to 1975, Ellis and his staff taught rational thinking as a preventive mental health program in addition to regular subjects at The Living School, a small private grade school housed in the Institute for Advanced Study in Rational Psychotherapy (now called the Albert Ellis Institute). The school prospered for several years, during which time the staff discovered that not only therapists but teachers could teach REBT principles in the classroom to improve children's emotional well-being.

Based on the effective thinking, feeling, and behaving strategies that were taught at The Living School, Knaus (1974) developed a curriculum that would educate children in the ABC's of REBT. Bedford (1974) wrote a short story emphasizing the connection between thinking, feeling, and behaving. Since then, REE-derived programs include Vernon's (1989a, 1989b) *Thinking, Feeling, Behaving* (Vernon, 1989a, 1989b, 1998c, 2006a, 2006b), *The Passport Program* (Vernon, 1998a, 1998b), and Bernard's You Can Do It! Education (youcandoiteducation.com.au) have been developed that teach children to develop critical thinking skills, differentiate between facts and assumptions, distinguish between thoughts and feelings, link thoughts and feelings, identify what leads to emotional upset, distinguish between rational and irrational beliefs, and learn to challenge irrational beliefs.

REBT in the form of its educational derivative rational emotive education (REE) has a long-standing presence in the field of school-based mental health programs and has always been used as a form of prevention, promotion, and intervention focused on young people and their problems (e.g., Knaus, 1974). Its focus has been on the elimination of the irrational beliefs of children and adolescents associated with emotional, behavioral, and achievement problems and the promotion of rational beliefs associated with social, emotional, and work competence. The research across four decades indicates that when REBT is used in schools with both clinical and non-clinical populations, it has a positive effect (e.g., DiGiuseppe, Miller, & Trexler, 1979; Gonzalez et al., 2004; Hajzler & Bernard, 1991; Mahfar, Noah, & Senin, 2019; Popa & Bochis, 2012; Steins & Haep, 2015).

As prevention, REE programs are employed in classrooms to help prevent the development of irrational beliefs and associated unhealthy emotions and behaviors. They help children of all ages recognize the self-defeating effects of irrational beliefs and the beneficial outcomes of rational beliefs. As well, when young people are equipped with emotional problem-solving skills including rational self-statements and disputing skills, they are able to diffuse potential problem situations that potentially can lead to more harmful outcomes.

As promotion, REBT-based programs are, again, being used with groups of young people with an eye to the strengthening of rational beliefs and self-management skills that help young people make the very most of their innate potential by helping them minimize unhealthy emotions, irrational beliefs, and to maximize their effort and well-being.

As intervention, REBT has a long track record and supportive research (e.g., Hajzler & Bernard, 1991) as a form of 1:1 and group interventions for young people with psychosocial and mental health problems (anxiety, low self-esteem, behavior problems). Apparently, REBT is being used more frequently with young people with internalizing than externalizing problems (Terjesen et al., 1999). When working with children who manifest internal or externalizing disorders, REBT practitioners recognize the need for multisystemic solutions encompassing the child's full ecology.

Rational-emotive education (REE) is uniquely suited for a prevention curriculum for several reasons: (a) the principles can be readily transferred into lessons that teach children the core REBT concepts; (b) it is a comprehensive approach, in that by identifying irrational beliefs that perpetuate the problem, children gain a better understanding of how to change their negative feelings and self-defeating behaviors; (c) a wide variety of cognitive behavioral methods are employed in delivering the lessons; (d) the concepts can be adapted to different age levels, ethnicities, and intelligence levels; (e) the principles emphasize helping children "get better" not just "feel better"; (f) it is a skills-oriented approach that equips children with cognitive, emotive, and behavioral strategies to apply to problems of daily living, both in the present and future.

Rational-emotive education (REE) is based on the assumption that it is possible and desirable to teach children how to help themselves cope with life more effectively. Specifically, the importance of preventing emotional disturbances by providing children with "tools" with which to cope is the basis of rational-emotive education. The core principles of REBT—that emotional problems result from faulty thinking about events rather than from the event itself and that these faulty, irrational thoughts can be disputed, resulting in more moderate, healthy feelings and productive behaviors—forms the basis of an REE program, along with the A-B-C-D-E-F paradigm and an understanding of the core irrational beliefs: self-downing, demanding, and frustration intolerance.

Unlike other emotional education programs, REE empowers recipients to take charge of their lives, first by understanding the connection between what they think, feel, and do, and then by learning that while they may not be able to change other people or the events in their lives, they can exercise control over themselves. Given the realities that many young people have to contend with, this pragmatic approach enables them to make changes that are within their control, which at the same time, will enhance the quality of their lives.

In the following sections, several ways of implementing REE will be described, followed by examples of REE lessons and further applications.

Implementing REE

There are four basic approaches to implementing an REE program: the informal approach (teachable moment), structured emotional education lessons, learning centers, and integration into the curriculum. Each has its merits. Optimally, all four approaches will be used, in addition to REBT concepts being practiced and modeled in the environment.

The Informal Approach

The basic assumption of this approach is that teachers and parents will seize "teachable moments" to introduce and reinforce rational thinking concepts. There are numerous ways in which this can be done: with the entire class, individually, or with small groups of children.

As an example, suppose that a teacher returns a test and it is obvious that almost all the children are upset with their low scores. At this point, the teacher could introduce rational thinking in the classroom setting by asking children what the score says about them: does it make them a better or worse person? Does this bad score mean that they will always do poorly on exams? Just because they did not do well on this test, does it necessarily mean they will not do well in the course? Is getting a bad score the worst possible thing that could ever happen to them? Raising disputations of this sort helps children avoid self-downing, awfulizing, and overgeneralizing. A next step could be to ask them what they could have done, if anything, to improve their score, which could result in appropriate goal setting for the next exam.

Similarly, this approach can be used with an individual. Selina, a fourth grader, frequently got upset when learning something new. She would throw down her pencil and tear up her paper and simply not finish the task. When the teacher approached her and asked her to explain what was wrong, Selina replied, "It's too hard—I'll never learn this." The teacher introduced some disputations: had she ever tried to learn anything before and succeeded? Just because something was hard, did it mean she should give up? Although Selina responded appropriately to these questions, she remained frustrated, so the teacher drew two talking heads. On the first one, she listed Selina's irrational beliefs: "This is too hard—I'll never learn this." On the second one, she helped Selina identify rational self-talk, such as "This is hard, but I just have to work harder to learn it; I don't like learning hard things, but I can stand it if I do a little at a time." The teacher instructed Selina to keep this visual inside her desk to use as a reminder when she felt frustrated and wanted to give up. As a homework assignment, she asked Selina to read *The Little Engine That Could* (Piper, 1986), a book that described how a little train chanted "I think I can, I think I can" as he tried to make it up a mountain and think about how this story applied to her situation.

The informal approach can also be used with small groups. For instance, as the teacher was walking through the hall, he noticed a group of young adolescents arguing with each other. As he approached the group, he heard all sorts of accusations being directed at one individual: "You're a horrible, selfish friend...you stole Katinka's boyfriend and we will never forgive you for it. We know you are the one who started all the rumors about us, and we are going to turn all the other girls against you so that no one in this class will ever speak to you again." The teacher wanted to diffuse the situation, so he pulled the group into an empty classroom and asked them to tell him more about the situation. As they talked, he began to challenge some of their assumptions: where was the evidence that this girl had started all the rumors? Did they know for a fact that she "stole" another's boyfriend? Did they have so much power that they could turn *everyone* against her? Forever is a long, long time—do they really believe that they will *never* speak to her again, or is it possible that they will eventually get over being so upset? These disputations seemed to help de-escalate their emotions and put the problem in better perspective, and eventually they reached a point where they could communicate more effectively about how they felt and listen to the other side of the story.

In each of these situations, if the teacher had not intervened, the problems would have compounded themselves and interfered with children's ability to concentrate in school. Furthermore, until the underlying beliefs are addressed, the problems would have perpetuated themselves. Nipping problems in the bud through this informal approach helps prevent this from occurring.

To use this approach, it is necessary to have a thorough understanding of the basic REBT principles and the disputation process. In addition, it is important to realize that while it might be easier to tell children how to feel or what to do to solve a problem, it is advisable that they be allowed to work things out for themselves, with proper guidance. Once they are able to dispute their irrational beliefs that will result in more moderate, healthy feelings, they are in a better position to look at alternatives and develop a plan to resolve the problem.

Structured REE Lessons

The second approach, the most structured of all, is a series of emotional education lessons that can be presented to a small group or to a total class of children. In contrast to subject-matter lessons, these lessons are typically not graded because the emphasis is on personal application of concepts. However, in this age of accountability, teachers can develop effective ways to measure whether or not the concepts have been attained, since skill acquisition is also an inherent part of the lessons.

Rational-emotive education lessons are typically experiential, with a good deal of student involvement and group interaction, which increases the likelihood that children will be engaged in the activity. Understandings are deduced from the use of such methods as simulations, games, role-playing, art activities, bibliotherapy, guided discussions, and music and writing activities. In addition, time is spent debriefing the lesson so that, through guided questions, children master the content.

REE Concepts

REE lessons are developed around the following basic concepts: self-acceptance, feelings, beliefs, and disputing beliefs (Vernon, 2004).

1. *Self-acceptance.* REE emphasizes the importance of developing a realistic self-concept, including accepting the notion of personal weaknesses as well as strengths. Learning that who a person is should not be equated with what he or she does is also a key component, as well as understanding that people are fallible human beings who make mistakes and must accept the fact that they are not perfect.
2. *Feelings.* A critical component of REE lessons is learning the connection between thoughts, feelings, and behaviors. Developing a feeling vocabulary, learning to deal with emotional overreactions, assessing the intensity of feelings, and distinguishing between healthy and unhealthy ways to express feelings are also important. Understanding that feelings can change, that the same event can result in different feelings depending on how the event is perceived, and that it is natural to have feelings are significant concepts.
3. *Beliefs.* A key component of REE is that there are two types of beliefs, rational and irrational. Irrational beliefs result in negative feelings that can lead to self-defeating behaviors. These irrational beliefs manifest themselves in the form of a basic "must" that falls into three main categories: self-demandingness, other-demandingness, and world-demandingness (Ellis, 1994). Self-demandingness refers to the idea that you must always perform well and win others' approval; and if you do not, you are incompetent, unworthy, and deserve to suffer. Other-demandingness implies that people with whom you associate must always treat you kindly, considerately, and fairly; and if they do not, they are unworthy, bad, rotten, and deserve to be punished. World-demandingness means that the conditions in which you live must be enjoyable, hassle-free, safe, and favorable; and if they are not, it is awful and horrible and unbearable. Rational beliefs are self-enhancing and result in moderate feelings that help people achieve their goals; they are realistic preferences that typically result in constructive behaviors (Dryden, 1999). The goal of the disputation process is to replace irrational beliefs with rational beliefs.
4. *Facts* vs. *Assumptions.* It is also important that children understand the difference between facts and assumptions. As concrete thinkers, children and many adolescents readily misconstrue events by failing to distinguish between a fact (she didn't sit by me) from assumptions (she's mad at me and doesn't want to be my friend). Because of their impulsive nature, it is all too common for young people to act on their assumptions and create more problems when others react to their overreaction.

5. *Disputing Beliefs.* The concept of disputing, a cornerstone of this theory, entails replacing irrational beliefs with rational beliefs in order to achieve a more sensible way of thinking, which in turn results in more moderate emotions and more self-enhancing behavior. The disputational process can take several forms: functional disputes, or questioning the practicality of the irrational beliefs (Vernon, 2004; Ellis & MacClaren, 1998); the Socratic approach, in which questioning gives clients insight into the irrationality of their thinking (Ellis & MacClaren, 1998); the didactic approach, where the differences between rational and irrational beliefs are explained (Ellis & MacClaren, 1998); empirical disputes, which help people evaluate the factual aspects of their beliefs; logical disputes, which enables people to see how illogical it is to escalate desires into demands and use of exaggeration or humor. These types of disputes can be taught directly to children in REE lessons or the concepts can be incorporated into lessons that teach children to apply the various types of disputations.

These basic concepts form the essence of the REE lessons, but it is critical that they be presented in accordance with the developmental level of the child. For example, it is appropriate to use the terms *rational* and *irrational* with older adolescents, but with younger children, the terms *sensible* and *insensible* would be easier for them to grasp. Likewise, younger children will not understand the concept of disputing unless it is presented in a very concrete manner, such as with the use of puppets in a dialogue, with one puppet being insensible and the other being sensible. Similarly, whereas adolescents can more readily understand the how irrational beliefs result in negative feelings and unproductive behaviors, younger children need to have these concepts presented in a very concrete method, such as making a paper chain to visually illustrate how insensible thoughts create negative feelings which result in poor behavioral choices.

It is also important to present the concepts in a sequential manner to assure greater mastery of the concepts. It is best to introduce these concepts in units. For example, the first unit might be self-acceptance, and all concepts pertaining to that would be introduced, followed by those relating to beliefs, and so forth. It is also advisable to have a sequential progression of lessons within the specific units so that concepts can be introduced and expanded on. For example, in a feelings unit, the distinction between healthy and unhealthy feelings precedes the more difficult concept that feelings come from thoughts. Likewise, when introducing beliefs, a first level would be to distinguish facts from beliefs before moving on to the notion of rational and irrational beliefs. In addition, the lessons should follow a similar structure, as subsequently described.

REE Lesson Plan Format

Having a well-developed lesson is essential, as is the notion of presenting the activities in developmentally appropriate formats to help children master the concepts. For example, rather than explain in a short lecture the difference between facts and assumptions, it is much more effective to engage students in identifying facts and assumptions in a game format similar to tic-tac-toe (Vernon, 1980) or to learn that everyone makes mistakes by attempting to juggle tennis balls (Vernon, 1989a). As previously mentioned, a wide variety of methods can be incorporated into REE lessons: games, simulations, role-playing, puppetry, music and art activities, writing and worksheet activities, drama, experiments, bibliotherapy, and rational-emotive imagery, for example (Bernard, 2001, 2018; Vernon, 1980, 1989b, 1998a, 1998b, 1998c).

A lesson should contain the following:

1. *Learning objectives.* It is important to have one or two learning objectives for each lesson. For example, in a unit on beliefs for second graders, a specific objective would be to identify the negative effects of demanding. For a sixth grader, a specific objective would be to identify the connection between thoughts and actions. The objectives should be stated in behavioral terms so that they can be measured and they should be developmentally appropriate for the age level. It is preferable, in delivering a sequential curriculum that there be separate objectives for each grade level.
2. *Stimulus activity.* This is the heart and soul of the lesson, where the concepts are introduced. The stimulus activity should be engaging and can assume a variety of formats as previously described. For example, an REE lesson on tease tolerance can be developed using art—children make a radio out of a cardboard box and write rational thoughts they can use to tune out teasing around a dial on the radio (Vernon, 2002, pp. 222–224). Art can also be used to help adolescents deal with depressed feelings. They can draw around their hand and in the palm, write down the things they are depressed about, and then identify rational coping self-statements on each finger to serve as a reminder about how to cope with depression (Vernon, 2002, pp. 131–132). Experiential activities can also be very engaging. Elementary children can be divided into two groups, procrastinators and non-procrastinators. They are to pretend that they are recruiting "members" to their club, so the procrastinators make a poster of all the good things about being a procrastinator, and the non-procrastinators do the same. Discussion follows about the advantages and disadvantages of procrastination (Vernon, 2002, p. 184). Adolescents can learn how to use rational thoughts to de-escalate anger by making a paper accordion, identifying thoughts about an anger-provoking incident on one level of the accordion sheet, and then writing a rational thought to counteract the irrational thought contributing to the anger on the next level of the accordion (Vernon, 2002, p. 167).

   It is advisable to use more concrete activities with younger children and gradually introduce more abstract lessons with adolescents. However, it is also important to be experiential and to use wide array of activities to maintain interest. The stimulus activity should take no more than half of the allotted time for the lesson, leaving time for discussion.
3. *Content and personalization questions.* Because a critical part of the lesson is the personal application of concepts, it is very important to allow sufficient time for discussion. Two types of questions provide the most effective debriefing: content questions, which focus on the cognitive concepts presented in the les-

son, and personalization questions, which involve applying the concepts to the child's own life. For example, in a lesson on rational thinking, the objective was to learn how to distinguish between rational and irrational thinking. The activity, for high school students, involved a short lecturette on the difference between rational and irrational thinking, followed by a worksheet, where students were asked to identify irrational beliefs in statements such as: My parents never let me do anything—everyone else has more freedom than I do; I can't stand it if my boyfriend breaks up with me—I'll never find anyone like him again. The content questions asked students to describe the difference between rational and irrational thinking and examples of key irrational beliefs. The personalization questions asked students if they were generally rational or irrational thinkers, what they would need to do to change the way they think in order to handle situations more effectively and how they can apply what they learned to their own lives (Vernon, 1998c).

4. Using this lesson plan format provides a basic structure, but at the same time, allows for flexibility and creativity in the actual design of the activity. The inclusion of both content and personalization questions achieves the objectives of emotional education programs: to present mental health concepts and to help students personally apply these to their own lives. The primary focus is prevention, with the hope that these concepts will reduce the frequency and intensity of future problems.

Considerations in Implementing Lessons

In conducting emotional education lessons, it is vital to establish an atmosphere of trust and group cohesion because children are encouraged to look at themselves, to share with others, to apply concepts to their own lives, and to learn from classmates with regard to emotional and behavioral adjustment. Sensitivity should be exercised, listening carefully to children's responses, supporting their struggles to gain new insights, and encouraging their attempts to acquire REE concepts.

It is also important to create an atmosphere where students respect each other's expression. The facilitator of the lesson has the responsibility for seeing that this minimal rule is respected so that children will feel comfortable in sharing. At the elementary level, this may not be a problem, but as adolescence approaches, students become more self-conscious and hesitant. A non-threatening classroom atmosphere helps to assure the success of the emotional education experiences.

As previously mentioned, assigning a grade to an REE lesson is not recommended because it is difficult to evaluate personal application of concepts, which is one of the significant components of an REE lesson. However, since the objectives are measurable, quizzes or other types of evaluation can be used to determine cognitive acquisition of concepts. For example, after presenting a lesson on the difference between facts and assumptions, the teacher could have students complete a short True/False quiz, identifying which statements were facts and which were assumptions.

It is very appropriate to ask students what they learned following a lesson or to assign homework as a follow-up to the lesson to help reinforce the concepts. After the lesson on facts and assumptions, a homework assignment for younger children could involve having them be "fact detectives," where they attempt to identify facts versus assumptions in their interactions with peers or siblings. Or, after a lesson on developing high frustration tolerance, middle-school students were asked to try something that had previously proven to be frustrating and to practice the examples of self-talk they had learned in the lesson to help them deal more effectively with their frustration.

Sample REE Lessons

There are numerous ways to introduce REE concepts. The following two lessons illustrate the lesson plan procedure. The first lesson is for elementary students to help them learn that people can feel differently about the same event based on what they think and the second is a self-acceptance activity for adolescents.

Face Your Feelings

Objective: To learn that people can feel differently about the same event.
Materials: Four paper plates per student; markers or crayons.
Stimulus Activity:

1. Ask students to draw faces on their paper plates to represent the following emotions: happy, sad, angry (mad), worried.
2. Explain that you will be reading some situations and that they are to think about how they feel when they experience a situation similar to the ones they are hearing about.
3. Read aloud each of the following situations, one at time, instructing students to respond by flipping up the face that illustrates how they would feel. Before reading another situation, note the different feelings that were portrayed and make a tally on the board.

Situations:

It is going to snow tonight.
Your younger cousins are coming to visit.
Your parents are taking you shopping after school.
Your teacher is keeping you in for recess.
You didn't get picked for the kickball game.
You are moving to a new reading group.
You might move to a different town and go to a different school.

Discussion:
Content Questions:

1. Did everyone respond to a given situation with the same feeling? If not, why do you think this happened?
2. Do you think that there is any situation in which all people would feel exactly the same? If so, what would be some examples?
3. Why do you think two people can feel differently about the same situation?

Personalization Questions:

1. Can you think of a time when you felt one way about something and your friend felt another way? (Encourage sharing of examples).
2. How do you think you should act if someone feels differently about a situation than you do?
3. What did you learn about feelings from this activity?

To the Leader:

In the discussion, emphasize that feelings vary based on what the person is thinking. Use examples to illustrate this process so that it is clear to the children.

Don't Soak It Up

Objective: To identify how to deal with criticism and put-downs which contribute to self-downing.

Materials: One sponge and a bucket of water, paper, and pencil for each student.

Stimulus Activity:

1. Introduce the activity by stating the objective of the lesson and asking for a volunteer.
2. Ask the volunteer to dip the sponge into the bucket and pull it back out. Discuss with the class what has happened to the sponge (it soaked up lots of water).
3. Next, explain that when people say negative things about us that often we "soak up" the negative words, just as in the demonstration, without examining the content of the message to see if in fact it is true. For example, if someone says that you are ugly and stupid, you need to look at the evidence, asking yourself if that is really true. If not, you don't have to "soak it up." Instead, you need to think about wringing out the sponge, getting rid of the put-downs or criticisms that aren't true.
4. Invite students to write down three recent examples of times they were absorbed by criticism or put-downs. Have them identify things they could say to themselves to avoid "soaking up" the negatives that lead to self-downing.
5. Invite students to share examples.

Discussion:

Content Questions:

1. What does the concept of "soaking it up" mean?
2. What can you do to avoid "soaking it up?"

Personalization Questions:

1. Are you someone who "soaks up the negative" often? If so, how do you feel when you do that? If not, how do you avoid soaking it up?
2. Suppose that some of the things others say about you are true—does that make you a bad person?
3. What did you learn from this lesson that you can apply to your life?

To the Leader:

Emphasize the importance of examining criticism to avoid excessive self-downing. Also stress that if some of it is true, it does not make you a bad person.

REE Learning Centers

Oftentimes elementary and middle-school teachers establish learning centers, where students work independently on activities to reinforce concepts presented in class or to introduce new ideas. REE activities can easily be incorporated into this type of format through worksheets, writing, or games. For example, Waters (1979) *Color Us Rational* stories lend themselves to a learning center activity. A copy of several of the stories can placed at the center, along with paper and pencil. After reading one or more of the stories, students are instructed to write a rational story based on one of their own experiences. Other good center activities involve having students write rational limericks or make rational bumper stickers or posters for their rooms, making up silly songs to help them deal with sad feelings, putting on rational puppet plays, or playing a game of hop scotch, where children have to identify rational self-talk to help them deal with anger or anxiety before jumping to the next space.

The teacher is limited only by his or her creativity in designing center activities. They should be engaging and able to be completed independently.

Integration into the Curriculum

Yet another approach to REE emotional education is to integrate the concepts into an existing subject-matter curriculum. When teaching literature, teachers could select and discuss stories that present characters solving problems rationally or expressing feelings in a healthy manner. Topics for themes could be related to self-awareness such as making mistakes, identifying strengths and weaknesses, and the prices and payoffs for perfection. Vocabulary and spelling lessons could include feeling-word vocabularies and definitions.

Social studies lessons could focus on personal and societal values and on a rational understanding of the concept of fairness as it applies to societal groups or to law and order, for example. Students could examine the rational and irrational practices of politicians, the difference between facts and assumptions in political campaigns, or the concept of high-frustration tolerance as it applies to political leaders.

Integration into the curriculum is less direct than a structured lesson, but it is a viable way of reinforcing rational concepts and making them an integral part of the school structure. Although it may seem awkward and forced initially, once teachers become more familiar with the REE concepts, they will find that integration becomes more natural.

You Can Do It! Education (youcandoiteducation.com.au)

I (Michael Bernard) am the Founder of You Can Do It! Education, a school-home collaborative social and emotional learning program that has been employed in 1000s of early learning centres, primary and secondary schools in Australia, and

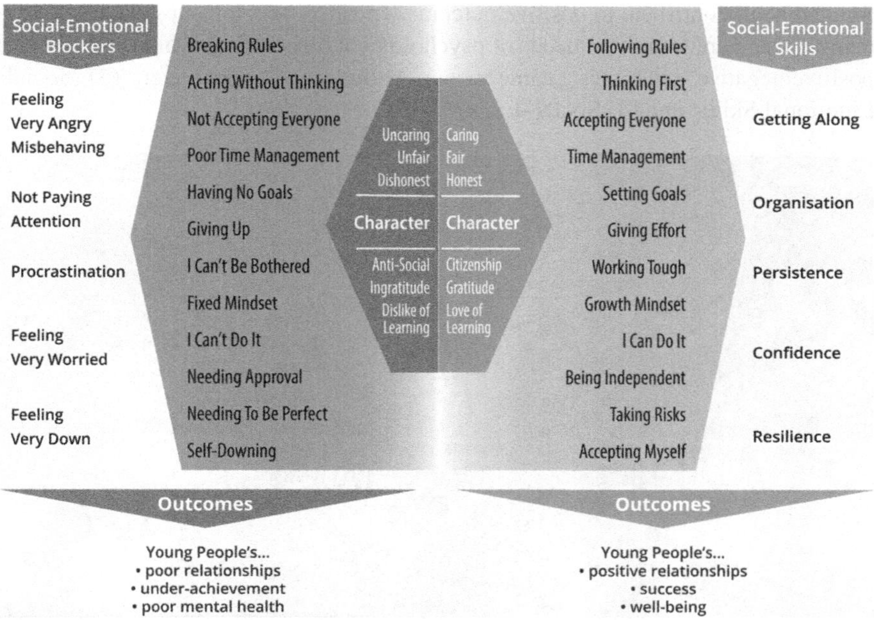

Fig. 20.1 You Can Do It! Education's Social–Emotional Learning Framework

in schools overseas. You Can Do It! Education has a central focus on developing the attitudes and social–emotional skills for young people of all ages. Published research indicates that when schools implement our programs, students become more resilient, confident, persistent, organized, and get along better—their engagement and achievement improves as does their relationship, behavior, and wellbeing (Fig. 20.1).

Today, over 1,000,000 students have participated in You Can Do It! Education programs introduced in over 4000 primary and secondary schools throughout Australia, New Zealand, England, the United States, and soon Europe.

You Can Do It! Education (YCDI!) (e.g., Bernard, 2013; Bernard, Vernon, Terjesen, & Kurasaki, 2013) derives largely from REBT/REE (e.g., Katsikis, Kostogiannis, Kassapis, Katsiki, & Bernard, 2018), intrinsic motivation theory, cognitive-behavior therapy, and positive psychology that identifies the psychological characteristics of young people that contribute to both negative and positive emotional, behavioral, relationship, and achievement outcomes. Research supporting YCDI's central propositions and effects are reported in the literature (Ashdown & Bernard, 2012; Bernard, 2006, 2008, 2017; Bernard & Walton, 2011; Markopolous & Bernard, 2015; Yamamoto, Matsumoto, & Bernard, 2017).

On the left in the dark orange side, we see (1) Negative Attitudes and (2) Under-developed Character (*values and strengths*) that create (3) Social–Emotional Blockers. All three elements contribute to negative student outcomes (poor relationships, under-achievement, and poor mental health). Additionally, the framework represents three positive elements of a young person's inner world, in lighter orange: (1) Positive Attitudes and (2) Character (*values, strengths*) and (3) Social-Emotional

Skills that all contribute to positive outcomes (positive relationships, success, well-being). There are four dimensions of psychological functioning, which contribute to positive/negative outcomes; namely, (1) Attitudes, (2) Character, (3) Social–Emotional Skills, and (4) Social–Emotional Blockers.

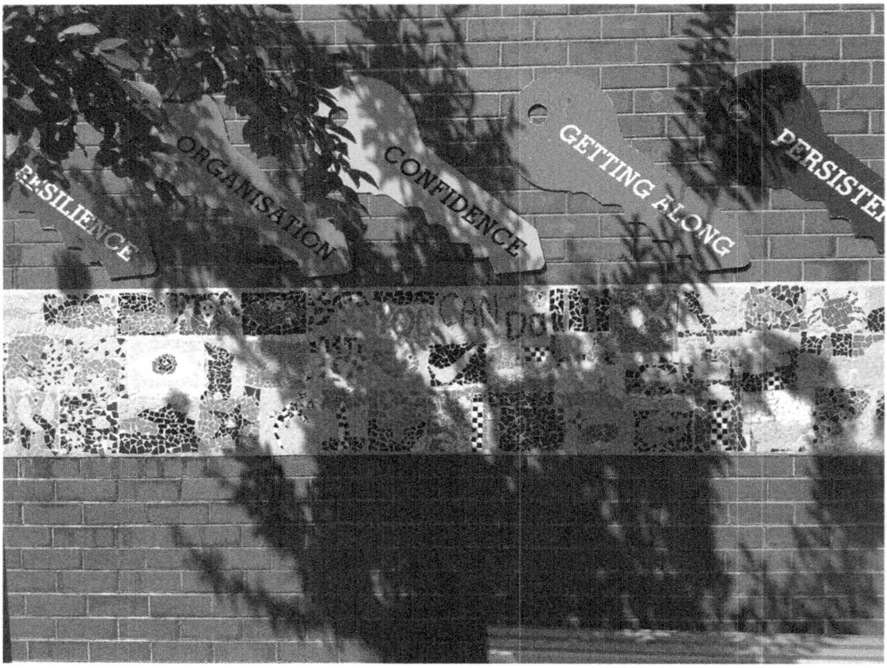

While YCDI! is most known as teaching five social–emotional skills (confidence, persistence, organization, getting along, resilience), "Attitudes" —many of which are Ellis' rational and irrational beliefs—nourish and supports the five SELs and are recognized as central and foundational to positive and negative outcomes in young people (Fig. 20.2).

This picture of an iceberg is a metaphor for central focus of You Can Do It! Education; attitudes. Students (and all humans) are like ice-bergs—the only part of the iceberg that we can see is the smallest part that sits above the water; the only part we can see in students are their behaviors (what they do and say). Below the waterline, where we cannot see (but can only guess at) lays the students' feelings and emotions—and it is how they feel that causes them to behave as they do (both positively & negative behaviors follow this model). Below their feelings, lays their thinking or self-talk—and it is what they say to themselves in their head (what they THINK) that causes their feelings, which causes their behavior. Lastly, at the very bottom of everyone's iceberg, lays the attitudes students hold about themselves and life around them. It is these, either positive or negative attitudes that cause students to think a certain way, which causes their feelings and finally their behavior (which of course, then results in outcomes, results, consequences.)

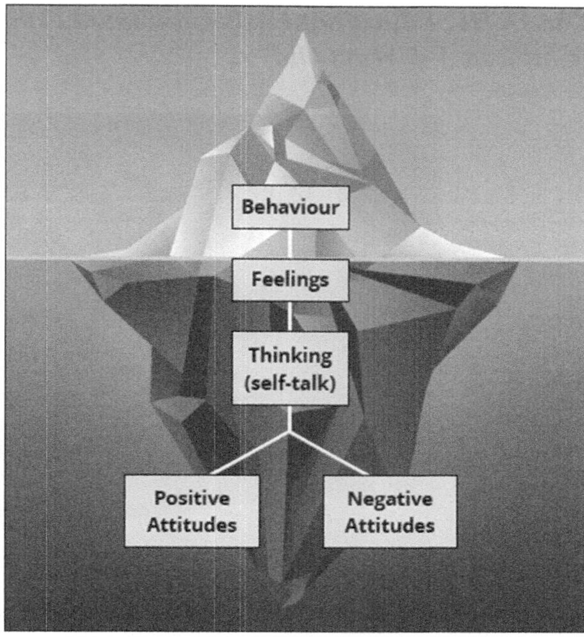

Fig. 20.2 Children are like icebergs

Teaching You Can Do It! Education

There are a number of school entry points for YCDI! These will be briefly reviewed including social–emotional learning curricula programs, integration in the classroom, school practices for building critical mass, helping children and adolescents overcome social–emotional difficulties and parent education).

Social–Emotional Learning Curricula

In 2018, four YCDI! curricula, new editions of existing programs, were released in an online, digital format. As a rule, these programs are taught by classroom teachers to intact classrooms. Lessons are timetabled to be taught once a week in 20–50 min sessions across each week of the school year. YCDI!'s SEL programs have been recognized as best-practice SEL program, by Beyond Blue/Be You, the Australian federal government's mental health initiative.

In all four programs, many lessons teach REE concepts and skills as described in the previous section of this chapter.

The YCDI! Education Early Childhood Program Achieve (Children 3–6 Years Old)

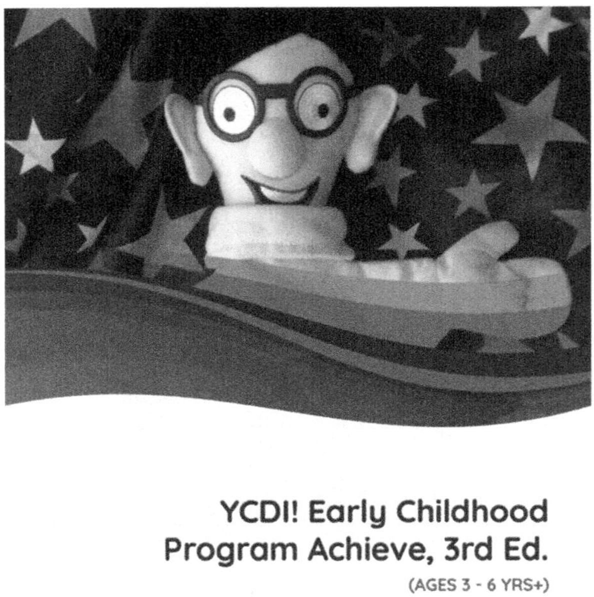

The new third edition of this extremely popular online digital program now includes specific suggestions for teaching young children 3–4 years of age. These suggestions appear within the 32 lesson plans. The program teaches the positive attitudes and social–emotional skills that develop young children's resilience, confidence, persistence, organization, and getting along. Two short animations introduce the young children to their new classmates: Ricky Resilience, Connie Confidence, Pete Persistence, Oscar Organisation, and Gabby Get Along who are also represented in five hand puppets, posters, and songs. The program includes a scope and sequence of 32 weekly lessons (8 lessons per school term) with each lesson consisting of learning intentions and success criteria. A parent education guide consisting of four parent education talks is also provided that demonstrates how parents can support SEL at home.

NEW *Program Achieve Primary (Grades 1–6)*

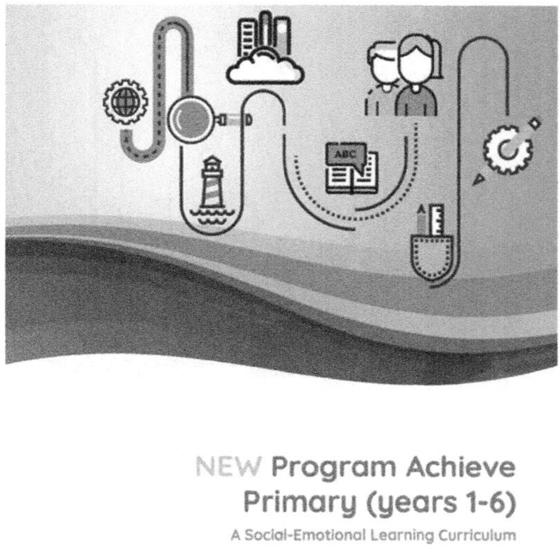

The NEW Program Achieve curricula (Primary) contain lessons that teach attitudes, values/character strengths and social–emotional skills for success, relationships, and well-being as well as for overcoming social–emotional blockers. A scope and sequence have been developed based on this framework covering eight lessons for each of four terms across years 1–6 (192 lessons). The 32 lessons at each year level are organized to be delivered across four terms and cover the following topics: (1). Achievement: Work Confidence (growth mindset), Persistence, Organisation, and Teamwork (2). Relationships: Values, Character Strengths, and Getting Along Skills (3). Well-being, Resilience, and Happiness (awareness, self-management, ABCs of emotions, cognitive restructuring, mindfulness) and (4). Social–Emotional Blockers: awareness and management of anger, not paying attention, procrastination, worry, feeling down. Each lesson begins with a statement of Learning Intentions and Success Criteria followed by a lesson plan that includes the following elements: (1) Engage students (2) Share learning intentions and success criteria (3) Explicit teaching (4) Student activities (5) Students demonstrate success criteria and reflect (6) Weekly goal setting challenge (7) Coaching points 4 week.

NEW *Program Achieve Primary (Grades 7–10)*

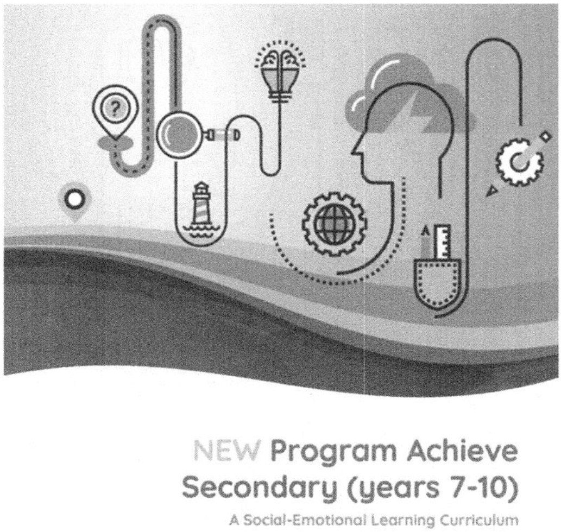

The NEW Program Achieve-Secondary is now available online providing teachers access to digital activity plans and downloadable Teacher Guides and Student Worksheets. This curriculum is designed to contain short, targeted activities delivered in 15–20 min periods during the busy timetabled secondary school day. The NEW Program Achieve-Secondary includes 32 activities to be taught to students in grades 7 and 8 and an additional 32 activities to be taught to students in years 9 and 10. The activities are organized to be delivered across four terms and cover the following topics (1) Achievement: Work Confidence (growth mindset), Persistence, Organization, and Teamwork (2) Relationships: Values, Character Strengths, and Getting Along Skills, (3) Wellbeing: Resilience and Happiness (self-awareness, self-management, ABCs, cognitive restructuring, mindfulness) (4) Social–Emotional Blockers: Anger, Not Paying Attention, Procrastination, Worry and Feeling Down (awareness and self-management) Activities take between 15 and 20 min of class time to present to students and can be offered flexibly throughout the school week in either Home Groups, personal and social development classes, or health and physical education.

The Successful Mind at School, Work, and Life (Grades 9–12)

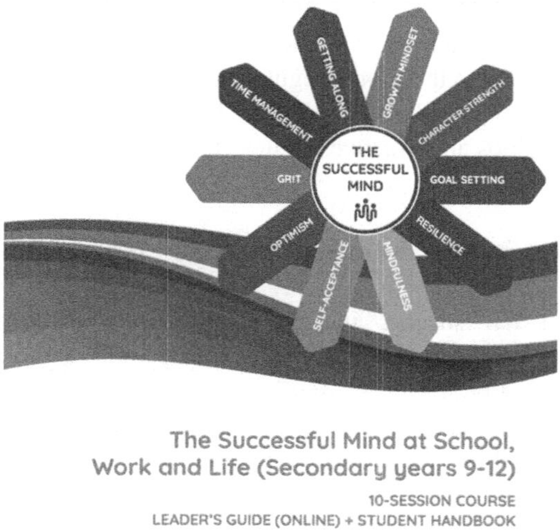

This 10-session course is designed for upper secondary students to prepare them for their final years in school, pre-employment and part-time work experiences, and for life beyond school. A distinctive feature of this course is its suitability to be delivered in career education classes with content linked to the CORE Skills for Work framework. The online Leader's Guide contains background information and a session plan needed to conduct each of the 10 sessions: (1) Growth Mindset (2) Character Strength (3) Goal Setting (4) Resilience (5) Mindfulness (6) Self-acceptance (7) Optimism (8) GRIT (9) Time Management (10) Getting Along The Student Handbook contains a variety of content, activity worksheets students complete during each session, a variety of tips and individual action plans completed after a session.

The You Can Do It! Classroom: Integration of Social and Emotional Learning

One of the biggest lessons learned from many years of experience is that for SEL curricula to have a maximum impact on young people's achievement and emotional well-being, the DSELs and positive attitudes (rational beliefs) need to be taught and reinforced in the classroom (and school) throughout the school year.

Just as teachers introduce their students to "classroom rules" and the academic standards that constitute the objectives of the curriculum early on in the school year, it is recommend that the 5 SELs and 12 Attitudes become part of the overall purpose of the class. It is recommended that teachers integrate the 5 SELs into the classroom ethos so that their students know that it is important for them to learn and apply them in their doing schoolwork, in their interpersonal relationships, and in managing their own emotions. One of the best practices for doing this is to display on the walls on a permanent basis examples of positive Habits of the Mind and negative Habits of the Mind and how they impact their emotions and behaviors in the classroom and refer to them on a regular basis.

The following steps can be taken by teachers to incorporate You Can Do It! Education into the ethos and practices of their classroom.

Step 1. Teach Students the Meaning of "Success" and "Well-Being"

Explain to students that "success" means doing the best you can in schoolwork and other areas of your life (art, sport, art, music, doing a job) and not feeling that you have to be the best to be a success. Explain to students that "Well-Being" means feeling happy and safe; having one or more friends; being engaged in schoolwork; and participating in school, home, and community activities. It also means that you do not feel very worried, down, or angry for long periods of time and that you do not make poor behavioral choices such as bullying or being late or absent from school or engaging in unhealthy behavior like drinking or smoking.

Step 2. Establish Students' Understanding of the Goals of You Can Do It! Education

Discuss with students how student success and well-being is *not* due to great parents, teachers, or super-intelligence although those things matter. What matters more and what has been discovered from scientific research are the different ways of thinking, feeling and behaving that people of all ages need to be successful and happy. Explain that you will not only be teaching students the academic curriculum but also a curriculum focused on teaching students the social–emotional skills they need to be all they can be and to flourish.

Step 3. Discuss the Definition of the Social–Emotional Skill Being Taught

(Example): Explain to students the following: "One of the characteristics of a successful person is Confidence. I'd like you to think about how you would define Confidence in relation to your classroom learning. Take a minute to bring to mind students you know who exhibit confidence when learning." In pairs or groups, ask students to prepare a "Y Chart" about Confidence. What does it look like (makes eye contact, puts hand up), sound like (I've been successful before, I've done hard things before, I'll have a go), feel like (motivated, enthusiastic, empowered)?

Have pairs or groups develop a definition of confidence, and then have students generate and display a class definition. Make sure that the definition includes important elements of Confidence as reflected in the definitions provided in YCDI reference material.

Step 4. Identify Examples of Behaviors to be Practiced that Reflect Use of SEL Skill Being Taught

(Example): Explain to students that one way they can increase their Confidence in classroom learning is to practice being Confident. The more they practice Confident behavior, the more Confident they will become. In pairs or small groups, have students discuss and identify examples of confident behavior in relation to their classroom and learning.

Have students generate a composite list of examples and display them in classroom. Make sure that the list includes examples of Confidence as found in YCDI reference material.

Step 5. Teach the Attitudes/Self-Talk that Support the 5 Social and Emotional Skills

(Example): Explain to students that a powerful influence over their Confidence in all situations is their thinking. You will explain that it is your "Thinking" about what "Happens" to you that determines your "Feelings" and "Behaving" including how confidently you feel and behave.

You can show students an illustration/image that shows how different ways of thinking (positive and negative) lead to differences in how Confident one feels and behaves when having a difficult assignment to do. Describe to students the positive Attitudes (ways of thinking/self-talk) that underpin the foundation of Confidence using a variety of images and definitions that can be found in YDCI resource materials. These are: Accepting Myself, Taking Risks, Being Independent, and I Can Do It. You can also contrast these with negative Habits of the Mind (ways of thinking) that hurt one's Confidence and lead to feeling anxious and down: Self Downing, Needing to Be Perfect, Needing Approval, and I Can't Do It.

Step 6. Use Behavior-specific Feedback to Acknowledge Students

When you catch a student practicing a behavior that reflects the SEL you are teaching, acknowledge the student verbally, non-verbally, or in a written comment (e.g., "You were confident." "You tried hard and did not give up. That's persistence." "Doesn't it feel good to be organized?" "You are getting along very well when working together." "You stayed calm in a difficult situation. That's resilience.").

School-Wide Practices for Building Critical Mass

In order for all students to strengthen their SELs—and this point is crucial—schools need to not only teach curricula like Program Achieve, they also need to provide students with opportunities to apply and practice what they are learning, receive recognition for applying what they have learned, and to hear from different people in different settings (e.g., assemblies, excursions) how SELs can help them to be successful and happy.

As an example, I (Bernard) remember visiting a secondary school that was teaching YCDI! to students in four different sessions at the beginning of the day. The students were learning the language but too many—especially the challenging students—were not putting what they were learning about into action. One afternoon, I sat in on a physical education class, the PE teacher was telling students about a forthcoming state-wide football competition they were to enter, and he handed out new uniforms. However, to my surprise and disappointment, he failed to mention how the team's performance would be enhanced by team members using their keys of confidence, persistence, organization, getting along, and resilience. So, I clearly saw the need for schools to build a critical mass of SEL practices in order to reach the minds and hearts of all students.

These practices serve to establish a culture within a school, so that SEL and YCDI! becomes just "the way we do things around here" and that even if some teachers and the school principal leaves, the culture is still embedded and long-lasting in the school ground, classrooms, and staff.

Here are examples of school-wide practices.

Visual Displays and Posters YCDI! Education is very visual. Schools acquire different YCDI! posters for display, and students (as well as parents) design visual reminders.

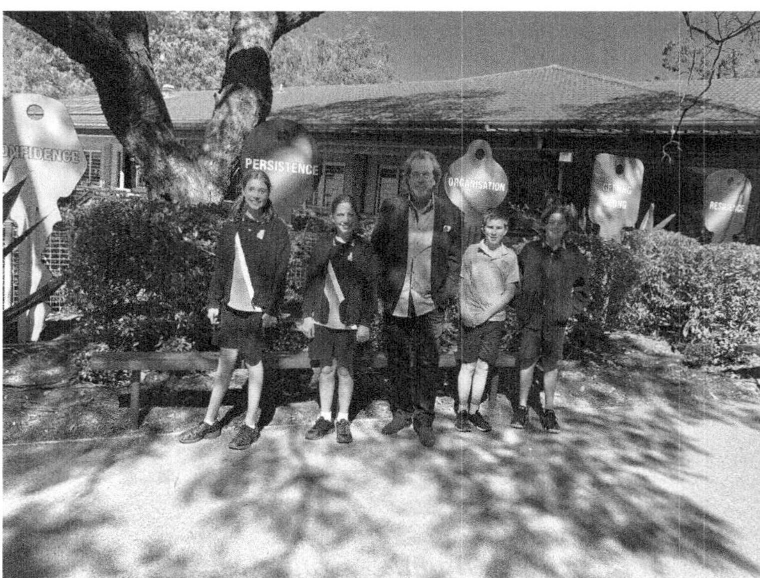

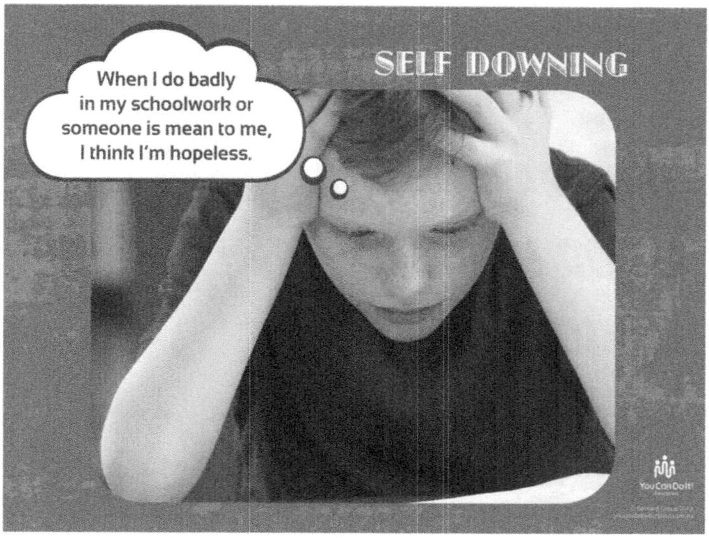
SELF DOWNING
When I do badly in my schoolwork or someone is mean to me, I think I'm hopeless.
YouCanDoIt!

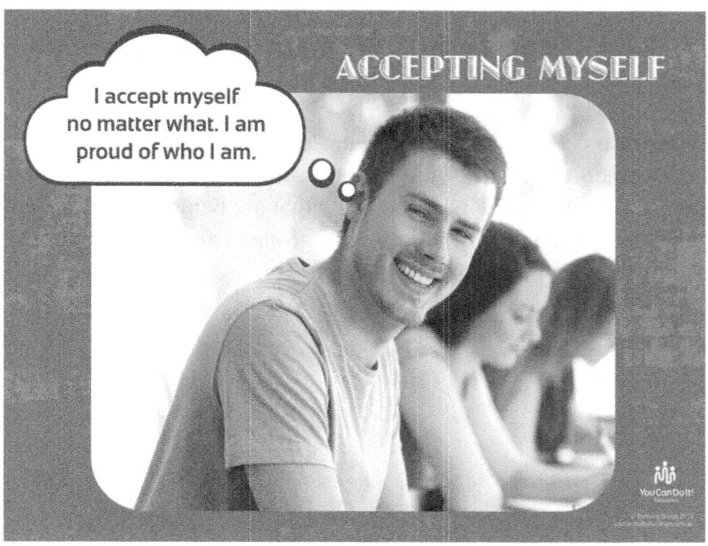
ACCEPTING MYSELF
I accept myself no matter what. I am proud of who I am.
YouCanDoIt!

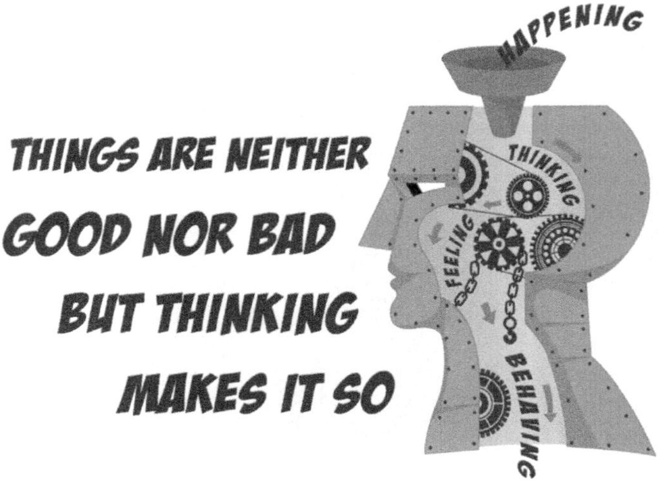
HAPPENING
THINGS ARE NEITHER
GOOD NOR BAD
BUT THINKING
MAKES IT SO
THINKING
FEELING
BEHAVING

Excursions There is no better place to help students see the relevance and usefulness of employing different attitudes and social–emotional skills is before, during and after excursions. Excursion leaders should prime students with those SELs that will help make the excursion fun and a great success.

School Assemblies School assemblies are excellent forums for principals/head teachers and others to address the school community on one or more of the Foundations and Positive Habits of the Mind that are being stressed in your school. Guest speakers' plays and other discussion groups can address the meaning and importance of the 5 Foundations and positive Habits of the Mind to student well-being, success and relationships.

Student Recognition Awards

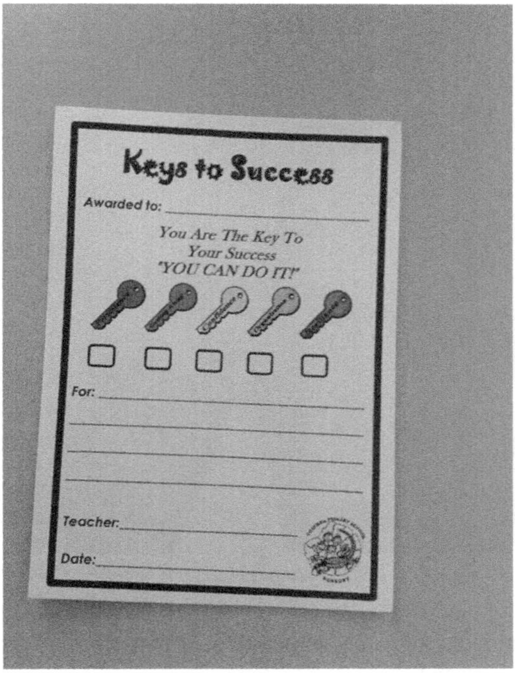

An excellent vehicle for bringing all students in a class/grade/year level of school "on board" is to award students recognition certificates for employing one or more of the 5 Foundations on a regular basis. Many schools present awards for achievement, citizenship, or "Student of the Month." It is recommended that awards for demonstrating characteristics consistent with the goals of YCDI be employed.

Helping Children and Adolescents Overcome Social-Emotional Difficulties

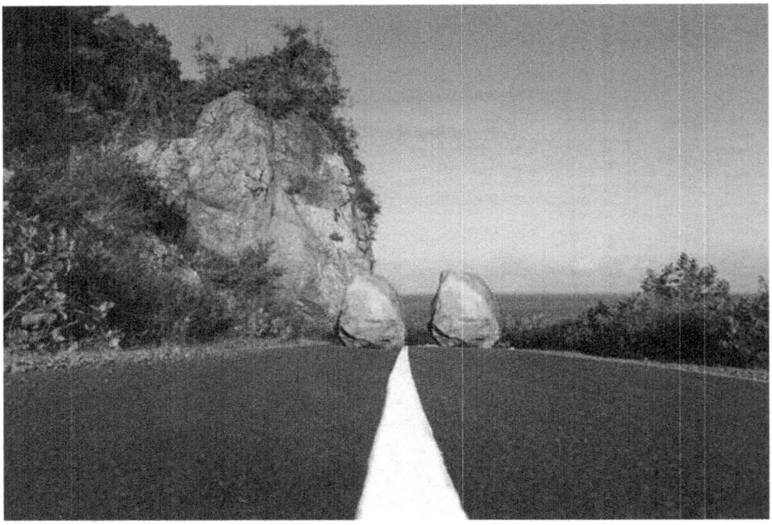

In YCDI! Education and in the Program Achieve curricula, social-emotional difficulties are referred to as 'blockers'. Social-emotional blockers can be conceived as blockers sitting in the road students take toward success and happiness. The goals of YCDI! Education in this area are three-fold: (1) helping students become aware of the existence of different blockers that everyone experiences to greater and lesser extents, (2) helping "normalize" for students the existence of blockers; meaning helping students accept their existence without thinking there is anything wrong or abnormal about them, (3) helping students develop a mindset that there are different things they can do to reduce the size of blockers – and to help themselves take the blocker off their road to success and happiness. The five blockers addressed in YCDI! include:

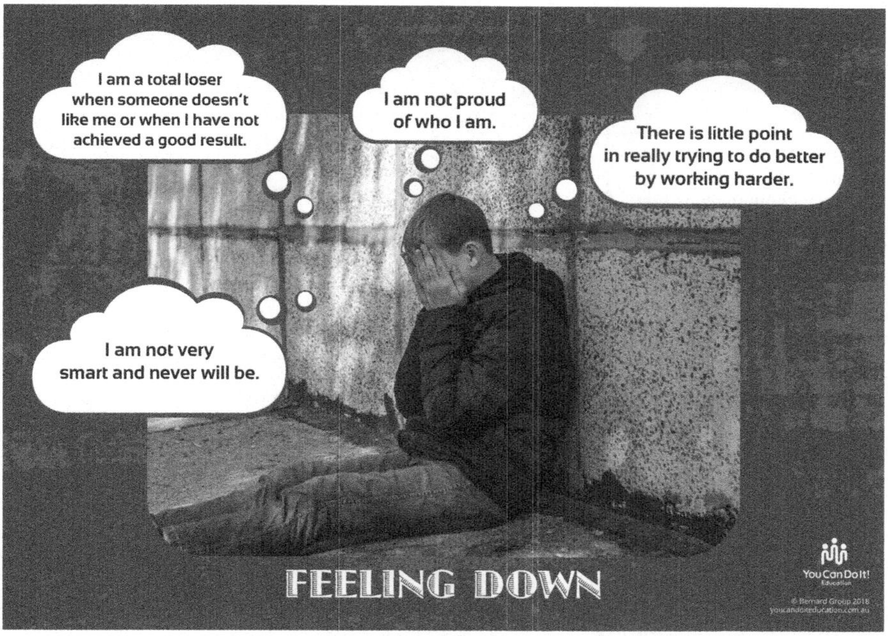
I am a total loser when someone doesn't like me or when I have not achieved a good result.
I am not proud of who I am.
There is little point in really trying to do better by working harder.
I am not very smart and never will be.
FEELING DOWN
YouCanDoIt! Education

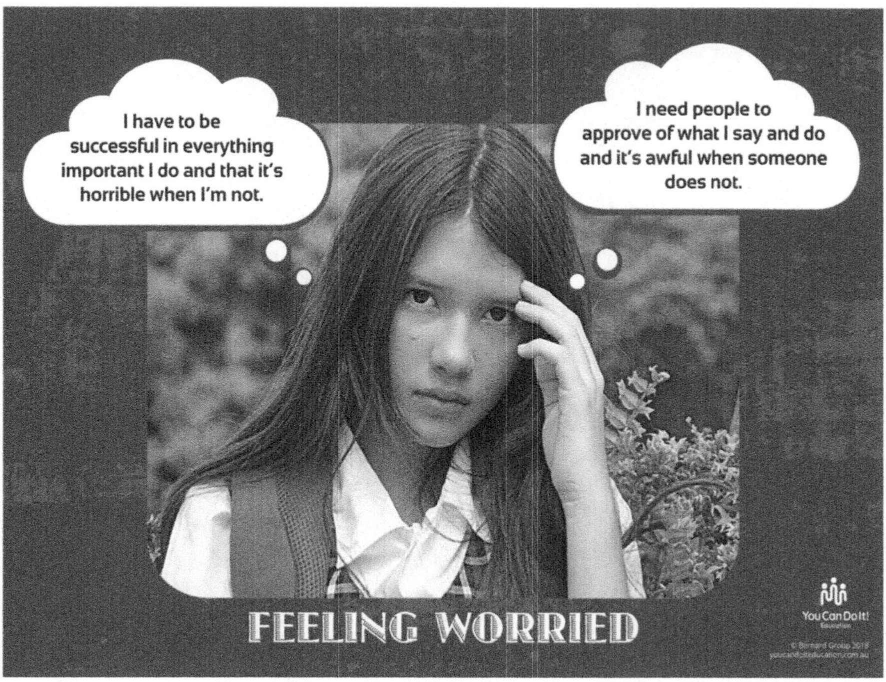
I have to be successful in everything important I do and that it's horrible when I'm not.
I need people to approve of what I say and do and it's awful when someone does not.
FEELING WORRIED
YouCanDoIt! Education

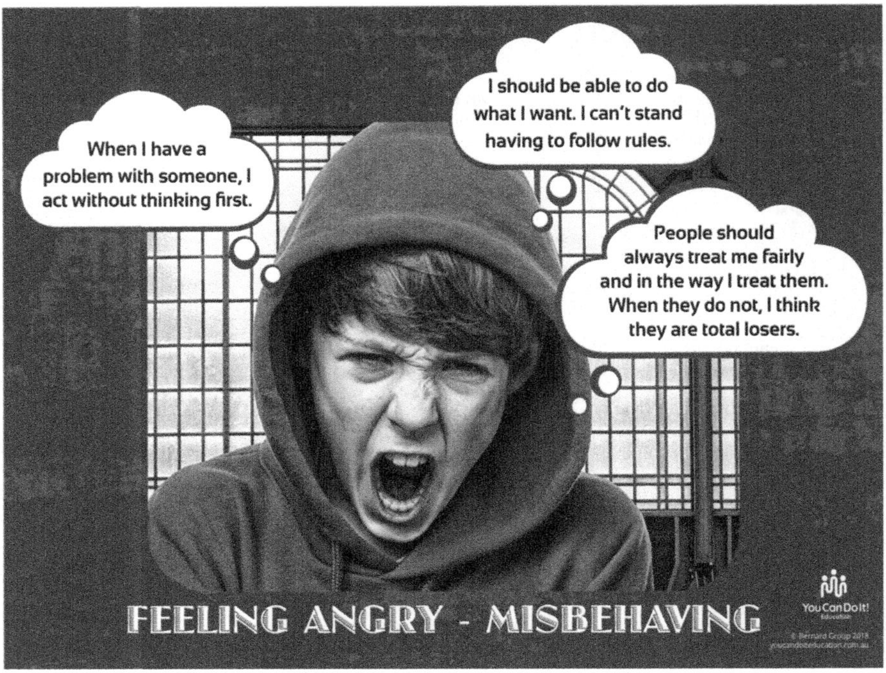
When I have a problem with someone, I act without thinking first.
I should be able to do what I want. I can't stand having to follow rules.
People should always treat me fairly and in the way I treat them. When they do not, I think they are total losers.
FEELING ANGRY - MISBEHAVING
You Can Do It!

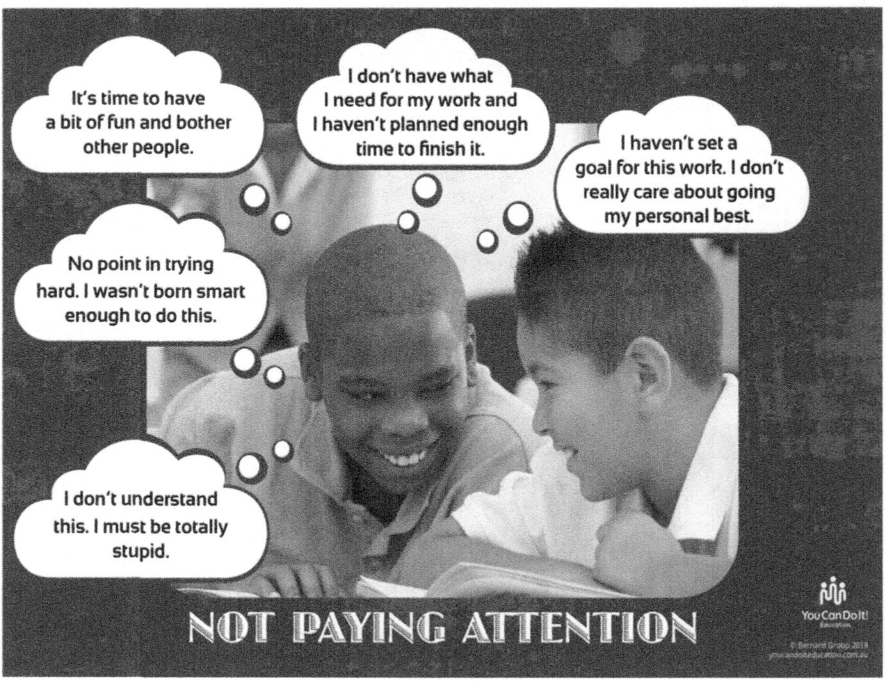
It's time to have a bit of fun and bother other people.
I don't have what I need for my work and I haven't planned enough time to finish it.
I haven't set a goal for this work. I don't really care about going my personal best.
No point in trying hard. I wasn't born smart enough to do this.
I don't understand this. I must be totally stupid.
NOT PAYING ATTENTION
You Can Do It!

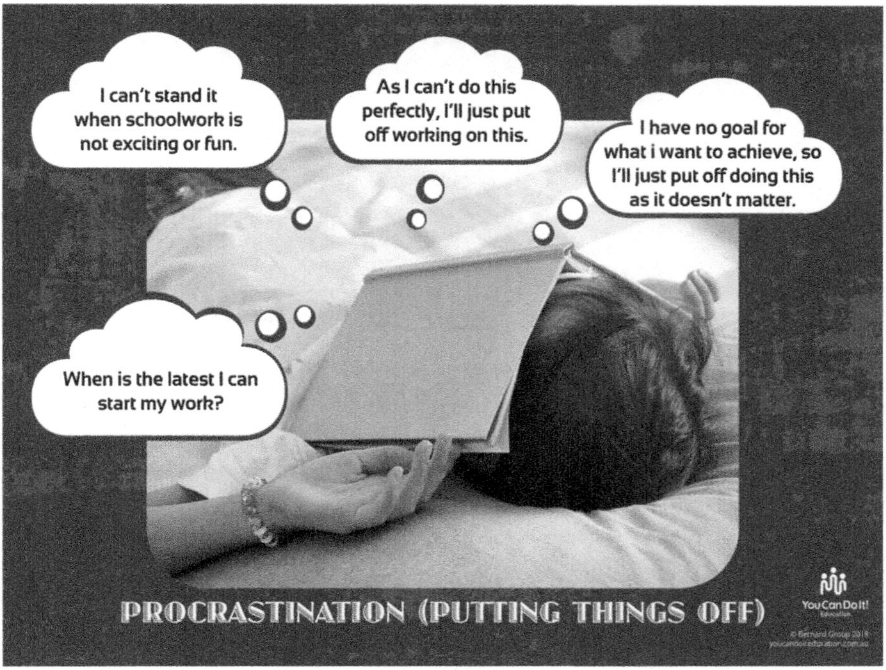
I can't stand it when schoolwork is not exciting or fun.
As I can't do this perfectly, I'll just put off working on this.
I have no goal for what i want to achieve, so I'll just put off doing this as it doesn't matter.
When is the latest I can start my work?
PROCRASTINATION (PUTTING THINGS OFF)
YouCanDoIt!

Here are some ways YCDI! helps students overcome blockers.

1. Normalize blockers. Indicate that everyone has one or more blockers from time to time. Having a blocker does not mean there is anything wrong with you.
2. Empower students to overcome blockers. Explain to students that throughout life (and in school), they will learn some things that can help them reduce blockers in size.
3. Employ lessons from *Program Achieve*. Lessons and activities exist at Years Levels 1–10 that explicitly teach students about the five social-emotional blockers and how they can be overcome.
4. Lessons and activities exist that explicitly teach students about Resilience and how to self-manage and stay calm when faced with difficulties and challenges using the ABCs of REBT and cognitive-restructuring negative to positive attitudes and self-talk.

In five of the lessons in Program Achieve (grades 1–6), students receive as handouts, five social-emotional lifesavers (see Worry Lifesaver below):

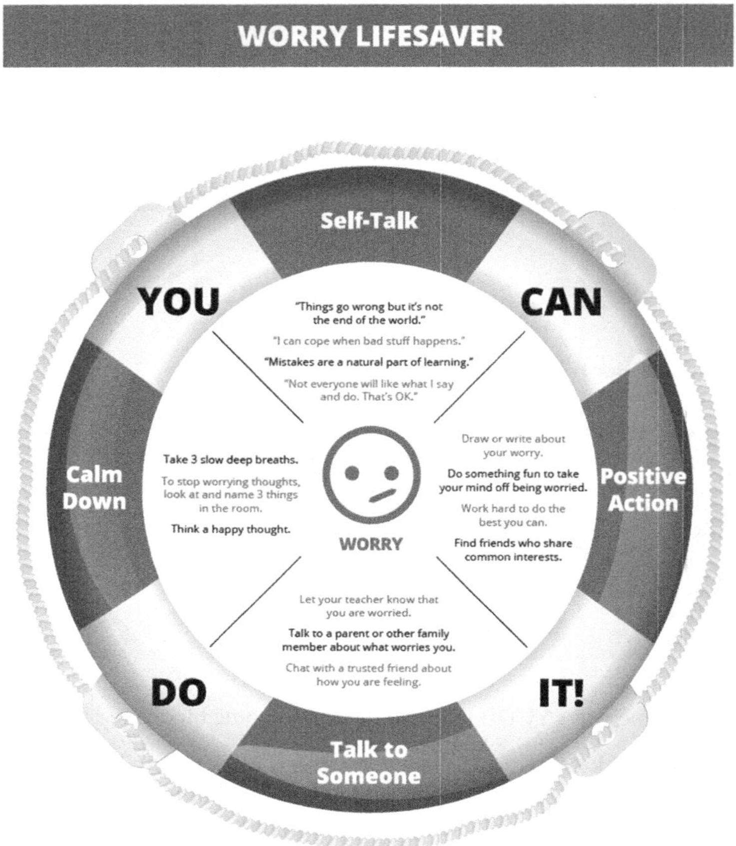

Parent Education

YCDI! Education has from its' inception been a school-home collaborative program recognizing the positive impacts parents can have on their children's school achievement and wellbeing. Our parent education programs have a focus on several topics related to effective parenting: (1) Stress management, (2) Parent effectiveness skills including relationship building, motivation and discipline and (3) Parents supporting their children's social–emotional skill development. This module introduces two YCDI! Education parent education programs, both based on the latest research on parent effectiveness.

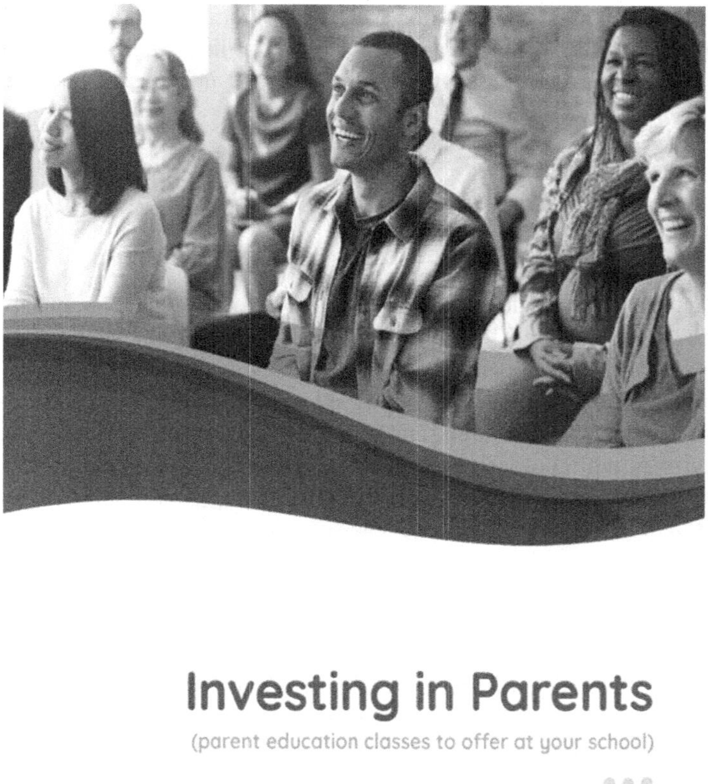
Investing in Parents
(parent education classes to offer at your school)

One program, *Investing in Parents*, is a set of 17 parent education classes (1–1.5 h) that can be offered at your school by a school leader, counselor, teacher or parent educator during or after school on a variety of parenting topics (e.g., authoritative parenting style, parent stress management and resilience, children's social-emotional learning at home).

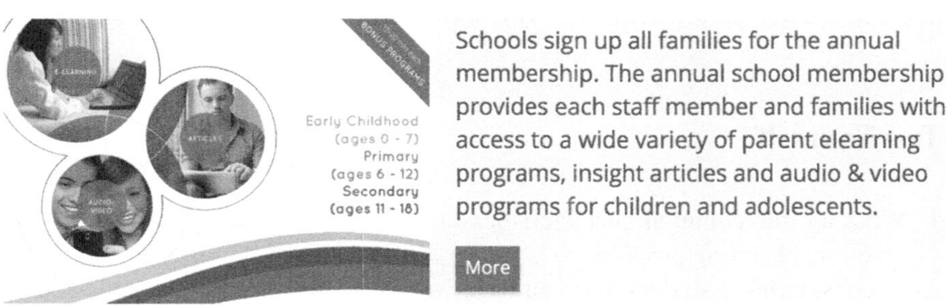

The other program is an on-line, digital program consisting of a variety of eLearning video-animated programs for parents, on-line articles on parenting and for older children and adolescents, inspirational and informative audio and video programs.

Conclusions

In the ideal world, approaches such as rational-emotive education and its' derivatives such as You Can Do It! Education would be routinely implemented in schools throughout the world in a systematic effort to enhance the emotional health of children. The major assumption of emotional education programs is that prevention is more effective than remediation, and that if we can teach children how to think rationally, they will approach both developmental and situational challenges in a healthier manner, which in turn will decrease the proliferation of self-defeating behaviors that far too many young people succumb to.

In order to effectively implement REE and YCDI, teachers and other school personnel must learn the theory and model it. Professionals need to continually challenge their own irrational thinking, getting rid of their demands that their job should always be easy, that their students should always behave perfectly, or that they will always be treated fairly. They must stop making overgeneralizations about student behavior or performance, avoid awfulizing about their work conditions, refrain from equating their own self-worth with their performance as a teacher; and force themselves to give up their demandingness that everything should come easily to their students. Until teachers themselves "walk the walk" and believe in the REBT principles, implementing REE and YCDI will not be as effective.

Although REE lessons appear to be an effective way to help children and adolescents approach life more successfully, rational thinking principles need to be an inherent part of every young person's experience. Adults are important models, and although it is difficult to develop a rational stance toward life when surrounded by irrationality in the world, every effort to teach rational principles, directly or indirectly, will help facilitate healthy emotional development.

Test Yourself

1. What are the common characteristics of a successful school-based social and emotional learning program?
2. In considering a student that you have worked with who has had some social-emotional difficulties, identify and consider the role of negative attitudes and under-developed character that create social-emotional blockers.
3. Positive or healthy habits of the mind are key to effective social–emotional development. In reflection of the classroom or schools where you may work with students, what creative strategies might you want to use to promote these positive habits?

References

Ashdown, D. M., & Bernard, M. E. (2012). Can explicit instruction in social and emotional learning skills benefit the social-emotional development, well-being, and academic achievement of young children? *Early Childhood Education Journal, 39*, 397–405.

Aspen Institute. (2019). *From a nation at risk to a nation of hope*. https://www.aspeninstitute.org/events/national-commission-final-report-release/.

Bedford, S. (1974). *Instant replay*. New York: Institute for Rational Living.

Bernard, M.E. (2001). *Program achieve: A curriculum of lessons for teaching students how to achieve success and develop social-emotional-behavioral well-being* (2nd ed., Vols. 1-6). Oakleigh, VIC (AUS): Australian Scholarships Group.

Bernard, M.E. (2006). It's time we teach social and emotional competence as well as we teach academic competence. *Reading and Writing Quarterly, 22*, 103–119.

Bernard, M. E. (2008). The effect of you can do it! Education on the emotional resilience of primary school students with social, emotional, behavioral and achievement challenges. *Proceedings of the Australian Psychological Society Annual Conference, 43*, 36–40.

Bernard, M. E. (2013). You Can Do It! Education: A social-emotional learning program for increasing the achievement and well-being of children and adolescents. In K. Yamasaki (Ed.), *School-based prevention education for health and adjustment problems in the world*. Tokyo: Kaneko Shobo.

Bernard, M. E. (2017). Impact of teaching attitudes and behaviors for learning on the reading achievement of students falling behind. *International Journal of Learning, Teaching and Educational Research, 16*, 51–64.

Bernard, M.E. (2018). *NEW program achieve (years 1-6; years 7-12). A social-emotional learning curriculum*. East Melbourne: The Bernard Group. https://youcandoiteducation.com.au/.

Bernard, M. E., Vernon, A., Terjesen, M., & Kurasaki, R. (2013). Self-acceptance in the educational and counseling of young people. In M. E. Bernard (Ed.), *The strength of self-acceptance. Theory, research and application* (pp. 155–192). New York: Springer Press.

Bernard, M. E., & Walton, K. E. (2011). The effect of you can do it! Education in six schools on student perceptions of wellbeing, teaching-learning and relationships. *Journal of Student Well-Being, 5*, 22–37.

DiGiuseppe, R., Miller, N.J., and Trexler, L.D. (1979). A review of rational-emotive psychotherapy outcome studies. In A. Ellis and J.M. Whiteley (Eds.), *Theoretical and empirical foundations of rational-emotive therapy*. Monterrey, CA: Brooks/Cole.

Dryden, W. (1999). *Rational emotive behavioural counselling in action* (2nd ed.). London: Sage.

Ellis, A. (1971). An experiment in emotional education. *Educational Technology, 11*, 61–64.

Ellis, A. (1972). Emotional education in the classroom: The living school. *Journal of Child Psychology, 1*, 19–22.

Ellis, A. (1994). *Reason and emotion in psychotherapy: A comprehensive method of treating human disturbances*. New York: Institute for Rational-Emotive Therapy.

Ellis, A., & MacClaren, C. (1998). *Rational emotive behavior therapy: A therapist's guide*. Atascadero, CA: Impact.

Gonzalez, J. E., Nelson, J. R., Gutkin, T. B., Saunders, A., Galloway, A., & Shwery, C. S. (2004). Rational emotive therapy with children and adolescents: A meta-analysis. *Journal of Emotional and Behavioral Disorders, 12*, 222–235.

Hajzler, D. J., & Bernard, M. E. (1991). A review of rational emotive outcome studies. *School Psychology Quarterly, 6*, 27–49.

Katsikis, D., Kostogiannis, C., Kassapis, S., Katsiki, A., & Bernard, M. E. (2018). Integrating social-emotional learning in schools: A proposal based on rational-emotive behavior education. *Effective Scientist-Practitioner, 1*, 19–45.

Knaus, W. (1974). *Rational emotive education: A manual for elementary school teachers*. New York: Institute for Rational Living.

Mahfar, M., Noah, S. M., & Senin, A. A. (2019). Development of rational emotive education module for stress intervention of Malaysian boarding school students. *Sage Open, 2019*, 1–16.

Markopolous, Z., & Bernard, M. E. (2015). Effect of the bullying: The power to cope program on children's response to bullying. *Journal of Relationships Research, 6*, 1–11.
Piper, W. (1986). *The little engine that could*. New York: Platt and Munk.
Popa, C., & Bochis, A. (2012). The effects of a rational emotive behaviour education program on the sociometric status and interpersonal perception modification of 9-10 year old Romanian pupils. *Procedia - Social and Behavioral Sciences, 46*, 5792–5796.
Steins, G., & Haep, A. (2015). Social learning and rational-emotive education: An exploratory investigation of students' perspective. *Psychology, 6*, 1096–1107.
Terjesen, M., Doyle, K., Rose, R., Sciutto, M., Iovine-Calabro, E., & Zampano, G. (1999). *REBT in the schools: A review and implications for school psychologists*. Poster presented at the 107th annual convention of the American Psychological Association (APA; Division 16). Boston, MA.
Vernon, A. (1980). *Help yourself to a healthier you*. Washington, DC: University Press of America.
Vernon, A. (1989a). *Thinking, feeling, behaving: An emotional education program for children*. Champaign, IL: Research Press.
Vernon, A. (1989b). *Thinking, feeling, behaving: An emotional education program for adolescents*. Champaign, IL: Research Press.
Vernon, A. (1998a). *The passport program: A journey through emotional, social, cognitive, and self-development, grades 1–5*. Champaign, IL: Research Press.
Vernon, A. (1998b). *The passport program: A journey through emotional, social, cognitive, and self-development, grades 6–8*. Champaign, IL: Research Press.
Vernon, A. (1998c). *The passport program: A journey through emotional, social, cognitive, and self-development, grades 9–12*. Champaign, IL: Research Press.
Vernon, A. (2002). *What works when with children and adolescents: A handbook of individual counseling techniques*. Champaign, IL: Research Press.
Vernon, A. (2004). *Counseling children and adolescents* (3rd ed.). Denver, CO: Love Publishing.
Vernon, A. (2006a). *Thinking, feeling, behaving: An emotional education curriculum for children (2nd ed.; Grades 1–6)*. Champaign, IL: Research Press.
Vernon, A. (2006b). *Thinking, feeling, behaving: An emotional education curriculum for adolescents (2nd ed.; Grades 7–12)*. Champaign, IL: Research Press.
Waters, V. (1979). *Color us rational*. New York: Institute for Rational Living.
Yamamoto, T., Matsumoto, Y., & Bernard, M. E. (2017). Effect of the cognitive-behavioral you can do it! Education program on the resilience of Japanese elementary school students: A preliminary investigation. *International Journal of Education Research, 86*, 50–58. https://doi.org/10.1016/j.ijer.2017.08.006

Chapter 21
REBT Coaching for Young People to Achieve Goals and Develop in Life

Demetris Katsikis and Chrysoula Kostogiannis

Introduction

Coaching young people without mental health issues to achieve greater success to flourish as well as to solve practical and emotional barriers to these outcomes is an emerging and promising field for preparing children and adolescents to develop in life. The main focus of coaching young people is to help them achieve personal, interpersonal, and social development goals through step-by-step guidance. Coaching younger populations can be viewed as a specific evidence-based method including an active process that helps them learn new attitudes and social–emotional skills for successful attainments, good health, and wellbeing (Katsikis, Kassapis, Kostogiannis, & Bernard, 2018). Given the persistent call from mental health scientists-practitioners to help today's youth establish healthy attitudes, stable character strengths, and long-term social–emotional and behavioral skills (e.g., Bernard, 2017, 2018; Collaborative for Academic, Social, Emotional Learning [CASEL], 2005; Durlak, Domitrovich, Weissberg, & Gullotta, 2016; Durlak, Weissberg, Dymnicki, Taylor, & Schellinger, 2011; Giant, 2014; Katsikis, Kostogiannis, Kassapis, Katsiki, & Bernard, 2018; Ratner & Yusuf, 2015; Sklad, Diekstra, Ritter, Ben, & Gravesteijn, 2012) coaching can efficiently serve and promote this purpose.

D. Katsikis (✉) · C. Kostogiannis
Institute for Rational-Emotive and Cognitive Behavior Therapy, Athens, Greece
e-mail: dkatsikis@recbt.gr

M. Bernard, M. D. Terjesen (eds.), *Rational-Emotive and Cognitive-Behavioral Approaches to Child and Adolescent Mental Health: Theory, Practice, Research, Applications*, https://doi.org/10.1007/978-3-030-53901-6_21

Definitions, Forms, and Roles of Coaching Young People

Typically, coaching children and adolescents involves one-to-one, small-group, group and classroom conversations focused on the enhancement of learning and development through increasing self, other, and life self-awareness as well as developing their sense of self and social responsibility (van Nieuwerburgh, 2012). Through Socratic or didactic questioning and coach–coachee mutual collaboration, the coach facilitates the self-directed learning of the young coachee, demonstrates active listening skills and empathy, and teaches a wide array of social–emotional skills and values in a supportive and motivational environment. The coach helps the coachees to: (a) set realistic goals, (b) follow specific steps toward these goals, (c) create a space or environment in which change occurs, (d) look for feedback and measure progress, (e) build self-awareness, (f) build self-confidence, (g) use internal resources and achieve resilience, (g) focus on their potential and their future, (h) create their own toolkit of resources and strategies to use at any time and be empowered to plan and (i) take steps on a path toward change and get support to move forward on their journey through life (Giant, 2014).

Coaching young people includes a wide range of applications for different developmental ages, stages, and populations following Piaget and Vygotsky's works (e.g., Costa, Garmston, Hayes, & Ellison, 2015; Karten, 2013) and involving different evidence-based approaches (e.g., Behavioral Coaching, Cognitive-Behavioral Coaching, Educational Leadership Coaching, Instructional Coaching, Literacy Coaching, Peer Coaching, Solution-Focused Coaching; for a review see Devine, Meyers, & Houssemand, 2013). Coaching children and adolescents can be *direct* (immediate work with the child or adolescent) and *indirect* (working with parents, teachers and important other persons in child's or adolescent's life) during coaching practice. (In this chapter, the author focuses on the direct coaching form with children and adolescents.)

Coaching younger populations can take place in different settings (e.g., private practice, school, community youth centers and related services, clinic, etc.) where safety and privacy are ensured. In out-of-school settings, coaching young populations is usually conducted by specialists trained in evidence-based theories and applications to younger populations (e.g., child psychologists and related counselors, sporting coaches, mentors, social workers, psychiatrists, other wellbeing specialists, etc.). In the school setting, coaching younger populations (for a related chapter see Katsikis, Kassapis, et al., 2018) can either be conducted by all trained school personnel (including parents), in case coaching is required and applied on a *schoolwide* basis, or by teachers and other school mental health specialists in case coaching is optional and applied on a *targeted assistance* basis.

The main role of the coach who directly works with younger populations is to encourage, facilitate, motivate, and enhance the coachee's attainments, health, and wellbeing by fostering self-directed tools, techniques, and creative means for personal growth and development (Green, Grant, & Rynsaardt, 2007). The coach helps kids and teens become active and directive agents of their own development and blossom academically, behaviorally, emotionally, professionally, and socially by acting as a catalyst, educator, facilitator, mentor, motivator, pedagogist, and life teacher. The effective coach establishes active coaching alliance and trust with the coachee; genuinely strives to help coachees construct meaning and attain goals; offers ample understanding, empathy, and respect; inspires confidence to the coachees and is proponent of direct responsible action, reflection, and learning. Following Ellis's model of 11 rational living principles (Bernard, 2011), coaches help young coachees establish: (a) self-interest balanced with (b) social interest, (c) self-direction, (d) unconditional self-acceptance, (e) tolerance of others, (f) good balance between short-term and long-term hedonism, (g) commitment to creative, absorbing activities and pursuits, (h) responsible risk-taking and experimenting, (i) high frustration tolerance and willpower, (j) effective problem-solving skills, and (k) scientific thinking and flexibility.

In schools, coaches may also act as (a) resource providers by expanding the coachees' use of academic skills to improve school performance and achievement, (b) insurers that young people implement their school tasks appropriately in a curriculum-based way (c) providers of optimal methodologies and best practices that the coachees can use to meet specific learning challenges, (d) supporters and facilitators of the coachee's active participation (e.g., observation, reflection, asking feedback, providing innovative ideas, etc.) in the class or the small group, (e) catalysts of change in current school practices that need revision and development in favor of students and (f) establishers of a health-related climate and environment in the school setting (Bernard, 2016a, 2016b; Killion, Harrison, Bryan, & Clifton, 2012).

Differences Among Coaching, Counseling, and Therapy

As Dryden (2011) points out, emotional and behavioral problems exist and may get in the way of productive coaching and, therefore, counseling, psychotherapy, and coaching can have some common grounds. Neenan and Palmer (2012) also stated, "We believe that some distinctions between therapy and coaching are overstated – therapy often gets dismissed as just repairing weakness and dysfunction, while coaching is focused on unlocking potential, improving performance, enhancing well-being and delivering results" (p. 3). Despite these fundamental viewpoints, the author reports explicit and specific differences among coaching young people and doing counseling or psychotherapy with the same populations. Main differences are reported in Table 21.1 (based on Freeman, personal communication, July 18, 2017; adapted, modified, and enriched by the author).

The main difference, then, between counseling or psychotherapy and coaching is that the latter is based on sanogenetic models of change that rely on preventive and proactive actions toward young people's development, goal achievement, and wellness (Katsikis, Kostogiannis, & Dryden, 2016). Additionally, the author would emphasize (a) the clear orientation of coaching to the future, (b) its' action orientation, (c) the inclusion of strengths-based approaches and (d) the prominent emphasis on goal attainment and wellbeing.

Table 21.1 Differences between coaching and counseling/psychotherapy fields

Child/adolescent Counseling or psychotherapy	Child/adolescent Coaching
Pathogenetic models	Sanogenetic models
Rehabilitation	Development
Emotional and problem-solving goals	Developmental goals
Mental health	Wellbeing
*Inter*vention and *re*action	*Pre*vention and *pro*action
Disorders, dysfunctions and problems (e.g., diagnostic and statistical manual of mental disorders, DSM-5; APA, 2013)	Issues, challenges and functions (e.g., international classification of functioning, disability and health, ICF; WHO, 2001)
Why are you the way you are?	*How* do you *change* from the way you are?
Session	Meeting
Patient, client	Coachee
Serve young people with disorders or dysfunctions	Serves a continuum of students' mental health (Bernard, 2018)
Clinic	Community (e.g., school, home, recreational settings)
Treatment	Management
Deficits, distortions, irrational beliefs	Strengths, accurate inferences, rational beliefs
Transference and counter-transference	Mutual collaboration based on trust
Resistance or defensiveness	Barriers, roadblocks, doubts, objections, disagreements, queries, questions towards development
From the past to present	From present to the future
Insight-oriented work	Action-oriented work
Work *through* personal issues	Work *around* personal issues

The author highlights that coaching young populations is an effective service for a continuum of student mental health from disorders to flourishing (Bernard, 2018; see Fig. 21.1).

Bernard (2018) has written: It seems to me that a school's mental health and well-being program should have a dual focus: (1) helping prevent and reduce students' social–emotional difficulties and mental health problems and (2) promoting students' positive well-being and flourishing. Programs and practices address the positive and negative dimensions of student mental health that can be represented on a continuum from −10 to +10. At −10 to −5 are those students with extreme mental health problems such as anxiety disorders, ADHD, eating disorders). From −5 to 0 are students with less severe social–emotional problems that block their well-being and success including worry, feeling down, and anger. From 0 to +5 are students without significant social–emotional difficulties but who have lesser to moderate degrees of positive well-being. +5 to 10 represent progressively well-adjusted students and those at the highest levels who are flourishing.

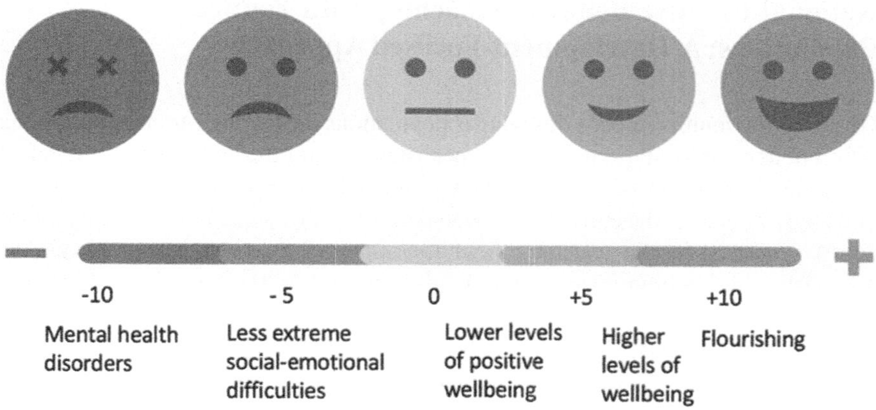

Fig. 21.1 Continuum of mental health to wellbeing: from disorders to flourishing (Bernard, 2018)

Following Bernard's continuum and adapting Dryden's work on which population can benefit the most from single-session work and very brief coaching procedures (Dryden, 2016), the author proposes that coaching can serve a wide array of younger populations including (a) young people who want to achieve goals and develop, (b) younger people with common, non-clinical, practical, or emotional problems, (c) younger people who view any kind of help (including coaching) as intermittent help through their different development stages, (d) younger people with clinical problems who want help with non-clinical problems.

Coaching: A Milestone for Young People

As a holistic initiative, coaching gives prominence to the human potential to flourish by strengthening the faculty of reason through active learning, goal setting, reflection, and action for goal achievement. The cultivation of reason during coaching process can promote self-responsibility through development of rational attitudes and beliefs. According to major Cognitive Behavior theories, like Rational-Emotive Behavior Theory (REBT), these attitudes and beliefs directly shape emotive, behavioral, and wellbeing factors in young populations (e.g., Bernard, 2018). Therefore, cultivation of rational attitudes and beliefs during coaching may foster abundance, art, beauty, mutual benevolence, communitarianism, culture, education, freedom, health, humanities, knowledge, peace, philosophy, pleasure, quality of life, life richness, satisfaction, safety, and science (see also Pinker, 2018). Focusing on the promotion of coaching young populations is a crucial step to provide children and adolescents with the social–emotional, behavioral, and wellbeing skills they need to flourish and develop in life.

Rational-Emotive Behavior Coaching with Younger Populations: A Development-Focused Approach

Given (a) the multiple needs of younger populations during their transitions among different developmental stages, (b) the persistent call for the betterment of students' social–emotional and behavioral health in the schools and community (Bernard, 2006, 2018), and (c) the current (e.g., Katsikis et al., 2016; Katsikis & Kostogiannis, 2016) synergies in the coaching field for applying evidence-based, integrative approaches in coaching younger populations, the author draws on Ellis's Rational-Emotive Behavior Theory (REBT) because of its extensive applications in the coaching field (Bernard & David, 2018).

REBT is the first and most comprehensive form of cognitive behavioral practice (CBT) (Bernard & Dryden, 2019; Dryden & Bernard, 2019; David, Lynn, & Ellis, 2010; Ellis, 1962, 1972, 1994, 2004; Ellis & Becker, 1982; Ellis & Dryden, 1997; Ellis & Harper, 1975) with wide applications in younger populations (Bernard, 2004, 2006; Ellis & Bernard, 2006; Knaus, 1974, 2001; Vernon, 1994, 2006a, 2006b, 2006c). REBC is the application of Ellis' REBT theory and practice to the coaching field (Bernard & David, 2018; Dryden, 2011, 2017; Katsikis et al., 2016).

Following Dryden (2017) and Katsikis et al. (2018), REBC in young populations can be (a) practical problem-focused, (b) emotional problem-focused, and (c) development-focused. The first two forms of coaching (practical and emotional-problem focused coaching) have been presented elsewhere regarding REBC in the schools (Katsikis et al., 2018) and, thus this chapter focuses on the development-focused REBC. This form of REBC focuses on strengths rather than overcoming problems and deficits like practical problem and emotional problem-focused REBC. The general goal of development-focused REBC is to help young populations establish happiness, success, and wellbeing by teaching them rational attitudes and related principles, skills, and values.

Development-Focused REBC Content. In the early and recent days of REBT, child psychologists, psychotherapists, teachers, and other child specialists present Rational-Emotive Education (Knaus, 1974, 2001) or Rational-Emotive Consultation (Vernon, 1994) on an individual, small group, group, or classroom basis in young populations (children, adolescents) and the accompanying adult populations (parents, teachers, school principals, etc.). Nowadays, a more comprehensive and developmental-focused approach that can be effectively used for development-focused REBC is based on the theory and practice of Michael Bernard's "You Can Do It! Education" (YCDI!; Bernard, 2013a, 2013b, 2018) programs. YCDI! programs include educational, coaching, and mentoring programs for younger populations from pre-K to 12th grade and can be effectively used during practical problem-focused, emotional-problem focused, and development-focused REBC with these populations. Recent research has established the effectiveness of YCDI! programs on development-focused (e.g., goal achievement, success, positive relationships, and wellbeing) and practical problem and emotional problem-focused REBC (e.g., betterment of various problematic behaviors and emotions; e.g., Ashdown &

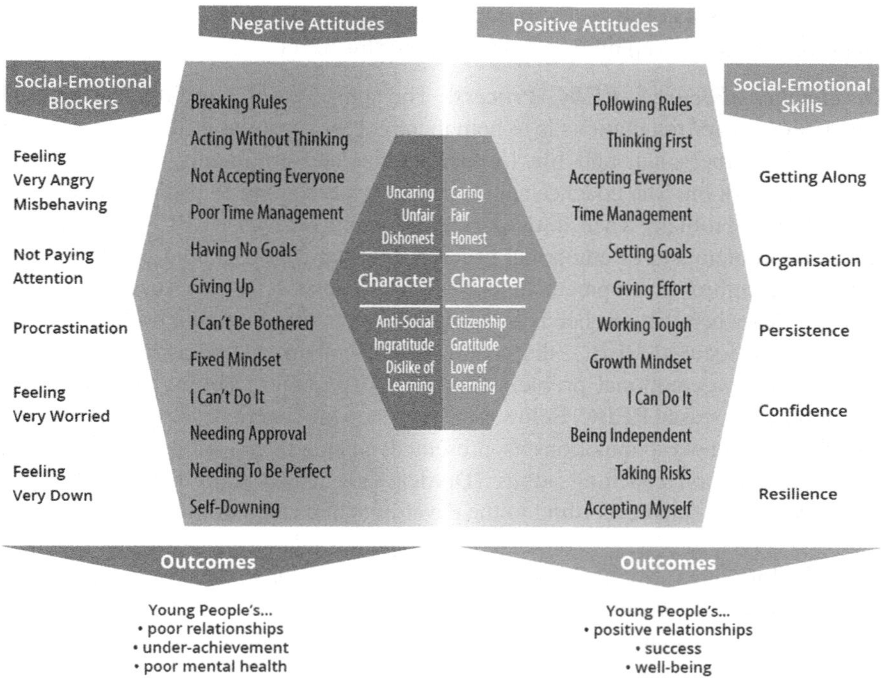

Fig. 21.2 Michael Bernard's social–emotional learning framework (Bernard, 2018)

Bernard, 2012; Bernard, 2017; Bernard & Walton, 2011; Markopoulos & Bernard, 2015; Yamamoto, Matsumoto, & Bernard, 2017).

The content of YCDI! Programs, including REBC, is based on the following social–emotional learning framework (see Fig. 21.2).

Regarding development-focused REBC content, the coach can include exercises and activities based on the right half section of the framework above. This section of Bernard's social–emotional learning framework addresses the positive aspects of the psychological functioning of young populations that lead to three positive outcomes, namely, positive relationships, success, and wellbeing (see outcomes in the right down section of the framework). To achieve these three outcomes, young people need to cultivate a range of positive character values and strengths (e.g., caring, fairness, honesty, citizenship, gratitude, love of learning), positive attitudes (e.g., compliance—following rules, thinking first—reflectivity, acceptance of everyone, time management, goal-setting, working tough—high frustration tolerance, growth mindset, I can do it!—optimism, self-acceptance) and five social–emotional skills (getting along, organization, persistence, confidence, resilience). The development-focused REBC coach can seek contents of these materials for explicit teaching and application in the YCDI! catalogue site (https://youcandoiteducation.com.au/blocks/androgogic_catalogue/index.php?c1=Schools&c2=Resources). Through discussions and activities pertaining to the positive attitudes section of Bernard's framework (character values and strengths, positive attitudes and social–emotional skills), the REBC coach helps the coachee(s) become aware, exercise, cultivate, empower, maintain, and ultimately, achieve her/his developmental goals.

Development-Focused REBC–Process. The purpose of development-focused REBC in younger populations is to help them get the most out of themselves in the personal, interpersonal, and life (home, school, and community) domains they choose to work on. The coachee should not be experiencing as primary a practical or emotional problem when initiating development-focused REBC and if s/he is, practical problem and/or emotional problem-focused REBC should be offered and completed before development-focused REBC starts. It is also strongly recommended that when the coachee is bringing a practical or emotional problem during development-focused REBC, the coach should embark temporarily on practical problem and/or emotional problem-focused REBC before getting back again to development-focused REBC. Below, a step-by-step process of development-focused REBC for younger populations is presented, adapted, and modified by related Dryden's work on coaching adults (Dryden, 2017). All steps below should be adapted and presented according to the developmental stage of the young coachee.

Step 1: Introduce Michael Bernard's Social–Emotional Learning framework including character strengths/values and positive attitudes as keys for goal achievement in terms of social–emotional skills and subsequent outcomes as the foundation for development-focused REBC.

- Help the young coachee to review the presence of social–emotional skills in her/his life through Bernard's surveys on social–emotional skills. Then discuss with the young coachee how s/he views her/his development including the role of strengths, values and attitudes in her/his current skills and outcomes, and the place of these skills and outcomes in her/his coaching experience).
- Help the young coachee decide how to use her/his strengths, values, and attitudes for goal achievement
  - Using strengths, values, and attitudes as broad goals in case the young coachee believes that they can be important *catalysts* for their development, the coach helps young coachees locate specific examples of the strengths, values, and attitudes from Bernard's framework through questions like "What goals or behaviors would you like to nominate that would indicate that you were more accepting others", for example.
  - Using strengths, values, and attitudes as specific *factors* in development-focused REBC. In this case, the young coachee first selects a goal that is important to her/him in terms of social–emotional skills and/or positive outcomes from the framework and then chooses either a value, a strength, or an attitude that will aid the pursuit of the goal. Here the young coachee reminds her/himself of the strength, the value, and/or the attitude from the framework while s/he is pursuing the goal. For example, consider a young coachee that selects to improve his/her confidence as a goal and then s/he chooses self-acceptance as the specific factor on which s/he has to work on to achieve the goal.

Step 2: Help the coachee to set goals. A good balance between goal *specificity* and goal *generality* to meet the developmental stages of younger populations (e.g., "I will know, when I do it") is important. Some strategies that will aid the goal-setting process are outlined below.

- Help the young coachee understand the characteristics of a development-focused goal. The coach helps the coachee to see that a good developmental goal is: (a) directive, including specific steps, (b) ongoing and long-term (without end-point), (c) when an end-point, this goal needs to be short-term, and (d) behavioral, translated into specific actions. Other goal typologies like SMART goals can also be used based on the philosophy of the coach.
- Help the young coachee to select a goal that the coachee wants to achieve rather than what others want her/him to achieve (unless both sides have equal goals).
- Help the young coachee to choose a goal from Bernard's framework (e.g., self-acceptance, confidence, etc.) and then translate it into behavioral action. If the young coachee has several developmental goals in mind, then help the coachee make a hierarchy of goals and select a target goal (the goal that the coachee wishes to pursue first) to start with.
- Help the young coachee to choose a goal that is personally meaningful to her/him and is not included in Bernard's or other frameworks used by the coach: Use other terms like "meaning", "purpose", "mission", "journey", "road", "importance", "fairy tale", or other developmentally appropriate terms that resonate with the young coachee. Although almost all goals have a pragmatic value for young people, they are less likely to persist in their pursuit unless they are underpinned by their personal values and strengths. For example, a child may say that finding more friends at school is a personally meaningful goal for her/him at the moment. This goal seems to be in the "getting along" category from Bernard's framework, but the young coachee is resonating more with the phrasing "finding more friends" than the former. Thus, in this case, the coach should help coachee make a behavioral plan on how to find more friends at school.
- Help the young coachee choose a goal that involves engaging with tasks that have intrinsic value for her/him. No matter how enjoyable the coaching tasks for the young coachee, s/he may avoid doing them because they may have not intrinsic merit for her/him. Therefore, the coach should help the young coachee do pleasant and/or unpleasant (but not harmful) tasks that are good for her/him to do because they will help her/him achieve what s/he wants.
- Help the young coachee to select a goal that s/he is prepared to integrate into her/his life. No matter how intrinsic, meaningful, or valued a goal is for the young coachee, if the latter cannot look at the place of this goal within the context of her/his life as whole, s/he will not pursue it. If the goal is highly valued by the young coachee but cannot, at present, be integrated into the coachee's life, the coach should invite her/him to think whether s/he wants to restructure her/his life to accommodate goal: If so, then the restructuring should take place to first accommodate the goal, if not, then the coach should invite the young coachee to select a goal that can be adapted into her/his life.

- Help the young coachee to choose an objective for which s/he is prepared to make sacrifices to achieve. If the young coachee is prepared to restructure her/his life to accommodate her/his valued developmental goal, then the coach helps the coachee to consider what changes s/he is prepared to make to do this. The more the young coachee is prepared to make selected sacrifices, the more s/he will be willing to pursue her/his desired goals. The coach should expel the implications for making the selected sacrifices on other people in the young coachee's life and, then it is important that these other people are told of the sacrifice so that they can decide to give or not give their consent or support to the subsequent change for the young coachee.

Step 3: Help the young coachee to design an action plan. When helping the coachee to set an action plan for reaching her/his development-based goal, it is crucial to:

- Help the young coachee to devise a clear method for determining the degree of accomplishment of her/his development-based goal. When the development-based goal is broad, it is important to remember that it has specific elements (e.g., the enactment of a specific resilience skill in a specific situation when the young coachee broadly desires to improve her/his resilience skills). These help the young coachee track her/his progress towards the broad goal. Once the young coachee has accomplished the goal, it is important to ask her/him how s/he will know precisely if s/he will go about maintaining it. This requires the REBC coach and the young coachee to work collaboratively and may involve using an existing or devising a customized measure of tracking the young coachee's progress towards the goal and her/his maintenance of the goal once achieved. Depending on the goal(s) and the wishes of the coachee, some goals may be evaluated in a more general, experiential-based ways instead of a more specific one.

- Help the young coachee to referent actions that s/he wishes to take to achieve the goal. The coachee should be guided to select actions that s/he already has the skills to perform (in case of a lack of skill, the coach collaborates with the coachee on how the latter is going to learn the skills, from whom and in which setting).
- Help the young coachee to build a realistic time schedule to achieve her/his goal. This schedule will be partly based on the length of the coaching contract and how many goals the coachee wishes to achieve during the REBC process. Once the coachee has determined the time schedule, s/he should be guided to allocate tasks to different time slots so that both coach and coachee know what to do by when and by what means. This schedule needs to be monitored and modified based on the coachee's actual experience of implementing the action plan.
- Ensure that the young coachee can apply the action plan into her/his life: The coachee commits her/himself to act at particular times that is convenient to her/him and in contexts that are accessible. If not the case, the coach should help the coachee to make modifications so that her/his action plan fits into her/his life.
- Motivate the young coachee to set a launch date to inform others (if the coachee wishes that). In case it resonates with the coachee, discuss what this might

involve and whether s/he wants to "go public" with this. If this does not appeal to the coachee, have her/him begin as s/he wishes.

Step 4: Help the young coachee implement the action plan. When the action plan is launched, the coach has to perform several tasks to help the coachee monitor and stay on course toward goal achievement.

- Encourage the coachee to use their selection of motivating or mediating variables from Bernard's social–emotional framework through a variety of selected REBC activities and techniques (see *Development-focused REBC – Content* above) related to the coachee's goal achievement. The coachee can learn to constantly remind her/himself frequently of the importance of the goal in her/his life (e.g., "I am doing this activity because I want to improve my getting along skills"). Or s/he can select a character strength, value, attitude, or skill to keep in mind while pursuing the goal. And s/he can directly work on specific handouts from Michael Bernard's YCDI! materials on specific character strengths, values, attitudes, skills, and outcomes. While doing several of these tasks, the coachee can be helped to either think that "doing this will help me be more creative in life" or deal with potential barriers by telling her/himself that "even if I fail today, I am not a failure. I am a fallible kid and I can learn from failure".
- Monitor the young coachee's implementation of the action plan. Sometimes, the time-based action schedule of the coachee will need to be changed in light of the coachee's experiences or changes. As such, it is crucial that the coach monitors her/his progress along the way. Such monitoring requires coach–coachee collaboration with parties both being clear about what the latter is going to do and reviewing what s/he did exploring potential discrepancies between plans and achievements. Any action plan changes should emerge out of the coachee's experiences of implementing it, and any barriers should be addressed.
- Help the young coachee to capitalize on her/his success when it is clear that s/he is doing well with respect to her/his action plan. There are two ways to do this: One way is to find out what the coachee has been doing that has brought about her/his progress and to suggest that s/he continues doing what is working for her/him. Another way is to encourage the coachee to think of ways that s/he can generalize what s/he has been learning from implementing her/his development-based goal to other relevant areas of her/his life where s/he would like to develop.
- Help the young coachee to maintain her/his gains once s/he has met her/his goal. For example, the coach can help the coachee, (a) identify and implement steps s/he will need to take and maintain her/his gains, (b) identify and deal with any barriers that might interfere with the maintenance strategies followed during REBC, (c) develop high frustration tolerance for boredom and discomfort that s/he might experience during the maintenance process, and (d) identify and deal with any vulnerability factors that, if faced, might lead them to experience lapses in the use of maintenance strategies which may affect the gains achieved from development-focused REBC.
- Help the coachee pursue other goals and generalize learning once s/he has shown evidence of maintaining their main development-based goal. Then, the coachee

is more prepared to pursue another relevant goal, and the coach can help her/him go through the same process with the new goal informed by the work that s/he has done on the first goal. As the coachee makes progress on the second goal, the coach can encourage her/him to look for patterns among the goals set at the beginning and use these patterns as s/he increasingly takes on the role of her/his own coach.

The more the REBC coach can help the young coachee to identify and use helpful patterns of strengths, values, attitudes, and skills, and acting from the work s/he has done on her/his goals, the more the former can help the latter to formalize these as self-development principles and generalize them across different life domains. These principles would include some of the character strengths and values, positive attitudes and social–emotional skills outlined in Bernard's social–emotional framework (put in the young coachee's own words). Other principles that fall outside this framework and they are endorsed as helpful by the coach in collaboration with the coachee during development-based REBC should also be considered.

Common Problems and Barriers during Development-Focused REBC

One of the many benefits of REBC is that it can help young populations prepare for and manage common developmental challenges and barriers or problems (Katsikis et al., 2018). Despite the flourishing effects of development-focused REBC, young populations may temporarily hinder their development toward goal achievement, good health, and wellbeing when they face internal and/or external challenges, issues, barriers, or problems during their development.

According to the social–emotional framework of Bernard (Fig. 21.2), children and adolescents may face five social–emotional blockers (feeling anger and misbehavior, not paying attention, procrastination, feeling very worried, feeling very down) because of 12 negative attitudes (non-compliance, impulsiveness, non-acceptance of others, poor time management, non-goal setting, giving up, low frustration tolerance, fixed mindset, pessimism, approval seeking, perfectionism, self-depreciation) and under-developed character values and strengths (lack of caring, unfairness, dishonesty, anti-sociality, ingratitude, disliking of learning) that can potentially lead them to poor outcomes like poor relationships, underachievement, and poor mental health.

Additionally, Vernon (2002, 2009c) has proposed a REBT model illustrating how irrational thinking of children and adolescents, their developmental level, and other situational factors may gradually derail their self, emotional, social, physical, and cognitive development and play a major role on how they respond to typical developmental problems. According to this model, irrational thinking like demandingness, awfulizing/overgeneralizing, low frustration tolerance and self-downing may interact (or not) with other situational factors (e.g., physical abuse, sexual abuse, alcoholism, death/AIDS disease, divorce, alternative family structures, homelessness, poverty, stepfamily, violence). All these factors may challenge younger populations when facing typical developmental issues in terms of belonging-rejection, competition, dating, fears, grades, relationships with parents, peer relations, puberty, sexual identity, sexuality, striving to be independent, sports performance, and transitions. If irrational thinking is intensively, frequently, and constantly interacting with the above situational factors during the aforementioned developmental issues, it may lead to more serious challenges and problems like substance abuse, criminal behavior, delinquent behavior, eating disorders, sexual acting out, gang involvement, self-mutilation, teen pregnancy, suicide, and violent behavior.

Although development-focused REBC is highly emerging and much promising in addressing the whole development of young populations, its central focus and purpose is not to directly address the above common barriers, challenges, or problems. In such cases, when the coachee faces a common barrier, challenge, or problem like the ones included in Bernard's and Vernon's models (except from the serious problems in Vernon's model), the coach should convert the development-focused REBC process into an emotional problem and/or practical problem-focused REBC process. While the development-focused REBC coachee may have neither experienced an emotional problem nor a practical problem that required professional help during the recent past, when facing either or both types of problems, it is time that the coach apply the appropriate REBC coaching process to help the coachee regulate her/his emotions (in case of an emotional problem) and/or find appropriate solutions to a practical problem (in case of a practical problem) and then resume the development-focused REBC process. This can be done several times during the development-focused REBC process provided that the coachee's emotional and/or practical goals during the respective REBC processes do not overshadow the development-based goals that have been set at the outset of the development-focused REBC process.

In case that (a) the emotional problem of the young coachee is of recent origin or occurs intermittently, (b) her/his emotional reactions lie within a mild to moderate range of distress, (c) the emotional problem is limited to a certain situation or aspect of the young coachee's life, (d) the young coachee is not defensive with respect to the problem, and (e) s/he is open to address and change the problem (Cavanagh, 2005), then the coach should temporarily change the focus of the REBC process from the development-focused goals to the emotional problem. Accordingly, the coach helps the young coachee locate an unhealthy negative (or unhealthy positive) emotion and teaches her/him how to use the ABCDEF model of REBT to deal effectively with the located unhealthy emotion by converting it to a healthy one. When the coachee deals effectively with her/his emotional problem, then the coachee resumes the development-focused REBC process.

Taking into account the same aforementioned prerequisites, if the young coachee appears with a practical problem that hinders her/his progress during development-focused REBC, the coach applies practical problem-focused REBC to help the coachee deal effectively with that problem. In this case, the young coachee is usually confused or tangled up with a practical issue or issues and needs clarity, solutions, and a problem-solving, step-by-step process which s/he hopes to get by talking things through with the coach but s/he is not emotionally distressed about the issue(s). If the young coachee does have an emotional problem about her/his practical issue, the former in REBC is generally tackled before the latter as the presence of the emotional problem will impede and distract the coachee from focusing on solving the practical problem. Given that the coachee is helped to deal effectively with her/his emotional problem (if any) about her/his practical problem through emotional problem-focused REBC, then the coach helps the young coachee with her/his practical problem by helping her/him apply effective REBT action methods like problem-solving, positive reinforcement, stimulus control, time-out, skills training, in vivo desensitization, and other acceptable behavioral methods. When the coachee deals effectively with her/his practical problem, then the coachee resumes the development-focused REBC process.

There is a wide array of exercises, activities, and techniques for the coach who turns from development-focused REBC to practical problem and emotional problem-focused REBC that can be found in Michael Bernard's YCDI! database and Ann Vernon's "Thinking, Feeling, Behaving" curricula (2006a, 2006b) and other related counseling and coaching resources for children and adolescents (Vernon, 2002, 2009c; Vernon & Barry, 2013). Through creative discussions and other counseling arts (e.g., activity-based experiential interventions, drama, literature, music, play and games, visual arts, expressive writing, etc.), the coach can help the young coachee during emotional problem and/or practical problem-focused REBC to effectively tackle issues of acting out, anger, anxiety, bullying, grief, guilt, lowered mood, perfectionism, performance and competition, procrastination, relationships, low self-acceptance, self-consciousness, self-downing, stress, low frustration tolerance, teasing, transitions, underachievement, and then resume to development-focused REBC.

In case that (a) the young coachee has serious, multiple, and complicated emotional and/or practical problems that exceed (in terms of time and energy spent during the coaching process) the developmental goals initially set by her/him at the outset of the development-focused REBC, (b) there is persistent resistance or high reluctance (and not temporary lack of collaboration) on the part of the young coachee, (c) initial efforts on the part of the coach to establish either development-focused, practical problem or emotional problem-focused REBC have failed and (d) the young coachee had several, non-successful coaching and/or therapeutic/counseling experiences in the past (especially non-successful REBT-related experiences), then the coach should refer the coachee for other or more intensive services (e.g., full biopsychosocial assessment, individual therapy, etc.).

A Case of Development-Focused REBC in a 14-Year-Old Boy Who Wished to Flourish in Terms of Confidence and Getting Along

Giannis is a 14-year-old boy that was referred to the author for "mental health services" (according to the written words of the body of referral). During the first meeting, Giannis and his parents expressed their concern about the former's recent lowered mood, lowered peer relations, and poorer school grades, but their main concerns was his lack of confidence and peer relationships. The ADHD Rating Scale-5 of DuPaul, Power, Anastopoulos, and Reid (parent and teacher versions) administrated through the body of referral had shown mild symptoms of inattention, while the rest of mental health assessments conducted showed no other significant problems. The family seemed to be cohesive and was highly collaborative with the author. The author asked Giannis and the parents what they would like to achieve (Giannis was asked individually and then the family as a whole about Giannis). Both Giannis and his parents said that they recognized his problems aforementioned problems but they were all feeling sad because they had still not found a mental health specialist that s/he would help Giannis develop as a person in personal, social, and school territories of his life. They both seemed to not want Giannis to take "psychotherapy" or "counseling" sessions because they, believed that his problems were pretty manageable by all members in the family (Giannis had a 17-year-old sister) and that they wished Giannis could find a person that would make a close, helping relationship with him and that this person would help him flourish as a person and achieve his goals in life despite his current difficulties.

Accordingly, the author introduced Giannis and his parents to the REBC coaching content and process by presenting them a PowerPoint on a big screen in his office related to the three REBC coaching types (development-focused, practical problem-focused, and emotional problem focused REBC) tailoring the importance of development-focusing coaching with their wish as expressed in their words during their meeting with the author. Giannis and his parents were totally in agreement with development-focused coaching, and they all signed a related contract with the author (Giannis and the parents were open to the number of coaching sessions. They said that they will be happy that Giannis take as many sessions as possible as soon as he achieves his goals).

During Step 1 of the development-focused REBC, the author introduced Giannis to Bernard's Social–Emotional Learning Framework including strengths/values, attitudes, and skills as milestones for goal achievement and holistic personal development. He helped Giannis to review the presence of social–emotional skills in his life (through school-related and generalized versions of Bernard's Personal Evaluation survey (Bernard, 2013b)). Giannis had lower scores in confidence and getting along. Then the coach helped Giannis learn how to use strengths, values, and attitudes for positive outcomes by highlighting the relations among these four elements.

During Step 2, the author helped Giannis to set goals by helping him understand the characteristics of a development-focused goal (directive, ongoing, broad with specific steps to act on) and select a goal from Bernard's framework that (a) had intrinsic value for him, (b) was currently based on Giannis's strength, (c) the tasks included in it had intrinsic value for him, (d) could be integrated in his life, and (e) he was prepared to make sacrifices to achieve it. Giannis chose confidence and getting along as areas to be empowered and then he decided three specific attitudes to achieve his goals, (a) growth mindset (for confidence) (b) self-acceptance (for confidence), and (c) non-approval seeking (for getting along).

Specifically, Giannis decided that his confidence would be empowered if he learned to play the violin and that this would be an important indicator of a growth mindset for him, because he wanted that from his childhood years but he had never stepped up. He also decided that confidence would be boosted if he accepts himself unconditionally each time he struggles with his homework or receives a lower grade school by endorsing the attitude, "I am Giannis and I accept myself no matter what I do and that's ok" (self-acceptance). Giannis also decided to practice getting along by continually telling and supporting his viewpoints in front of his peers' disapprovals by endorsing the mindset that "I can continue supporting my own viewpoint despite important other peers' disapproval".

These goals had intrinsic value for Giannis because *he* wanted to achieve them (he also said that his parents would agree with these goals). Giannis chose these goals, because they were based on two "fundamental", as he said, character strengths and values from Bernard's framework (accepting himself and being independent, regarding the goal of confidence and being caring and honest regarding the goal of getting along). He selected these goals because they had a special meaning in his current life and because he highly valued them as important prerequisites for a better adolescence. He also stated that he was fully prepared to undertake the tasks included to achieve these goals and that he was ready to make sacrifices despite possible barriers like lower self-acceptance, lower frustration tolerance, and possible rejections of his viewpoints from others at school. Giannis decided to begin with confidence and the growth mindset marker (to learn how to play the violin).

During Steps 3 and 4, the author helped Giannis design an action plan and implement it. Giannis came up with the following action plan to learn how to play the violin: (a) buy a violin, (b) find a place to rehearse or use a section of his house's basement as a rehearsal room, (c) find a trained violin teacher that he is comfortable with, (d) arrange a series of lessons, (e) devise a practice schedule, and (f) join a band or orchestra when competent to play. The author helped Giannis to devise a 6-point scale for measuring his goal above. For example, if Giannis buys a violin, finds a place to rehearse, finds a violin teacher, and arranges a series of lessons, his score will be 4, because he will have achieved the 4 out of the 6 actions included in his action plan.

With respect to confidence and getting along and their selected markers (self-acceptance and non-approval seeking, respectively), Giannis was given an array of age-appropriate activities and exercises from Michael Bernard's book *The You Can Do It! Education Mentoring Program* (Bernard, 2013b).

Regarding the self-acceptance attitude "I am Giannis and I accept myself no matter what I do and that's ok" that Giannis wanted to empower to achieve more confidence, the author helped him through YCDI! activities (a) define "real" confidence (through self-acceptance), (b) identify degrees of his confidence, (c) list confidence building blocks (successful achievements in the past, possible barriers on achieving new things, positive thinking that he had learned from past achievements), (d) build confidence self-talk, (e) establish and boost confidence self-talk, (f) list personal strengths and weaknesses, (g) exercise on unconditional self-acceptance, h) learn that taking responsible risks and making mistakes is not so bad, and (i) make individual action plans for implementing his chosen risks.

Regarding the non-approval seeking attitude "I can continue support my own viewpoint despite important other peers' disapproval" that Giannis wanted to empower to achieve better getting along, the author helped him through YCDI! activities (a) define "real" getting along (mutual cooperation, sharing of experiences, and doing creative stuff all together), (b) cooperate with other people, (c) resolve conflicts by discussion rather than fights, (d) manage state anger, (e) show tolerance of other peers' characteristics and disapprovals, and (f) react to difficult people and pressure situations in a positive way.

Special attention was given to Giannis in terms of maintaining his effort during each step of the above action plan: Each time Giannis was fulfilling a step or an activity, he was responsible to tick an appropriate box including each step or activity and "go public" with this success to his parents, the author, and his favorite friends. Also, the author ensured that Giannis had the skills to enact the tasks that each goal included: A trained violin teacher would evaluate Giannis's potential to become a violin player and the author examined data from the full psychoeducational assessment that was conducted with Giannis from the body of referral (indeed, Giannis had average or above average abilities, school achievement, and social–emotional–behavioral skills). The author also ensured that Giannis could apply the action plans and the activities administered with convenience in all contexts selected to be applied (home and school). Throughout Step 3, Giannis was reminded by the author to keep his selected character strengths/values, positive attitudes, social–emotional skills to the front of his mind when designing and implementing his action plan and the subsequent activities/exercises. Indeed, Giannis had convinced himself to constantly thinking that "doing all this will help me be more creative in life".

Giannis implemented his action plan and activities/exercises as above but found it difficult to find a rehearsal room having to travel half an hour per day to find an appropriate place to rehearse the violin. However, he persisted with this and eventually found a peer neighbor who had a big enough empty basement that he and his parents could make it available for 2 hours of violin rehearsals per day.

Giannis also faced an issue with two of his peers when they made fun of him while he was stating his viewpoints during recess and the author used emotional problem-focused REBC to help him deal with his emotions of anger and shame which led him to stop trying his getting along activities for 1 week. As Giannis was becoming more familiar with the development-focused REBC content and process, he was able to use it to good effect that he resumed his getting along activities and behavioral exposures after addressing his emotions of anger and shame and asserting himself with his peers.

All in all, Giannis attended 24 sessions and achieved greater confidence and getting along by increasing his average scores on these subscales in Bernard's related instrument (his confidence scores from 11 out of 25 in the pre-test to 22 out of 25 in the post-test and his getting along scores from 9 out of 25 in the pre-test to 23 out of 25 in the post-test based on a 5-point Likert scale from "never" to "very often"). Not only did he start learning and advancing in violin but he also was thinking, feeling, and behaving more in self-acceptance and non-approval seeking terms based on his observations and his parents' observations. He also capitalized on these successes on learning basic piano skills, expanding unconditional acceptance to others (besides himself) and making more friends without being pre-occupied on their viewpoints or disapprovals about him as a person.

The development-focused REBC process closed with the author helping Giannis maintain his gains once he met his goals. Thus, the author observed that Giannis had a lot of grit and passion along the way and helped him cultivate these two elements through further activities and exercises from Bernard's mentoring resources book. The author also helped Giannis more with high frustration tolerance exercises to help him reinforce his assertive (instead of his older passive or mildly assertive) actions toward his peers when peer disapproval was getting in his way. The author also met with Giannis's parents where they highlighted the importance of maintaining Giannis's progress by monitoring how effectively he applies his newly acquired skills and cautioned Giannis and his parents to be alert for possible barriers, challenges, and vulnerabilities that might lead him to experience lapses.

The author gave Giannis a certificate of development-focused REBC graduation and proposed to him that they will have three follow-up coaching sessions (in a month, in 3 months, in 6 months) to see if learning was maintained and generalized and if Giannis would like to pursue other relevant or totally new goals. The author encouraged Giannis and his parents to look for patterns among the goals set at the beginning and use these patterns as he was increasingly taking on the role of his own coach.

Conclusion

Development-focused REBC can stand alone, as a self-sufficient service, integrating other REBC types (and other mental health services) on the road to personal goal achievement and happiness of younger populations.

Development-focused REBC can become a paradigm shift in mental health practice moving the mentality from diagnosis and disorders or problems to wellbeing, flourishing, and getting the most out of all (young) people.

Development-focused REBC with its cutting-edge theoretical, research, and practice is already transforming the way we see and apply effective services in younger populations.

Development-focused REBC is gradually becoming the catalyst toward integrative mental health services and rational education of children across the whole mental health continuum, from mental health disorders to flourishing, by reminding us of the common goal that all responsible mental health services strive for today: self, other, and life happiness.

Test Yourself

1. How would you differentiate the clinical approach of REBT from development-focused REBC?
2. Identify three of the common barriers toward implementing development-focused REBC?
3. What role do strengths, values, and attitudes playing in REBC?

References

American Psychiatric Association. (2013). *Diagnostic and statistical manual of mental disorders* (5th ed.). Arlington, VA: Author.

Ashdown, D. M., & Bernard, M. E. (2012). Can explicit instruction in social and emotional learning skills benefit the social-emotional development, well-being, and academic achievement of young children? *Early Childhood Education Journal, 39*(6), 397–405.

Bernard, M. E. (2004). *The REBT therapist's pocket companion for working with children and adolescents*. New York: Albert Ellis Institute.

Bernard, M. E. (2006). It's time we teach social-emotional competence as well as we teach academic competence. *Reading and Writing Quarterly, 22*(2), 103–119.

Bernard, M. E. (2011). *Rationality and the pursuit of happiness: The legacy of Albert Ellis*. New York: Springer.

Bernard, M. E. (2013a). You Can Do It! Education: A social-emotional learning program for increasing the achievement and well-being of children and adolescents. In K. Yamasaki (Ed.), *School-based prevention education for health and adjustment problems in the world*. Tokyo, Japan: Kaneko Shobo.

Bernard, M. E. (2013b). *The You Can Do It! Education mentoring program* (2nd ed.). Oakleigh, VIC: Australian Scholarships Group.

Bernard, M. E. (2016a). *Stress management for teachers and principals*. Oakleigh, VIC: Australian Scholarships Group.

Bernard, M. E. (2016b). Beliefs and teacher stress. *Journal of Rational-Emotive & Cognitive-Behavior Therapy, 34*(3), 209–224. https://doi.org/10.1007/s10942-016-0238-y

Bernard, M. E. (2017). Impact of teaching attitudes and behaviors for learning on the reading achievement of students falling behind. *International Journal of Learning, Teaching and Educational Research, 16*(8), 51–64.

Bernard, M. E. (2018). NEW program achieve (years 1–6; years 7–12). In *A social-emotional learning curriculum*. East Melbourne, VIC: The Bernard Group. Retrieved from https://youcandoiteducation.com.au/

Bernard, M. E., & David, O. A. (Eds.). (2018). *Coaching for rational living: Theory, techniques and applications*. Cham, Switzerland: Springer.

Bernard, M. E., & Dryden, W. (Eds.). (2019). *Advances in REBT: Theory, practice, research, measurement, prevention and promotion*. Cham, Switzerland: Springer.

Bernard, M. E., & Walton, K. (2011). The effect of You Can Do It! Education in six schools on student perceptions of well-being, teaching, learning and relationships. *Journal of Student Wellbeing, 5*(1), 22–37.

Cavanagh, M. J. (2005). Mental-health issues and challenging coachees in executive coaching. In M. J. Cavanagh, A. M. Grant, & T. Kemp (Eds.), *Evidence-based coaching: Theory, research and practice from the behavioural sciences* (pp. 21–36). Bowen Hills, QLD: Australian Academic Press.

Collaborative for Academic, Social, and Emotional Learning (CASEL). (2005). *Safe and sound: An educational leader's guide to evidence-based social and emotional learning (SEL) programs*. Chicago: Author.

Costa, A. L., Garmston, R. J., Hayes, C., & Ellison, J. (2015). *Cognitive coaching: Developing self-directed leaders and learners*. Lanham, MD: Rowman & Littlefield.

David, D., Lynn, S., & Ellis, A. (Eds.). (2010). *Rational and irrational beliefs. Implications for research, theory, and practice*. New York: Oxford University Press.

Devine, M., Meyers, R., & Houssemand, C. (2013). How can coaching make a positive impact within educational settings? *Procedia-Social and Behavioral Sciences, 93*, 1382–1389.

Dryden, W. (2011). *First steps in using REBT in life coaching*. New York: Albert Ellis Institute.

Dryden, W. (2016). *When time is at a premium: Cognitive-behavioural approaches to single-session therapy and very brief coaching*. London: Rationality.

Dryden, W. (2017). *A practical guide to rational emotive behavioural coaching*. Hove, UK: Routledge.

Dryden, W., & Bernard, M. E. (Eds.). (2019). *REBT with diverse client problems and populations*. Cham, Switzerland: Springer.

Durlak, J. A., Domitrovich, C. E., Weissberg, R. P., & Gullotta, T. P. (Eds.). (2016). *Handbook of social and emotional learning: Research and practice*. New York: Guilford.

Durlak, J. A., Weissberg, R. P., Dymnicki, A. B., Taylor, R. D., & Schellinger, K. B. (2011). The impact of enhancing students' social and emotional learning: A meta-analysis of school-based universal interventions. *Child Development, 82*(1), 405–432.

Ellis, A. (1962). *Reason and emotion in psychotherapy*. Secaucus, NJ: Lyle Stuart.

Ellis, A. (1972). Emotional education in the classroom: The living school. *Journal of Clinical Child Psychology, 1*(3), 19–22.

Ellis, A. (1994). *Reason and emotion in psychotherapy* (Rev. updated ed.). New York: Birch Lane.

Ellis, A. (2004). Why rational-emotive behavior therapy is the most comprehensive and effective form of behavior therapy. *Journal of Rational-Emotive & Cognitive-Behavior Therapy, 22*(2), 85–92.

Ellis, A., & Becker, I. (1982). *A guide to personal happiness*. North Hollywood, CA: Wilshire.

Ellis, A., & Bernard, M. E. (Eds.). (2006). *Rational emotive behavioral approaches to childhood disorders: Theory, practice and research*. New York: Springer.

Ellis, A., & Dryden, W. (1997). *The practice of rational-emotive behavior therapy*. New York: Springer.

Ellis, A., & Harper, R. A. (1975). *A new guide to rational living*. North Hollywood, CA: Wilshire.

Giant, N. (2014). *Life coaching for kids: A practical manual to coach children and young people to success, well-being and fulfilment*. London: Jessica Kingsley.

Green, L. S., Grant, A. M., & Rynsaardt, J. (2007). Evidence-based life coaching for senior high school students: Building hardiness and hope. *International Coaching Psychology Review, 2*(1), 24–32.

Karten, T. J. (2013). *Inclusion coaching for collaborative schools*. Thousand Oaks, CA: Corwin.

Katsikis, D., Kassapis, S., Kostogiannis, C., & Bernard, M. E. (2018). Coaching in schools. In M. E. Bernard & O. A. David (Eds.), *Coaching for rational living* (pp. 397–412). Cham, Switzerland: Springer.

Katsikis, D., & Kostogiannis, C. (2016, June). School rational-emotive behavior coaching (S-REBC): Preliminary data and suggested applications. Paper presented at the 2nd International Congress of Cognitive Behavioral Coaching (2nd ICCBC), Athens, Greece.

Katsikis, D., Kostogiannis, C., & Dryden, W. (2016). A rational-emotive behavior approach in life coaching. *Journal of Evidence-Based Psychotherapies, 16*(1), 3–18.

Katsikis, D., Kostogiannis, C., Kassapis, S., Katsiki, A., & Bernard, M. E. (2018). Integrating social-emotional learning in schools: A proposal based on rational-emotive behavior education. *Effective Scientist-Practitioner, 1*(1), 19–45.

Killion, J., Harrison, C., Bryan, C., & Clifton, H. (2012). *Coaching matters*. Oxford, UK: Learning Forward.

Knaus, W. J. (1974). *Rational-emotive education: A guide for elementary school teachers*. New York: Institute for Rational Living.

Knaus, W. J. (2001). *Rational emotive education*. Retrieved September 10, 2009, from http://jinder.se/pdf/ebooks/Rational_Emotive_Education.pdf

Markopoulos, Z., & Bernard, M. E. (2015). Effect of the bullying: The power to cope program on children's response to bullying. *Journal of Relationships Research, 13*(6), 1–11.

Neenan, M., & Palmer, S. (Eds.). (2012). *Essential coaching skills and knowledge. Cognitive behavioural coaching in practice: An evidence based approach*. New York: Routledge.

Pinker, S. (2018). *Enlightenment now: The case for reason, science, humanism and progress*. London: Allen Lane.

Ratner, H., & Yusuf, D. (2015). *Brief coaching with children and young people: A solution focused approach*. Hove, UK: Routledge.

Sklad, M., Diekstra, R., Ritter, M. D., Ben, J., & Gravesteijn, C. (2012). Effectiveness of school-based universal social, emotional, and behavioral programs: Do they enhance students' development in the area of skill, behavior, and adjustment? *Psychology in the Schools, 49*(9), 892–909.

van Nieuwerburgh, C. (Ed.). (2012). *Coaching in education: Getting better results for students, educators and parents*. London: Karnac.

Vernon, A. (1994). Rational-emotive consultation: A model for implementing rational-emotive education. In M. E. Bernard & R. DiGiuseppe (Eds.), *Rational emotive consultation in applied settings* (pp. 129–148). Hillsdale, NJ: Lawrence Erlbaum.

Vernon, A. (2002). *What works when with children and adolescents: A handbook of individual counselling techniques*. Champaign, IL: Research Press.

Vernon, A. (2006a). *Thinking, feeling, behaving: An emotional education curriculum for children* (2nd ed.; grades 1–6). Champaign, IL: Research Press.

Vernon, A. (2006b). *Thinking, feeling, behaving: An emotional education curriculum for adolescents* (2nd ed.; grades 7–12). Champaign, IL: Research Press.

Vernon, A. (2006c). Depression in children and adolescents: REBT approaches to assessment and treatment. In A. Ellis and M. Bernard (Eds.), *Rational-emotive behavioral approaches to childhood disorders: Theory, practice and research* (pp. 212–231). New York: Springer.

Vernon, A. (2009a). Rational-emotive behavior therapy. In A. Vernon & T. Kottman (Eds.), *Counseling theories: Practical applications with children and adolescents in school settings* (pp. 153–184). Denver, CO: Love Publishing.

Vernon, A. (2009b). Applications of rational-emotive behavior therapy with children and adolescents. In A. Vernon (Ed.), *Counseling children and adolescents* (4th ed., pp. 175–202). Denver, CO: Love Publishing.

Vernon, A. (2009c). *More what works when with children and adolescents: A handbook of individual counselling techniques*. Champaign, IL: Research Press.

Vernon, A., & Barry, K. L. (2013). *Counseling outside the lines: Creative arts interventions for children and adolescents – individual, small group and classroom applications*. Champaign, IL: Research Press.

World Health Organization. (2001). *International classification of functioning, disability and health*. Geneva, Switzerland: Author.

Yamamoto, T., Matsumoto, Y., & Bernard, M. E. (2017). Effect of the cognitive-behavioral You Can Do It! Education program on the resilience of Japanese elementary school students: A preliminary investigation. *International Journal of Education Research, 86*, 50–58. https://doi.org/10.1016/j.ijer.2017.08.006

Chapter 22
Rational Emotive Parent Education

Oana Alexandra David

Overview of the Chapter

This chapter presents an approach to parent education based on the Cognitive-Behavioral and Rational Emotive Behavioral Therapy (REBT) approach. The chapter addresses the following questions:

- How did REBT contribute to the parent education field?
- What is the focus of REBT-based parent education?
- How well does REBT parent education work, for whom and how?
- What are the recent developments in the field and how are they connected with the trends in the parenting education field?

Parenting

Parenting refers to the process of child-rearing and includes all the endeavors that parents make to socialize their children (e.g., emotions, cognitions, behaviors, values). Effective parenting (i.e., positive parenting; Eisenberg et al., 2005) is characterized by high levels of warmth, involvement, positive discipline, and consistent practices. Dysfunctional or sub-optimal parenting refers to characteristics such as lack of warmth, hostility, negativity, conflict, and harsh discipline or neglect.

Parenting and parent–child relationship are considered to contribute in essential ways to child mental health (see Ryan, O'Farrelly, & Ramchandani, 2017 for a

---

O. A. David (✉)
Department of Clinical Psychology and Psychotherapy,
Babes-Bolyai University, Cluj-Napoca, Romania
e-mail: oanadavid@psychology.ro

M. Bernard, M. D. Terjesen (eds.), *Rational-Emotive and Cognitive-Behavioral Approaches to Child and Adolescent Mental Health: Theory, Practice, Research, Applications*, https://doi.org/10.1007/978-3-030-53901-6_22

review). It has been found that inconsistent, harsh, or insensitive parenting contribute to the development of externalizing or internalizing disorders in children (e.g., Repetti, Taylor, & Seeman, 2002). Causal connections have been found in longitudinal studies between ineffective or suboptimal parenting and children's emotional and social development, physical health, and academic attainment (e.g., Waylen, Stallard, & Stewart-Brown, 2008).

Given the fact that many of the parents report using dysfunctional practices such as hostility, resentment, and hitting or shouting and that the origins of many mental health problems lie in childhood, it becomes essential that parents receive support in improving their skills. Indeed, parent education programs have been developed based on the premise that parenting can be improved. Parent education refers to preventative and systematic programs aimed at teaching parents effective parenting skills as a means for promoting better child adjustment and preventing child psychopathology (Fine, 1980).

Parent education has many variations in terms of characteristics (Britto, Ponguta, Reyes, & Karnati, 2015), including their approach (attachment based, systemic, behavioral, or cognitive-behavioral), format (e.g., group, individual, self-administered, media) or settings where they are delivered (e.g., community, clinic, home-based or combination), etc.

Rational-Emotive Behavior Therapy (REBT) is a form of Cognitive-Behavior Therapy (CBT) that conceptualizes the quality of parenting and parent education with a focus on irrational and rational cognitions as essential determinants of parent emotions and behaviors. Thus, REBT parent education aims to teach parents rational parenting beliefs and differentiates itself from other CBT parent education programs (e.g., Incredible Years curricula) based on its primary focus on helping parents first address their emotional problems associated with parenting difficulties.

The REBT Theory of Parenting

REBT was founded by Albert Ellis in 1955, which was originally named Rational Therapy and later changed to Rational Emotive Behavioral Therapy (Ellis, 1994). The main assumptions of REBT are that emotional suffering is determined largely by irrational (rigid, extreme) beliefs and that humans need to use scientific methods to test their thinking and consequently their irrational beliefs into rational ones. The ABC model synthetizes these assumptions and is the cornerstone of the REBT, and thus to its parent education application.

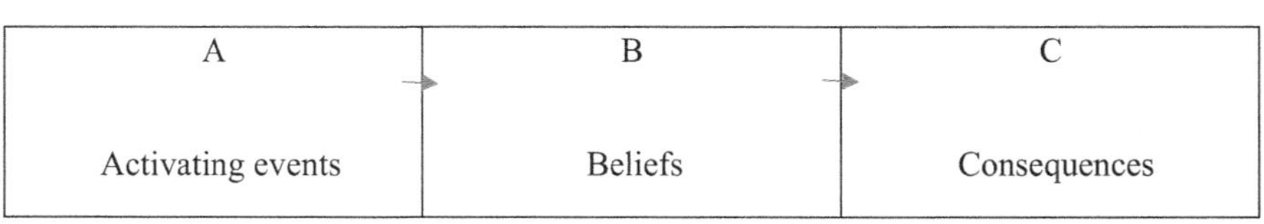

In his theory, (Ellis 1962, 1991, 2003; Ellis & Bernard 2006) conceptualized irrational beliefs as rigid beliefs that are inconsistent with reality, illogical, and unhelpful in reaching long-term goals. Thus, in this model, parental reactions to child noncompliance (the C; e.g., anger and yelling) is caused not by child's misbehavior (the A) but by his or her irrational beliefs about it (the Bs; e.g., "Children must be obedient").

Bernard and Joyce (1984) described the main irrational beliefs that are causing parents to experience dysfunctional negative emotions, such as anger, depression, anxiety, or guilt. These emotions are called dysfunctional since they are interfering with the use of effective parenting strategies. The main form of irrational beliefs is demandingness (DEM) which refers to absolutistic should of the person regarding self, others, and life. Awfulizing (AWF) refers to exaggerated negative evaluations of circumstances, self or others. Frustration intolerance (FI) refers to believing that things that are frustrating cannot be tolerated. Global evaluation (GE) refers to individuals evaluating their worth based on specific attributes or behaviors. Rational beliefs in turn refer to flexible beliefs that are consistent with the empirical reality are logical and helpful in terms of supporting the people in reaching their long-term goals. The rational alternative to DEM is preferences (PRE) which refer to acknowledge that own wishes and making efforts to reach them but not demanding that they happen. Badness (BAD) is the rational alternative to AWF that acknowledged the badness of negative events but does not exaggerate to make them a catastrophe. Frustration tolerance (FT) is the rational alternative to FI that refers to the belief that one can stand the frustration faced. Unconditional acceptance of self, others, and life is the rational alternative to GE that refers to give up global evaluations based on arbitrary criteria and evaluate only behaviors as good or bad.

In Table 22.1 shows how various types of irrational beliefs are related to specific emotions and how their corresponding rational beliefs are related to functional negative emotions.

Table 22.1 Illustration of the connection between IBs, emotions, and parenting when confronted with negative As

Dysfunctional parenting		Rational parenting	
Irrational beliefs	Dysfunctional negative emotions	Rational beliefs	Functional negative emotions
"I cannot stand being disobeyed"	Anger	"I do not like being disobeyed but I can stand it"	Annoyance
"I am a bad parent"	Guilt	"I have made faults with my children"	Remorse
"It is awful not to be respected"	Anxiety	"It is bad not to be respected but is not awful"	Concern
"I am worthless since I have failed as a parent"	Depression	"I have made mistakes but this does not reflect on my value"	Sadness

How REBT Conceptualizes Parenting Styles

Ellis has described in his book *How to Raise an Emotionally Healthy, Happy Child* (Ellis, Wolfe, & Moseley, 1966) how irrational beliefs determine dysfunctional parenting and how irrational beliefs are transmitted to children. In Hauck (1967), has proposed in his book called *The Rational Management of Children* the concept of rational parenting that stayed as foundational for the REBT-based parent education field. He identified four styles of parenting and their underlying cognitive mechanisms, namely the unkind and not firm style, the unkind and firm style, the kind and not firm style, and the kind and firm style.

The unkind and not firm parenting style is a neglectful and irrational parenting style since it lacks both affectionate or positive interactions and consistent limit setting. Parents using this style are uninvolved and do not use behavioral control strategies. Children of parents that use this parenting style are at great risk for antisocial and defiant behavior.

The unkind and firm style is a dysfunctional parenting style characterized by low levels of warmth and high demands from the parent. Parents using this style are setting excessively strict rules and are focused mainly on the faults of their children. Irrational beliefs that determine the use of unkind and firm parenting style are related to the control domain: DEM: "Children need to obey authority", "I must be in charge", FI: "I cannot stand to be disobeyed", GE: "Not being obeyed means that I am a failure", AWF: "It is awful not to be obeyed". Children of parents that use this style have often approval DEM and are anxious and submissive.

The kind and not firm parenting style is a dysfunctional parenting style characterized by high levels of warmth and low demands from the parent, corresponding to the permissive parenting style of Baumrind (1967). Parents using this style are warm to their children but pose little demands on children, and when setting limits are inconsistent in following them through. Irrational beliefs that determine parents to use the kind and not firm parenting style are related to approval demands based on the following processes: DEM: "I must be approved by my children", FI: "I cannot stand to see my children complain", GE: "I am a bad parent if I frustrate my children", AWF: "It is awful to frustrate my child". Children of parents that use the kind and not firm parenting style have FI to rules or hard working and low responsibility.

The kind and firm style is the rational parenting style characterized by high levels of warmth and high levels of demands from the parent. Parents using this style are involved in positive interactions with their children and are able to set and maintain firm rules. The kind and firm parenting style is supported by parents' rational beliefs such as unconditional self and child acceptance.

In a study that we conducted (Gavita, David, & DiGiuseppe, 2014), we documented that global evaluation in the form of self-downing (e.g., "I am a bad parent") is a proximal determinant of parent anger.

The essential role that unconditional acceptance plays in rational parenting was emphasized by Ellis (Ellis et al., 1966) and is discussed in detail in the chapter *Self-acceptance and raising children* (David & DiGiuseppe, 2016). According to

Ellis, one of the most valuable things that parents can teach children is not to rate people by their actions, possessions, status, or traits in terms of their self-worth. For example, parents can learn in REBT parent education self-acceptance and then teach it by explaining to the child that she/he can dislike another person's traits but needs to avoid judging the whole of the person as bad. It is important that the parent internalizes unconditional acceptance to be able to model it and verbalize it to their children in critical events.

Parent Education Programs

REBT parent education is a preventative program focused primarily on equipping parents with skills to manage their parental distress and, in a second step, to adopt rational parenting. Thus, the main mechanism for change is targeting parental cognitions based on the ABC model and learning the rational parenting style. The priority that REBT parent education gives in intervention to the emotional difficulties of the parents is based on research supporting significant differences in the outcomes for such an initial focus (see Gavita & Joyce for a review; see also Gavita, David, & Joyce, 2011).

There are a series of sequences in the REBT parent education and which reflect the ABC model of REBT (Joyce, 1995, 2006):

1. Assessment of the initial level of parent and child functioning, considering relevant variables, such as child mental health, parenting style, parent beliefs, parent emotions. Specific tools were developed for the assessment of these variables, such as the Parent Anger Scale (Gavita, DiGiuseppe, David, & DelVecchio, 2011; see Appendix 1), or the Parent Rational and Irrational Beliefs Scale (Gavita et al., 2011; see Appendix 2). The same assessment is implemented at the end of the parent intervention and ideally at follow-up.
2. Teaching parents the ABCs of managing their emotional distress;
3. Familiarizing parents with rational beliefs and reinforcing their practice;
4. Teaching parents the rational parenting style and effective parenting practices;
5. Teaching parents on how to use rational-emotive methods for dealing with children's emotional problems.

There are a few REBT parent education programs that were developed and tested, and in the next section, their contents, structure, and evidence base will be described.

Rational Parent Education

Rational Parent Education was the first curricula that was developed by Marie Joyce (1995) based on initial efforts to adapt REBT to parenting (e.g., Berger, 1983). The structure of this curricula reflect the stages presented above and is segmented in four sections: (1) Psychoeducation on the ABC model and assessment of emotional distress; (2) Introducing the kind and firm parenting style and reinforcing rational thinking; (3) Rational problems solving about children's emotional and behavioral difficulties; and (4) Educating rational thinking in children.

Efficacy of the Rational Parent Education was tested (Joyce, 1995) in a quasi-experimental study that included 48 parents. Parents were distributed in the Rational Parent Education condition or the control wait-list condition. Significant improvements were obtained in the Rational Parent Education group for parent irrational beliefs, anger, and guilt after the program compared to the control group. Moreover, measures at 10-month follow-up showed improvements in child behavior problems and GE.

SOS Help for Parents

SOS Help for Parents is a REBT self-help parenting education curricula developed by Lynn Clark (1996a, 1996b). The program consists of child management skills assessment, video education and vignettes, self-help books, forms and handouts. The program dedicates one of the self-help books to helping parents deal with emotional difficulties and the second to helping parents deal with child behavioral difficulties, each of them being accompanied by video contents. Resources are either for counseling and mental health professionals or for parents.

The program builds around three basic child-rearing rules and four major child-rearing errors to be avoided by parents which are explained in both the video and the self-help books. The three child-rearing rules reinforced by the program are: (1) Reward good behavior; (2) Do not reward bad behavior; and (3) Correct bad behavior. Parent positive disciplining strategies are built around the rules and consist of effective use of rewards, effective instructions, consequences, ignoring, and time-out. The four major child-rearing errors to be avoided by parents are: (1) failure to reward good behavior; (2) Accidentally rewarding of bad behavior; (3) Accidentally punishing good behavior; and (4) Failing to correct bad behavior when mild corrections are needed.

The SOS Help for Parents curricula was tested in two separate studies. One of the studies (Khowaja et al., 2016) was a pilot investigation of the program in a brief 6-week format. Fifty-seven mothers of preschool children from Pakistan participated in this study and were distributed to the parent education group or control group which consisted of information about child care. Results showed significant improvements in parenting in the parenting education group compared to the control group, in terms of laxness and over-reactivity. Another study (Gavita et al., 2011) has investigated this program in a 10 sessions format in preventing externalizing disorders in school-aged children. Positive results were found for parents' distress, parenting, and externalizing symptoms in children.

Rational Positive Parenting Program

The Rational Positive Parenting Program (rPPP) was developed by Oana David (David & DiGiuseppe, 2016; Gavita, 2011) and builds upon the aforementioned sequences and parent education programs, which are integrated in a comprehensive format and complimented with innovative components, such as "psychological pills"/rational statements or rational cartoons (see www.retman.ro) to generalize rational thinking and coach it for children. Structure and contents of the full format rPPP are presented in Table 22.2.

The rPPP can be delivered in three formats: full-length, short version, and an online format. The full-length (10 weekly sessions) and short versions (4 sessions) of rPPP are held using a group format. The program is using experiential strategies, handouts, video vignettes, and monitoring forms (see Appendix 3).

The rPPP is most well documented REBT parent education, its efficacy being tested in many rigorous trials, in all its formats. The full-length 10 sessions rPPP was tested in both the prevention and treatment of child externalizing symptoms in 130 preschool and school-aged children. It was compared to a cognitive-behavioral standard education program and results showed that both improved parenting, but rPPP brought more generalized improvements for child externalizing symptoms and longer term outcomes (David, David, & Dobrean, 2014). Moreover, the mechanism of change in the rPPP was found to be parental distress and parenting (David, 2014), which supports the REBT theory.

The efficacy of the short version of the rPPP was tested when working with placement parents. Ninety-seven foster parents were included in the study, which were distributed in the rPPP or a wait-list. Results showed that the parent education was effective in improving parent distress and child behavior problems. In another trial (Gavita & Calin, 2013), the self-help rPPP was found effective in the prevention of both externalizing and internalizing symptoms in children.

Table 22.2 Structure of the rPPP program

Sessions 1–3	Assessment and psycho-education on the ABC model. managing parental distress. Consolidating parent rational beliefs and introducing the rational parenting style.
Sessions 4–5	Positive relationship with the child as foundation skill. using rewards-based tools and effective limit-setting.
Sessions 6–7	Strategies for managing noncompliant behavior (e.g., time-out).
Sessions 7–10	Effective communication and problem-solving skills. Assessment, maintenance of gains, and termination issues.

Advances in REBT Parent Education

A major current focus in psychotherapeutic and prevention sciences is increasing accessibility to interventions, targeting relevant risk factors, and increasing their efficacy based on a precision medicine approach. In this vein, REBT parent education programs were adapted to be implemented online.

The rPPP was extended with an online version based on eight sessions that makes use of interactive exercises, videos, and forms. Innovative components are based on the emotion regulation framework and momentary ecological assessment by integrating it with the mobile PsyPills app (David & David, 2019). The PsyPills app allows parents to access personalized "psychological pills" when in distress and receive personalized rational thinking strategies that were found effective. Another innovative tool incorporated is gaming and implicit attention bias modification for parents. The game is aimed at training parents' attention towards positive faces and can be used in the beginning of the parent education by the parents that have difficulties disengaging from negative patterns of interactions.

Contents of the online rPPP are the following: Module 1—I want to be a rational positive parent!; Module 2—Rational parenting: managing stress; Module 3—Rational parenting: unconditional parenting; Module 4—Positive parenting and rewards; Module 5— Limit setting; Module 6—Managing child behaviors; Module 7—Effective communication and praise; Module 8—Problem solving. Efficacy of the online rPPP was recently tested in a trail and its efficacy was documented for parenting and improving parent–child positive interactions (David, Capris, & Jarda, 2017). Building on the contents of the online rPPP, the mobile app *Rational Parenting Coach – REThink parenting!* was recently developed (David, 2019) and it capitalizes on the CB-REB phases of intervention, but also personalizes the parent education based on an initial assessment of parenting styles, parent distress, and child difficulties (see Fig. 22.1). Moreover, the app offers the possibility to use strategies when needed, based on an ecological momentary assessment and monitoring.

Another online parent education program that can be accessed online is YCDI! Positive Parent Program (https://www.youcandoiteducation.com.au/parents/) which is part of the You Can Do It! Education program developed by Michael Bernard and Patricia Bernard. YCDI Parents focuses on three main areas: Positive Parents (e.g., being a positive role model, managing stress), Effective Parents (e.g., effective discipline and relationship skills), and Positive Children (e.g., developing children's resilience and positive character). The program uses an e-learning format where the parent receives information related to the topic of each module.

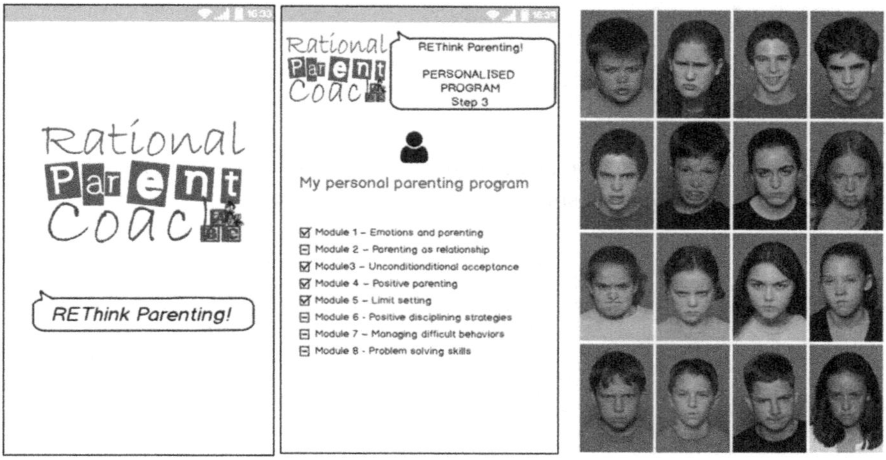

Fig. 22.1 The Rational Parenting Coach mobile app

Conclusions

REBT Parent education has brought important contributions to the more general parent education field and at the same time has meaningfully extended the applications of RE-CBT. Comprehensive curriculums have been developed which have been documented in rigorous studies and found effective in the prevention of child psychopathology. REBT parent education is unique not only for its focus but also given the integration of recent advancements in clinical cognitive sciences and technologies.

"Test Yourself" Questions

1. While all parenting education programs focus on assisting parents in improving parenting skills, what is the primary focus of REBT-based parent education?
2. REBT parent education focuses on teaching parents rational parenting. What cognitions are determining parents to adopt a kind and not firm parenting style?
3. There are a few REBT parent education programs that were developed. Which are the four phases of intervention that are common to all?

Appendix 1

Parent Anger Scale

Instructions: At one time or another, most parents feel angry. For each of the following items, circle the response that best describes you.

1	2	3	4	5	6
Less than once a month	About once a month	About once a week	Several days a week	Every day	Several times a day

1. Even though I hold it in and do not show it, I get angry with my child.	1	2	3	4	5	6
2. I get angry and break or throw away some of my child's things.	1	2	3	4	5	6
3. I get angry and cannot stop thinking about the way my child behaved.	1	2	3	4	5	6
4. I get angry and have a problem controlling my behavior toward my child.	1	2	3	4	5	6
5. I get angry with my child.	1	2	3	4	5	6
6. I get angry with my child and feel like throwing things, slamming doors, or banging the table.	1	2	3	4	5	6
7. I get angry with my child and I feel like spanking or hitting my child.	1	2	3	4	5	6
8. I get angry with my child and I spank, slap, or hit my child.	1	2	3	4	5	6
9. I get angry with my child and throw things, slam doors, or bang the table.	1	2	3	4	5	6
10. I get so angry with my child that I cannot control my behavior.	1	2	3	4	5	6
11. I get so angry with my child that I do not do things that I know my child wants me to do.	1	2	3	4	5	6
12. I get so angry with my child that I feel my blood boil.	1	2	3	4	5	6
13. I get so angry with my child that I feel my muscles get tight.	1	2	3	4	5	6
14. I get so angry with my child that I grab or push my child.	1	2	3	4	5	6
15. I get so angry with my child that I just want to make the tension go away.	1	2	3	4	5	6
16. I get so angry with my child that I say mean things, use bad language, curse, or insult my child.	1	2	3	4	5	6
17. I get so angry with my child that I scream or yell at my child.	1	2	3	4	5	6
18. I lose control of my anger with my child.	1	2	3	4	5	6
19. I resent the time and energy I put into parenting.	1	2	3	4	5	6
20. I think my anger with my child is justified because of the way my child behaves.	1	2	3	4	5	6
21. I think that I have a harder job being a parent than other people.	1	2	3	4	5	6
22. I think that my child deserves to be punished for misbehaving.	1	2	3	4	5	6
23. I use my anger to get my child to behave.	1	2	3	4	5	6
24. When I feel angry with my child, I boil inside, don't show it, and keep things inside of me.	1	2	3	4	5	6
25. When I get angry with my child, I feel like saying mean things to my child.	1	2	3	4	5	6
26. When I get angry with my child, I feel like screaming or yelling at my child.	1	2	3	4	5	6
27. When I get angry with my child, I tell relatives and friends so they will know how bad my child has behaved.	1	2	3	4	5	6

28. I lose my temper with my child about:

    1. almost nothing.
    2. only one thing.
    3. two or three things.
    4. several things.
    5. many things.
    6. almost everything.

29. When I get angry with my child, I stay angry for:

    1. only a few minutes.
    2. less than 1 hour.
    3. about 1–2 hours.
    4. several hours.
    5. about 1–2 days.
    6. several days.

30. On average how angry do you get at your child?

    1. Not at all angry.
    2. Somewhat angry.
    3. Mildly angry.
    4. Moderately angry.
    5. Very angry.
    6. Extremely angry.

Appendix 2

Parent Rational and Irrational Beliefs Scale (P-RIBS)

Name: Today's Date: _/_/___

Age:___ Sex: Male or Female (circle one) Date of Birth: _/_/___

General instructions: This scale has two parts. Please follow the specific instructions as follows.

Part 1

Instructions: Please think about a situation when your child(ren) disobey or disrespect you. Try to recall the thoughts that you have had in such situations. When faced with adverse situations, some parents tend to think that situation absolutely must be the way they want (in terms of *absolute must*). In the same situation, other people think in *preferential terms* and *accept* the situation, even if they want very much that those situations do not happen. In light of these possibilities, please estimate how much the statements below represent the thoughts that you have in such situations.

	Strongly disagree	Disagree	Neutral	Agree	Strongly agree
1. My child absolutely must respect and obey me.	1	2	3	4	5
2. If my child disobeys me, it doesn't mean that I am a worthless person.	1	2	3	4	5
3. I think it is awful to be disobeyed by my own child.	1	2	3	4	5
4. If my child disobey me, it means that I am worthless.	1	2	3	4	5
5. It is unbearable to be disobeyed by my own child.	1	2	3	4	5
6. I am always optimistic about my future.	1	2	3	4	5
7. I can stand when my child disobeys me, although it is difficult for me to tolerate it.	1	2	3	4	5
8. It is important for me to keep busy.	1	2	3	4	5
9. I really do not want my child to disobey me, but I realize and accept that things do not have to always be the way I want them to be.	1	2	3	4	5
10. It is unpleasant and unfortunate to be disobeyed by my own child, but it is not terrible.	1	2	3	4	5
11. When my child disobeys me, I think that they are bad, worthless, or condemnable.	1	2	3	4	5
12. When my child disobeys me, I accept them as being worthwhile despite her/his poor behavior.	1	2	3	4	5

Part 2

Instructions: Please think about a situation when your child(ren) disobey or disrespect you. Try to recall the thoughts that you have had in such situations. When faced with adverse situations, some parents tend to think that situation absolutely must be the way they want (in terms of *absolute must*). In the same situation, other people think in *preferential terms* and *accept* the situation, even if they want very much that those situations do not happen. In light of these possibilities, please estimate how much the statements below represent the thoughts that you have in such situations.

	Strongly disagree	Disagree	Neutral	Agree	Strongly agree
13. I absolutely must be a good parent.	1	2	3	4	5
14. If I am not a good parent, it doesn't mean that I am a worthless person.	1	2	3	4	5
15. I think it is awful to be a bad parent.	1	2	3	4	5
16. If I am not a good parent, it means that I am worthless.	1	2	3	4	5
17. It is unbearable to think of myself as a bad parent.	1	2	3	4	5
18. I am always optimistic about my future.	1	2	3	4	5
19. I can stand to be a bad parent.	1	2	3	4	5
20. It is important for me to keep busy.	1	2	3	4	5
21. I really do want to be a good parent, but I realize and accept that I may not always be as good at parenting as I want to be.	1	2	3	4	5
22. It is unpleasant and unfortunate to be a bad parent, but it is not terrible.	1	2	3	4	5
23. When my child disobeys me, I think that my child is bad, worthless, or condemnable.	1	2	3	4	5
24. When my child disobeys me, I accept him/her as being worthwhile.	1	2	3	4	5

Appendix 3

The ABC worksheet

A Activating event What happened?	B Beliefs	C Consequences How did you feel? (emotional, physiological, behavioral) How intense? 1-10
E.g., My child misbehaved.	He should obey to my requests.	Anger, 7 Harsh punishment

Bank account of unconditional accepting and validating statements (child and partner)

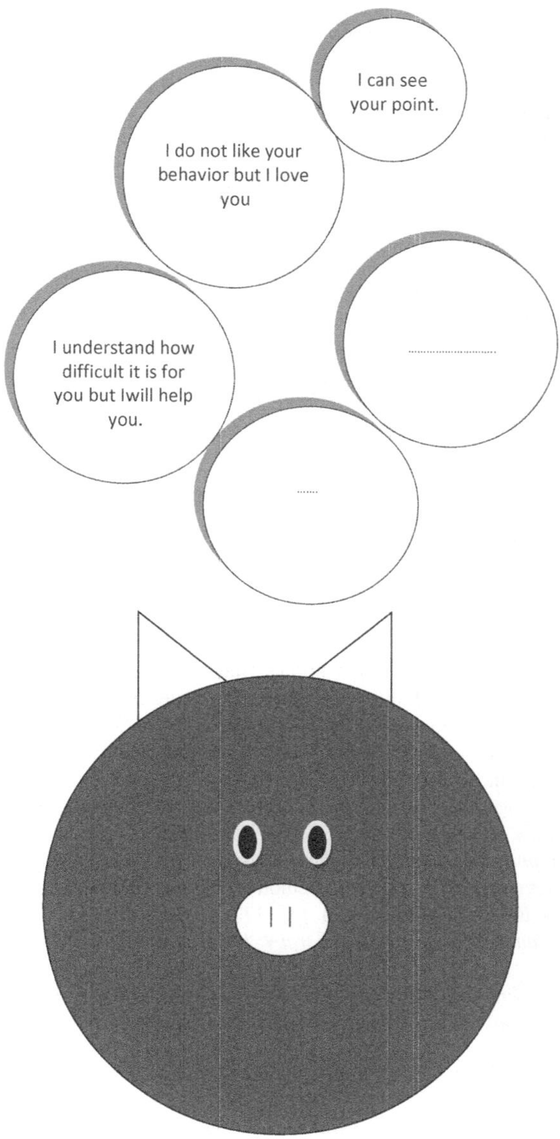
I can see your point.
I do not like your behavior but I love you
I understand how difficult it is for you but Iwill help you.
…………………………
……

References

Baumrind, D. (1967). Child care practices anteceding three patterns of preschool behavior. *Genetic Psychology Monographs, 75*(1), 43–88.

Berger, A. (1983). *The role of irrational cognitions in the phenomenology of anger and guilt in parents of disturbed children* (Unpublished Ph.D. Dissertation). Hofstra University, July, 1983.

Bernard, M. E., & Joyce, M. R. (1984). *Rational-emotive therapy with children and adolescents*. New York: Wiley.

Britto, P., Ponguta, L. A., Reyes, C., & Karnati, R. (2015). *A systematic review of parenting programmes for young children in low and middle income countries*. UNICEF.

Clark, L. (1996a). *SOS help for emotions. Managing anxiety, anger and depression*. Bowling Green, KY: Parents Press & SOS Programs.

Clark, L. (1996b). *SOS help for parents. A practical guide for handling common everyday behavior problems*. Bowling Green, KY: Parents Press & SOS Programs.

David, O. A. (2014). The rational positive parenting program for child externalizing behavior: Mechanisms of change analysis. *Journal of Evidence-Based Psychotherapies, 14*(1), 21–38.

David, O. A. (2019). The rational parenting coach app: REThink parenting! A mobile parenting program for offering evidence-based personalized support in the prevention of externalizing and internalizing disorders in children. *Journal of Evidence-Based Psychotherapies, 19*(2), 97–108.

David, O. A., Capris, D., & Jarda, A. (2017). Online coaching of emotion-regulation strategies for parents: Efficacy of the online rational positive parenting program and attention Bias modification procedures. *Frontiers in Psychology, 8*, 500. https://doi.org/10.3389/fpsyg.2017.00500

David, O. A., & David, D. (2019). Managing distress using mobile prescriptions of psychological pills: A first 6-month effectiveness study of the PsyPills app. *Frontiers in Psychiatry, 10*, 201.

David, O. A., David, D., & Dobrean, A. (2014). Efficacy of the Rational Positive Parenting program for child externalizing behavior: can an emotion-regulation enhanced cognitive-behavioral parent program be more effective than a standard one?. *Journal of Evidence-Based Psychotherapies, 14*(2), 21–38.

David, O. A., & DiGiuseppe, R. (2016). *The rational positive parenting program*. New York: Springer International Publishing.

David, O. A. & Podina, I. (2014). Positive Attentional Bias as a Resilience Factor in Parenting. Implications for Attention Bias Modification Online Parenting Interventions. In S. Ionescu, M. Tomita, S. Cace (Eds.), *Volume of the 2nd World Congress on Resilience "From person to society"* (pp. 425–428). Bologna: Medimond International Proceedings.

Eisenberg, N., Zhou, Q., Spinrad, T. L., Valiente, C., Fabes, R. A., & Liew, J. (2005). Relations among positive parenting, children's effortful control, and externalizing problems: A three-wave longitudinal study. *Child Development, 76*(5), 1055–1071.

Ellis, A. (1962). *Reason and emotion in psychotherapy*. New York: Lyle Stuart.

Ellis, A. (1991). The revised ABCs of rational-emotive therapy (RET). *Journal of Rational-Emotive & Cognitive-Behavior Therapy, 9*(3), 139–172.

Ellis, A. (1994). *Reason and emotion in psychotherapy: Expanded and revised edition*. Secaucus, NJ: Birch Lane.

Ellis, A. (2003). Similarities and differences between rational emotive behavior therapy and cognitive therapy. *Journal of Cognitive Psychotherapy: An International Quarterly, 17*(3), 225–240.

Ellis, A., & Bernard, M. E. (Eds.). (2006). *Rational emotive behavioral approaches to childhood disorders*. New York: Springer.

Ellis, A., Wolfe, J., & Moseley, S. (1966). *How to raise an emotionally healthy, happy child*. New York: Crown.

Fine, M. J. (1980). *Handbook on parent education*. Academic Press.

Gavita, O. A. (2011). *Evidence-based parent programs for child disruptive behavior*. Unpublished doctoral dissertation, Babes-Bolyai University, Cluj-Napoca.
Gavita, O. A., & Calin, A. (2013). Retman rational stories versus rational parenting program for the treatment of child psychopathology: Efficacy of two formats of rational-emotive behavior therapy. *Journal of Cognitive and Behavioral Psychotherapies, 13*(1), 33–52.
Gavita, O. A., David, D., & DiGiuseppe, R. (2014). You are such a bad child! Appraisals as mechanisms of parental negative and positive affect. *Journal of General Psychology, 141*(2), 113–129.
Gavita, O. A., DiGiuseppe, R., David, D. & DelVecchio, T. (2011). The development and validation of the Parent Rational and Irrational Beliefs Scale. *Procedia of Social and Behavioral Sciences, 30*, 2305–2311.
Hauck, P. (1967). *The rational management of children*. New York: Libra.
Joyce, M. R. (1995). Emotional relief for parents: Is rational-emotive parent education effective? *Journal of Rational Emotive Behavior Therapy, 13*(1), 55–75.
Joyce, M. R. (2006). A developmental, rational emotive-behavioral approach for working with parents. In A. Ellis & M. E. Bernard (Eds.), *Rational emotive behavior approaches to childhood disorders*. New York: Springer.
Khowaja, Y., Karmaliani, R., Hirani, S. A., Khowaja, A. R., Rafique, G., & McFarlane, J. (2016). A pilot study of a 6-week parenting program for mothers of pre-school children attending family health centers in Karachi. Pakistan. *International Journal of Health Policy and Management, 5*(2), 91–97.
Repetti, R. L., Taylor, S. E., & Seeman, T. E. (2002). Risky families: Family social environments and the mental and physical health of offspring. *Psychological Bulletin, 128*(2), 330–366.
Ryan, R., O'Farrelly, C., & Ramchandani, P. (2017). Parenting and child mental health. *London Journal of Primary Care, 9*(6), 86–94. https://doi.org/10.1080/17571472.2017.1361630
Waylen, A., Stallard, N., & Stewart-Brown, S. (2008). Parenting and health in mid-childhood: A longitudinal study. *European Journal of Public Health, 18*(3), 300–305. https://doi.org/10.1093/eurpub/ckm131

Chapter 23
Teacher Stress Management Using Rational Emotive Behavior Therapy

Oksana Huk and Camille Bernstein

The aim of this chapter is to provide an overview of both the research literature on teacher stress as well as provide practical strategies on how to prevent and address it using Rational Emotive Behavior Therapy (REBT). First, a definition for stress is provided along with how it may present itself among teachers. Causes of teacher stress and consequences that arise from it are then discussed. Stress may arise from within the teacher or from factors in the school, and similarly, stress can have a detrimental effect on the teachers, students, and the school community. Next, looking through the lens of REBT, research on how teacher irrational beliefs relates to stress is discussed, and then practical examples of how to recognize these beliefs and attempt to modify them utilizing various consultative models are given. The final sections of this chapter explore how REBT can currently be used for professional development to modify teacher stress along with suggestions for future directions for how REBT can be employed in schools.

The term stress among teachers is conceptualized differently within the research literature (Skaalvik & Skaalvik, 2016). At times it refers to "stressors" related to working as a teacher, like completing paperwork, and at other times it refers to the unpleasant affective feeling one can experience as a result from working (Skaalvik & Skaalvik, 2016, p. 1786). To date, there is not one working definition for stress (Skaalvik & Skaalvik, 2016), but common definitions refer to the negative and unpleasant affective experience (Kyriacou, 2011; Skaalvik & Skaalvik, 2016) that results from an inability to cope (DiGiuseppe, Doyle, Dryden, & Backx, 2013; Kyriacou, 2011; Lazarus & Folkman, 1987) with an imbalance of

O. Huk (✉)
Psychology Department, Iona College, New Rochelle, NY, USA
e-mail: ohuk@iona.edu

C. Bernstein
Psychology Department, The Hagedorn Little Village School, New Rochelle, NY, USA

M. Bernard, M. D. Terjesen (eds.), *Rational-Emotive and Cognitive-Behavioral Approaches to Child and Adolescent Mental Health: Theory, Practice, Research, Applications*, https://doi.org/10.1007/978-3-030-53901-6_23

overwhelming demands and minimal protective factors (Demerouti, Bakker, Nachreiner, & Schaufeli, 2001; Kyriacou, 2011; Lazarus & Folkman, 1987).

As a profession, teaching is regarded as one that is highly stressful (Johnson et al., 2005). There has been scholarly interest in teacher stress, burnout, and coping mechanisms spanning several decades, with literature reviews ranging back to the 1970s (Brunsting, Sreckovic, & Lane, 2014). The topic of teacher stress has also been studied on an international basis including but not limited to Romania (Clipa, 2017), Ireland (Buckley, Abbott, & Franey, 2017), Kosovo (Shkëmbi, Melonashi, & Fanaj, 2015), Italy (Pepe & Addimando, 2013), and Turkey (Mohamed, 2018). Within the United States, a study conducted by Herman, Hickmon-Rosa, and Reinke (2018) found that within a sample of 121 elementary school teachers, 93% fell into groups that experienced high levels of stress, leaving only 7% to be classified as well-adjusted.

Factors Leading to Teacher Stress

Teacher Demographics

Years of experience working as a teacher has been shown to be related to stress, job satisfaction, and turnover. Teachers who are younger and with fewer years of teaching experience are more likely to leave the profession than are older teachers (Mack, Johnson, Jones-Rincon, Tsatenawa, & Howard, 2019). In contrast, responses to interviews among 30 teachers nearing retirement in Norway indicated that weekends and vacations were enough time for younger teachers to feel ready to return to work; whereas older teachers took more sick time, work leave, or retired earlier. Interestingly, research examining gender, race, and stress results in inconsistent results (Bernard, 2016; Castro, Quinn, Fuller, & Barnes, 2018; Haberman, 2005).

School Characteristics

Student Behavior

Student misbehavior occurs frequently in classrooms, with teachers managing student misbehavior daily (Clunies-Ross, Little, & Kienhuis, 2008). Student behavior has been shown to be one of the most significant stressors for all teachers (McCormick & Barnett, 2011). Behavior can take different forms and is often reported differently throughout research (Aloe, Shisler, Norris, Nickerson, & Rinker, 2014). Alter, Walker, and Landers (2013) created nine categories of challenging behaviors and surveyed 800 teachers to identify those that were most problematic and occurred most frequently. They identified the following behaviors as most to least problematic: "off-task, verbal disruption, verbal aggression, noncompliance, out of seat, physical aggression, physical disruption, self-stimulatory, and isolation/no social interaction" (p. 57). When analyzing data from 664 elementary and secondary teachers from British Columbia and Ontario, Collie et al. (2012) found that teachers reported less stress related to student behavior as well as higher levels of teaching efficacy and job satisfaction when their students exhibited more positive behaviors and greater motivation.

Workload and Working Conditions

According to the National Education Association (2018), a teacher's contracted workday is 7 hours. However, teachers often spend significant portions of time completing tasks outside their contracted hours. Hansen and Sullivan (2003) identified working conditions in educational settings, such as an "increased workload, longer working hours, and low salaries [to] all contribute to high levels of employee stress that may lead to absences due to stress-related illnesses, impairment of coworker relationships, and feelings of hopelessness or disillusionment" (p. 620).

Accountability

School accountability has also been shown to be a factor in teacher attrition, as a larger proportion of teachers in schools rated as low or acceptable in performance were more likely to leave the profession than teachers in schools rated as exemplary. Teachers in the "intend to leave" group noted that they "perceived teachers to be 'punished' for poor school accountability ratings" as compared to teachers who indicated they were more likely to remain in the profession (Mack et al., 2019, p. 8). One such factor that may be used in school accountability ratings is high-stakes testing. Teachers also reported feeling pressure from the potential consequences of these tests on students, including the possibility of attending summer school, grade retention, and possibly feeling anxiety transferred from teachers. Ryan et al. (2017) found that test-based accountability significantly predicted stress, attrition, and burnout when analyzing survey responses from 1866 teachers. In a survey of 708 teachers in Florida, 22.5% of teachers reported feeling stress from the pressure of high-stakes tests, with one participant describing high-stakes testing as "cruel and unusual punishment for both the students and the teachers" (Jones & Egley, 2004, p. 20). Teachers also reported feeling pressure from the potential consequences of these tests on students, including the possibility of attending summer school, grade retention, and possibly feeling anxiety transferred from teachers.

Perceptions of Support from Administration

Perception of support from the administration has been shown to protect teachers from stress, burnout, and turnover (Skaalvik & Skaalvik, 2011) while increasing job satisfaction (Skaalvik & Skaalvik, 2011). According to Haberman (2005), perceiving that administration is not supportive is the second biggest job-related stressor for teachers, after student misbehavior.

In contrast, Cancio, Albrecht, and Johns (2013) surveyed 408 special education in the US teachers and found they felt supported when administration demonstrated that they were trusted professionals, provided opportunities for growth, provided guidance and feedback, and showed that they are worthy of concern.

Consequences of Teacher Stress

Teacher stress is a widespread problem that leads to negative consequences for teachers (McEwen & Sapolsky, 2006; Souza, Sousa, Belísio, & Azevedo, 2012), students (Roorda, Koomen, Split, & Oort, 2011), and school systems (Miller, 2012). When teachers are stressed, they may experience physical and psychiatric symptoms (McEwen & Sapolsky, 2006). They also have higher rates of absenteeism (Miller, 2012), attrition (Ronfelt, Loeb, & Wyckoff, 2012), occupational burnout (Rudow, 1999), and turnover (Rudow, 1999). Students of stressed teachers are more likely to have reduced academic performance and effects on their engagement achievement (Roorda et al., 2011). Finally, school systems are faced with higher monetary costs when they have to replace teachers who may leave the profession or retire early as a result of feeling stressed (Greenberg, Brown, & Abenavoli, 2016). Teacher stress has been found to predict the amount of negative relationships teachers may have with students (Yoon, 2002). This is important as the type of teacher–student relationship developed has been shown to impact school avoidance, self-directedness, and participation in the classroom (Birch & Ladd, 1997), as well as the aforementioned impact on students' engagement and achievement (Roorda et al., 2011). It is at least possible that teachers may refer more students when feeling more stressed. For example, it is possible that stress may result in the development of irrational beliefs (i.e., a lower frustration tolerance for student behavior and/or insistence that students *must* behave in a certain way), which may, in turn, result in more referrals to practitioners such as school psychologists, counselors, and social workers.

Irrational Beliefs and Teacher Stress

Currently, REBT identifies four irrational beliefs: demandingness, frustration tolerance, awfulizing, and global evaluations of human worth. Bernard (1990) modified these beliefs for teachers to more closely reflect their work: self-downing, authoritarian attitudes toward students, attitudes toward the school organization, and low frustration tolerance. Self-downing refers to the belief that teachers' self-worth is contingent upon their performance as a teacher. Authoritarian attitudes toward students refer to the belief that students should behave a certain way and punished if they do not. Low frustration tolerance refers to the thought that one simply cannot tolerate feeling frustrated or tolerate situations associated with this frustration. Finally, attitudes toward the school organization refers to the idea that that the administration should listen to their ideas about how things should be done.

Research suggests that teachers' thoughts are predictive of their negative affect, with each belief leading to different outcomes. Low frustration tolerance has been shown to be the strongest predictor of teacher stress (Bermejo-Toro & Prieto-Ursúa, 2006; Bernard, 1990, 2016; Popov, Popov, & Damjanovic, 2015) and has been associated with burnout, depression, somatization, anxiety (Bermejo-Toro & Prieto-Ursúa, 2006), and emotional exhaustion (Huk, Terjesen, & Cherkasova, 2019). Self-downing has been shown to predict overall stress (Bernard, 2016) and lack of personal accomplishment (Huk et al., 2019). Authoritarian attitudes were found to correlate with stress, burnout, sense of personal accomplishment, interpersonal sensitivity, paranoid ideation (Bermejo-Toro & Prieto-Ursúa, 2006), and depersonalization (Huk et al., 2019). Irrational attitudes toward the organization have been shown to be related to overall stress, anxiety, depression (Popov et al., 2015), and total burnout (Huk et al., 2019). Finally, the greater overall total irrational beliefs endorsed by teachers has been related to greater stress experienced by teachers (Bernard, 2016).

The Use of REBT in School Consultation

One of ways school practitioners (i.e., school psychologists) may support teachers and students is through the use of consultation. "Consultation within the human service professions represents an indirect model of delivering educational and mental health services whereby a professional with specialized experience (i.e., consultant) and a staff member (i.e., consultee) work together to optimize the functioning of a client in the staff member's setting" (Erchul & Sheridan, 2014, p. 3). As the focus of this chapter is the school setting, the consultant in this case is the school practitioner, the consultee is the teacher, and the client is the student. REBT is a multifaceted intervention that can take several forms. Due to limitations of working within a school system, such as large caseloads and time constraints, it is important that the focus of consultation remains the improvement of functioning of the student. In order to increase the skills of the teacher, the practitioner may work individually with the teacher and/or provide workshops to groups of teachers during the course of the school year. These workshops may provide the practitioner with the opportunity to introduce the language, concepts, and strategies of REBT while working individually with teachers may provide opportunities throughout the year to reinforce these concepts. It is important to note that while practitioners can implement strategies to reduce teachers' stressors within schools, they cannot always directly modify them. For instance, practitioners can work with teachers through consultation and classroom observation to create behavioral intervention plans to help modify student behavior through evidenced-based strategies, but it is also important to help teachers think differently about their stressors rather than trying to modify each one. While school-based practitioners are available to provide emotional support to teachers during the consultation process, the primary role of the practitioner during a school-based consultation session is to provide indirect support to students by working with teachers, rather than providing direct mental health support to teachers and individuals who may be experiencing significant mental distress. Sheridan and Cowan (2004) identify two goals in school-based consultation "(1) the short-term goal of resolving the students' presenting difficulties (i.e., remedial intervention) and (2) the long-term goals of preventing future similar challenges and improving the consultees' problem-solving skills (i.e., a preventive approach)" (p. 614). Bramlett and Murphy (1998) note that skills such as reflective listening, friendliness, empathy, openness, flexibility, and efficiency are crucial in developing the consultant–consultee relationship. While regularly scheduled consultation sessions are ideal, time constraints and workload are often barriers to adding multiple consultation sessions into an already full schedule. Practitioners may wish to ensure that teachers know they are welcome to come to their office at any time that is convenient for them to discuss concerns. Consultation in schools may realistically take the form of teachers seeking out support when a problem arises. Since consultation with teachers may sometimes only realistically take the form of one or two sessions, it is important to keep both the aforementioned short-term and long-term goals referenced by Sheridan and Cowan (2004) in mind. By incorporating evidence-based behavior strategies as well as REBT techniques into a consultation session, the consultant may be able to touch upon both goals while working within a system wrought with time constraints and large workloads. It is important to assess whether the teacher needs help with a practical problem (e.g., learning classroom management strategies), or an emotional problem (e.g., feeling anxious about working with a student who behaves poorly), or a combination of both.

Bernard and DiGuiseppe (2000) describe Rational Emotive Behavioral Consultation (REBC) as a collaborative process with the goal of the "reduction in the intensity, duration, and frequency of extreme emotions that may prevent consultees from solving existing practical problems" (pp. 337–338). Bernard and DiGuiseppe (2000) posit that these intense emotions may prevent consultees, such as teachers, from effectively implementing strategies to address a problem and that the consultee's irrational beliefs must be addressed in order to increase the effectiveness of the consultation process. REBC may be implemented in both individual and group formats. Consultants, such as school practitioners, may assist consultees in lessening the extreme negative emotions they feel and understanding the role of irrational beliefs in their emotional reactions to adverse events. For example, a teacher experiencing difficulty with a student may not effectively implement a behavior intervention plan if he or she is experiencing very intense emotions. As practitioners, we can help teachers change their emotions by teaching them how to modify their thoughts. Doing so may make it easier for teachers to implement plans, thereby helping change students' behaviors and further reduce the teachers' stress.

The principles of REBT have also been combined with those of Bandura's Social Cognitive Theory in Rational Emotive–Social Behavioral Consultation (RE-SB) to address both teachers' irrational beliefs and efficacy beliefs. Warren and Baker (2013) also provide suggestions for the implementation of RE-SB on an individual basis. During individual sessions, the consultant should (1) identify the problem, (2) determine the consultant's feelings and behaviors, (3) determine thoughts that led to these feelings and behaviors, (4) address and challenge maladaptive thoughts, and (5) help the consultant model rational thoughts and adaptive emotions and behaviors (p. 8). Through personal experiences, we have found that in order to effectively help teachers, one must be seen as a trustworthy individual, must be able to develop alliance and rapport with the teacher, and must be willing to validate the teachers' concerns and emotions before starting the consultative work. As teachers self-refer to practitioners for consultative services, they may feel wary of approaching or confiding in a practitioner who s/he does not trust or feel comfortable with.

Therapeutic Alliance and Building Trust

According to Tschannen-Moran and Hoy (2000), trust can be conceptualized as an integration of five concepts: reliable, competent, honest, open, and benevolent. People gain reputations for how trustworthy they are, and once someone is seen as not being trustworthy, it can be very hard to change this perception. Benign or neutral actions taken by someone who is seen as not trustworthy are often interpreted as "suspicious" (p. 550); whereas even unfavorable actions taken by someone who is trusted often will not drastically harm the relationship.

Practitioners are advised to attempt to begin building trust when first starting work in a school. Schools tend to be political places, and information, whether factual or fictitious, may spread across a school building quickly. While teachers may find collecting data on students burdensome, they tend to easily convene and discuss data they collected on newly hired individuals (e.g., what time they come to work, what shoes they wore, where/whether they take lunch, if they smoke, what kind of car drive, etc.) Some ways to build trust include following: honoring commitments (including completing tasks they agreed to complete), ensuring that those tasks are completed well and accurately, maintaining honesty with those around them, communicating openly and professionally with their co-workers, and demonstrating warmth with others. A particularly important way to build trust is to avoid gossiping in school systems (Tschannen-Moran & Hoy, 2000). Teachers will likely feel more comfortable speaking openly with practitioners if they are assured that information they share about student behavior, possible frustrations with other staff members, and/or information they heard about other employees will not be repeated and that they will not be judged for sharing the information.

Trust is also a key component of the development of rapport. According to West et al. (2017), rapport is necessary to build a relationship with an individual, and it requires reciprocity. They further note that in order to develop rapport, trust, empathy, and mutual respect are needed. It would be advisable that professionals begin the initial stages of rapport building by assuring that information discussed will remain confidential, barring legal exceptions, to assist in developing an atmosphere of trust. Initial stages of rapport building may also include allowing time for teachers to express negative emotions they may be experiencing prior to immediately attempting to implement strategies to "fix" an issue. By allowing teachers to express their emotions, professionals may be able to validate teachers' experiences as well as gain an understanding of teachers' underlying thought processes and possible irrational beliefs. On occasions where teachers require on-going consultation, the professional may wish to associate their office with positive experiences by creating a relaxing and positively reinforcing atmosphere.

Assessing Teacher Emotions

When teachers seek consultative services, it is important to help them identify what feeling they are experiencing as well as be clear that feeling badly in a healthy way can sometimes be helpful too. Suppose a teacher is crying as she tells you about a student who is misbehaving in a class. These tears can be the result of feeling sad, depressed, anxious, concerned, etc. Knowing the emotion helps the practitioner and teacher pave the way to uncovering the belief leading to the emotion. Additionally, if teachers know the emotion they are experiencing, they can learn to implement REBT strategies themselves. The practitioner can use statements like, "It sounds like you are feeling anxious. Is that right?" Be cautious when hearing emotions like "Overwhelmed" which can refer to any emotion (e.g., depressed, anxious, etc.). Sometimes clients have a difficult time naming their feeling. In these cases, it may be helpful to ask them what action they want to take.

Example:
Teacher: [crying]
Practitioner: What are you feeling?
Teacher: I don't know
Practitioner: What do you want to do?
Teacher: I want to punch something
Practitioner: Do you think you're feeling angry?

Assessing Antecedent Events

After assessing and validating the teachers' emotions, ensure to adequately assess their description of the stressor. A teacher saying, "He was completely disruptive" can mean that the student called out a few times or threw a desk. It is important to not make assumptions and instead to operationalize the problem. During this assessment, it may be helpful to consider the teacher's work experience. Consider a teacher who has been working for 20 years. Each year this teacher has had 20 students in her class. Now she tells you that she has a student who is the "most disrespectful student she has ever seen." At face value, out of 400 students, this student is the most disrespectful. That is important information! It is helpful to know if the student is really the most disrespectful student out of 400 same-aged peers or if the teacher is using colorful language.

Example:

Teacher: Timmy was out of control. He completely disrupted my entire class and that can't ever happen again!

Practitioner: That sounds incredibly difficult. We can certainly make sure that everyone stays safe and that you're able to conduct your lessons.

Teacher: It was! He was all over the place! He was impulsive and aggressive.

Practitioner: I can see why you're so upset. You mentioned that Timmy was impulsive and aggressive. Talk to me about his impulsivity, what did it look like? Was he out of his seat? Climbing on furniture? Running around the room?

Teacher: He was running across the room in front of me as I was trying to teach a group lesson.

Practitioner: Ok, what about the aggressive behaviors you mentioned?

Teacher: While he was running, he tried to hit several staff members.

Assessing Teacher Irrational Beliefs

After teachers describe their stressor and feelings, the practitioner can assess the beliefs they endorse. Prompts as simple as, "What was going through your head when that happened?" or "Tell me what you're thinking about all of this," can be used. Once an irrational belief is uncovered, the practitioner can dispute it by asking how helpful it is to think that way, asking for the evidence to support the belief, or exploring the logic behind the belief.

Low Frustration Tolerance (LFT)

Teachers often manage high workloads, and depending on the school, prep times vary. Additionally, they also have obligations in their personal lives that they are responsible for, which takes time and effort; even taking a break to use the bathroom can present challenges. Practitioners may hear statements like "I just can't take this anymore!" It is helpful to first acknowledge their situations are challenging and uncomfortable with statements like, "I know. It is really hard. That sounds really frustrating!" While their situations are challenging, teachers claiming that they cannot stand it rather than they strongly dislike it likely leads to an unhealthy emotion. A more helpful thought for teachers would be, "As much as I dislike this, I can stand it/tolerate it." Other strategies that can be useful is reminding the teacher of his or her past accomplishments dealing with difficult situations. For example, a practitioner may say something like, "I know this is incredibly difficult, but I know you can handle it, because I remember when you (fill in: did something really hard)." Additionally, it may be helpful to work with the teacher on practically solving whatever problem they "cannot stand". For example, if the teacher "cannot stand" how much work she has, it may be helpful to learn time management skills, prioritizing tasks, or when feasible learning to let some things go until the next day.

Another strategy is use of the Catastrophe scale to dispute exaggerating or awfulizing. In this exercise, consultees are asked to call to mind feeling upset by a particular person or situation and rate how bad that was on a scale from 0 to 100, with a rating of 90–100 indicating a true catastrophe (Bernard & DiGuiseppe, 2000, p. 345). A disclaimer: Sometimes situations are truly awful and using the catastrophe scale is not appropriate or helpful. Consider a teacher reporting feeling depressed after a student passed away from substance abuse. Using the catastrophe scale and trying to modify the teacher's belief about this incident to being bad but not awful can potentially be very harmful for the teacher. Instead, validate the teacher's emotions and experiences. It may be helpful to discuss action steps for the teacher to involve herself with an agency that prevents substance abuse among children. It is also possible that the best way to support a teacher may be providing referrals to outside sources, such as a therapist, to address any significant, ongoing concerns, or negative emotions.

Example:

Teacher: I can't take it anymore. I have so much work! In addition to all the grading I have, meetings this week, writing up goals, I have to take care of everything at home too! I just can't catch a break, and I'm so unbelievably tired.

Practitioner: I'm sorry that sounds really hard.

Teacher: It is. It's awful! Practitioner: I get that it's bad, and it sounds really bad, but is it *awful*? On a scale of 1–10, where 10 is the most awful thing that could ever happen, how *awful* would you say it is?

Teacher: It's definitely a 15!

Practitioner: No, 10 is as high as you can go. Ten is the most awful.

Teacher: Fine, it's a 10.

Practitioner: OK, so let's suppose all of this work is at a 10, where would you place, oh, I don't know, a plane crash?

Teacher: Ugggh, OK. So, it's not AWFUL like that. That's a 10. This would be more like a 7, but it really stinks.

Practitioner: Yes, yes, it really does! It is bad, and I get that it is bad, but how is this helping us to come up with a solution?

Self-Downing

When teachers endorse self-downing, we can help teachers separate their value as a human being from their work as a teacher. Practitioners may hear statements like, "I just feel like such an idiot that I can't get this right," when referring to helping a student. The goal is to help teachers change their thoughts from, "I'm really worthless, because I cannot get this student to learn" to "I really want this student to learn this material, but even if he doesn't, I am still a worthwhile human being."

Additionally, it may be helpful to explore any solutions to address practical problems. For example, if a teacher is reporting thinking she is worthless because she cannot teach well, it may be helpful to look into professional development or requesting observations and feedback from peers or supervisors to improve her skills. It would be important to still separate her views of her skills from her perception of self-worth, but it may be worth trying to improve her skillsets. It may also help to remind teachers of external factors that may impact a students' ability to learn, such as home environment, parent involvement, cognitive ability, etc.

If a teacher endorses self-downing, first help teacher acknowledge that working with students is not easy. If it were easy everyone would do it. Other strategies that may be helpful are to remind the teacher of past accomplishments with students or point out the teacher's strengths in other areas or to ask if they would say the same thing to a friend or co-worker. For example, "If your coworker came to you telling you a student in her class was not learning, you would tell her she's an idiot?" The teacher is likely to respond with an emphatic, "No! Of course not!" The practitioner can then begin exploring how to differentiate one's global rating of self from their competence at their job.

The Self-Acceptance Exercise may also help to facilitate this discussion. This exercise assists in disputing self-downing beliefs by writing positive and negative characteristics. Part of the circle involves identifying positive and negative aspects of a person's role at work, in this instance, positive and negative aspects of their role as a teacher. Other areas of the circle involve the positive and negative aspects of other areas of the person's life. This facilitates a discussion regarding how logical it is to base feelings of self-worth on one feature written in the circle (Bernard & DiGuiseppe, 2000, p. 345).

Example:

Practitioner: I can see how upset you are that Sally failed a second math test.

Teacher: Yes! I even reviewed the material with her. I'm a horrible teacher.

Practitioner: It sounds very stressful to base your entire teaching career over two tests (*At this part of the consultation, the practitioner may wish to take out the Self-Acceptance Exercise*). This circle shows us there are positive and negative aspects we all have in our jobs, but that we are more than just our jobs. I heard you say that you feel like you failed Sally as a teacher due to two math tests, so we can write "Students occasional fail an exam". Have the teacher write this in an area of the circle with a "–". It may be helpful to remember that sometimes students have difficulty with a subject despite a teacher's best efforts. Can you tell me a time where a student was successful with you?

Teacher: Well, Joseph was struggling with spelling, but we made spelling words into songs and he got a 90% on his next test.

Practitioner: That's very creative! Ask the teacher to write "creativity in lessons" in an area of the circle with a "+". I can see how busy everyone is in this school! It seems like there's much more to being a teacher than directly working with the students!

Teacher: Oh you wouldn't believe it! There's so much work outside of the classroom.

This may be how the conversation progresses to identifying additional positive and negative aspects of teaching, such as lesson planning, time management, and contact with parents, as well as how progressive the consultation is to other areas of the teacher's life such as the other possible roles as parent, volunteer, etc.

Authoritarian Attitudes Toward Students

When teachers endorse this belief, we can help them by validating their experience and then modifying their thoughts to a preference. For example, changing their thoughts from, "Students should always be respectful and behave appropriately," to "I wish students would behave better, but I can stand it when they don't," or, "I wish students behaved better, but no one can behave perfectly 100% of the time", When a teacher endorses this belief, first acknowledge how difficult it can be to work with students who behave unfavorably. It is also helpful to gain a global viewpoint of the student and a realistic view of student's strengths and weaknesses.

A practical problem-solving tool here may be to address the teacher's classroom management skills. As student behavior has been identified as a source of stress for teachers, it is logical to provide teachers with knowledge of techniques to manage behavior within the classroom. In a review of the literature, Simonsen, Fairbanks, Briesch, Myers, and Sugai (2008) identified 20 evidence-based practices. These practices were then grouped within five features of classroom management. The first feature involves the maximization of structure which incorporates the amount of teacher-directed activity and the physical arrangement of the classroom. The second feature is to post, teach, review, monitor, and reinforce expectations which also incorporate active supervision. The third feature involves actively engaging students in observable ways. This considers the rate of opportunities for students to respond, the use of response cards direct and computer-assisted instruction, class-wide peer tutoring, and guided notes. The fourth factor encompasses the use of a continuum of strategies for responding to appropriate behaviors. These strategies include specific and/or contingent praise, class-wide group contingencies, behavioral contracting, and token economies. The fifth and final factor involves the use of a continuum of strategies to respond to inappropriate behavior, including error corrections, performance feedback, differential reinforcement, planned ignoring with contingent praise and/or instruction of classroom rules, response cost, and time out from reinforcement (pp. 353–357).

Example:

Teacher: I really don't know what to do anymore! Charlie just won't listen.

Practitioner: What's going on?

Teacher: He won't sit still and keeps calling out in class. I've told him numerous times to stop, but he won't.

Practitioner: I can see how both of those behaviors disrupt the classroom. With these types of behaviors, it may be helpful to "catch him being good" by praising him for raising his hand rather than calling out and give him a turn or let him be a "special helper" when you see him sitting nicely in his chair.

Teacher: I shouldn't have to reward him for doing what he's supposed to be doing! He's in school, he's supposed to sit and listen.

Practitioner: Yes, sitting and listening are the expectations for students, but some children may have some inherent difficulty sustaining attention and regulating themselves. Yes, it would be really nice if he was doing these things, but given that he has not been listening, how is it helpful for us to say that he should be? Let's see if some of these strategies may assist in lessening some of these disruptive behaviors and increase Charlie's success with sitting and listening.

Attitudes Toward the School Organization

Teachers are often faced with policy changes and new rules and regulations from both administration and state regulatory agencies. In personal experience, teachers are rarely involved in decision-making processes at school or given the opportunity to provide feedback to administration. During consultation sessions with teachers, practitioners may often hear statements such as "What were they thinking? This isn't practical for a classroom!" or "When do they expect me to implement this? Just another thing to do. Why don't they ask us what we think?" While teachers' sources of frustration are valid, the rigid belief that administration should listen to their ideas about how things should be done rather than it would be preferable to ask teachers their opinions are where their negative emotion may change from adaptive to maladaptive. This particular belief presents challenges for the practitioner, because they likely share the same administration. Additionally, depending on the practitioner's title, they may be seen as part of the administration, part of the staff, or both. Thus, practitioners are advised to validate the teacher's experiences while being thoughtful about their responses. Teachers are likely to feel more connected if the practitioner sides with them, but realistically speaking, it might not be possible to do so. It may also be helpful to work with the teacher on building assertiveness skillsets on how to speak up to the administration appropriately.

Example:

Teacher: I can't believe she's asking me to this! I already have so much to do, and this is a complete waste of my time.

Practitioner: [listening/comforting nod].

Teacher: I am so angry! It's not even that she asks me to do this, but she doesn't care that I have over 20 years of experience in the classroom. When I tried to tell her that it didn't make sense to do things this way, she didn't even listen to what I had to say. That might make sense in a college classroom from a textbook, but this is real life and it won't work!

Practitioner: OK. I know this is hard, and you already have a lot to do.

Teacher: Yes! I do!

Practitioner: What would help you right now?

Teacher: Honestly, I'm not really sure. I guess I have to do it, but I don't want to.

Practitioner: I know. That's pretty clear. It would be nice if your suggestions were considered, but it sounds like that's not an option right now. Do you think there is a reason she is asking you to do it this way?

Teacher: I don't know. She thinks it is how you are supposed to do it.

Practitioner: Is it worth trying to complete this task as it was outlined to you and then providing feedback afterwards? Maybe, given all of your experience, you can find really creative ways to make it better, and that your feedback will be more welcomed if you try to make it work first? What do you think?

Teacher: I guess that's possible. What if she still doesn't listen to my opinion?

Practitioner: She might not, and that would stink, but does it really take away from how much experience you have or the lessons you've learned over the years?

Ending the Session

At the end of every session, it may be helpful to have the teacher repeat the new rational belief in his or her own words. Doing so helps the teacher formulate this type of thinking for herself, and it also allows the practitioner to check for understanding. There have been times where clients have shared new irrational beliefs at this time rather than a rational belief, and it is good for the practitioner to know this before the client leaves to rectify it.

Additionally, following the consultative session, it would be wise for professionals to continue to practically support teachers by remaining visible within the school building and "checking in" with teachers regarding both students' behavior and performance, as well as teachers' well-being. Professionals may stop by a classroom to quietly observe or simply send an email asking not just about classroom behavior but also on the teachers' well-being. Through personal experience, even a simple, "I heard you the other day, and I wanted to follow up with you on this matter," can make someone feel supported. Also, asking the individual specifically, "How can I help you?" or "How can I best support you?" can be powerful techniques.

REBT in Professional Development

As with REBC, Warren and Baker (2013) indicate that RE-SB may also be applied in both group and individual formats. Group sessions may be proactively conducted during teachers' scheduled in-service trainings to provide behavioral management strategies, interventions to assist with teacher–student relationships, or to provide information on relevant topics such as "the ABC Model, the influence of efficacy beliefs, and the impact of observational learning on students" (p. 7). For example, most schools have professional development days prior at the beginning of the school year. During this time, presentations on various topics are presented to school staff.

One such topic may be the introduction of REBT and how it applies to teachers in a school setting. Topics may include a brief overview of REBT, rational vs. irrational beliefs, and how these beliefs may specifically manifest in school systems. Time may also be allotted for an introduction to specific strategies to target these irrational beliefs and/or developing practical skills. For instance, one such session can include a combination of REBT and classroom management skills. The beginning of the session can provide psychoeducation on the utility of feeling healthy negative feelings versus unhealthy negative feelings when it comes to effectively teaching. Teachers can share challenging incidents they have experienced with their students as well as what they were thinking during these times. Practitioners can use these examples as an opportunity to question the teachers whether if they thought differently, they may have felt differently, and thus behaved differently and ultimately helped change the students' behaviors. Chances are, teachers are likely to feel comforted and engaged by hearing their colleagues share similar experiences, thoughts, and feelings. The next part of the in-service could then focus on practical classroom management strategies, where teachers can share what gets in their way of implementing these strategies. In other words, teachers may offer that they feel too annoyed or angry to provide reinforcement to a student for behaving well when the student behaved so poorly earlier in the day. The group can then work together to dispute any irrational beliefs (e.g., they shouldn't have to provide reinforcement) and think of new effective beliefs that can be used in the same situation. Finally, role plays could be a helpful technique where teachers could practice thinking these new beliefs together.

By providing an overview of these topics at the beginning of the school year, this may serve as a point of reference throughout the year as needed during consultation with teachers. Not only does this provide an awareness that one's beliefs may influence one's emotions, but it also allows the consultant to work more efficiently within the school by providing this information to all teachers at once rather than on an individual basis as the need may arise. Group formats may also be used in response to problematic situations that arise over the course of the school year. In these sessions, the consultant may facilitate discussions with teachers and the sessions may be focused on the collaborative development of problem-solving strategies. In fact, through personal experiences, these sessions seem to be the most helpful when teachers honestly communicate their experiences and beliefs. For example, when teachers adamantly try to convince you how awful it is when they have too much on their plate, it serves as a great opportunity to practice using disputes together. As always, during these times, validating that their experience as stressful and that feeling badly in a healthy way can be useful and tends to be well received.

Future Directions for the Use of REBT with Teachers

School systems present a myriad of professional challenges for teachers as well as opportunities for both professional and personal growth. By creating a more supportive working environment, teachers may be able to increase their knowledge of practical problem-solving skills to decrease sources of stress (i.e., behavior management skills to reduce occurrences of student misbehavior) and also increase their knowledge of emotional problem-solving skills (i.e., REBT strategies to decrease maladaptive negative beliefs).

Changing the climate of any workplace is a difficult undertaking. It involves shifts in policies as well as shifts in thinking from all employees: teacher's assistants, lead teachers, practitioners, administration, etc. The implementation of change often begins at the administrative level. Practitioners may be in a unique position to have the opportunity to meet with administrators and provide evidence regarding the use of REBT strategies in a school setting and discuss ways to incorporate this philosophy into the culture. For example, as previously mentioned, schools often provide in-service workshops in the beginning of the school year and additional workshops throughout the year. Practitioners are often asked to provide these workshops, often regarding evidence-based behavior management strategies. They may wish to discuss conducting a workshop regarding REBT at the beginning of the school year to begin the shift in helping teachers and school staff distinguish rational versus irrational beliefs. This workshop may then serve as a reference point during future meetings with teachers.

While an introduction to REBT through a workshop may serve as a useful starting point, the exposure to, and reinforcement of, these strategies is important over the course of the school year. Teachers decorate their classrooms with motivational quotes, educational materials, and classroom rules for students. They may consider creating a poster or two of motivational quotes and perhaps a visual of an REBT strategy, such as the self-acceptance exercise, as a reminder that a negative event such as student misbehavior, an overdue report, or an upset parent is only one aspect of their day. These events should be balanced with all of the positive aspects of their job performance such as a well-planned lesson, a thank you note from a parent, and a student who mastered a new skill.

Practitioners play a vital role in ensuring that the language used in REBT and the evidence-based strategies remain in use. During consultation sessions with teachers, practitioners should remember that the issues teachers bring to the consultation session may have both a behavioral component (i.e., student misbehavior) as well as an emotional component (i.e., frustration, anger, disappointment, etc.) In order to ensure that all components of a problem are being addressed, practitioners may wish to have sheets with REBT strategies such as the catastrophe scale and self-acceptance exercise available in their offices for use. The practitioner should also consider leaving time during the consultation session to address teachers' maladaptive thoughts. As time constraints often pose challenges to ongoing consultation, practitioners may wish to ask the teacher about his or her schedule to set up a time to either "pop-in" to the classroom or schedule another consultation session at a time that is convenient for the teacher. Furthermore, practitioners may also be in a unique position to increase teachers' self-esteem and feelings of support within the school by informing administrators via email when students benefit from strategies implemented by the teacher or when parents provide positive feedback regarding their child's performance or about the teachers themselves.

Future research should continue to explore the degree to which teacher perceptions modify their stress and burnout levels. Similarly, research should examine what factors relate to teacher engagement, the antithesis of burnout. Furthermore, intervention research can examine the degree to which providing teachers with an REBT framework helps them both manage their stress levels as well as increase other constructs like their self-efficacy or competence as a teacher.

"Test Yourself" Questions

1. One factor contributing to teachers' experiences of stress is student misbehavior within their classrooms. What strategies may teachers consider using proactively to reduce occurrences of student misbehavior? What strategies may teachers consider using after the occurrence of misbehavior?
2. Teachers may experience stress from a number of factors that are out of their control (i.e., high-stakes testing, demographic factors, administrative support, etc.) From an REBC perspective, how might one provide intervention to assist teachers in lessening their experiences of stress associated with factors that cannot be controlled?
3. How might practitioners incorporate the use of both REBT strategies and practical skill development into their everyday practice?

References

Aloe, A. M., Shisler, S. M., Norris, B. D., Nickerson, A. B., & Rinker, T. W. (2014). A multivariate meta-analysis of student misbehavior and teacher burnout. *Educational Research Review, 12*, 30–44. https://doi.org/10.1016/j.edurev.2014.05.003

Alter, P., Walker, J., & Landers, E. (2013). Teachers' perceptions of students' challenging behavior and the impact of teacher demographics. *Education and Treatment of Children, 36*(4), 51–69. https://doi.org/10.1353/etc.2013.0040

Bermejo-Toro, L., & Prieto-Ursúa, M. (2006). Teachers' irrational beliefs and their relationship to distress in the profession. *Psychology in Spain, 10*, 88–96.

Bernard, M., & DiGuiseppe, R. (2000). Advances in the theory and practice of rational-emotive behavioral consultation. *Journal of Educational and Psychological Consultation, 11*(3&4), 333–355. https://doi.org/10.1207/S1532768XJEPC113&4_04

Bernard, M. E. (1990). *Taking the stress out of teaching*. Melbourne, VIC: Collins Dove.

Bernard, M. E. (2016). Teacher beliefs and stress. *Journal of Rational Emotive and Cognitive Behavior Therapy, 34*(1), 209–224. https://doi.org/10.1007/s10942-016-0238-y

Birch, S., & Ladd, G. (1997). The teacher–child relationship and children's early school adjustment. *Journal of School Psychology, 35*(1), 61–79. https://doi.org/10.1016/S0022-4405(96)00029-5

Bramlett, R., & Murphy, J. (1998). School psychology perspectives on consultation: Key contributions to the field. *Journal of Educational and Psychological Consultation, 9*(1), 29–55. https://doi.org/10.1207/s1532768xjepc0901_2

Brunsting, N. C., Sreckovic, M. A., & Lane, K. L. (2014). Special education teacher burnout: A synthesis of research from 1979 to 2013. *Education and Treatment of Children, 37*(4), 681–711. https://doi.org/10.1353/etc.2014.0032

Buckley, D., Abbott, D., & Franey, J. (2017). An exploration of Irish teachers' experiences of stress. *Irish Journal of Applied Social Studies, 17*(1), 28–47. https://doi.org/10.21427/D7M71K

Cancio, E. J., Albrecht, S. F., & Johns, B. H. (2013). Defining administrative support and its relationship to the attrition of teachers of students with emotional and behavioral disorders. *Education and Treatment of Children, 36*(4), 71–94.

Castro, A., Quinn, D. J., Fuller, E., & Barnes, M. (2018). *Policy brief 2018-1: Addressing the importance and scale of the U.S. teacher shortage.* Retrieved July 5, 2019 from the University Council of Education Administration Website: http://www.ucea.org

Clipa, O. (2017). Teacher stress and coping strategies. In O. Clipa (Ed.), *Studies and current trends in science of education* (pp. 120–128). Suceava, Romania: LUMEN Proceedings. https://doi.org/10.18662/lumproc.icsed2017.14

Clunies-Ross, P., Little, E., & Kienhuis, M. (2008). Self-reported and actual use of proactive and reactive classroom management strategies and their relationship with teacher stress and student behaviour. *Educational Psychology, 28*(6), 693–710. https://doi.org/10.1080/01443410802206700

Collie, R., Shapka, J. D., & Perry, N. E. (2012). School climate and social-emotional learning: Predicting teacher stress, job satisfaction, and teaching efficacy. *Journal of Educational Psychology, 104*(4), 1189–1204. https://doi.org/10.1037/a0029356

Demerouti, E., Bakker, A., Nachreiner, F., & Schaufeli, W. (2001). The job demands-resources model of burnout. *Journal of Applied Psychology, 86*(3), 499–512.

DiGiuseppe, R., Doyle, K., Dryden, W., & Backx, W. (2013). *A practitioner's guide to rational-emotive therapy* (3rd ed.). New York: Oxford University Press.

Erchul, W. P., & Sheridan, S. M. (2014). Overview: The state of scientific research in school consultation. In W. P. Erchul & S. M. Sheridan (Eds.), *Handbook of research in school consultation* (2nd ed., pp. 3–17). New York: Routledge.

Greenberg, M. T., Brown, J. L., & Abenavoli, R. M. (2016). *Teacher stress and health effects on teachers, students, and schools* (Social and Emotional Learning). University Park, PA: Edna Bennett Pierce Prevention Research Center, Pennsylvania State University.

Haberman, M. (2005). Teacher burnout in black and white. *The New Educator, 1*, 153–175. https://doi.org/10.1080/15476880590966303

Hansen, J., & Sullivan, B. A. (2003). Assessment of workplace stress: Occupational stress, its consequences, and common causes of teacher stress. In J. Wall & G. R. Walz (Eds.), *Measuring up: Assessment issues for teachers, counselors, and administrators* (pp. 611–622). Greensboro, NC: ERIC Counseling and Student Services Clearinghouse.

Herman, K. C., Hickmon-Rosa, J., & Reinke, W. (2018). Empirically derived profiles of teacher stress, self-efficacy, and coping and associated student outcomes. *Journal of Positive Behavior Interventions, 20*(2), 90–100. https://doi.org/10.1177/1098300717732066

Huk, O., Terjesen, M. D., & Cherkasova, L. (2019). Predicting teacher burnout as a function of school characteristics and irrational beliefs. *Psychology in the Schools, 56*(5), 792–808. https://doi.org/10.1002/pits.22233

Johnson, S., Cooper, C., Cartwright, S., Donald, I., Taylor, P., & Millet, C. (2005). The experience of work-related stress across occupations. *Journal of Managerial Psychology, 20*(2), 178–187. https://doi.org/10.1108/02683940510579803

Jones, B. D., & Egley, R. J. (2004). Voices from the frontlines: Teachers' perceptions of high-stakes testing. *Education Policy Analysis Archives, 12*(39). Retrieved July 25, 2019 from: http://epaa.asu.edu/epaa/v12n39/

Kyriacou, C. (2011). Teacher stress: From prevalence to resilience. In J. Langan-Fox & C. L. Cooper (Eds.), *Handbook of stress in the occupations* (pp. 161–173). Cheltenham: Edward Elgar.

Lazarus, R. S., & Folkman, S. (1987). Transactional theory and research on emotions and coping. *European Journal of Personality, 1*(3), 141–169. https://doi.org/10.1002/per.2410010304

Mack, J. C., Johnson, A., Jones-Rincon, A., Tsatenawa, V., & Howard, K. (2019). Why do teachers leave? A comprehensive occupational health study evaluating intent-to-quit in public school teachers. *Journal of Applied Biobehavioral Research, 24*(1), 1–13. https://doi.org/10.1111/jabr.12160

McCormick, J., & Barnett, K. (2011). Teachers' attributions for stress and their relationships with burnout. *International Journal of Educational Management, 25*, 278–293.

McEwen, B., & Sapolsky, R. (2006). Stress and your health. *The Journal of Endocrinology & Metabolism, 91*(2), E2. Retrieved from: https://academic.oup.com/jcem/article/91/2/E2/2843213#

Miller, R. (2012). *Teacher absence as a leading indicator of student achievement: New national data offer opportunity to examiner cost of teacher absence relative to learning loss* [PDF file]. Washington, DC: Center for American Progress. Retrieved from: https://www.scribd.com/document/108763845/Teacher-Absence-as-a-Leading-Indicator-of-Student-Achievement

Mohamed, T. (2018). Sources of occupational stress among teachers: A field of study for teachers working in Libyan schools in Turkey. *International Journal of Academic Research in Economics and Management Sciences, 7*(1), 1–15. https://doi.org/10.6007/IJAREMS/v7-i1/3856

National Education Association. (2018). *Teacher compensation: Fact vs. fiction*. Retrieved July 4, 2019, from the National Education Association website: www.nea.org/home/12661.htm

Pepe, A., & Addimando, L. (2013). Comparison of occupational stress in response to challenging behaviours between general and special education primary teachers in northern Italy. *International Journal of Special Education, 13*, 11–23.

Popov, S., Popov, B., & Damjanovic, R. (2015). The role of stressors at work and irrational beliefs in the prediction of teacher stress. *Primjena Psihologija, 8*(1), 5–23.

Ronfelt, M., Loeb, S., & Wyckoff, J. (2012). *How teacher turnover harms student achievement* (CALDER No. 70). Washington, DC: American Institutes for Research.

Roorda, D. L., Koomen, H. M. Y., Split, J. L., & Oort, F. J. (2011). The influence of affective teacher-student relationships on students' school engagement and achievement: A meta-analytic approach. *Review of Educational Research, 81*(4), 493–529. https://doi.org/10.3102/0034654311421793

Rudow, B. (1999). Stress and burnout in the teaching profession: European studies, issues, and research perspectives. In R. Vandenberghe & A. M. Huberman (Eds.), *Understanding and preventing teacher burnout* (pp. 38–58). Cambridge: Cambridge University Press.

Ryan, S. V., von der Embse, N. P., Pendergast, L. L., Saeki, E., Segool, N., & Schwing, S. (2017). Leaving the teaching profession: The role of teacher stress and educational accountability policies on turnover intent. *Teaching and Teacher Education, 66*, 1–11. https://doi.org/10.1016/j.tate.2017.03.016

Sheridan, S. M., & Cowan, R. J. (2004). Consultation with school personnel. In R. T. Brown (Ed.), *Handbook of pediatric psychology in school settings* (pp. 599–616). Mahwah, NJ: Lawrence Erlbaum Associates Publishers.

Shkëmbi, F., Melonashi, E., & Fanaj, N. (2015). Workplace stress among teachers in Kosovo. *SAGE Open, 5*(4), 1–8. https://doi.org/10.1177/2158244015614610

Simonsen, B., Fairbanks, S., Briesch, A., Myers, D., & Sugai, G. (2008). Evidence-based practices in classroom management: Considerations for research to practice. *Education and Treatment of Children, 31*(3), 351–380. https://doi.org/10.1353/etc.0.0007

Skaalvik, E. M., & Skaalvik, S. (2011). Teachers' feeling of belonging, exhaustion, and job satisfaction: The role of school goal structure and value consonance. *Anxiety, Stress & Coping, 24*(4), 369–385. https://doi.org/10.1080/10615806.2010.544300

Skaalvik, E. M., & Skaalvik, S. (2016). Teacher stress and teacher self-efficacy as predictors of engagement, emotional exhaustion, and motivation to leave the teaching profession. *Creative Education, 7*(13), 1785–1799. https://doi.org/10.4236/ce.2016.713182

Souza, J. C. D., Sousa, I. C. D., Belísio, A. S., & Azevedo, C. V. M. D. (2012). Sleep habits, daytime sleepiness and sleep quality of high school teachers. *Psychology & Neuroscience, 5*(2), 257–263. https://doi.org/10.3922/j.psns.2012.2.17

Tschannen-Moran, M., & Hoy, W. K. (2000). A multidisciplinary analysis of the nature, meaning, and measurement of trust. *Review of Educational Research, 70*(4), 547–593. https://doi.org/10.3102/00346543070004547

Warren, J., & Baker, S. (2013). School counselor-consultation: Enhancing teacher performance through rational emotive-social behavioral consultation. In *Ideas and research you can use: VISTAS 2013*. Retrieved from: https://www.counseling.org/knowledge-center/vistas/by-year2/vistas-2013/docs/default-source/vistas/school-counselor-consultation-enhancing-teacher-performance

West, K., Hoessler, C., Bennetch, R., Ewert-Bauer, T., Wilson, M., Beaudoin, J.-P., et al. (2017). *Educational development guide series: No. 2. Rapport-building for educational developers*. Ottawa, ON: Educational Developers Caucus.

Yoon, J. (2002). Teacher characteristics as predictors of teacher-student relationships: Stress, negative affect, and self-efficacy. *Social Behavior and Personality, 30*(5), 485–494. https://doi.org/10.2224/sbp.2002.30.5.485

Chapter 24
Applications of Rational-Emotive and Cognitive-Behavior Technologies with Children and Adolescents

Daniel O. David, Silviu A. Matu, and Roxana A. I. Cardos

Introduction

Cognitive-behavior therapy (CBT), including rational emotive-behavior therapy (REBT) as one of its main pillars, has experienced two major revolutions in the last two decades. One is related to the proliferation of the evidence-based approach as a way of testing and proving the efficacy and the scientific status of psychological interventions, using rigorous methodology such as randomized clinical trials (David & Montgomery, 2011). The second revolution, which we will discuss extensively in this chapter, is related to the integration between psychological interventions and technology, which has been reflected in both research and practice in the clinical field, including for children and adolescents. It is important to mention that the integration of technology into psychotherapy has not taken a separate path from the evidence-based approach, meaning that technological developments have been ana-

The original version of this chapter was revised. The correction to this chapter is available at https://doi.org/10.1007/978-3-030-53901-6_25

D. O. David (✉)
Department of Clinical Psychology and Psychotherapy/The International Institute for the Advanced Studies of Psychotherapy and Applied Mental Health, Babeş-Bolyai University, Cluj-Napoca, Romania

Department of Oncological Sciences, Icahn School of Medicine at Mount Sinai, New York, NY, USA
e-mail: danieldavid@psychology.ro

S. A. Matu · R. A. I. Cardos
Department of Clinical Psychology and Psychotherapy/The International Institute for the Advanced Studies of Psychotherapy and Applied Mental Health, Babeş-Bolyai University, Cluj-Napoca, Romania
e-mail: silviu.matu@ubbcluj.ro; roxana.cardos@ubbcluj.ro

M. Bernard, M. D. Terjesen (eds.), *Rational-Emotive and Cognitive-Behavioral Approaches to Child and Adolescent Mental Health: Theory, Practice, Research, Applications*, https://doi.org/10.1007/978-3-030-53901-6_24

lyzed with the same rigor and using the same criteria which required compelling empirical evidence to prove their utility (e.g., Fodor et al., 2018).

Although there are numerous innovations that have driven the technological revolution in children's and adolescents' mental health treatment, we will group them under three main categories: (a) computer, internet, and mobile-based applications; (b) virtual reality applications; and (c) robotic-based applications.

Classical CBT and REBT, understood as an unmediated face-to-face interaction between a client and a therapist or a counselor, has four main components: (1) assessment, (2) case formulation, (3) intervention techniques, and (4) therapeutic relationship (Beck, 2011; Ellis & Dryden, 1997). The first three components can be summarized as collecting information about the client's problems, offering the client a good understanding of his/her problems from a psychological and clinical perspective, and guiding the client in identifying the steps that he/she has to follow in order to overcome those problems (APA Presidential Task Force on Evidence-Based Practice, 2006). These components are mainly related to *information exchanges* between the client and the therapist. Computer, internet, and mobile applications cover the main purpose of gathering relevant information about the client and offer personalized and clinically informed guidance on how to manage emotional and behavioral problems, all done using a computer or mobile phone connected to the internet, from anywhere the client might be at a certain moment, most of the times in contexts that are inaccessible to the mental health specialist, such as a client's home (Andersson, Carlbring, Ljótsson, & Hedman, 2013).

Virtual reality (VR) applications require special technological tools (i.e., goggles) in order to experience a three-dimensional (3D) artificial environment that was developed to mimic a real one as good as technology allows it and which is somehow relevant to the problem of the client. The therapist observes how the client reacts or performs in that environment (conducts assessment) and/or teaches the client new ways of reacting and behaving in this situation, for example by helping him/her to change the irrational/dysfunctional beliefs he/she holds in relation to the (virtual) activating event (David, Matu, & David, 2013). Augmented reality (AR) is a similar technology that blends reality with artificial elements, instead of immersing the client in a fully virtual environment. The clinical rationale behind immersing the client in the computer generated environment in order to conduct assessment or to provide intervention is the fact that such experiences are more ecological than many of the classical means to conduct assessment or intervention (e.g., relying on self-reports of the client about past events; Rizzo & Kim, 2005), and many times classical methods cannot be performed in real-life situations (e.g., the therapist can't fly with the patient and demonstrate to him/her how to perform exposure and to restructure irrational beliefs).

The integration of robotic-based applications into psychotherapy is related to interactions between a client and a robot agent in which (a) the robot covers at least some of the functions that are regularly performed by a therapist, (b) the presence of the robot facilitates the goals of the intervention, or (c) the robot performs some actions that are not regularly performed by the therapist but have a clinical utility (David, Matu, & David, 2014). For example, an emerging topic in the literature on children suffering from Autism Spectrum Disorders (ASD) is the use of robots in order to facilitate learning and social communication, as research shows that these children are attracted to robots and they are expressing social behaviors toward them. Moreover, they are more likely to interact with other humans if this interaction is mediated by a robot (Kim et al., 2013).

The integration of technological tools into psychotherapy offers some important advantages over the classical means of delivering mental health services, by making them more accessible (e.g., accessing therapist guidance from anywhere, at any time), more ecological (e.g., teaching clients to identify and change their beliefs as they are directly confronted with a virtual activating event) and facilitate therapeutic interaction (e.g., using robotic agents for children with ASD) or other kind of interaction with therapeutic benefits (e.g., robotic toys or pets).

In the following section, we will analyze the applications within each of the three categories that we have previously delimited: computer, internet, and mobile-based applications; virtual reality applications; and robotic-based applications. We will discuss the available evidence that supports the use of these applications when working with children and adolescents, in order to have an understanding of their scientific status. We will also offer some detailed examples within each category that are relevant for children and adolescent populations.

Using Technology to Enhance REBT Interventions for Children and Adolescents

Computer, Internet, and Mobile-Based Applications

Computer, internet, and mobile-based application are becoming a common presence in the field of CBT (they are often called iCBT), and several of them have been developed using an REBT framework. iCBT have been proposed as a way to increase access to evidence-based psychological intervention (Andersson, 2010). They differ not only by the technological tool that is used to deliver them but also by the degree to which they allow the interaction between the client and the therapist. This level of interaction stretches from direct interaction using audio-video communication over the internet (Stefan & David, 2013), to *self-help* interventions that do not imply any kind of interaction between user and clinician (Titov et al., 2013). Self-help interventions offer information to the clients about the problems they are confronted with and guides them through a series of techniques derived from the face-to-face protocols that are meant to reduce their symptoms.

The intervention could also be delivered through game-like applications, in order to increase engagement, especially in the case of children (Kearns, 2015). Information is presented to the clients in different formats, such as text, videos, and animations. Self-help interventions might also provide some form of feedback to the users, based on his/her activity, although this feedback is generated automatically, based on the user's activity and the algorithms programmed in the system (e.g., feedback related to the user improvements on assessment instruments).

Other forms of intervention offer direct and asynchronous interaction between the client and the therapist (*guided self-help*), meaning that they interact via emails or messages that allow them to exchange information, to give and receive feedback; however, the communication is not instantaneous (Andersson et al., 2013). There are also *blended* intervention, which combine face-to-face sessions (or sessions offered via teleconference) with computer/internet/mobile interventions. In this case, the client gets initiated into the intervention by the therapist, and then follows the exercises and techniques indicated by the self-help intervention offered with the help of technology (Kenter et al., 2015).

Meta-analytic studies support the efficacy of iCBT for various conditions, especially for depression and anxiety disorders for children (Păsărelu, Andersson, Bergman Nordgren, & Dobrean, 2017; Vigerland et al., 2016) populations, and indicate that the use of these applications is equally effective as classical interventions. Applications that include some form of interaction between the client and the clinician, even if the interaction is asynchronous, tend to be more effective (Baumeister, Reichler, Munzinger, & Lin, 2014; Titov, Andrews, Choi, Schwencke, & Mahoney, 2008). Users of guided applications report some form of therapeutic alliance, even if there is no synchronous interaction with the therapist (Andersson et al., 2012). However, the ratings made by therapist on the therapeutic alliance seem to be more relevant than those made by the client (Vernmark et al., 2019). The fact that we have consistent evidence does not mean, however, that any commercially available application on the internet or in the mobile application stores have been tested and proven to be effective (see Sucala et al., 2017).

We will describe two applications that offer good examples of the integration between technology and REBT. One is a gamified application that targets emotional symptoms in youths and the last one is focused on improving parenting skills.

REThink Therapeutic Game (http://psychotherapy.psiedu.ubbcluj.ro/national-research-grants/the-rethink-online-therapeutic-game/)

A recent and expanding strategy for increasing children's and adolescents' access to mental health care is the use of therapeutic computer games (Institute of Digital Media and Child Development Working Group on Games for Health, 2016; Kearns, 2015). Therapeutic games are games with non-entertainment goals (Ceranoglu, 2010) that make use of the fascination that children and teenagers have for electronic games, in order to deliver mental health prevention or intervention programs. As computer games are the most frequent and popular form of entertainment among adolescents (Horne-Moyer, Moyer, Messer, & Messer, 2014), they represent an appealing tool to reach youth population. As computers, smartphones, and tablets are becoming even more ubiquitous, the use of computerized games found its way into clinical care of youth (Ceranoglu, 2010). Serious, therapeutic games have been developed to facilitate psychotherapeutic interventions for children and adolescents, and there is already research indicating that they can be effective in addressing a variety of mental health symptoms (Horne-Moyer et al., 2014). Recent studies highlight the need for more theory-based, evidence-based therapeutic serious games, with clearly specified intervention protocols, that can be used for preventing mental disorders in children and adolescents.

The REThink game was developed (David, Cardoş, & Matu, 2019a, 2019b), as a prevention tool that promotes emotion regulation skills in children and adolescents. The game aims to help children and adolescents (aged between 10 and 16 years) learn healthy psychological strategies for coping with distress. REThink is anchored in the Rational-Emotive and Behavioral Education (Ellis & Bernard, 2006; REBE), a preventive approach derived from REBT, which focuses on helping children and adolescents change their unhelpful patterns of thinking, as well as their unhealthy behaviors and emotions, in order to prevent psychopathology. REBE has proved to be efficient in mental health promotion among non-clinical populations of children and adolescents (Gonzalez et al., 2004; Trip, Vernon, & McMahon, 2007).

REThink is an interactive adventure game with seven levels. Each of the seven levels of the game corresponds to a certain step in the REBE approach. The game takes place in multiple areas of planet Earth that are under the power of a maleficent character (*Irrationalizer*) that promotes irrationality. At the end of the game, the player has to save the inhabitants of the planet from the powers of irrational characters. The game includes a main character, RETMAN. RETMAN is a comic book character developed at the Albert Ellis Institute in New York in the 1970s in order to disseminate the principles of REBT theory to the general population in a fun and attractive manner. The initial book (Merrifield & Merrifield, 1979) had Albert Ellis as a main character depicted as an unconventional superhero therapist teaching other people how to live rationally. This idea was later adapted in Romania for children and adolescents, and RETMAN (http://psychotherapy.psiedu.ubbcluj.ro/meet-retman/the-retmagic-of-retman/) became the main character of a series of rational stories, rational comics, and cartoons (David, 2010) in which he assisted children to overcome negative dysfunctional emotions (depression, anxiety, and anger), by changing irrational beliefs. In the REThink game, RETMAN has five friends (*Preferilizer*, *Ponderancer*, *Toleraser*, *Acceptableizer*, *Optimizer*) that help him in his missions. Each of these friends represents a rational way of thinking (i.e., preferences beliefs). *Irrationalizer* is RETMAN's and player's enemy, who promotes irrational thinking together with his servants (*Necessitizer*, *Awfulizer*, *Frustralizer*, and *Discourager*), which represents irrational way of thinking (i.e., demandingness beliefs). RETMAN and his helpers' mission is to support the player to teach people from Earth to be more rational, more functional, and happier. Each level has various degrees of complexity, which increases as the player progresses in the game. The scenario of the game focuses on seven objectives, represented by the seven levels: Level 1—identifying the emotional reactions and differentiating between functional and dysfunctional emotions; Level 2—identifying beliefs that underly emotional responses. Level 3—identifying the relation between beliefs, emotions, and behaviours. Level 4—changing irrational cognitions into rational cognitions; Level 5—learning problem-solving skills; Level 6—learning relaxation skills; Level 7—consolidating previous skills and learning happiness skills.

Outcomes of a randomized clinical trial (David, Cardos, & Matu, 2019a) indicated that the REThink game had a positive impact as a prevention program for emotional and depressive symptoms. Also, REThink improved children's ability to regulate their emotions. Results indicated that REThink is efficacious for preventing emotional problems in children and adolescents and for promoting emotional awareness and control, with implications for building resilience. Results of the mechanisms of change analysis (David, Cardos, & Matu, 2019b) indicated that changes in irrational beliefs mediated the effect of the REThink intervention on depressive mood and distress, as contrasted with the control group. Age was not a significant moderator, which indicates that the game was equally effective for children and adolescents. Given its accesability, REThink is a valuable evidence-based prevention tool for emotional problems in youth.

Online Rational Positive Parenting Program

The Rational Positive Parenting Program (rPPP; David & DiGiuseppe, 2016; Gavita, David, Bujoreanu, Tiba, & Ionutiu, 2012; David, 2019) represents an evidence-based REBT parenting program developed in order to teach parents emotion-regulation skills and positive parenting strategies. rPPP has scientific support for its full-length (David, David, & Dobrean, 2014), short-length (Gavita et al., 2012), face-to-face and self-help (Gavita & Calin, 2013), online (David, Capris, & Jarda, 2017) and mobile formats (David, 2019), for improving parents' emotion regulation skills, which also act as mechanisms for child outcomes (Gavita, David, & DiGiuseppe, 2014).

The online version of the rPPP consists of eight modules (David & DiGiuseppe, 2016). Parents are coached to stimulate good behavior, to assess family rules, to implement a reward and negative consequences system, to solve problems, to cope with specific child-related situations, and to transmit efficiently to their children all the things they learned (David & DiGiuseppe, 2016). Beside the sessions, parents have to complete a series of homework tasks, which facilitate the transfer of skills and strategies into everyday contexts. The online version (David et al., 2017) integrates in the intervention attention bias modification procedures (ABM) and "psychological pills". Attention bias modification implies a computerized emotion-regulation procedure based on deployment of attention, in order to implicitly train the parents flexibly allocate their attention to stimuli in the environment. Functional reappraisal statements are offered to the parents in order to regulate a dysfunctional emotion. The efficacy of the online format of the rPPP was tested in a randomized clinical trial (David et al., 2017) and proved to be effective in improving emotional and attitutindal outcomes, with high effect sizes, for both parents, and children.

VR Applications

Experiencing a 3D VR environment requires special devices, such as a head mounted display (HMD) or a room where images are projected on multiple walls, also called a CAVE system. The interaction with the virtual environment is done using multiple gadgets, such as controllers, or trackers for head, body and hand position, that translate the movements of the users from the real world into the virtual world (Schultheis & Rizzo, 2001). Additional sensorial channels such as sounds or scents can also be added to the virtual experience. Better quality of the projected images, more naturalistic interfaces for interacting with the environment, and stimulations on multiple sensorial channels, all increase the presence of the user, meaning that he/she is more likely to experience the virtual environment as if it is a real environment (Cummings & Bailenson, 2016).

VR applications have been used for the treatment of various mental health conditions. The specific psychological mechanisms that are targeted through the integration of this technology and the case formulation will depend largely on the symptomatology of the client although there are some communalities. The best-documented application in the literature is the use of VR for conducting exposure treatment for anxiety disorders, also called *Virtual Reality Exposure Therapy* (VRET; Rothbaum, Hodges, & Kooper, 1997). Following behavioral case formulation, the patient is exposed gradually to the feared stimuli until habituation has been reached and the patient feels tolerable levels of anxiety (Krijn, Emmelkamp, Olafsson, & Biemond, 2004). The clinical rationale for using this type of exposure strategy is that it can be safely performed inside the therapist's office, without the need to conduct exposure in real-life condition that might be threatening (e.g., developing a panic attack while being exposed to heights) or might be affecting confidentiality (e.g., flying with a patient that has flight anxiety and teaching him how to perform block safety behaviors; Szentagotai, Opris, & David, 2010). Several reviews and meta-analyses have indicated that these interventions are effective in treating anxiety disorders and that their effects are comparable to classic interventions (Opriş et al., 2012; Powers & Emmelkamp, 2008) Moreover, given that some phobic patients might be reluctant to follow treatment knowing that it requires real-life exposure, it has been suggested that VRET might be more appealing to them, because the feared stimuli are presented only in VR. VR has been used for treating children suffering from spider phobia, school phobia, and social phobia, following the principles of graduate exposure (for a review see, Bouchard, 2011).

We will now describe one VR application that has the highest relevance for this chapter. The application presents a VR system for the assessment and treatment of Attention Deficit Hyperactivity Disorder (ADHD).

Virtual Classroom Application for Children with ADHD

This application was developed by the Institute for Creative Technologies from the University of Southern California and by Digital MediaWorks Inc., in order to offer an ecological and valid assessment for ADHD (Rizzo et al., 2006) in children. The system uses a HMD device to project the child in a virtual environment simulating a classroom where he/she is being seated at a pupils desk and is required to follow an activity that is similar to those that he/she would do in a regular day at school (read the letter or words that are written on the blackboard). The environment embeds a virtual teacher and several virtual classroom mates. The clinician can manipulate the material that is being presented to the child on the blackboard and can ask the child to complete different tasks, such as reporting the moment when a specific letter is being presented. The clinician can also manipulate several distractors that might appear in a classroom environment, such as the sounds coming from the street or a paper plane that is being thrown by a colleague. Based on the correct responses and the errors of the child in following the instructed task and the degree to which he/she gets distracted by other stimuli in the environment, a behavioral performance index can be calculated which could be indicative for attention deficits or hyperactivity symptoms. Moreover, the HMD device, which is tracking the head movements of the user in order to adjust the point of view and to offer a realistic experience, can provide additional quantitative data about the head movements of the child during the task. This information can also be used to assess the degree of hyperactivity. The rationale behind the development of such a system and using it for the assessment of ADHD is the fact that such an assessment has much more ecological validity than classical paper-and-pencil test used to measure attention. Even computerized tasks that translate the classical tests into a digital version lack ecological validity, as most of the times there is less correspondence between the way in which the predictor is assessed (i.e., the test) and the context in which we want to predict behavior (i.e., real-life scenario).

Psychometric research has shown that children with ADHD perform more poorly than typically developing children on an attention task in the Virtual Classroom (Parsons, Bowerly, Buckwalter, & Rizzo, 2007). They identified less targets, reported more incorrect targets, were more distracted by irrelevant stimuli, and showed higher levels of body and head activity during the task. Subsequent research confirmed the initial results and indicated that the assessment performed with Virtual Classroom is equivalent to standard measures of attention (Neguț, Jurma, & David, 2017).

This application can also be used for the treatment of ADHD, being a promising application for future integration of REBT assessment and treatment principles when working with ADHD populations. The ecological context in which the behavior of the child can be observed makes the application a useful training environment for the child's parents and teachers. During therapy sessions, while the child is immersed in a virtual task, the caregivers can observe the behavior of the child and practice under the supervision of the therapist how to apply different reinforcement strategies to reward adaptive behaviors or to correct maladaptive behaviors that emerge during the task (Anton, Opris, Dobrean, David, & Rizzo, 2009).

Robotic-Based Applications

The integration of robotic-based applications into psychotherapy is related to interactions between a client and a robot agent in which (a) the robot covers at least some of the functions that are regularly performed by a therapist, (b) the presence of the robot facilitates the goals of the intervention, or (c) the robot performs some actions that are not regularly performed by the therapist but have a clinical utility (David, Matu, et al., 2014). This tasks can be performed by robots built with the purpose of interacting with human beings and are called social robots. They can be defined as an artificial system that can simulate the way in which we interact with other humans (e.g., simulate verbal and non-verbal language) or with other living beings (e.g., simulate the interaction with a pet). The physical instantiation of the robot is not a necessary condition, as they could be virtual and presented via a computer display (David, Matu, et al., 2014). For example, a virtual avatar of a therapist can monitor the evolution of remitted patients that suffered from depression by verbally asking questions about their mood and can also provide therapeutic support by guiding patients through simple cognitive restructuring techniques (Pagliari et al., 2012). In this case, the artificial agent takes the role of the therapists while also simulating the way the client and therapist interact and the interaction is done in the home of the patient. As a second example of using robotic agents in psychotherapy, an emerging topic in the literature on children suffering from Autism Spectrum Disorders (ASD) is the use of robots in order to facilitate learning and social communication, as research shows that these children are attracted to robots and they are expressing social behaviors toward them. Moreover, they are more likely to interact with other humans if this interaction is mediated by a robot (Kim et al., 2013). Finally, robots have already been used for many years as companions (as robotic toys and robotic pets) for children and elderly in order to provide a source of positive interactions and emotions (Broadbent, Stafford, & MacDonald, 2009). In this final case, the robot does not perform a role that is commonly assumed by the therapist, but the interaction with the robot has some therapeutic benefits.

Robotic agents can be integrated into psychotherapy in three different ways (see David, Matu, et al., 2014): (a) as a *robo-therapist*, the robot performs several of the activities that are regularly performed by the clinician, such as performing assessment, offering a case formulation and guidance through the intervention; (b) as a *robot-mediator*, the presence of the robot is required because it engages the client, increases the efficacy of the intervention, and/or the effects of the intervention are visible sooner compared to situation in which the robot is not present; (c) as a *robo-assistant*, the robot performs several activities that are not regularly performed by the clinician (e.g., performing pleasant activities with the patient at home) but have a clinical utility.

There are few examples in the literature that cover the robot-therapist role, probably due to the complexity of developing artificial agents capable of performing a vast array of clinical activities.

The robo-mediator role is specific to children that have been diagnosed with ASD. Several studies (for a review see Diehl, Schmitt, Villano, & Crowell, 2012) have indicated that children with ASD are enjoying interacting with robotic agents, they are responsive to the social cues initiated by the robots, and express social behaviors towards robots, and do so to a greater extent than situations in which they are interacting with another human or with a non-responsive toy. Given these results, intervention studies have integrated robotic agents in the treatment in order to offer children cues to perform various social behaviors and to reinforce good performance. In a common scenario, the robot gives the child a verbal and non-verbal instruction (e.g., indicates an object by pointing and says "look"). If the child follows the instruction, then the robot will give the child a positive social feedback, or if it fails to follow the instruction, it will encourage him/her to try again (David, Costescu, Matu, Szentagotai, & Dobrean, 2018). Positive results have been found across multiple outcomes, such as prosocial behaviors in younger populations (Vanderborght et al., 2012), joint attention (Simut, Vanderfaeillie, Peca, Van de Perre, & Vanderborght, 2016), and turn taking in collaborative play scenarios (David, Costescu, Matu, Szentagotai, & Dobrean, 2019). It is important to have in mind that much of this research has used single-case designs or small samples, and not all children report these patterns of improvement. More research is needed to understand which children benefit the most from the interaction with the robot.

Finally, the robo-assistant role is specific to different robotic agents that have been used to reduce hospitalized children's distress levels and support their well-being (Moerman, van der Heide, & Heerink, 2019). A recent systematic review (Moerman et al., 2019) suggests that different robotic agents used in a hospital context may have a positive impact on children adjustment to the hospital environment and their emotional state. However, it is necessary to further determine how to integrate the use of robotic agents in the hospital activities and procedures. We will now describe in more detail two examples of integrations between REBT and robotic technology.

Reducing Distress in Children Using Robo-RETMAN as a Robo-therapist

We have presented earlier the RETMAN character that has been used to promote REBT principles in several ways, such as comics, stories, and the REThink game. For smaller children, two versions of RETMAN have been developed as sensorized robotic toys allowing them to interact with the robot and learn some basic principles of REBT/REBE. One version (for preschool children) depicts the character as a friendly plush toy, while the other as an action figure (for school-age children). In both cases, the child uses a set of radio-frequency identification cards depicting different dysfunctional emotions (depression, anxiety, anger) which he/she can place them near the sensor of the robot in order to ask RETMAN for help in dealing with these emotions. RETMAN than offers the child a rational psychological pill adapted to his/her emotional state and to the typical type of problems that children of that age might be confronted with. Empirical research shows that children benefit more in terms of reduction of dysfunctional emotions and irrational beliefs when they receive the rational statement offered by the robot before a stressful situation than when the same statement is simply read to them (David & David, 2013). Moreover, the use of the robot showed positive effects even when compared to watching a set of cartoons that were developed to target the same type of dysfunctional emotions by modeling more rational beliefs (David & David, 2013; David, David, & Vanderborght, 2013).

Assessing and Restructuring Irrational Beliefs in Children with ASD Using a Robot-Mediator Approach

We have previously described the ways in which robotic agents have been used as mediators of the intervention in the treatment of children with ASD. Most of the previous work has been done mainly in a behavioral approach (focusing on reinforcements for adaptive behaviors); however, there are some examples where the robot was used as a mediator using an REBT/REBE approach, both for assessment and intervention. In one study (Costescu, Vanderborght, & David, 2016), the robot Keepon (Kozima, Michalowski, & Nakagawa, 2009) was used to provide false negative feedback on a simple puzzle to a group of children diagnosed with ASD and a group of healthy controls. Keepon is a small robot resembling a yellow snowman that is capable of flexing its body in order to imitate some basic human expressions, like approval or disapproval, but it is not able to move otherwise. After being promised a valuable reward that was conditioned on completing the puzzle and receiving a positive feedback from the robot, both groups received negative feedback from the robot and were observed in terms of their emotional expression (functional vs. dysfunctional), verbal utterance, and behavioral responses (adaptive responses such as seeking comfort vs. disruptive reaction such as aggressivity). The intensity of experienced emotions was also measured using a visual representation. The children were given new opportunities to solve similar puzzles and the researchers measured the frequency of using the same strategy or trying to change it in order to receive a positive feedback. Verbalizations that children made after negative feedbacks were coded by trained observers and the frequency of rational and irrational statements contained by their utterances was measured. The results indicated that ASD children more frequently used statements that contained demandingness and awfulizing but not statements that indicated low frustration tolerance or global evaluations. Also, ASD children expressed more frequently emotions that fell under the dysfunctional category, while typically developing children expressed more emotions that fell under the functional category. ASD children also manifested more disruptive behaviors and made use more frequently of the same strategy to solve the puzzle (for more details see, Costescu et al., 2016). These results suggest that irrational beliefs are relevant constructs that can be studies even in this population, where cognitive approaches are less frequently used. Also, they point to the idea that robotic agents can represent relevant interaction partners which can stimulate activating events allowing the assessment, and perhaps the intervention on relevant cognitions.

Indeed, in a subsequent study, the same authors (Costescu et al., 2017), used the Keepon robot to teach children with ASD basic REBE concepts, such as the distinction between functional and dysfunctional emotions and between rational and irrational beliefs. The study was a randomized trial, allocating ASD children to either the 6-sessions group format intervention or to a group that followed the regular treatment schedule (treatment as usual). The robot offered social reinforcements to children by positive or negative feedback, contingent on their performance on tasks that were designed to test their understanding of the ABC model (Ellis, 1994). Functional and dysfunctional emotions, rational and irrational beliefs, as well as adaptive behaviors were coded based on their responses to 15 hypothetical negative social situations (vignettes). The results indicated positive results favoring the REBE intervention on the frequency of rational beliefs (but not irrational beliefs) stated by the children, as well as on the intensity of negative emotional experiences. This brief intervention offers a good example on how to integrate robotic technology into educational activities for ASD children using an REBT framework.

Discussion: How to Integrate Technological Applications Into Practice

The integration of technology with psychotherapy has changed the way we think about mental health services. The idea that psychological interventions have to rely on the direct and unmediated contact between the therapist or counselor and the client has now become less essential. There are several advantages that the technological tools have brought to the field of children and adolescents' psychological interventions. First, and perhaps the most important, is the fact that they have extended youth access to evidence-based psychological services. Not only that the child/adolescent can access such services from anywhere there is an internet connection, but mental health services are becoming more cost-effective, and their economic burden on patients and health systems can be lowered (e.g., Podina, Mogoase, David, Szentagotai, & Dobrean, 2016). The fact that a therapist can now refer some young people to online/mobile tools for at least some components of the intervention (e.g., learn how to practice a particular technique) also means that the therapist can now work with more young people and address the unmet needs for mental health care (Grist, Porter, & Stallard, 2017). The integration of robots in the treatment of ASD would allow a therapist to rethink the treatment plan so that some basic skills could be trained by the robotic agent, while the clinician can focus on other essential components of the intervention.

A second advantage brought by technological tools to the psychological interventions used with children and adolescents is the fact that they can make psychotherapy and counseling more attractive to patients. Computerized and online interventions can get rid of the stigma associated with entering a clinician's office. VR exposure can make the treatment more appealing to young people that are reluctant to be confronted with the phobic stimuli (e.g., social anxiety). Integrating robotic agents into behavioral treatments of children with ASD might increase their engagement and interest for the intervention. The use of therapeutic games such as REThink or the use of robo-RETMAN can make REBT/REBE interventions more engaging and appealing to children with emotional disorders.

Third, as we have pointed across the chapter, the use of technology can help to extend or support the work of the therapist in contexts in which he/she does not have access in a classical approach. The use of internet and mobile applications can offer support to the children/adolescent in critical moments and increase the chances of using successfully the strategies that were taught by the clinician. Similarly, robotic agents, like robo-RETMAN, can support children and adolescents in regulating their dysfunctional emotions and practice rational thinking between sessions.

Finally, technology could also enhance the efficacy of psychological interventions for children and adolescents. For example, identifying and restructuring irrational beliefs and practicing rational alternatives might have better effects if these steps are performed in VR, having direct access to the stream of thoughts that are activated by the critical event. In the case of robots, engaging ASD children in the treatment might also enhance learning and lead to better therapeutic outcomes. However, such improvements in the efficacy of the interventions have yet to be proven by rigorous empirical research.

We conclude this section by trying to answer a question that is frequent among REBT practitioners working with children and adolescents: "Can I use technology in my practice if I haven't been specifically trained to do so?". We answer this question by stating that the integration with technology is not a new form of psychotherapy (David, Matu, et al., 2013). As we have pointed out, the same treatment components targeting the same psychological mechanisms are also engaged by technologically enhanced interventions. Thus, any clinician that has a good understanding of the technological tools that we have presented can integrate them into their regular practice.

Concluding Remarks

The integration of technology in REBT offers new opportunities for supporting younger clients overcomes the problems they are confronted with. We have described several applications and discussed how they could improve clinical practice. Although many of these applications have been extensively tested, some of them still need consistent empirical investigation in order to prove their efficacy and evidence-based status. Moreover, some of the applications presented here have been tested extensively on adult population, but few studies have focused on children and adolescents (e.g., most of VR applications), and more research is needed in those areas.

REBT has been on the forefront of these technological developments and has been the basis for the development of several evidence-based applications. However, there are many areas with great potential that have only been explored at this point. The use of robots to identify and restructure irrational beliefs in children with ASD is an interesting avenue, which might extend the applicability of REBT interventions to a population that has not been commonly in its focus. The same is also true for VR as a tool to assess and tackle irrational beliefs of younger clients.

In the future, over 10 years, we expect that common REBT practices with younger populations will be more focused on the use of technology within the psychotherapeutic/counseling and clinical assessment processes. By integrating the theoretical foundations with innovative ways of delivering effective services, REBT will maintain its status as an up-to-date evidence-based intervention. We consider that future REBT technological tools will facilitate real-time monitoring and the delivery of personalized therapeutic interventions. Thus, the benefits of future digital technologies can be used to improve the effectiveness of REBT therapies and to develop young people's access to these interventions. We expect that, in the future, REBT specialists will increasingly focus on developing and testing technology-based prevention programs. We believe that this strategy is one of the best to prevent mental disorders in adulthood, but also one of the least used today, because of access barriers. Delivering psychological prevention programs by technological means can fill these practical and research gaps and can develop young people's access to mental health prevention programs. Regarding the future of REBT programs for children and adolescents, we expect that the development of the technological domain will lead to the development of different evidence-based technology-based REBT programs for youth population. We expect that the REBT research field will start to keep up with technological development in terms of testing new developed tools.

The use of technology could help disseminate REBT principles and practice to multiple populations and contexts, and thus have a wide impact on promoting rationality and mental health of children and adolescents.

Test Yourself

1. What are some of the advantages and limitations of integrating technological tools into psychotherapy?
2. In consideration of youngsters and their parents that you have worked with, how might a program like the Rational Positive Parenting Program, RoboRETman, or REThink been beneficial to promote emotion regulation and positive behaviors?
3. What are some strategies that you think you can consider to allow you to implement technology within your clinical practice?

References

Andersson, G. (2010). The promise and pitfalls of the internet for cognitive behavioral therapy. *BMC Medicine, 8*(1), 82–86. https://doi.org/10.1186/1741-7015-8-82

Andersson, G., Carlbring, P., Ljótsson, B., & Hedman, E. (2013). Guided internet-based CBT for common mental disorders. *Journal of Contemporary Psychotherapy, 43*(4), 223–233. https://doi.org/10.1007/s10879-013-9237-9

Andersson, G., Paxling, B., Wiwe, M., Vernmark, K., Felix, C. B., Lundborg, L., et al. (2012). Therapeutic alliance in guided internet-delivered cognitive behavioural treatment of depression, generalized anxiety disorder and social anxiety disorder. *Behaviour Research and Therapy, 50*(9), 544–550. https://doi.org/10.1016/j.brat.2012.05.003

Anton, R., Opris, D., Dobrean, A., David, D., & Rizzo, A. (2009). Virtual reality in rehabilitation of attention deficit/hyperactivity disorder: The instrument construction principles. In *2009 Virtual Rehabilitation International Conference* (pp. 59–64). Piscataway, NJ: IEEE.

APA Presidential Task Force on Evidence-Based Practice. (2006). Evidence-based practice in psychology. *American Psychologist, 61*(4), 271–285. https://doi.org/10.1037/0003-066X.61.4.271

Baumeister, H., Reichler, L., Munzinger, M., & Lin, J. (2014). The impact of guidance on Internet-based mental health interventions: A systematic review. *Internet Interventions, 1*(4), 205–215. https://doi.org/10.1016/j.invent.2014.08.003

Beck, J. S. (2011). *Cognitive therapy: Basics and beyond*. New York: Guilford press.

Bouchard, S. (2011). Could virtual reality be effective in treating children with phobias? *Expert Review of Neurotherapeutics, 11*(2), 207–213. https://doi.org/10.1586/ern.10.196

Broadbent, E., Stafford, R., & MacDonald, B. (2009). Acceptance of healthcare robots for the older population: Review and future directions. *International Journal of Social Robotics, 1*(4), 319–330. https://doi.org/10.1007/s12369-009-0030-6

Ceranoglu, T. A. (2010). Video games in psychotherapy. *Review of General Psychology, 14*(2), 141–146. https://doi.org/10.1037/a0019439

Costescu, C. A., Vanderborght, B., & David, D. O. (2016). Beliefs, emotions, and behaviors-differences between children with ASD and typically developing children. A robot-enhanced task. *Journal of Evidence-Based Psychotherapies, 16*(2), 221–237.

Costescu, C. A., Vanderborght, B., & David, D. O. (2017). Robot-enhanced CBT for dysfunctional emotions in social situations for children with ASD. *Journal of Evidence-Based Psychotherapies, 17*(2), 119–132.

Cummings, J. J., & Bailenson, J. N. (2016). How immersive is enough? A meta-analysis of the effect of immersive technology on user presence. *Media Psychology, 19*(2), 272–309. https://doi.org/10.1080/15213269.2015.1015740

David, D. (2010). *Retmagia şi minunatele aventuri ale lui Retman. Poveşti raţionale pentru copii şi adolescenţi (Retmagic and the wonderful adventures of Retman. Stories for children and adolescents)*. Cluj-Napoca, Romania: RTS Cluj.

David, D., Matu, S. A., & David, O. A. (2013). New directions in virtual reality-based therapy for anxiety disorders. *International Journal of Cognitive Therapy, 6*(2), 114–137.

David, D., Matu, S. A., & David, O. A. (2014). Robot-based psychotherapy: Concepts development, state of the art, and new directions. *International Journal of Cognitive Therapy, 7*(2), 192–210.

David, D., & Montgomery, G. H. (2011). The scientific status of psychotherapies: A new evaluative framework for evidence-based psychosocial interventions. *Clinical Psychology: Science and Practice, 18*(2), 89–99. https://doi.org/10.1111/j.1468-2850.2011.01239.x

David, D. O., Costescu, C. A., Matu, S., Szentagotai, A., & Dobrean, A. (2018). Developing joint attention for children with autism in robot-enhanced therapy. *International Journal of Social Robotics, 10*(5), 595–605. https://doi.org/10.1007/s12369-017-0457-0

David, D. O., Costescu, C. A., Matu, S., Szentagotai, A., & Dobrean, A. (2019). Effects of a robot-enhanced intervention for children with ASD on teaching turn-taking skills. *Journal of Educational Computing Research, 58*(1), 29–62.

David, O. A. (2019). The Rational Parenting Coach app: REThink parenting! A mobile parenting program for offering evidence-based personalized support in the prevention of child externalizing and internalizing disorders. *Journal of Evidence Based-Psychotherapy, 19*(2), 1–19.

David, O. A., Capris, D., & Jarda, A. (2017). Online coaching of emotion-regulation strategies for parents: Efficacy of the online rational positive parenting program and attention bias modification procedures. *Frontiers in Psychology, 8*, 500. https://doi.org/10.3389/fpsyg.2017.00500

David, O. A., Cardoş, R. A., & Matu, S. (2019a). Is REThink therapeutic game effective in preventing emotional disorders in children and adolescents? Outcomes of a randomized clinical trial. *European Child & Adolescent Psychiatry, 28*(1), 111–122. https://doi.org/10.1007/s00787-018-1192-2

David, O. A., Cardoş, R. A., & Matu, S. (2019b). Changes in irrational beliefs are responsible for the efficacy of the REThink therapeutic game in preventing emotional disorders in children and adolescents: Mechanisms of change analysis of a randomized clinical trial. *European Child & Adolescent Psychiatry, 28*(3), 307–318. https://doi.org/10.1007/s00787-018-1195-z

David, O. A., & David, D. (2013, July). *State efficacy of CBT delivered by a new robot (RETMAN) promoting emotional resilience in children.* Paper presented at the 7th World Congress of Behavioural and Cognitive Therapies, Lima, Peru.

David, O. A., David, D., & Dobrean, A. (2014). Efficacy of the rational positive parenting program for child externalizing behavior: Can an emotion-regulation enhanced cognitive-behavioral parent program be more effective than a standard one? *Journal of Evidence-Based Psychotherapies, 14*(2), 159–178.

David, O. A., David, D., & Vanderborght, B. (2013, September). *The efficacy of the RETMAN robot versus cartoons in helping children manage exam anxiety.* Poster presented at the 43rd Annual Congress of the European Association for Behavioral and Cognitive Therapies, Marrakech, Marocco.

David, O. A., & DiGiuseppe, R. (2016). *The rational positive parenting program.* Cham, Switzerland: Springer International Publishing.

Diehl, J. J., Schmitt, L. M., Villano, M., & Crowell, C. R. (2012). The clinical use of robots for individuals with autism spectrum disorders: A critical review. *Research in Autism Spectrum Disorders, 6*(1), 249–262. https://doi.org/10.1016/j.rasd.2011.05.006

Ellis, A. (1994). *Reason and emotion in psychotherapy*. New York: Citadel Press.

Ellis, A., & Bernard, M. E. (2006). *Rational emotive behavioral approaches to childhood disorders*. New York: Kluwer Academic\Plenum Publishers.

Ellis, A., & Dryden, W. (1997). *The practice of rational emotive behavior therapy*. New York: Springer publishing company.

Fodor, L. A., Coteț, C. D., Cuijpers, P., Szamoskozi, Ş., David, D., & Cristea, I. A. (2018). The effectiveness of virtual reality based interventions for symptoms of anxiety and depression: A meta-analysis. *Scientific Reports, 8*, 10323. https://doi.org/10.1038/s41598-018-28113-6

Gavita, O. A., & Calin, A. (2013). Retman rational stories versus rational parenting program for the treatment of child psychopathology: Efficacy of two formats of rational- emotive behavior therapy. *Journal of Cognitive Behavioral Psychotherapy, 13*, 33–52.

Gavita, O. A., David, D., Bujoreanu, S., Tiba, A., & Ionutiu, D. R. (2012). The efficacy of a short cognitive–behavioral parent program in the treatment of externalizing behavior disorders in Romanian foster care children: Building parental emotion-regulation through unconditional self-and child-acceptance strategies. *Children and Youth Services Review, 34*(7), 1290–1297. https://doi.org/10.1016/j.childyouth.2012.03.001

Gavita, O. A., David, D., & DiGiuseppe, R. (2014). You are such a bad child! Appraisals as mechanisms of parental negative and positive affect. *Journal of General Psychology, 141*(2), 113–129. https://doi.org/10.1080/00221309.2013.874971

Gonzalez, J. E., Nelson, J. R., Gutkin, T. B., Saunders, A., Galloway, A., & Shwery, C. S. (2004). Rational emotive therapy with children and adolescents a meta-analysis. *Journal of Emotional and Behavioral Disorders, 12*(4), 222–235. https://doi.org/10.1177/10634266040120040301

Grist, R., Porter, J., & Stallard, P. (2017). Mental health mobile apps for preadolescents and adolescents: A systematic review. *Journal of Medical Internet Research, 19*(5), e176.

Horne-Moyer, H. L., Moyer, B. H., Messer, D. C., & Messer, E. S. (2014). The use of electronic games in therapy: A review with clinical implications. *Current Psychiatry Reports, 16*(12), 520. https://doi.org/10.1007/s11920-014-0520-6

Institute of Digital Media and Child Development Working Group on Games for Health. (2016). Games for health for children – current status and needed research. *Games for Health Journal, 5*(1), 1–12.

Kearns, C. (2015). Prescription play: A primer on innovative use of video games technology in healthcare. *Journal of Visual Communication in Medicine, 38*(3–4), 152–163. https://doi.org/10.3109/17453054.2015.1100981

Kenter, R. M., van de Ven, P. M., Cuijpers, P., Koole, G., Niamat, S., Gerrits, R. S., et al. (2015). Costs and effects of Internet cognitive behavioral treatment blended with face-to-face treatment: Results from a naturalistic study. *Internet Interventions, 2*(1), 77–83. https://doi.org/10.1016/j.invent.2015.01.001

Kim, E. S., Berkovits, L. D., Bernier, E. P., Leyzberg, D., Shic, F., Paul, R., et al. (2013). Social robots as embedded reinforcers of social behavior in children with autism. *Journal of Autism and Developmental Disorders, 43*(5), 1038–1049. https://doi.org/10.1007/s10803-012-1645-2

Kozima, H., Michalowski, M. P., & Nakagawa, C. (2009). Keepon. *International Journal of Social Robotics, 1*(1), 3–18. https://doi.org/10.1007/s12369-008-0009-8

Krijn, M., Emmelkamp, P. M., Olafsson, R. P., & Biemond, R. (2004). Virtual reality exposure therapy of anxiety disorders: A review. *Clinical Psychology Review, 24*(3), 259–281. https://doi.org/10.1016/j.cpr.2004.04.001

Merrifield, C., & Merrifield, R. (1979). *Call me RetMan and have a ball: Comic book.* New York: Inst Rational Emotive Therapy.

Moerman, C. J., van der Heide, L., & Heerink, M. (2019). Social robots to support children's well-being under medical treatment: A systematic state-of-the-art review. *Journal of Child Health Care, 23*(4), 596–612. https://doi.org/10.1177/1367493518803031

Neguț, A., Jurma, A. M., & David, D. (2017). Virtual-reality-based attention assessment of ADHD: ClinicaVR: Classroom-CPT versus a traditional continuous performance test. *Child Neuropsychology, 23*(6), 692–712. https://doi.org/10.1080/09297049.2016.1186617

Opriş, D., Pintea, S., García-Palacios, A., Botella, C., Szamosközi, Ş., & David, D. (2012). Virtual reality exposure therapy in anxiety disorders: A quantitative meta-analysis. *Depression and Anxiety, 29*(2), 85–93. https://doi.org/10.1002/da.20910

Pagliari, C., Burton, C. D., McKinstry, B., Szentagotai, A., David, D., Serrano-Blanco, A., et al. (2012). Psychosocial implications of avatar use in supporting therapy for depression. *Annual Review of Cybertherapy and Telemedicine, 181*, 329–333. https://doi.org/10.3233/978-1-61499-121-2-329

Parsons, T. D., Bowerly, T., Buckwalter, J. G., & Rizzo, A. A. (2007). A controlled clinical comparison of attention performance in children with ADHD in a virtual reality classroom compared to standard neuropsychological methods. *Child Neuropsychology, 13*(4), 363–381. https://doi.org/10.1080/13825580600943473

Păsărelu, C. R., Andersson, G., Bergman Nordgren, L., & Dobrean, A. (2017). Internet-delivered transdiagnostic and tailored cognitive behavioral therapy for anxiety and depression: A systematic review and meta-analysis of randomized controlled trials. *Cognitive Behaviour Therapy, 46*(1), 1–28. https://doi.org/10.1080/16506073.2016.1231219

Podina, I. R., Mogoase, C., David, D., Szentagotai, A., & Dobrean, A. (2016). A meta-analysis on the efficacy of technology mediated CBT for anxious children and adolescents. *Journal of Rational-Emotive & Cognitive-Behavior Therapy, 34*(1), 31–50. https://doi.org/10.1007/s10942-015-0228-5

Powers, M. B., & Emmelkamp, P. M. (2008). Virtual reality exposure therapy for anxiety disorders: A meta-analysis. *Journal of Anxiety Disorders, 22*(3), 561–569. https://doi.org/10.1016/j.janxdis.2007.04.006

Rizzo, A. A., Bowerly, T., Buckwalter, J. G., Klimchuk, D., Mitura, R., & Parsons, T. D. (2006). A virtual reality scenario for all seasons: The virtual classroom. *CNS Spectrums, 11*(1), 35–44.

Rizzo, A. S., & Kim, G. J. (2005). A SWOT analysis of the field of virtual reality rehabilitation and therapy. *Presence: Teleoperators & Virtual Environments, 14*(2), 119–146.

Rothbaum, B. O., Hodges, L., & Kooper, R. (1997). Virtual reality exposure therapy. *Journal of Psychotherapy Practice & Research, 6*(3), 219–226.

Schultheis, M. T., & Rizzo, A. A. (2001). The application of virtual reality technology in rehabilitation. *Rehabilitation Psychology, 46*(3), 296–311.

Simut, R. E., Vanderfaeillie, J., Peca, A., Van de Perre, G., & Vanderborght, B. (2016). Children with autism spectrum disorders make a fruit salad with Probo, the social robot: An interaction study. *Journal of Autism and Developmental Disorders, 46*(1), 113–126. https://doi.org/10.1007/s10803-015-2556-9

Stefan, S., & David, D. (2013). Face-to-face counseling versus high definition holographic projection system. Efficacy and therapeutic alliance. A brief research report. *Journal of Cognitive & Behavioral Psychotherapies, 13*(2), 299–307.

Sucala, M., Cuijpers, P., Muench, F., Cardoş, R., Soflau, R., Dobrean, A., et al. (2017). Anxiety: There is an app for that. A systematic review of anxiety apps. *Depression and Anxiety, 34*(6), 518–525. https://doi.org/10.1002/da.22654

Szentagotai, A., Opris, D., & David, D. (2010). Virtual reality in evidence-based psychotherapy. In J.-J. Kim (Ed.), *Virtual reality* (pp. 445–468). InTech. https://doi.org/10.5772/13130

Titov, N., Andrews, G., Choi, I., Schwencke, G., & Mahoney, A. (2008). Shyness 3: Randomized controlled trial of guided versus unguided Internet-based CBT for social phobia. *Australian and New Zealand Journal of Psychiatry, 42*(12), 1030–1040.

Titov, N., Dear, B. F., Johnston, L., Lorian, C., Zou, J., Wootton, B., et al. (2013). Improving adherence and clinical outcomes in self-guided internet treatment for anxiety and depression: Randomised controlled trial. *PLoS One, 8*(7), e62873. https://doi.org/10.1371/journal.pone.0062873

Trip, S., Vernon, A., & McMahon, J. (2007). Effectiveness of rational-emotive education: A meta-analytical study. *Journal of Cognitive Behavioral Psychotherapy, 7*, 81–93.

Vanderborght, B., Simut, R., Saldien, J., Pop, C., Rusu, A. S., Pintea, S., et al. (2012). Using the social robot probo as a social story telling agent for children with ASD. *Interaction Studies, 13*(3), 348–372. https://doi.org/10.1075/is.13.3.02van

Vernmark, K., Hesser, H., Topooco, N., Berger, T., Riper, H., Luuk, L., et al. (2019). Working alliance as a predictor of change in depression during blended cognitive behaviour therapy. *Cognitive Behaviour Therapy, 48*(4), 285–299. https://doi.org/10.1075/is.13.3.02van

Vigerland, S., Lenhard, F., Bonnert, M., Lalouni, M., Hedman, E., Ahlen, J., et al. (2016). Internet-delivered cognitive behavior therapy for children and adolescents: A systematic review and meta-analysis. *Clinical Psychology Review, 50*, 1–10. https://doi.org/10.1016/j.cpr.2016.09.005

Correction to: Applications of Rational-Emotive and Cognitive-Behavior Technologies with Children and Adolescents

Daniel O. David, Silviu A. Matu, and Roxana A. I. Cardos

Correction to:
Chapter 24 in: M. Bernard, M. D. Terjesen (eds.), *Rational-Emotive and Cognitive-Behavioral Approaches to Child and Adolescent Mental Health: Theory, Practice, Research, Applications*, https://doi.org/10.1007/978-3-030-53901-6_24

The original version of this chapter was published with the family name of the author as 'Silviu'. This has been now updated as 'Matu'. The chapter has been now corrected.

The updated version of the chapter can be found at
https://doi.org/10.1007/978-3-030-53901-6_24

M. Bernard, M. D. Terjesen (eds.), *Rational-Emotive and Cognitive-Behavioral Approaches to Child and Adolescent Mental Health: Theory, Practice, Research, Applications*, https://doi.org/10.1007/978-3-030-53901-6_25

Index

M. Bernard, M. D. Terjesen (eds.), *Rational-Emotive and Cognitive-Behavioral Approaches to Child and Adolescent Mental Health: Theory, Practice, Research, Applications*, https://doi.org/10.1007/978-3-030-53901-6

S

Y

The manufacturer's authorised representative in the EU is Springer Nature Customer Service Centre GmbH, Europaplatz 3, 69115 Heidelberg, Germany. If you have any concerns regarding our products, please contact ProductSafety@springernature.com

Printed and bound by CPI Group (UK) Ltd, Croydon, CR0 4YY
30/09/2026
02225505-0017